Textbook of Periodontology for Undergraduate Students

According to AAP 2018 Classification

AF659879

Textbook of Periodontology for Undergraduate Students

According to AAP 2018 Classification

Devinder Singh Kalsi MDS
Professor
Former Principal and Head,
Department of Periodontology
BJS Dental College and Research Institute
Ludhiana, Punjab, India

Parul Kalsi BDS
Former Lecturer
Department of Periodontology
BJS Dental College and Research Institute
Ludhiana, Punjab, India

CBSPD

CBS Publishers & Distributors Pvt Ltd

New Delhi • Bengaluru • Chennai • Kochi • Kolkata • Lucknow • Mumbai
Hyderabad • Jharkhand • Nagpur • Patna • Pune • Uttarakhand

Disclaimer
Science and technology are constantly changing fields. New research and experience broaden the scope of information and knowledge. The authors have tried their best in giving information available to them while preparing the material for this book. Although all efforts have been made to ensure optimum accuracy of the material, yet it is quite possible some errors might have been left uncorrected. The publisher, the printer and the authors will not be held responsible for any inadvertent errors or inaccuracies.

Textbook of
Periodontology
for Undergraduate Students

According to AAP 2018 Classification

ISBN: 978-93-5466-815-9

Copyright © Authors and Publisher

First Edition: 2025

All rights reserved. No part of this book may be reproduced or transmitted in any form or by any means, electronic or mechanical, including photocopying, recording, or any information storage and retrieval system without permission, in written, from the authors and the publisher.

Published by Satish Kumar Jain and produced by Varun Jain for

CBS Publishers & Distributors Pvt Ltd
4819/XI Prahlad Street, 24 Ansari Road, Daryaganj, New Delhi 110 002, India
Ph: 011-23289259, 23266838 Website: www.cbspd.com
e-mail: delhi@cbspd.com

Corporate Office: 204 FIE, Industrial Area, Patparganj, Delhi 110 092, India
Ph: 011-4934 4934 Fax: 011-4934 4935 e-mail: publishing@cbspd.com; publicity@cbspd.com

Branches

- **Bengaluru:** Seema House 2975, 17th Cross, K.R. Road, Banasankari 2nd Stage, Bengaluru 560 070, Karnataka, India
  Ph: +91-80-26771678/79 Fax: +91-80-26771680 e-mail: bangalore@cbspd.com
- **Chennai:** 7, Subbaraya Street, Shenoy Nagar, Chennai 600 030, Tamil Nadu, India
  Ph: +91-44-26680620, 26681266 Fax: +91-44-42032115 e-mail: chennai@cbspd.com
- **Kochi:** 42/1325, 1326, Power House Road, Opposite KSEB, Power House, Ernakulum 682 018, Kochi, Kerala, India
  Ph: +91-484-4059061–65, 67 Fax: +91-484-4059065 e-mail: kochi@cbspd.com
- **Kolkata:** 147, Hind Ceramics Compound, 1st Floor, Nilgunj Road, Belghoria, Kolkata 700 056, West Bengal, India
  Ph: +91-33-25633055/56 e-mail: kolkata@cbspd.com
- **Lucknow:** Basement, Khushuma Complex, 7 Meerabai Marg (behind Jawahar Bhawan), Lucknow 226 001, UP, India
  Ph: +91-522-4000032 e-mail: tiwari.lucknow@cbspd.com
- **Mumbai:** PWD Shed, Gala No. 25/26, Ramchandra Bhatt Marg, Next to JJ Hospital Gate No. 2, Opp. Union Bank of India, Noorbaug, Mumbai 400 009, Maharashtra, India
  Ph: +91-22-66661880/89 e-mail: mumbai@cbspd.com

Representatives

- **Hyderabad** 0-9885175004
- **Jharkhand** 0-9811541605
- **Nagpur** 0-8692091830
- **Patna** 0-9334159340
- **Pune** 0-9664372571
- **Uttarakhand** 0-9716462459

Printed at: Magic International Pvt. Ltd., Greater Noida, UP, India

to

---

our loving parents

Dr PS Kalsi and Mrs JP Kalsi
and
Er JR Wadhwa and Mrs Kamal Wadhwa

and also to our wonderful children
Meher and Arjan

Foreword

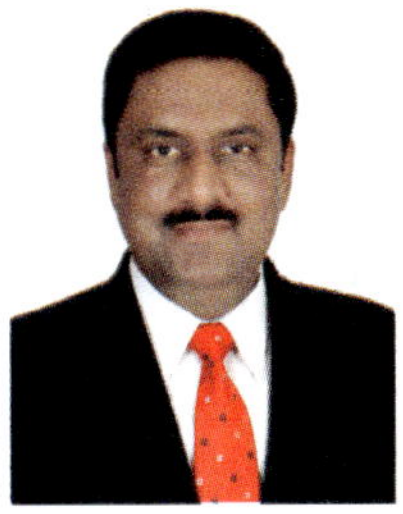

"There is no such thing as a 'periodontal patient,' as all patients with natural teeth have a periodontium." — Dr Glickman

We at times need to remind ourself of the above statement to know the true importance of periodontology in our daily practice. Probably no other specialty of dentistry has an all-encompassing effect on all fields of dentistry as periodontology. Dental surgeons, for several reasons, sometimes however, tend to overlook this fact and confine themselves to the 'task at hand' without managing a patient's periodontal needs adequately.

Periodontology is a seemingly simple but in reality, a vast and complicated subject. Its numerous different, yet intricately interlinked topics and concepts can be difficult to understand and memorize. Often many textbooks on periodontology, though well written, fail to attract a student's attention for being too voluminous. Teachers are in agreement that such 'great but bulky texts' are difficult to understand, memorize and often overwhelm the student into 'inaction'. Students justifiably feel lost and abandoned without access to good educational matter written in simple and student-friendly language.

Apparently, the authors have written this textbook keeping all this in mind. This textbook 'talks directly to the student' and explains what is important and why. It presents knowledge and concepts in a related and simple way. The text is amazingly easy to understand and concise but complete in all aspects. Topics have been so arranged that they act like building blocks that help conceptual learning and build connections between them. Diagrams are thoughtfully drawn and labelled to make the learning easier. Photographs speak volumes for the concept at hand. Keeping with recent developments, the entire text has been written according to the latest and in vogue, 2018 classification of periodontal and peri-implant diseases and conditions. This textbook is also unique due to its emphasis on the importance of a patient-centered approach to learning. What more could one ask for?

Although this textbook would be useful for all undergraduate students of dentistry, but it can also serve as an ideal handbook for postgraduate students and clinicians as well. I congratulate the authors for writing this masterpiece and I am sure, this textbook will find wide acceptance and will benefit both students and practitioners of dentistry.

Chandigarh

Puneet Girdhar MDS FICD
Joint Director, Medical Education and Research, Punjab
Joint Director (Incharge Dental), Department of Medical Education and Research, Punjab
Joint Director (Incharge Ayurveda), Department of Medical Education and Research, Punjab
Registrar, Punjab Dental Council, Mohali
Registrar, Punjab Nursing Council, Mohali
Former Member, Dental Council of India
Immediate Past National President, Indian Dental Association (Head Office)

Preface

With the introduction of the 2018 classification of periodontal and peri-implant diseases and conditions, the subject of periodontology and its concepts have undergone a drastic change. Renewed focus is now laid on preserving the health of the periodontium by early diagnosis and preventing initiation and worsening of periodontal diseases. All students of dentistry aiming to be successful practitioners should therefore not only learn intricacies of periodontal treatment but should also learn and master the art and technique of oral examination with uncompromising attention to detail. These notions were kept in mind while writing this textbook.

Due diligence and effort have been made to present the essential and critical topics of periodontology in a simple, flowcharted and 'to the point' manner. Thus, the information presented in this book is an all-inclusive review of the most essential and clinically relevant recent knowledge on basic concepts (*Chapters 1–5*), etiology and pathology (*Chapters 6–12*), planning, diagnosis and nonsurgical therapy (*Chapters 13–16*) and surgical therapy, inter-disciplinary relationships, supportive periodontal therapy and dental implants (*Chapters 17–22*). Commonly asked theory questions have been given at the end of each chapter.

To keep the reader engaged and related to the text at all times, a new idea of a continuous column with commonly asked viva questions running all along the text has been developed and used. These questions are placed in a way so as to precisely point to the section of text where the information related to the question is present. The aim is to help the student understand the underlying scientific concepts better. To help the reader attain and retain more information related to the running text, additional and background information has been presented in separate boxes titled 'Clinical Utility and Short Answer'. Clinically useful facts that are critical to the topic and patient management have been presented in boxes titled 'Alert'. Series of these two boxes contains information that when read additionally or as related information, adds to the understanding of the topic. Presented this way, the information that is indirectly related to the topic at hand does not 'clutter' the reader's mind but contributes immensely in building concepts and learning of the subject.

The authors are sure that dental students will be much better prepared in the subject of periodontology due to this effort by them.

Devinder Singh Kalsi
Parul Kalsi

Acknowledgments

Condensing the sea of information available on each topic of periodontology to fit the requirements of an undergraduate student was a tough task. To accomplish all this and put our ideas and concepts into words, lines and paragraphs and then to organize these in a flowcharted collection of topics in different chapters was not easy. We feel specially blessed to have completed this mammoth task in a short while.

We wish to express our gratitude to all our teachers from whom we have learnt the wonderful subject of periodontology and other dental subjects. Our gratitude also goes to our numerous colleagues for their constant support that has helped us grow as professionals. Special mention must be made here of Drs Ashish Jain, Rajan Gupta, Nymphea Pandit, Gautami, Rajinder Sharma, Shikha Tiwari and Vishakha. We remain especially indebted to Drs Ranjan Malhotra, Viniti, Shalini Gugnani, Kanteshwari Kummathali, Manik Sharma and Vandana for providing us that extra impetus time and again which proved crucial in shaping this book. This textbook has also been molded by the several suggestions and challenging questions posed by our students over time. The need for writing this textbook in its unique style particularly arose to satisfy the quest of knowledge of many such students. We remain indebted to all of them.

We are thankful to Mr SK Jain (CMD) and Mr Varun Jain (Director) CBS Publishers & Distributors Pvt Ltd, New Delhi, for their support in publishing this textbook. Appreciation is also due to Mr YN Arjuna (Senior Vice President—Publishing, Editorial and Publicity) and the able team of professionals under him for designing the impressive layout of this textbook.

Our family has stood by us during ups and downs and has cooperated by sacrificing time and attention that was rightfully theirs, during the writing of this textbook. We appreciate the constant guidance of Dr PS Kalsi a renowned author of several internationally acclaimed books on organic chemistry during the writing of this textbook. Without his help and support, this task would have been impossible. We are thankful to Dr Maninder Sokhey, who has always provided us unending professional support that has gone a long way in making us successful clinicians. Our children, Dr Meher Kalsi, MS, SR Neurosurgery, RML Hospital, New Delhi and Arjan Singh Kalsi, a computer enthusiast bring unmeasurable love and fulfillment into our lives. These have helped us pursue our academic interests, including this textbook, with zeal and vigor.

Devinder Singh Kalsi
Parul Kalsi

Contents

Chapter

1

Periodontology and Periodontics: An Introduction

Periodontology is the study of supporting tissues of teeth and implants in health and of diseases and conditions that affect them. The word periodontology is derived from greek words: 'peri' meaning around and 'odontos' meaning tooth. There are four supporting tissues of teeth: gingiva, alveolar bone, periodontal ligament and cementum; they are collectively called periodontium. ***Clinical practice*** of periodontology is called ***Periodontics***. A dental surgeon who practices periodontology is called a periodontist.

◂ *What is the difference between periodontology and periodontics?*

◂ *What is periodontium?*

Teeth and implants work together as connected units in an individual's dentition. Therefore a good knowledge of their supporting (*periodontal*) tissues is important for maintaining an adequately functioning dentition. Periodontology is one of the many specialties of dentistry. As all dental specialties are interlinked, thorough knowledge of each one of these is necessary to be a successful clinician. This is important even if a clinician prefers to restrict his/her practice to a specific dental specialty. From this point of view, periodontal health is important for success of any and all dental treatments. Afterall, of what use will a well-made bridge or restorative crown, perfect RCT, ideal orthodontic treatment, etc. be, if all these are done on teeth (*dentition*) that are mobile and not likely to adequately function or last for a reasonable time to justify cost and effort involved in treatment.

Periodontal treatment not only improves health of the dentition but it has also been proven to have a positive impact on an individual's systemic health. Periodontal health (*treatment*) also has a huge positive role in management of several systemic diseases and conditions. As both oral and systemic health and disease have an impact on each other, all dental specialties (*especially periodontology*) and medical specialties are therefore interrelated and interdependent.

Periodontal diseases have been known to occur in humans since ancient times. Ancient texts of Ayurveda, Ebers Papyrus, etc. have sections on oral health and treatment of gingival disease. Albucasis, an arabic physician who lived in middle ages not only documented the importance of calculus in etiology of periodontal disease but also designed a set of scalers for removal of calculus.

Modern periodontology has been developing rapidly since the 17th century. Several clinicians including Pierre Fauchard, John Hunter, Antony van Leeuwenhoek and many others are credited for development of a systematic approach to diagnose periodontal disease and its treatment. Pierre Fauchard (*considered to be the father of modern dentistry*), designed and developed periodontal instruments and the technique of scaling. In the 19th century, John W. Riggs recognized the importance of plaque and calculus in etiology of periodontitis and promoted maintenance of good oral hygiene to prevent it. Riggs was the first well-known clinician to restrict his practice to periodontics (*periodontitis was called 'Riggs' disease' at that time*). Major developments in understanding of periodontal health and treatment of periodontal disease occurred in the 20th century due to untiring

◂ *Name some clinicians who have contributed in development of periodontology in the past.*

◂ *What is Riggs disease?*

efforts of Drs Gottlieb, Orban, Widman, Neumann, Glickman, Waerhaug and their contemporaries.

Today, periodontology and periodontics continue to advance at a rapid pace due to clinical and research work of clinicians across the world. However, several details related to periodontal disease and its treatment are yet not known; a lot of work is presently being done to develop better understanding of periodontal disease and its treatment.

Chapter

2

Gingiva

A healthy periodontium is important for health and long-life of teeth. Understanding of normal features of periodontal tissues forms the basis of understanding of periodontal disease. Therefore, good knowledge of normal features or periodontal tissues is important for diagnosis and periodontal treatment.

PERIODONTAL TISSUES

Periodontal tissues are supporting structures of teeth. They are collectively referred to by the term ***periodontium*** (*perio–around; dontium–tooth*). There are ***four*** periodontal tissues:

◂ *How many periodontal tissues are there?*

1. Gingiva (*soft tissue*)
2. Periodontal ligament (*soft tissue*)
3. Alveolar bone (*hard tissue*)
4. Cementum (*hard tissue*)

Gingiva is discussed in this chapter whereas periodontal ligament, alveolar bone and cementum are discussed in chapter 3. Gingiva is masticatory mucosa—a type of oral mucosa.

ALERT!

Types of oral mucosa

◂ *What are the types of oral mucosa and its keratinization?*

There are ***three*** types of oral mucosa:

1. Masticatory mucosa
   a. Gingiva (*covered by keratinizing epithelium*)
   b. Hard palate mucosa (*covered by keratinizing epithelium*)
2. Specialized mucosa
   Dorsum of the tongue (*specialized for perceiving taste; covered by keratinizing but specialized epithelium containing taste buds*).
3. Lining mucosa (*covered by* ***non-keratinizing*** *epithelium*).

CLINICAL UTILITY AND SHORT ANSWER

Does masticatory mucosa (gingiva and hard palate mucosa) help in mastication?

No, only teeth masticate food. Masticatory mucosa only bears the impact of frictional forces of masticated food as it rubs past the gingiva and the hard palate during mastication. Masticatory mucosa is keratinized and is present on gingiva and hard palate.

GINGIVA

Gingiva surrounds and is attached to necks of teeth. A standard line diagram (Fig. 2.1) is used to depict a part of the periodontium in cross section.

Parts of Gingiva

Gingiva has ***three*** parts (Fig. 2.2):

◂ *What are the other names of free gingiva?*

1. Free gingiva (*also called—marginal* **or** *crestal gingiva*)

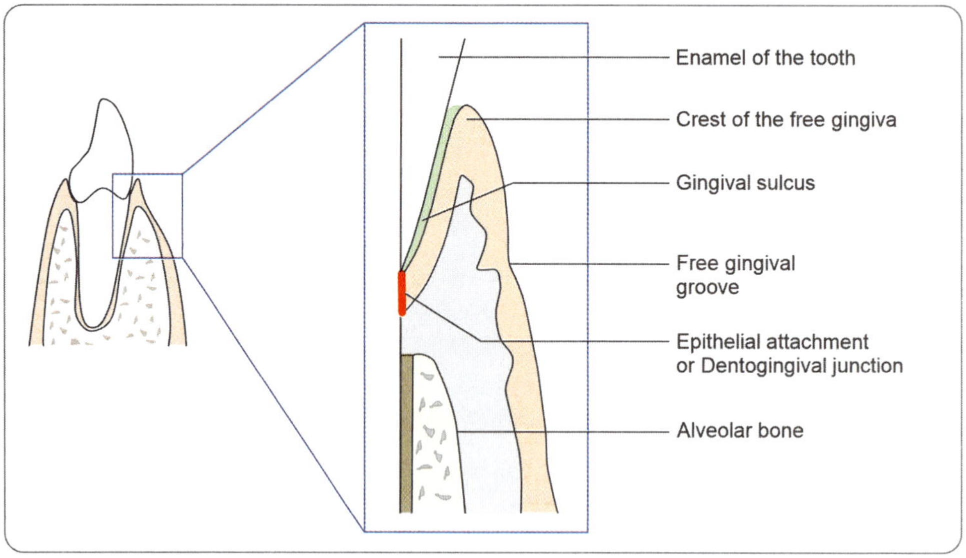

Fig. 2.1: Standard line diagram commonly used to depict a part of the periodontium in cross section

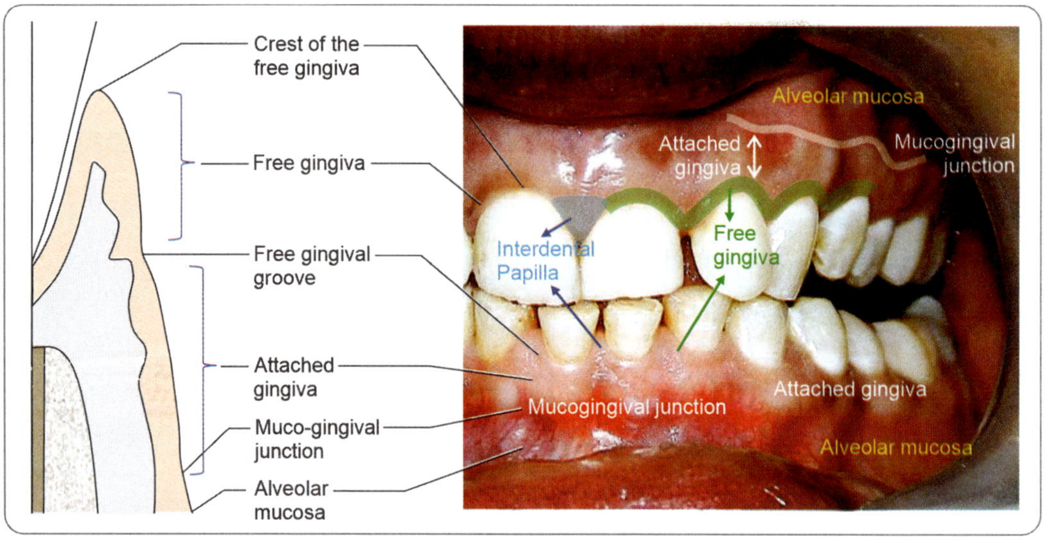

Fig. 2.2: Parts and anatomical landmarks of gingiva (*partially marked*) and corelation between clinical and histological landmarks and boundaries.

2. Attached gingiva
3. Interdental papilla (*also called interdental gingiva*).

Free Gingiva (*also called marginal* **or** *crestal gingiva*)

1. It is the coronal-most part of gingiva (Fig. 2.2).
2. It is not attached to the underlying tooth surface.

How does the free gingiva form the gingival sulcus? ▶

3. It surrounds the tooth like a collar and attaches to the tooth surface ***after*** folding inwards to create a pouch-like cavity called ***gingival sulcus***.
4. Free gingiva forms the ***soft tissue wall*** of the sulcus.

Is free gingival groove present in all individuals? ▶

5. Free gingiva is continuous with attached gingiva. A shallow 1 mm wide ***free gingival groove*** forms the clinical boundary between free and attached gingiva (Figs 2.2 and 2.3). Free gingival groove is present at the same level as the base of sulcus but can only be seen in **50%** of the population.

What type of epithelium lines the free gingiva? ▶

6. Free gingiva is lined by stratified squamous ***keratinizing*** epithelium on the ***oral/buccal and lingual/palatal surfaces*** and by stratified squamous ***non-keratinizing*** epithelium (*sulcular epithelium*) on the ***sulcular*** side (Fig. 2.12).

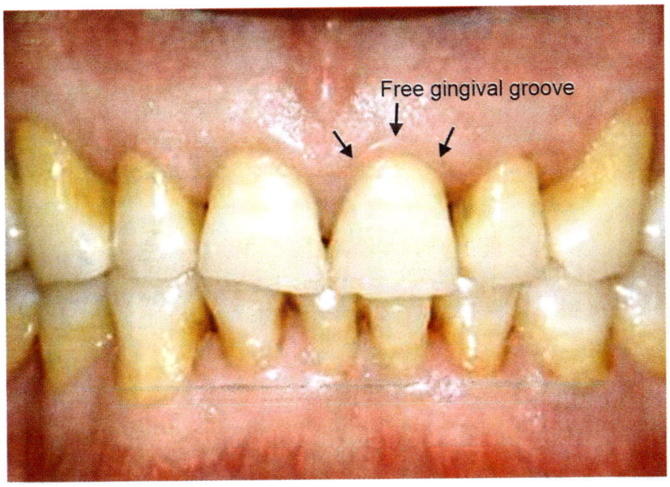

Fig. 2.3: Free gingival groove. It forms boundary between free and attached gingiva. As it is present at the same level as base of sulcus, the free gingival groove is a good indicator of level of base of sulcus and sulcus depth.

Gingival Sulcus

Gingival sulcus is a 'V' shaped pouch-like cavity (*shallow crevice/fissure*) formed by inward folding of free gingiva while attaching to tooth surface. The gingival sulcus extends from crest of gingiva to junctional epithelium (Fig. 2.4).

◂ *The gingival sulcus extends between which two anatomical landmarks?*

Depth of Gingival Sulcus

1. Depth of the normal gingival sulcus is ***variable***. It normally varies between ***0.5–3.0 mm*** **(*average depth is 1.8–2.0 mm*)**.
2. In a previously treated case of periodontitis that is now clinically healthy, a sulcus depth of ***4 mm*** is considered to be normal if there is no bleeding on probing at that site (*2018 classification*).
3. The ***ideal depth*** of the gingival sulcus is ***0 mm***.

◂ *What is the normal depth of gingival sulcus?*

◂ *What is the ideal depth of the gingival sulcus?*

Width of Gingival Sulcus

1. The gingival sulcus is ***very narrow*** because healthy free gingiva is very ***firmly adapted*** around the necks of teeth.
2. Due to this reason, sometimes, a periodontal probe cannot be inserted into it. If a periodontal probe is forced into the sulcus, it can cause tearing of free gingiva and pain (Fig. 2.5). However, microorganisms can easily enter and survive in the gingival sulcus.

◂ *Why is it difficult to insert a periodontal probe into a healthy sulcus?*

CLINICAL UTILITY AND SHORT ANSWER

Why does a sulcus that is more than 2 mm deep have greater chance of developing periodontitis?

- Periodontitis is caused by plaque microorganisms.
- The plaque microorganisms are kept in check by natural physical cleansing mechanisms of the oral cavity and body's immune system. These are supported by instituted physical cleansing mechanisms, e.g. tooth brushing, flossing, etc.
- However, toothbrushing and flossing are practically ineffective in maintaining health of the sulcus after a depth of 2–3 mm.
- Therefore, maintenance of a healthy sulcus is difficult if the depth of the sulcus is more than 3 mm. In some cases, sulci up to 4 mm can be normal but such cases are however not common.
- A diseased sulcus is called a pocket. Any factor that leads to increased plaque deposition will favour deepening of the gingival sulcus and its conversion to periodontal pocket.

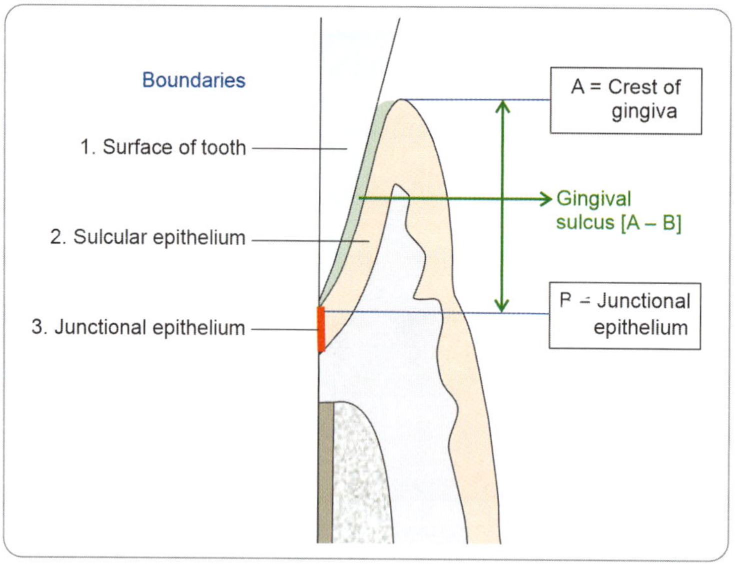

Fig. 2.4: Boundaries of the gingival sulcus (*green-shaded area*)

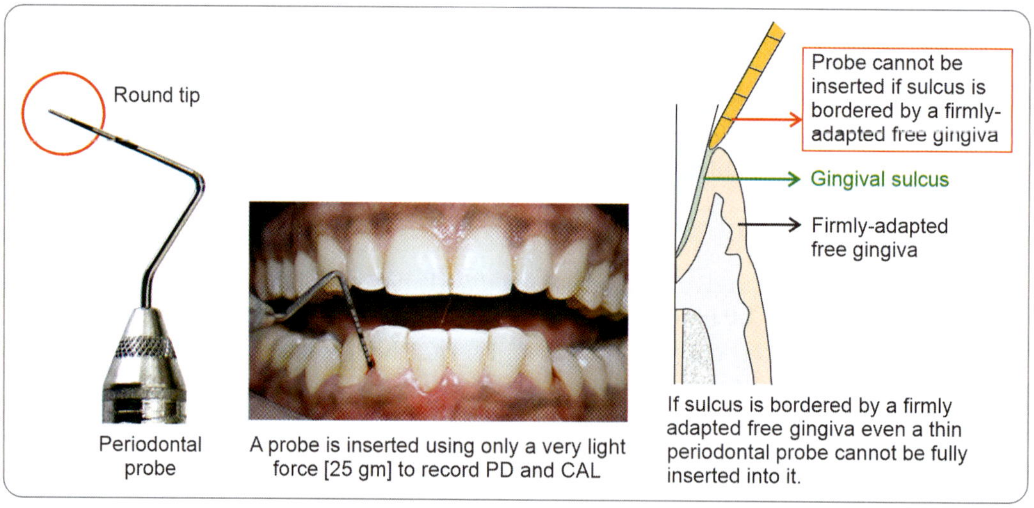

Fig. 2.5: Probing to record clinical probing depth. Probing is done with a periodontal probe that has a round and blunt tip (*end*). Sometimes firm and tightly adapted free gingiva does not allow easy insertion of a periodontal probe without tearing the gingiva.

Boundaries of Gingival Sulcus

The sulcus has *three* boundaries (Figs 2.4 and 2.12)

1. **Inner side**—surface of tooth.
2. **Outer side**—sulcular epithelium of free gingiva.
3. **Base**—coronal most cells of junctional epithelium.

Which cells make the base of the sulcus? ▶

How to measure depth of gingival sulcus or pocket

There are *two* ways of measuring depth of a sulcus and pockets (*in periodontitis sulcus is called a pocket*):

What is PD? ▶

How much pressure should be used for probing? ▶

Does PD tell us the current or past status of disease? ▶

I. **Clinical sulcus depth:** Sulcus or pocket depth measured with a periodontal probe is called ***probing sulcus depth or pocket depth*** (*PD*) (Fig. 2.5). For this, a probe is inserted into the sulcus under ***light*** pressure (*approximately 0.25 Newton force, i.e. 25 gm force*) till ***light*** resistance is felt and measurement on the probe is noted. PD tells us the ***current*** status of disease or health at a particular site. William's probe, WHO probe (*it has a 0.5 mm ball tip*), etc. are commonly used periodontal probes. Naber's probe is curved probe used for probing furcations of multirooted teeth (*Fig. 13.8*). Clinical PD is ***more*** than histological depth (Fig. 2.6).

II. **Histological:** In a ***histological*** section, distance from crest of free gingiva to base of sulcus (*coronal most cells of the junctional epithelium*) is called histological sulcus depth. Histological depth is ***less*** than clinical PD (Fig. 2.6).

◂ *Which is larger—clinical or histological sulcus depth?*

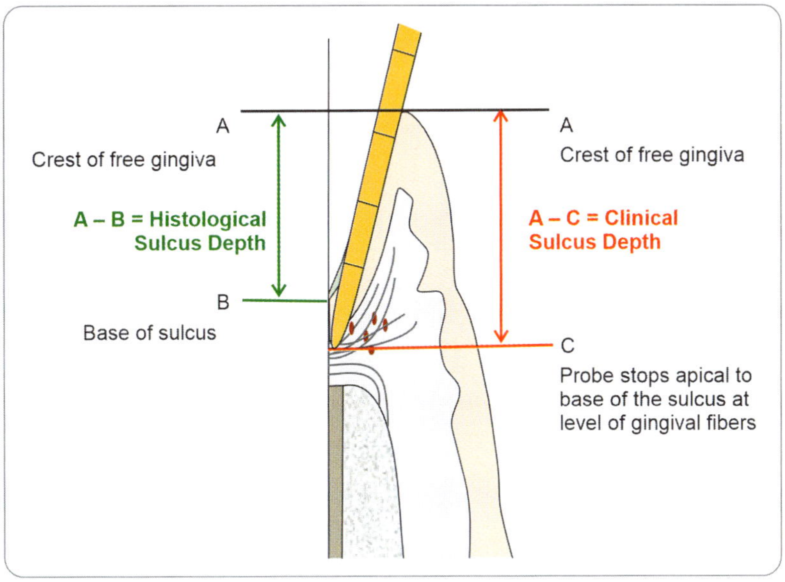

Fig. 2.6: Difference between histological and clinical sulcus depth

CLINICAL UTILITY AND SHORT ANSWER

Why clinical probing depth (PD) is always more than the histological sulcus depth?

For recording PD, a periodontal probe is inserted into the sulcus under slight pressure till a light resistance is felt (*approximately 0.25 Newton force, i.e. 25 gm force*). Because junctional epithelium at base of the sulcus is nonkeratinized, it does not provide any feelable resistance to the probe tip. Therefore, in spite of such light probing pressure, the probe tip penetrates through the base of the sulcus and stops only when resistance is provided to it by the fibers of the dento-gingival fiber group (Fig. 2.6). Thus, recorded clinical probing depth is more than the histological depth.

CLINICAL UTILITY AND SHORT ANSWER

How can you know the correct probing pressure?

25 grams force is approximately the force needed to cause a ***slight*** depression and blanching in the bulb of the thumb of finger when pressed with a probe tip.

CLINICAL UTILITY AND SHORT ANSWER

Why sulci or pockets' depths cannot be measured with an explorer instead of a probe?

◂ *Why explorer cannot be used for recording PD?*

An explorer has a sharp tip (*end*) while a periodontal probe has a rounded tip (Figs 2.5 and 13.7). In contrast to the probe, the tip of an explorer being sharp will penetrate easily and more into the gingival tissues (*perhaps stop at crest of the alveolar bone*) and record a greater probing pocket depth (*PD*). An explorer is used to detect hard tissue defects only.

CLINICAL UTILITY AND SHORT ANSWER

What is clinical attachment level (*CAL*) or clinical attachment loss (*CAL*)?

◂ *What is CAL?*

- The distance from cemento-enamel junction (*CEJ*) to tip of the probe that has been inserted into the sulcus/pocket for taking a probing depth is called Clinical attachment level (Fig. 2.7).
- As CAL quantifies periodontal attachment loss, it is also called clinical attachment loss.
- CAL is zero if base of the sulcus is coronal to the CE junction, i.e. there is no periodontal loss or recession (Fig. 2.21, diag. 1).
- CAL is a measure of total (*past + present ongoing*) periodontal destruction that has occurred due to periodontitis whereas PD tells us the present-day status of periodontitis.

◂ *What does CAL tell us: The current or past status of disease?*

What is the difference between CAL and PD? ▸

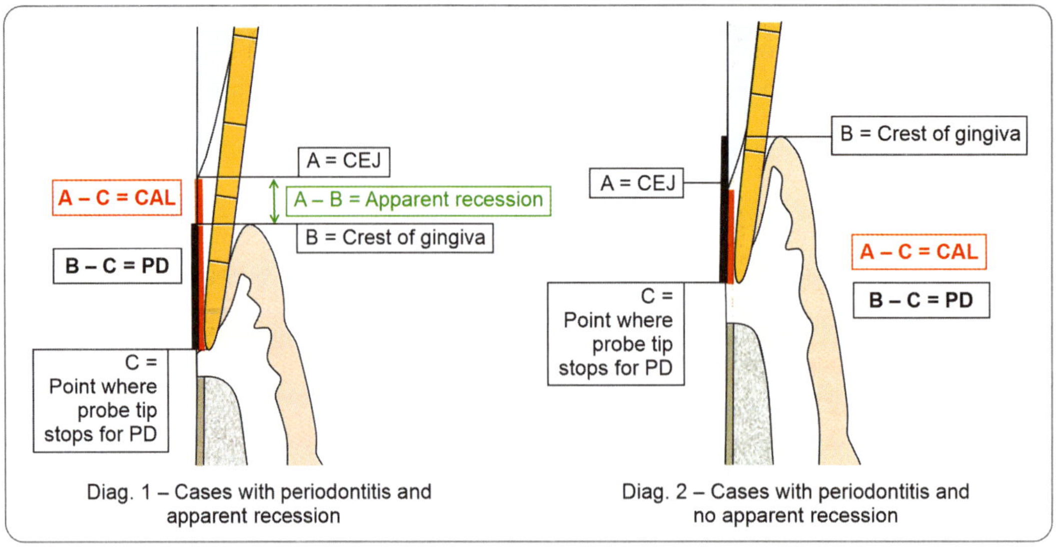

Fig. 2.7: Clinical attachment level (*CAL*) *vs* probing depth

CLINICAL UTILITY AND SHORT ANSWER

When and why can recorded CAL and PD be inaccurate? ▸

Why are CAL measurements not accurate in some cases?

In some subjects, the healthy free gingiva is so firmly adapted to the tooth that insertion of a probe to the base of the sulcus is not possible. This leads to recording of lesser than actual PD and CAL measurements (Fig. 2.5).

In other cases, if the gingiva is inflamed or excess probing pressure is used the probe gets pushed apically to the crest of the bone. In such cases, recorded CAL and PD are more.

CLINICAL UTILITY AND SHORT ANSWER

Which local and systemic factors cause periodontitis and lead to deepening of sulcus?

As the sulcus deepens, it becomes diseased (*periodontitis*); it is then called a pocket. Factors that cause deepening and conversion of the sulcus to a pocket are:

- Increased plaque deposits
- Inadequate natural cleansing, e.g. soft diet, improper tooth contours, etc. and plaque control mechanisms, e.g. faulty tooth brushing, etc.
- Systemic factors leading to xerostomia, (*decreased salivary flow*), decreased immunity, e.g. in diabetes, etc.
- Malocclusion (*makes plaque control difficult*)
- Iatrogenic factors, e.g. overhanging defective restorations, open proximal contacts, etc.

Contents of Gingival Sulcus

What is present in a sulcus and pocket? ▸

a. Food debris
b. Saliva and its constituents like salivary mucin, etc.
c. Gingival crevicular fluid and its constituents
d. Plaque microorganisms and their products
e. Desquamated epithelial cell
f. Leukocytes (*primarily neutrophils*)
g. Pus
h. As the sulcus converts to a pocket, calculus may also be seen.

Gingival Crevicular Fluid (GCF)

What is GCF? ▸

A sticky, colourless fluid called gingival crevicular fluid (*GCF*) is present in the gingival sulci and periodontal pockets. It is an ***inflammatory exudate*** and is produced in response to plaque microorganisms and other factors producing inflammation, e.g. physical injury, etc.

As rate of production and flow of GCF increases with increasing of intensity of inflammation, GCF is therefore increased in gingivitis and periodontitis (*pocket formation*).

◂ *Is GCF production more in pockets? Why?*

Constituents of GCF

◂ *What are the contents and functions of GCF?*

1. Cells: Epithelial, WBCs and microorganisms.
2. Organic compounds: Carbohydrates, proteins (*immunoglobulins, etc.*), lipids, etc.
3. Metabolic and bacterial products: Prostaglandins, endotoxins, antibacterial factors, etc.
4. Enzymes and enzyme inhibitors: Alkaline phosphatase, proteolytic enzymes, lysozymes, etc.

Functions of GCF

1. Controlling microorganisms in the sulcus/pocket by:
   a. Flushing-out microorganisms and debris.
   b. Providing a medium in which anti-microbial immune compounds and cells can exist in the sulcus/pocket.
2. Adhesion of free gingiva to the tooth due to its stickiness.

Measuring Rate of Flow of GCF

◂ *How is rate of flow of GCF measured?*

GCF is produced in very ***small*** quantity. It can therefore only be collected by ***special*** equipment. Methods of collection of GCF are:

1. **Absorbing filter paper strips:**
   i. **Intra-sulcular:** Absorbing strip is inserted into the sulcus either only till the entrance or all the way to the bottom of the sulcus. This is the most commonly used method.
   ii. **Extra-sulcular:** Strips are overlaid and adapted on surface of the gingiva and the tooth thereby bridging over the gingival sulcus.

   After the strips are wet with GCF, the rate of flow of GCF can be known by analyzing the strips in three ways:
   i. It is stained with ninhydrin and the area of the stained portion of the paper strip is measured.
   ii. Paper strips are weighed before and after collection of GCF. The increase in weight is co-related to volume of GCF produced.
   iii. An electronic device, e.g. periotron can be used. The strip is inserted into the *periotron* which gauges the wetness of the paper strip and gives a digital reading.
2. **Collecting the GCF in micropipettes (*microcapillaries*).**
3. **Sulcular washing methods:** A known volume of specially prepared solution is flowed into the sulcus and then re-aspirated from the sulcus itself using a collection needle. The entire collected fluid (*prepared solution + GCF*) is then measured and analyzed.
4. **Pre-weighed absorbent-twisted threads:** Pre-weighed absorbent threads can be tied at the necks of teeth at the free gingival margin or inserted into the sulcus/pocket and allowed to absorb GCF. The threads are then weighed to know increase in weight after a set interval of time. The increase in weight can be co-related to volume of GCF produced.

CLINICAL UTILITY AND SHORT ANSWER

What is the clinical significance of GCF?

Increase in rate of flow of GCF is directly proportional to severity of gingival inflammation (*gingivitis and periodontitis*).

ALERT!

Tetracycline is an antibiotic of choice for treating periodontitis because:

- It is a broad-spectrum antibiotic.
- Concentration of tetracycline in GCF is ***8–10*** times more than that in the blood. This high concentration of tetracycline makes it very effective in killing plaque microorganisms in the pocket.
- Tetracycline is used only in ***addition*** to scaling and root planing and other surgical techniques to treat some cases of periodontitis. It must ***not*** be routinely used for treating periodontitis or gingivitis.

◂ *What is the concentration of tetracycline in GCF?*

◂ *Why is tetracycline a drug of choice in treating periodontitis?*

What are the anatomical landmarks at coronal and apical extents of attached gingiva?

What type of epithelium covers the attached gingiva?

ATTACHED GINGIVA

The attached gingiva is a ***non-movable*** part of gingiva. It is firmly bound to underlying cementum of the root and periosteum of the alveolar bone. It extends from base of the sulcus/free gingival groove to the mucogingival junction (*free gingival groove forms at the level of base of the sulcus on oral aspect of gingiva*) (Figs 2.2 and 2.8). Attached gingiva is covered by stratified squamous ***keratinizing*** epithelium (Fig. 2.12).

What are the boundaries of attached gingiva?

Is an anatomical boundary present between attached gingiva and palatal mucosa?

Boundaries of Attached Gingiva (Fig. 2.8)

- Free gingiva on the coronal side.
- Alveolar mucosa on the apical side.
- On the ***palatal*** side, ***no*** anatomical boundary exists between attached gingiva and palatal mucosa. Here attached gingiva gradually blends ***unnoticeably*** with the palatal mucosa (*which is similar to attached gingiva*).

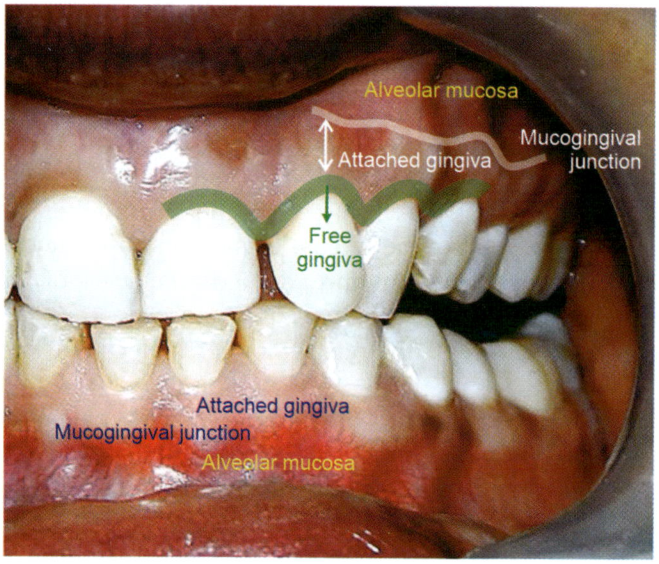

Fig. 2.8: Attached gingiva and its boundaries

What is mucogingival junction?

CLINICAL UTILITY AND SHORT ANSWER

What is alveolar mucosa?

- Alveolar mucosa covers the alveolar process (Figs 2.2 and 2.8).
- It is situated apical to attached gingiva and is separated from it by the mucogingival junction.
- Alveolar mucosa is not present on the palate.
- It is dark red in colour, movable and elastic.
- It is lined by non-keratinizing epithelium.

CLINICAL UTILITY AND SHORT ANSWER

Which areas of gingiva are keratinized (*covered by keratinizing epithelium*)?

1. Attached gingiva,
2. Interdental papilla's facial surface
3. Palatal mucosa (Figs 2.9 and 2.12).

What is the difference between attached gingiva and keratinized gingiva?

Is the width of attached gingiva same as that of keratinized gingiva?

CLINICAL UTILITY AND SHORT ANSWER

Is keratinized gingiva same as (*equal to*) attached gingiva?

No. Attached gingiva is only one constituent of keratinized gingiva. Both free and attached gingivae are keratinized, i.e. total width of keratinized gingiva is a sum of width of free gingiva and attached gingiva. Width of attached gingiva is therefore ***lesser*** than width of the keratinized gingiva (Fig. 2.9).

Functions of Attached Gingiva

1. As attached gingiva is firmly attached to underlying bone, it provides support to the unattached free gingiva.
2. As the attached gingiva is ***immovable,*** it absorbs the physical pull from the movable alveolar mucosa (*due to facial muscles*) and prevents it from reaching the free gingiva.
3. If the attached gingiva does not dissipate/buffer this pulling force, the free gingiva will get pulled down (*apically*) every time we open our mouth, stretch our lips, drink, speak, etc. Constant downward and outward pulling of the free gingiva and gaping of the gingival sulcus will enable ***food impaction*** in the sulcus and can cause ***gingival recession***.

◂ *Why is an adequate zone of attached gingiva necessary for gingival health?*

4. Being keratinized and firmly bound, it is strong enough to bear the force exerted by food during mastication (*as food passes over it*) and thus prevents injury to the underlying connective tissue.
5. Attached gingiva is firm in consistency and is firmer than free gingiva and alveolar mucosa. It therefore acts as a barrier to spread of inflammation from superficial to deeper periodontal tissues.
6. In periodontitis, an adequate zone of attached gingiva is believed to stop/reduce rate of increase of pocket depth (*PD*).
7. Dental implants having adequate attached gingiva around their necks are less likely to have peri-implantitis compared to ones having inadequate or no attached gingiva.

◂ *Why is it preferable to place dental implants in areas having adequate zone-attached gingiva?*

Width of Attached Gingiva

- The width of attached gingiva is a range, and this varies from ***1 mm to 4.5 mm***. It may be as high as 9 mm in some areas of the mouth in some patients.

◂ *What is the width of attached gingiva?*

- ***Maximum*** width of attached gingiva is found in ***incisor regions*** of both upper and lower jaws (*4.0–4.5 mm approximately*).
- ***Minimum*** width is found in ***premolar*** regions of both upper and lower jaws (*1.8–2.0 mm approximately*).

◂ *Where are the maximum and minimum widths of attached gingiva found?*

CLINICAL UTILITY AND SHORT ANSWER

Is width of attached gingiva constant throughout life?

- No.
- In ***totally disease-free*** gingival units, the width of attached ***gingiva increases slightly*** with ***increasing age***. In fact, it is significantly wider in 40–50-year age group than in 20–30-year age group.
- Increase in width of the attached gingiva occurs at the coronal end due to supra eruption or passive eruption (*apical deposition of cementum after the tooth has reached the occlusal plane*). The apical end of the attached gingiva, i.e. the muco-gingival junction does not shift and remains ***stationary*** throughout life.
- Decrease in width of attached gingiva occurs in periodontitis.
- Width of attached gingiva can be increased by mucogingival surgery (*see Chapter 19*).

◂ *Does width of attached gingiva change with age?*

How Much Width of Attached Gingiva is Considered Adequate/Ideal?

- Studies have ***not*** determined the minimum width (*in millimeters*) of attached gingiva required for its proper functioning, i.e. preventing pull from alveolar mucosa from reaching the free gingiva. Many times, it has been found that attached gingiva of narrower width performs this function adequately whereas one of broader width fails to do so.
- It is therefore accepted that—***attached gingiva of any width, however small, if is performing its function effectively, is adequate.*** Conversely, if attached gingiva is not performing its function effectively, attached gingiva at that particular area is inadequate.

◂ *How much width of attached gingiva is needed for its adequate functioning?*

◂ *Is adequacy of attached gingiva dependent on its width?*

◂ *Can attached gingiva of lesser width be adequate while that of a greater width inadequate?*

How to Measure Width of Attached Gingiva

The attached gingiva extends from base of sulcus/free gingival groove to the mucogingival junction. The width of the attached gingiva can be measured in the following ways:

1. *Clinical Measurement*

How is attached gingiva measured?

i. If free gingival groove is clearly visible, measure the distance from free gingival groove to mucogingival junction to know width of the attached gingiva **(Fig. 2.9, Z)**.

ii. If free gingival groove is ***not*** visible, subtract depth of the sulcus (*PD*) from distance between crest of free gingiva and mucogingival junction **(Fig. 2.9, X–Y = Z)**.

iii. Iodine staining: This method helps to clearly demarcate non-keratinized alveolar mucosa from the keratinized gingiva. ***Non-keratinized*** alveolar mucosa takes a brown stain (*as it has glycogen*) when diluted Schiller's or Lugol's solution is applied to it. The keratinized parts of the gingiva (*attached gingiva + free gingiva*) do ***not*** stain with these solutions. The unstained, i.e. total keratinized epithelium is measured and the depth of the sulcus is subtracted from this measurement to know the width of the attached gingiva (*same as in point* (*ii*) *above*).

2. *Rolling the Alveolar Mucosa*

Does rolling of attached gingiva help in finding width of attached gingiva?

This is more a method of identifying the mucogingival junction than it is a method of measuring the width of the attached gingiva. For this, the alveolar mucosa is pushed in the coronal direction with the side of a periodontal probe. This helps to clearly demarcate the muco-gingival junction and width of attached gingiva can then be calculated as described earlier (*point # ii above*).

3. *Histological Measurement*

In a histological section, the attached gingiva extends from the base of the sulcus to the mucogingival junction.

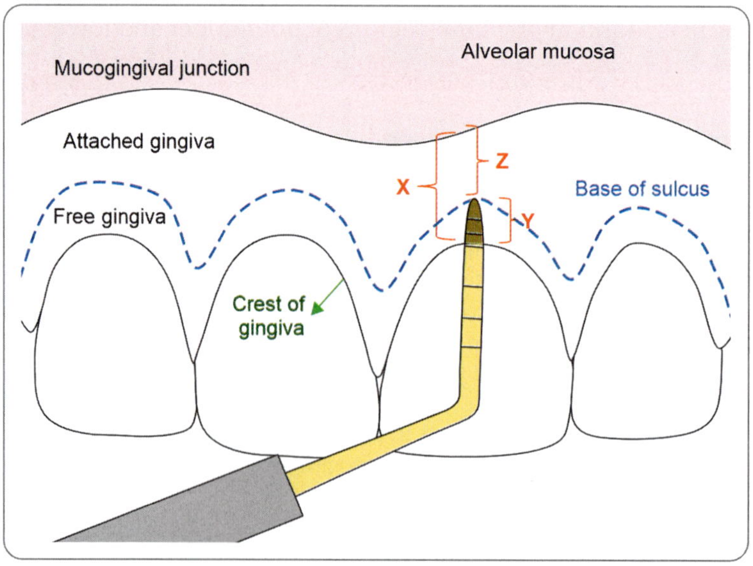

Fig. 2.9: Clinical measurement of width of attached gingiva and keratinized gingiva. Measurement of width of attached gingiva is done in three steps: Step 1—Measure the distance from crest of free gingiva to mucogingival junction (*X*). Step 2—Measure depth of sulcus (*Y*). Step 3—Subtract depth of sulcus (*Y*) from distance between crest of free gingiva and mucogingival junction (*X*) to know width of attached gingiva ($X - Y = Z$). Keratinized gingiva is the distance from crest of free gingiva to mucogingival junction (*X*).

How can you check adequacy of attached gingiva?

How to Know if Present Width of Attached Gingiva is Adequate or Not

This can be done in the following ways:

1. *Tension Test*

◂ *What is tension test?*

- For this, lip/cheek (*alveolar mucosa*) opposite the attached gingival unit being tested, is lightly pulled out.
- If the attached gingiva is adequate, pull from alveolar mucosa will not reach the free gingiva, therefore the free gingiva will ***not*** move or blanch when the test is being performed. In such cases attached gingiva is adequate and tension test is pronounced negative (Fig. 2.10).
- If on the other hand, free gingiva ***moves or shows blanching***, this means pull from alveolar mucosa reached the free gingiva (*which means attached gingiva did not absorb this pull*). Hence in such cases, attached gingiva is inadequate and tension test is positive (Fig. 2.10).
- In some borderline cases, where clear-cut results are not seen, the pull from alveolar mucosa can be slightly increased by lightly pressing the alveolar mucosa (*just apical to the mucogingival junction*) with the back of an instrument handle or side of a periodontal probe.

2. *Rolling the Alveolar Mucosa*

- This test can identify ***major*** inadequacies of the attached gingiva only.
- For this, alveolar mucosa is pushed in coronal direction with the side of a periodontal probe. If rolling the alveolar mucosa causes a very noticeable movement of the crest of free gingiva, attached gingiva is inadequate and the test is positive.

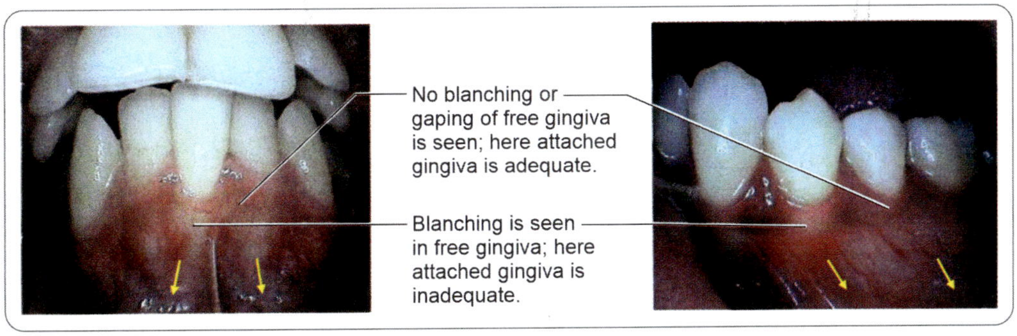

Fig. 2.10: Tension test. It is performed to gauge adequacy of attached gingiva

INTERDENTAL PAPILLA

Interdental papilla is that part of the gingiva which is present in the interdental space between two adjoining teeth of the same arch.

◂ *What is interdental papilla?*

- **Shape of interdental papilla is variable**
  - **When seen from buccal and lingual aspect**, in both ***anterior*** and ***posterior*** teeth ***having tight interdental contacts***, the interdental papilla is ***triangular*** (***pyramidal***) in shape (Figs 2.2 and 2.11, diags A and B).
  - In teeth with open contacts (*diastema*) and teeth with good contacts but with receded gingivae, interdental papilla is ***rounded***. In such cases, interdental papillae follow contour of the underlying alveolar bone (Fig. 2.11, diags C and D).
  - **When seen from mesial or distal aspect,** in posterior teeth that have wide contact areas, the interdental papilla grows around the contact area and has a ***'tent'*** like shape (*this creates two distinct papillae, i.e. one each on buccal and palatal or lingual sides around the contact area*). The ***depression*** between buccal and lingual/palatal interdental papillae is called ***interdental col*** (Fig. 2.11, diag. B, red line).
- The ***interdental col*** of the interdental papilla is lined by stratified squamous ***non-keratinizing*** epithelium (Fig. 2.11, diag. B, red line).
- The oral (*buccal and the lingual*) surfaces of interdental papilla are covered by stratified squamous ***keratinizing*** epithelium.

◂ *What is the shape of interdental papilla in teeth with tight interdental contacts?*

◂ *What is the shape of interdental papilla in teeth with open interdental contacts?*

◂ *What is interdental col?*

◂ *What type of epithelium lines the interdental papilla?*

CLINICAL UTILITY AND SHORT ANSWER

What is a 'col'? What is the clinical importance of interdental col?

'Col' is a ***mountaineering*** term for a valley like depression between two mountains. When seen from the proximal side, the buccal and lingual papillae in posterior teeth with wide interdental contact areas, appear as two small mountains and the depression between them appears like a valley between peaks of the buccal and lingual/palatal papillae. The depression in the interdental papilla is therefore called interdental col.

The interdental col area is lined by stratified squamous ***non-keratinizing*** epithelium. Because when compared to keratinizing epithelium, non-keratinizing epithelium is a weaker barrier (*defense*) against ingress of microorganisms, ***interdental col is a point of start of periodontitis*** **(Fig. 2.11, diag. B, red line)**.

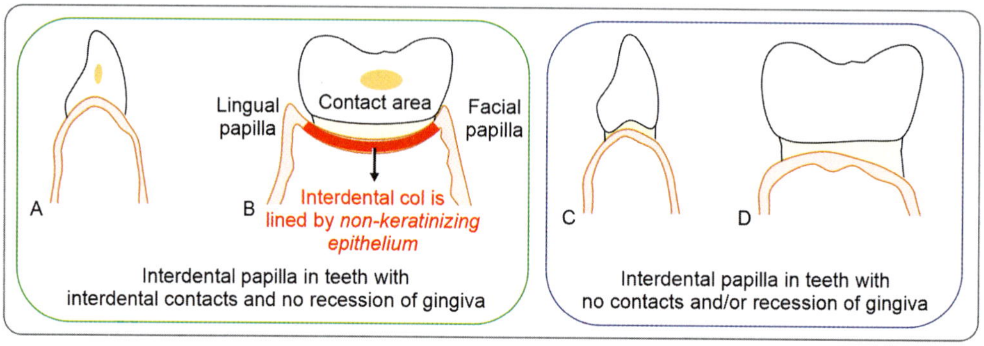

Fig. 2.11: Interdental papilla in anterior and posterior teeth

CLINICAL UTILITY AND SHORT ANSWER

Which different types of epithelia cover gingiva?

What is the difference between keratinized and parakeratinized epithelia? ▸

Epithelium of gingiva is of stratified squamous type and may be:

1. **Keratinized: 15%**
2. **Parakeratinized: 75%** (*parakeratinized epithelium is similar to keratinized epithelium; in this, the cells of the top layers retain pyknotic nuclei and the granular layer is not identifiable histologically*).
3. **Non-keratinized: 10%**

Three zones of epithelium can be identified in gingiva **(Fig. 2.12)**:

1. Outer epithelium (*buccal and lingual epithelia*) **(*keratinized or parakeratinized*)**
2. Sulcular epithelium **(*non-keratinized*)**
3. Junctional epithelium **(*non-keratinized*)**.

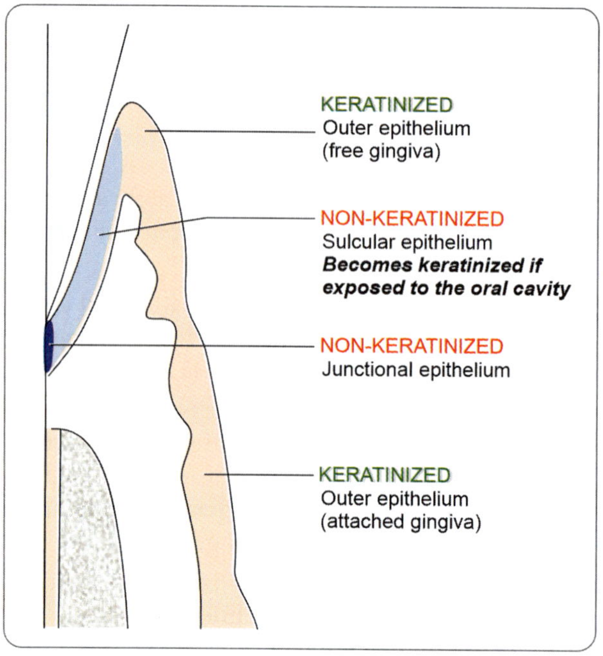

Fig. 2.12: Distribution of keratinized and non-keratinized epithelium in gingiva

CLINICAL UTILITY AND SHORT ANSWER

Describe the connective tissue underlying gingiva.

- It is mostly composed of type I collagen, ground substance and mucopolysaccharides.
- Collagen, elastin and reticulin fibres, blood and lymph vessels, nerves and different cells, e.g. WBCs are present in it.
- Connective tissue under the epithelium ***determines*** whether the epithelium will be keratinized or non-keratinized.

◄ *Does the connective tissue determine keratinization of epithelium?*

CLINICAL UTILITY AND SHORT ANSWER

What is keratinization?

Keratinization is a process by which cells of basal layer of the epithelium move superficially to end up in keratin layer on surface of the epithelium. As basal cells move to the superficial layers, they flatten, and show increase in number of tonofilaments and intercellular junctions. They also lose their nuclei and production of keratohyaline granules occurs in their cytoplasms. Keratinized epithelium has ***four*** layers:

1. Basal layer or Stratum basale.
2. Spinous or Prickle cell layer or Stratum spinosum.
3. Granular layer or Stratum granulosum.
4. Keratin layer or Stratum corneum.

◄ *Name the layers of keratinizing epithelium?*

What is the function of keratinization?

Keratinization is a defensive process. Disease-producing microorganisms enter tissues through intercellular spaces, which are weak spots in epithelium's defense. During the process of keratinization, keratin is deposited within the epithelium cells and intercellular spaces, this seals the intercellular spaces and makes them impermeable (*microorganisms now cannot enter through these*). In addition to this, cells of the top layer, i.e. stratum corneum get flattened and get arranged in overlapping layers. As a result, microorganisms trying to gain entry into the deeper tissues through keratinized epithelium, are physically stopped by a number of such impermeable cell layers that have impermeable intercellular spaces. This makes keratinized epithelium a strong line of defense against microbial infections. Keratinization also makes epithelium much more resistant to abrasive/frictional forces. Thus, skin and masticatory mucosa, being lined by keratinizing epithelium, can bear physical, abrasive, frictional, chemical and thermal insults easily.

◄ *How is keratinization protective in nature?*

The ***nonkeratinized*** epithelium covers lining mucosa of oral cavity and is a weaker line of defense against ingress of microbes. Nonkeratinized epithelial surfaces are however, more sensitive, pliable and elastic. Non-keratinizing epithelium has ***three*** layers:

1. Stratum basale
2. Stratum intermedium
3. Stratum superficiale.

◄ *Name the layers of non-keratinizing epithelium.*

Cells of Gingival Epithelium

Several types of cells are found in the epithelium. These include epithelial cells, fibroblasts, melanocytes, macrophages, mast cells, neutrophils, lymphocytes, plasma cells (*B lymphocytes that produce antibodies*), eosinophils, Langerhan's cells, Merkel cells, etc.

◄ *Name the different types of cells in the oral epithelium.*

CLINICAL UTILITY AND SHORT ANSWER

Why are cells of inflammation (*neutrophils, lymphocytes, etc.*) present even in clinically healthy and normal gingiva?

As plaque microorganisms are ***always*** present in gingival sulcus, defensive cells like neutrophils, lymphocytes are also always present to kill and control spread of these microorganisms and prevent them from causing gingivitis and periodontitis.

◄ *Explain why inflammatory cells are present even in healthy gingiva?*

CLINICAL UTILITY AND SHORT ANSWER

How is gingival pigmentation produced?

What are Melanocytes, Melanophages (*melanophores*) and Melanosomes (*premelanosomes*)?

Gingival epithelium has a brown pigment called melanin. This pigment imparts brown colour to the gingiva. Melanin is produced within melanocytes (*that are present in the basal and spinous layers of the*

(*Contd.*)

◄ *What causes brown colour of gingiva?*

◄ *Where is melanin produced?*

epithelium) and then expelled out of its body. These melanin granules are then phagocytosed (*eaten*) by keratinocytes of the epithelium; such keratinocytes are called melanophages or melanophores. The melanin in the melanophages imparts brown colour to the gingiva.

Pigmentation is therefore produced and is present within layers of the epithelium only.

Why must entire width of epithelium be removed for depigmentation of gingiva? ▸

Clinical importance: *If depigmentation of gingiva (whitening of gingival colour) has to be done, the entire epithelium must be surgically removed (excised). However, this reduction in intensity of brown colour of the gingiva (depigmentation) is temporary and pigmentation usually recurs after some time (about a year or so).*

In which layers of gingival epithelium are melanocytes present? ▸

Melanocytes synthesize melanin (*brown pigment that imparts colour to skin and the oral mucus membrane*). They are present in the basal and spinous layers of the epithelium.

Melanophages (*melanophores*): After melanin granules are synthesized, they are expelled from the melanocyte. These melanin granules are phagocytosed by keratinocytes. Such keratinocytes are called melanophages or melanophores (*keratinocytes are epithelial cells which produce keratin*).

Melanosomes or Premelanosomes: These are granules in melanocytes that contain tyrosinase. tyrosinase hydroxylates tyrosin to dihydroxyphenylalanine, which in turn is converted to melanin.

Turnover Rate of Gingival Cells

In how many days do new cells replace old gingival epithelium? ▸

New cells are needed to replace older ones after they are shed off. The turnover rate of the cells of the gingiva in young individuals is 5–6 days, this increases to 10–12 days in older individuals. Mitotic rates (*cell division rates*) are ***maximum*** in ***sulcular epithelium*** cells and ***minimum*** in ***attached gingiva*** cells. Mitotic rates are ***maximum*** in ***morning***, and ***lowest*** in ***evening***.

Basement Membrane of the Oral Epithelium

The basement membrane joins the epithelium to the underlying connective tissue.

- Under a light microscope basement membrane appears to be structure-less. It does not stain with the H–E (*hematoxylin–eosin*) stain but stains brightly with the PAS (*periodic Acid-Schiff*) method.
- Under the electron microscope, this structure less band is 400 Å thick (*1 angstrom unit* = 10^{-8} *cm*) and is seen to be made of two distinct layers (*lamina*):

Name layers of basement membrane. ▸

1. **Basal lamina:** It is further comprised of two layers:
   i. **Lamina lucida:** It is 45 nm (*1 nm* = 10^{-9} *cm*) thick, clear layer ***adjoining*** the epithelium.
   ii. **Lamina densa:** It is 50 nm thick layer that is darker in appearance and is present between lamina lucida and connective tissue of gingiva.

   Anchoring fibrils and filaments of basal lamina bind the epithelium to the underlying connective tissue. The basal lamina and the anchoring fibrils are produced by the epithelial cells.
2. **Reticular lamina** (*lamina reticularis*).

CLINICAL UTILITY AND SHORT ANSWER

What are the functions of the basement membrane?

- The basement membrane attaches the epithelium to the underlying connective tissue.
- It acts like a physical barrier that prevents ingress of microorganisms from epithelium into connective tissue.
- Malignant cells from malignancies starting in epithelium are also prevented from entering connective tissue and spreading by the basement membrane in early stages of such malignancies (*such malignancy restrained to the epithelium is called carcinoma in-situ*).
- It is selectively permeable, i.e. it allows diffusion of nutrients, metabolites and gases across it.

Gingival Connective Tissue

What is lamina propria? ▸

The gingival connective tissue is also called the ***lamina propria***; it is composed of two layers:

Name layers of lamina propria ▸

1. Papillary layer (***adjacent*** *to the epithelium*).
2. Reticular layer.

Fibers of Gingiva

There are three types of fibers in the gingiva: ***collagen, reticulin,*** and ***elastin***. Collagen fibers are the most ***abundant***.

Gingival Fibers (Collagen Fibers of Gingiva) (Fig. 2.13)

These are also called the ***gingival*** fibers. They provide physical support to the gingiva, give it its firm consistency and are primarily made up of ***Type I collagen***. They are arranged in different fiber groups:

◂ *Name different gingival fiber groups.*

1. **Dentogingival** (*also called as Gingivo-dental group*): They run from cementum of tooth's root to gingiva. These are further of 3 types:
   a. Fibers which run towards crest of gingiva.
   b. Those which run towards middle region of gingiva.
   c. Ones which end near outer surface of periosteum of alveolar bone **(*same as* 5)**.
2. **Alveogingival group:** These run from crest of alveolar bone towards center and crest of the gingiva.
3. **Circular group:** They encircle the tooth and run around it in a circular fashion like a ring within gingival connective tissue.
4. **Transseptal group:** They run interproximally between two adjacent teeth of the same arch (*cementum of one tooth root to that of the adjoining one*).
5. **Dentoperiosteal group (*same as* 1 c):** They fan out from cementum of tooth's root towards periosteum of alveolar bone.
6. **Semicircular fibers:** These attach to cementum of a tooth's root on one of its proximal surfaces just apical to the C-E junction and traverse around the same tooth lingually or buccally to attach on opposite proximal surface of the same tooth.
7. **Transgingival fibers:** They originate on proximal surface of one tooth root, go around and across the facial or lingual surface of the adjacent (*2nd*) tooth and then diagonally traverse the interdental space between 2nd and the next adjacent tooth (*3rd tooth*) to end on the interproximal surface of the 3rd tooth in the same arch.
8. **Interpapillary group:** These run in faciolingual direction in interdental papilla and provide support to the interdental papilla.

◂ *Which fiber group is similar to dentoperiosteal group?*

◂ *Do fibers of transgingival insert on the same tooth on which they originate?*

◂ *In which direction do fibers of the interpapillary group run?*

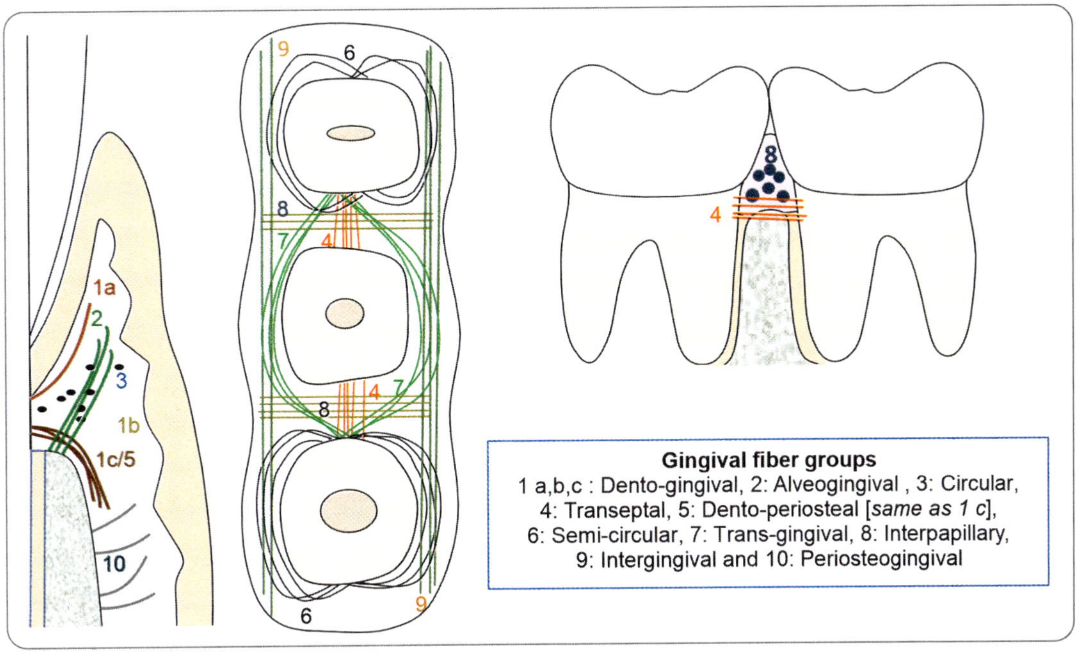

Fig. 2.13: Gingival connective tissue fibers

Which fiber groups provide support primarily to the attached gingiva? ▸

9. **Intergingival group:** These run parallel to the dentition (*dental arch*) in the attached gingiva. These are present on both facial and lingual surfaces and provide support and firmness to attached gingiva.
10. **Periosteogingival fibers:** They extend from periosteum of alveolar bone to the attached gingiva.

Functions of Gingival Fibers

What is the importance of gingival fibers? ▸

1. Gingival fibers ***stabilize*** all parts of the gingiva. They keep free gingiva firmly adapted to the tooth. Gingival fibers also attach the attached gingiva to the underlying tooth and bone. A firmly adapted free gingiva helps maintain integrity of the DG junction.
2. They impart firmness to gingiva and thus ***prevent*** tearing, injury and stripping of gingiva during mastication. In this way they provide indirect stability to the tooth.

CLINICAL UTILITY AND SHORT ANSWER

What is the other name for dentoperiosteal group of gingival fibers?
Gingivodental fibers extend from the root surface to the periosteum of the alveolar bone (*within the gingiva*). Dentoperiosteal fibers are also called gingivodental fibers by some authors.

What is the difference between semicircular and circular group fibers?
Semicircular group fibers originate from a proximal surface of a tooth's root and run either buccally or lingually to attach to the other proximal root surface of the same tooth.
Circular group fibers ***do not*** attach onto the root of a tooth on any surface. They run around the tooth in the gingival connective tissue.

What is the difference between transseptal and transgingival fibers?
Both these group of fibers run interproximally. The transseptal group runs between two adjacent teeth, whereas the transgingival group starts from a tooth (1st) goes across the 2nd tooth to attach onto the interproximal surface of the 3rd tooth.

What is Gingival ligament?
All fiber groups of the gingiva are collectively called as gingival ligament.

DENTO-GINGIVAL (*DG*) JUNCTION

The point of union where gingiva attaches to the tooth is called DG junction (Fig. 2.1, red line). DG junction is made by:

What comprises DG junction? ▸

1. **Junctional epithelium (*JE*) or attachment epithelium.**
2. **Epithelial attachment.**
   - It is the basal lamina of junctional epithelium (*produced by cells of the JE*) that fixes junctional epithelium to tooth surface.
   - Epithelial attachment acts like an organic ***glue*** to attach cells of JE to tooth.
   - Some organic strands also provide physical union with the tooth surface. In addition to this, strength of DG junction is increased by gingival group fibers. They help in keeping the marginal gingiva and therefore the JE tightly adapted and joined to the tooth surface.
   - The DG junction is ***unique*** because such a junction between a soft and a hard tissue (*gingiva and tooth*) that is mediated by a basal lamina is ***not*** found anywhere else in the human body.

Why is DG junction unique? ▸

Junctional Epithelium (*JE*) or Attachment Epithelium

Is JE keratinized or nonkeratinized? ▸

What are the dimensions of JE? ▸

What is the relation of JE to sulcular epithelium? ▸

1. The junctional epithelium is ***non-keratinizing*** (Fig. 2.12).
2. It is ***3–4*** cell layers thick and is present all around the tooth.
3. JE is ***0.25–1.35 mm in length*** and may have ***3–20*** layers.
4. It forms the attachment apparatus of gingiva to tooth (*therefore it is also called attachment epithelium*).
5. JE is continuous with the sulcular epithelium (*present coronal to JE*).
6. Turnover rate of the cells of the JE is between ***1–6 days***.

ALERT!

Write some important clinical considerations of JE.

- The JE is the ***weakest*** link in defense of gingiva.
- This is so because it is non-keratinized.
- Intercellular junctions in the JE are few and not very tight, intercellular spaces are wider and easily penetrable by bacteria.
- JE is just 3–20-cell thick.
- As sub-epithelial blood vessels lie just under the JE and are only a few cells away from surface of the epithelium where bacterial plaque collects (*in the sulcus*), bacteria can enter the subepithelial vessels under the JE easily. From here, infection can spread to deeper periodontal tissues to cause gingivitis and periodontitis.

◂ *Why is JE the weakest link in defense of gingiva?*

CLINICAL UTILITY AND SHORT ANSWER

What is dentogingival unit?

Gingival connective fibers and JE are collectively called dentogingival unit.

What is the difference between dentogingival junction and dentogingival unit?

- Dentogingival junction is the junction or area of union between gingiva and tooth.
- Strength of dentogingival junction is reinforced by gingival connective tissue fibers.
- As gingival connective tissue fibers and JE work collectively towards maintaining the dentogingival junction, gingival connective tissue fibers and JE are collectively called the dentogingival unit.

Blood Supply and Lymphatic Drainage of Gingiva

- Gingiva receives its blood supply from lingual, facial and maxillary arteries. Local area arterial supply comes from (Fig. 2.14):
  1. Supra-periosteal vessels running ***vertically*** over buccal and lingual surfaces of periosteum of the alveolar bone supply overlying gingiva (Fig. 2.14, black arrows).
  2. Vessels emerging from crest of the interdental bone supply overlying interdental gingiva.
  3. Vessels at coronal end of periodontal ligament spill out to supply overlying gingiva.
- ***No*** blood vessel extends into epithelium. Epithelium receives its nutritional supply by diffusion across basement membrane into the connective tissue.
- Veins run ***close*** to arteries.
- **Lymphatic drainage** of gingiva goes to:
  1. **Submandibular nodes** (*from buccal maxillary gingiva and lingual and buccal mandibular gingivae of premolars and molars*).
  2. **Submental nodes** (*from anterior mandibular gingiva*).
  3. **Jugulodigastric nodes** (*from posterior parts of oral cavity including gingiva of third molars*).

◂ *In which direction do blood vessels supplying the gingiva run?*

◂ *Do blood vessels enter epithelium?*

◂ *What is the lymphatic drainage of the gingiva?*

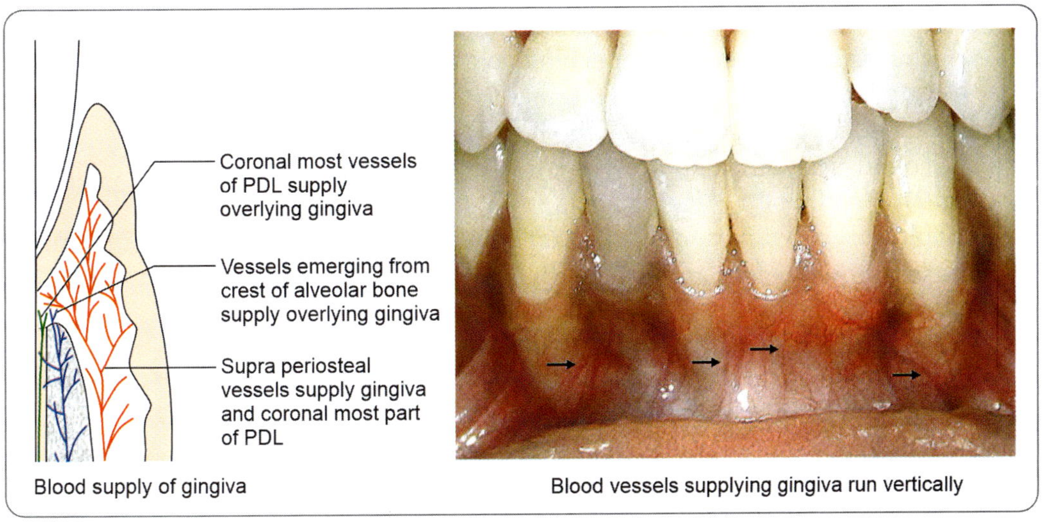

Fig. 2.14: Blood supply of gingiva

CLINICAL UTILITY AND SHORT ANSWER

How do cells of the epithelium receive nutrition if no vessels enter epithelium?

All metabolic requirements of epithelial cells are met by diffusion through basement membrane. To provide enough metabolic exchange, basement membrane is folded to increase its surface area. This folded basal lamina also provides additional physical strength to help epithelium bear physical forces.

CLINICAL UTILITY AND SHORT ANSWER

What is the clinical importance of fact that gingival vessels run vertically? ▸

In which direction do blood vessels supplying the gingiva run?

Blood vessels supplying the gingiva run ***vertically*** **(Fig. 2.14)**. Therefore, as far as possible, incisions in the gingiva and alveolar mucosa should be designed and placed vertically to minimize cutting of these blood vessels. Doing so will reduce bleeding and maintains maximum blood supply to healing tissue post operatively.

Nerve Supply of the Gingiva

What is the nerve supply of the gingiva? ▸

The major nerves supplying the gingiva are: Maxillary nerve, posterior, middle and anterior superior alveolar nerve, nasopalatine nerve, greater palatine nerve, lingual nerve, buccal nerve and mental nerve.

NORMAL CLINICAL FEATURES OF GINGIVA

The word ***'normal'*** implies ***clinically healthy gingiva*** (*clinical absence of gingival inflammation caused by gingivitis or periodontitis*). The following clinical features of the gingiva are assessed to diagnose health or disease status of the gingiva:

I. Color
II. Contour
III. Consistency
IV. Surface texture
V. Position
VI. Size
VII. Shape.

I. Colour of Gingiva

Is colour of gingiva same in all individuals? ▸

Colour of only ***marginal*** and ***attached*** gingiva is assessed. Colour of normal gingiva is ***different*** in different individuals and is ***related*** to the individual's skin colour.

- Colour of gingiva varies from ***light pink*** to ***dark brown***.

Why is it improper to say that colour of gingiva is coral pink? ▸

- Traditionally, colour of gingiva has been described to be 'coral pink' which is a brownish-pink colour. However, in every day practice, this is ***not*** found to be true. Wide variation in colour of gingiva is seen in normal gingiva of heathy individuals. Therefore, gingiva may be of:
  - Diffused light pink colour **(Fig. 2.15, diag. 1)**
  - Pink colour interlaid with brown patches (*patchy melanin pigmentation*) **(Fig. 2.15, diag. 2)**
  - Dark pink colour with bands of diffused light melanin pigmentation **(Fig. 2.15. diag. 3)**
  - Diffused brown colour interlaid with pink patches devoid of melanin **(Fig. 2.15, diag. 4)**.

In which individuals is the gingiva dark pink and brown? ▸

- Gingiva is generally of pink colour interlaid with brown patches or dark-brown colour interlaid with pink patches in coloured individuals (*dark coloured skin*). It is light pink in white races and albinos.

In which individuals is the gingiva light pink in colour? ▸

- It is therefore more appropriate to say that the ***base colour*** of gingiva is ***coral pink*** and this shows several variations due to other (*'add-on'*) factors, e.g. melanin pigmentation, etc. in different individuals and races.

What is the colour of alveolar mucosa? ▸

- The alveolar mucosa has a dull dark red color.

CLINICAL UTILITY AND SHORT ANSWER

What is coral pink color?

It is a brown–orange shade of pink. Corals are sea animals of brownish-orange colour. As base colour of gingiva closely resembles the colour of such corals, the gingiva's colour is described as coral pink color.

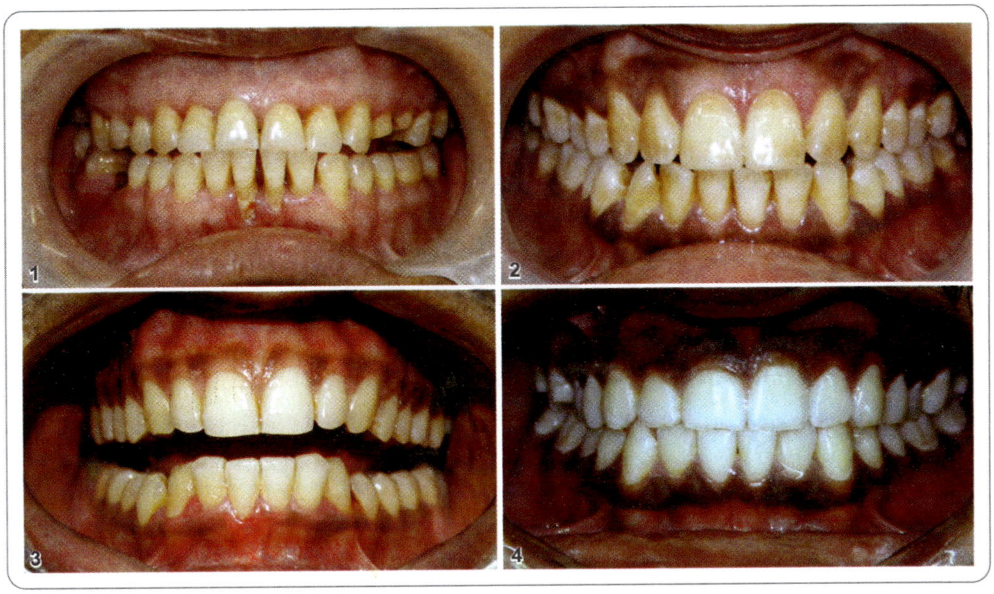

Fig. 2.15: Base colour of gingiva is coral pink and shows several variations due to 'add-on' factors like melanin pigmentation, etc. in different individuals. The alveolar mucosa has a dull dark red color.

Factors on Which Colour of Gingiva Depends

- **Degree of vascularity:** Greater the vascularity (*blood supply*), redder the color. Higher number of vessels supplying the area and/or increased blood supply due to vascular dilatation (*e.g. acute inflammation, i.e. acute gingivitis, etc.*) increases supply of oxygenated blood to the gingiva. This imparts a red color to the gingiva.
  Stasis of blood (*in chronic inflammation, i.e. chronic gingivitis and periodontitis*) causes reduction of oxygen in blood (*cyanosis*). This imparts a ***bluish*** colour to gingiva (*venous blood is blue while arterial blood is red*). If stasis occurs, the color of the gingiva changes to magenta, maroon, burgundy, etc. colours.

◂ *How does inflammation in gingiva affect its colour?*

- **Thickness of epithelium:** Greater the thickness of the epithelium, lighter will be the colour and vice-versa.
- **Degree of keratinization:** Greater the keratinization, lighter will be the color. If there is extreme hyperkeratinization, the gingiva will appear white.

◂ *How do thickness of epithelium and degree of keratinization affect colour of gingiva?*

- **Degree of pigmentation (*melanin*):** Melanin pigment imparts a brown color to the gingiva. Higher melanin pigmentation results in darker coloured gingiva. Melanin pigmentation can be in patches or diffused.

II. Contour of Gingiva

◂ *What is the contour of normal gingiva?*

- The clinically healthy gingiva has a ***'knife edge' deflecting*** and ***scalloped*** or ***arcuate contour*** (*series of semi-circles or arcs*) (*Fig. 2.16, deflecting contour-blue arrow, scalloping shown as yellow line*).
- If tooth surface is prominent (*convexity of tooth surface is increased*), the arcuate pattern or scalloping of overlying gingiva increases and the gingival crest is placed at a more apical level, e.g. on the labial surface of teeth in labio-version (Fig. 2.17, blue arrows) and vice-versa (Fig. 2.17, red arrows).

◂ *Is root prominence related to gingival contour?*

- As scalloping of gingiva increases, marginal gingiva gets thinner (Fig. 2.17, blue arrows); if on the other hand, scalloping decreases, i.e. becomes flatter, marginal gingiva becomes blunt, rounded and bulbous (Fig. 2.17, red arrows).

◂ *Is degree of scalloping of gingiva related to thickness of marginal gingiva?*

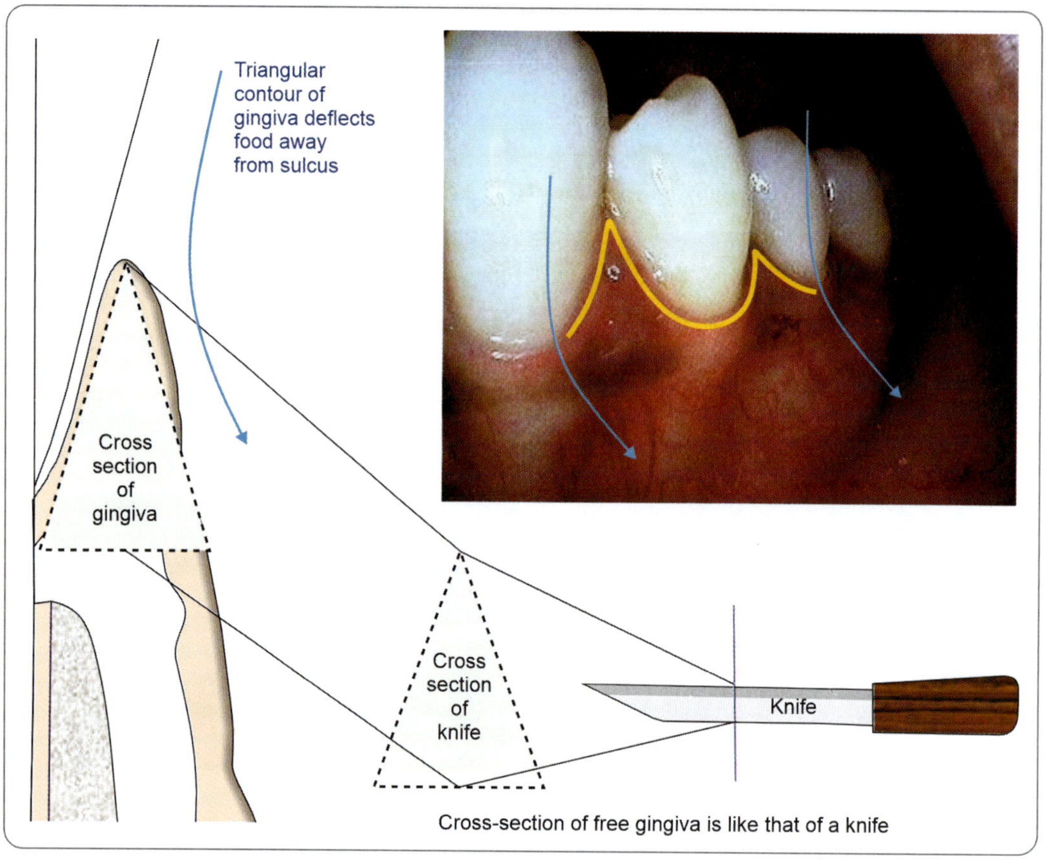

Fig. 2.16: Knife-edge deflecting contour of free gingiva deflects food away from the sulcus.

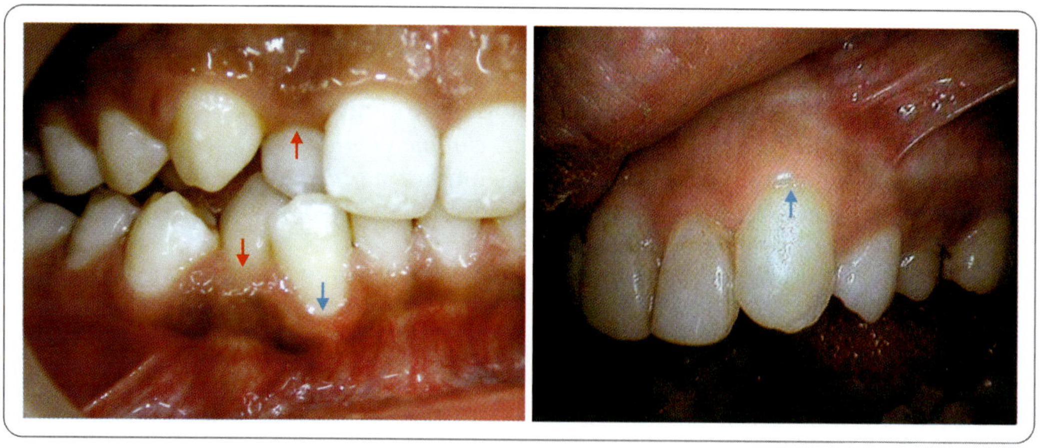

Fig. 2.17: Gingival margin is relatively more coronal, flatter and rounded in teeth that are in linguo-version (*red arrows*). Gingival margin is relatively more apical, thin and accentuated in teeth that are prominent or in labio-version (*blue arrows*).

CLINICAL UTILITY AND SHORT ANSWER

Why is knife-edge deflecting contour considered normal and bulbous and flat gingival contour abnormal?

How does knife-edge deflecting contour of the gingiva help in maintaining gingival health? ▶

Deflecting gingival contour of gingiva deflects food away from the sulcus during mastication of food. As food impaction into sulcus is one of the causes of periodontitis (*food debris is source of nutrition for bacteria*), therefore, a knife-edge deflecting gingival contour prevents periodontitis and is normal.

On the other hand, bulbous gingival contour does not completely deflect food away from the sulcus and leads to some food impaction into the sulcus. Therefore, gingiva with bulbous contours has more chances of having periodontitis and it therefore, has lesser chances of being remaining healthy. Bulbous contours are thus unhealthy.

III. Consistency (*Feel*) of Gingiva

- Clinically healthy gingiva has a ***firm*** and ***resilient*** consistency (*resiliency is tendency to bounce back to original shape after deforming force has been lifted*).
- The firm and resilient consistency of the gingiva is due to its healthy connective tissue. Gingival fibers contribute also to this.
- Resiliency of the gingiva is markedly reduced or even lost if gingiva is inflammed (*gingivitis and periodontitis*); here gingiva becomes soft and shows pitting after application of pressure.

◂ *What is the normal consistency of gingiva?*

◂ *What causes loss of consistency of gingiva?*

IV. Surface Texture of Gingiva

- Gingiva has a stippled or orange peel-like surface texture, i.e. it is minutely lobulated and pitted just like an orange peel (Fig. 2.18, blue arrows).
- Stippling is an adaptive mechanism. It reinforces epithelium to bear frictional and shearing forces of food as it rubs past the gingiva during mastication.
- Stippling is ***noticeable*** in only **40–50%** of individuals (Fig. 2.18, red arrow). It is ***absent*** in young children below 5 years of age and in older people. Stippling (*if was present*) disappears in inflammatory diseases of the gingiva, *e.g.* gingivitis and periodontitis. Stippling may be very fine and may therefore not be easily identifiable.
- Stippling is more clearly seen after drying the surface of the gingiva and viewing it in natural or diffused shadow-less light of a dental unit.

◂ *What is the normal surface texture of gingiva?*

◂ *What is the use of stippling?*

◂ *Is stippling present in all individuals?*

◂ *What is the best way to see stippling?*

CLINICAL UTILITY AND SHORT ANSWER

Which parts of the gingiva are stippled?

1. When present, stippling is ***identifiable*** on ***attached gingiva*** and ***center of the interdental papilla***. Facial gingival surfaces are more prominently stippled.
2. The ***free gingiva*** is ***not*** stippled (*even if stippling is present on attached gingiva and interdental papilla*).

◂ *Where is stippling present on the gingiva?*

◂ *Which part of the gingiva does not show stippling?*

CLINICAL UTILITY AND SHORT ANSWER

What is the average diameter of gingival pits?

On an average, pits on the stippled gingiva have a ***diameter*** of **50 microns** (*1 micron = 10^{-6} m*).

CLINICAL UTILITY AND SHORT ANSWER

Why should one dry the gingiva before viewing gingival stippling?

Gingival stippling is lost when gingiva is inflamed (*gingivitis and periodontitis*). When gingiva is wet with saliva, saliva flows into the pits on the gingival surface and forms a smooth mirror-like film over gingiva. If viewed wet, the otherwise pitted gingival surface then appears smooth. As a smooth gingival surface can be a sign of gingivitis and periodontitis, a stippled (*i.e. healthy gingiva*) but wet gingival surface may therefore be incorrectly diagnosed as gingivitis or periodontitis (*instead of healthy gingiva*). Gingiva must therefore be dried before deciding on its surface texture.

◂ *Why is presence of stippling likely to be missed if surface of gingiva is wet?*

CLINICAL UTILITY AND SHORT ANSWER

What is the difference between pitting on pressure and pitted (stippled) surface?

The ***pitted*** or ***stippled surface*** of gingiva is a ***normal*** feature of the clinically healthy gingiva. ***Pitting on pressure*** is a clinical sign which if present indicates the presence of **edema** in the gingiva, i.e. it is a sign of gingivitis and periodontitis. The sign pitting on pressure, can be demonstrated in an edematous (inflamed) gingiva by pressing lightly, for a short while, on the ***marginal*** and ***attached gingiva***, with the side of a dental probe and then noticing any pitting the instrument leaves behind.

◂ *How is pitting produced by pressure different from pits seen on stippled gingival surface?*

ALERT!

Degree of keratinization and coarseness/prominence/degree of stippling are related.

Epithelium with a coarse/more prominent stippling generally exhibits a higher degree of keratinization. Both, i.e. degree of keratinization and coarseness/prominence/degree of stippling increase and decrease simultaneously.

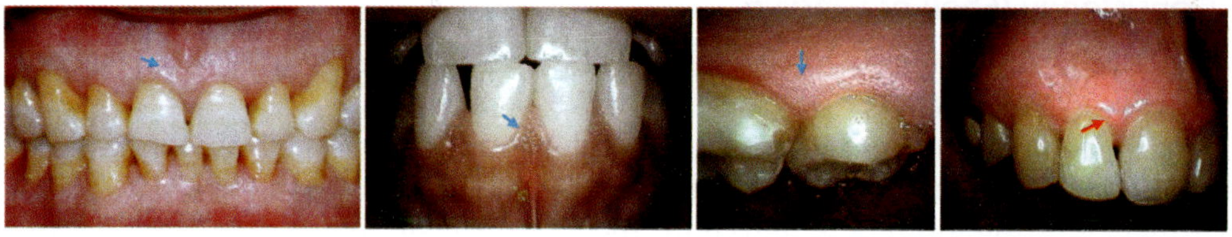

Fig. 2.18: Gingiva has stippled surface; only attached gingiva and central portions of interdental papilla are stippled (*blue arrows*). Stippling is very fine or is totally absent in 50% cases (*red arrow*).

V. Normal Position of Gingiva

What is location of gingival landmarks in relation to CE junction in normal gingiva? ▸

Position of the gingiva is decided by relating the position and location of gingival landmarks to the CE junction of a tooth. ***Normal*** position of gingiva is characterized by presence of:

- Gingival crest on enamel, slightly coronal to the CE junction **(Fig. 2.19, diag. 1)**.
- Base of sulcus coronal or at level of CE junction **(Fig. 2.19, diag. 1)**.

What is the implication of presence of base of sulcus on the anatomical root? ▸

- If base of the sulcus migrates apical to CE junction onto the cementum, this, is considered to be due to past or ongoing ***periodontitis*** (*irrespective of position of the crest of gingiva which may lie on enamel*) **(Fig. 2.19, diag. 3)**.

Exception: In case tooth is prominent, i.e. out of the curve of the arch, (*e.g. canines, viewed from buccal side*), all gingival landmarks are normally located more apically on the root. Only in such cases, if PD (*probing depth*) is less than 3 mm, presence of base of sulcus and crest of gingiva on the cementum is considered normal (*2018 classification—reduced periodontium due to tooth position; see Fig. 10A.3*) **(Figs 2.20, diags 1 and 2, 2.21 diag. 2)**.

For diagnosing clinical condition of gingiva (*normal vs abnormal*), which is more important—position of the crest of free gingiva, position of base of sulcus or depth of sulcus?

All three parameters are equally important and are used to decide normalcy and clinical health of gingiva.

- Healthy gingiva must ideally have both crest of gingiva and base of sulcus on enamel, i.e. coronal to CE junction, sulcus depth of less than 3 mm and must have normal clinical features (*as described in previous section of this chapter*) **(Figs 2.2 and 2.21. diag. 1)**.
- If crest of the gingiva lies on a tooth's crown but base of the sulcus lies on the cementum, this is abnormal **(Figs 2.19, diag. 3)**. As described above, the only exception to this rule are teeth with 'reduced periodontium due prominent tooth position' (*2018 classification*) **(Figs 2.20, diags 1 and 2, and 2.21, diag. 2)**.

When is presence of base of sulcus on the cementum considered normal? ▸

- According to the 2018 classification, reduced periodontium may also be seen in a ***treated*** case of periodontitis. Here, clinical gingival health on a reduced periodontium is characterized by location of base of sulcus on the cementum, i.e. apical to the CE junction, PD (*probing depth*) of less than 4 mm with no bleeding on probing (*4 mm sulcus depth is only **allowed** in previously **treated** and clinically healthy cases of periodontitis; for all other cases, normal gingiva must have sulcus depths of **less** than 3 mm*).
- Clinically healthy gingiva exhibits normal gingival clinical features and absence of bleeding on probing, erythema, edema and other symptoms of gingivitis.

CLINICAL UTILITY AND SHORT ANSWER

How do we decide health status of gingiva if gingival landmarks are present on root in cases of reduced periodontium (*2018 classification*)?

According to the 2018 classification of gingival and periodontal diseases, presence of gingival landmarks on root (*reduced periodontium*) may be because of:

1. Prominent tooth position, crown lengthening, etc. Here ***clinical*** gingival health is characterized by less than 3 mm PD **(Fig. 2.20, diags 1 and 2 and Fig. 2.21, diag. 2)** and ***absence*** of bleeding on probing, gingival erythema, edema and other symptoms of gingivitis.
2. In a case of past periodontitis that has now been successfully treated, ***clinical*** gingival health is characterized by less than 4 mm PD **(Fig. 2.20, diag. 3)** and ***absence*** of bleeding on probing, erythema, edema and other symptoms of gingivitis.

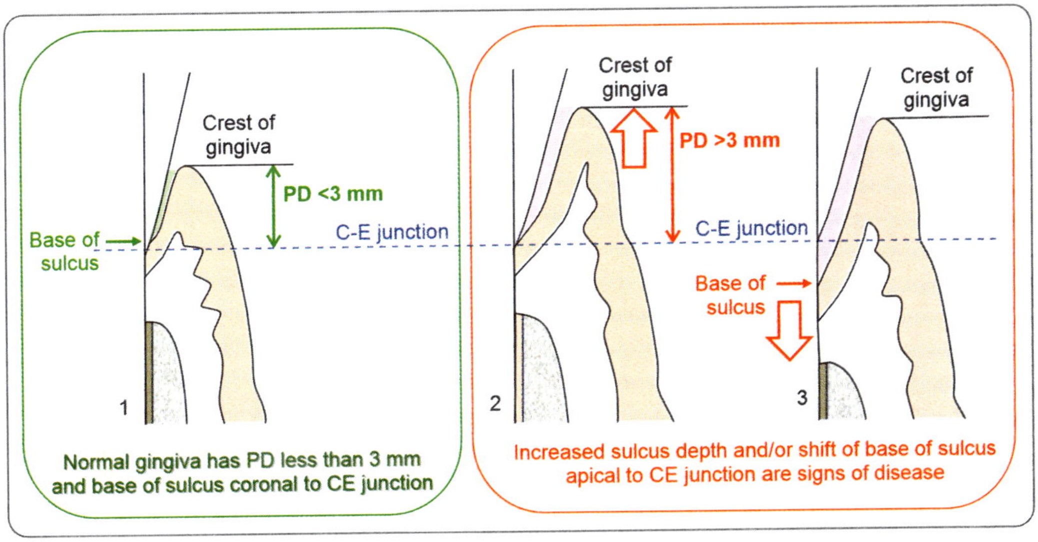

Fig. 2.19: When crest of gingiva is located on enamel, both probing sulcus/pocket depth (*PD*) and location of base of sulcus are taken into account for judging gingival normalcy.
In normal gingiva, both gingival crest and base of sulcus must be located at/coronal to the CE junction (*diag. 1, green arrow*) and sulcus depth (*PD*) must be less than 3 mm (*diag. 1 green double arrow*). If sulcus depth (PD) is more than 3 mm (*diag. 2 red double arrow*) and/or base of sulcus is apical to CE junction (*diag. 3, red arrow*) these are abnormal.

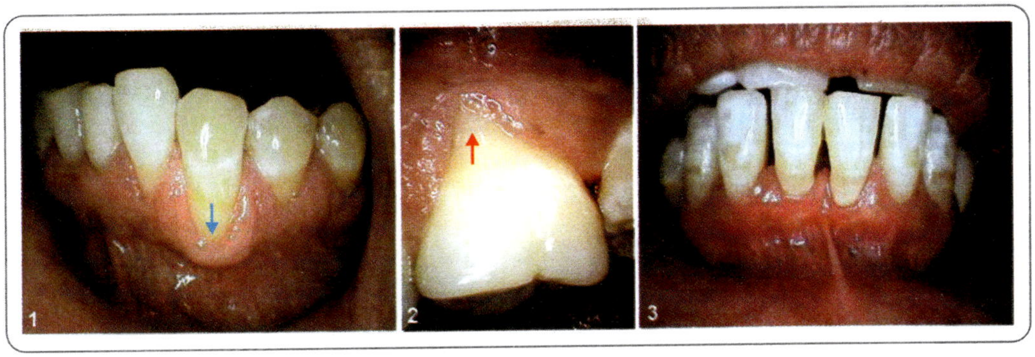

Fig. 2.20: Reduced periodontium due to prominent position of the tooth (*diag.1, blue arrow*), prominent root of multirooted tooth (*diag. 2 red arrow*) and in a successfully treated case of periodontitis (*diag. 3*).

VI. Size of Normal Gingiva

The normal size of the gingiva ***cannot*** be described in physical terms. While deciding on size, i.e. whether it is normal or abnormal, the following have to be kept in mind:

1. Normal-sized gingiva will exhibit normal clinical features.
2. Although gingiva can increase in size (*due to increase in its bulk*), reduction in size below the 'normal' size is ***not*** possible.

◂ *Describe the size of normal gingiva?*

The following can be safely assumed from the above facts:

1. Gingiva is considered to be of normal size if there is no overt increase in size.
2. Gingiva which is not normal will usually be enlarged.
3. Increase in size also alters other normal clinical characteristics of gingiva.

Thickness of Gingiva

Clinically two types of normal gingival thicknesses have been described:

1. Thick gingival biotype **(Fig. 2.22, diag. A)**.
2. Thin gingival biotype **(Fig. 2.22, diag. B)**.
    - Thin gingival biotype is associated with narrow zone of keratinized gingiva and with small teeth.

◂ *Is thickness of gingiva related to width of keratinized gingiva?*

- Thick gingiva is associated with broad zone of keratinized gingiva and wider teeth.
- Females usually have thin gingiva while males usually have thick gingiva.

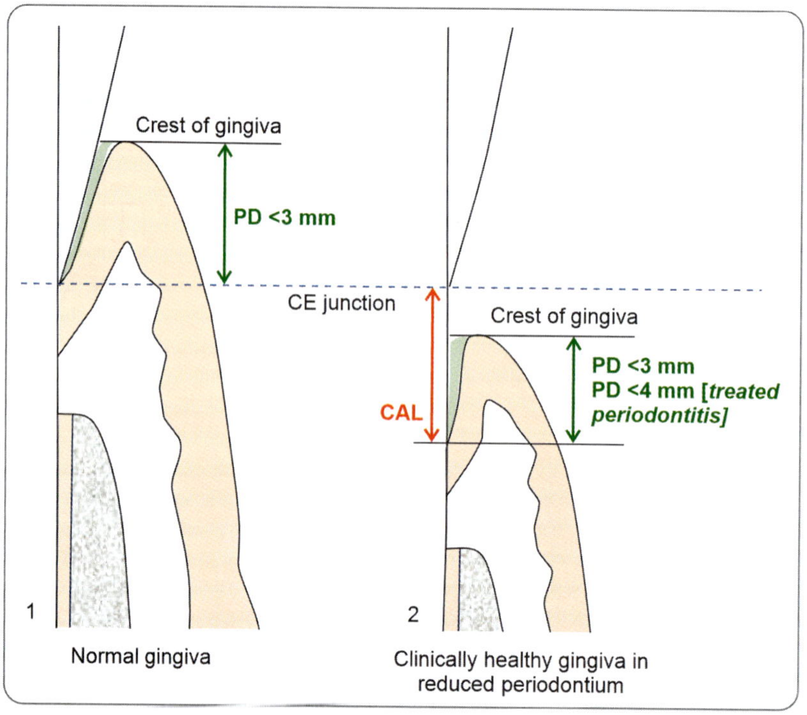

Fig. 2.21: Clinical health in normal and reduced periodontium (*CAL due to prominent position of tooth or periodontitis*) is characterized by sulcus depths of less than 3 mm (*diag. 1 and 2 green double arrow*) and absence of bleeding on probing, redness, edema and other symptoms of gingivitis.

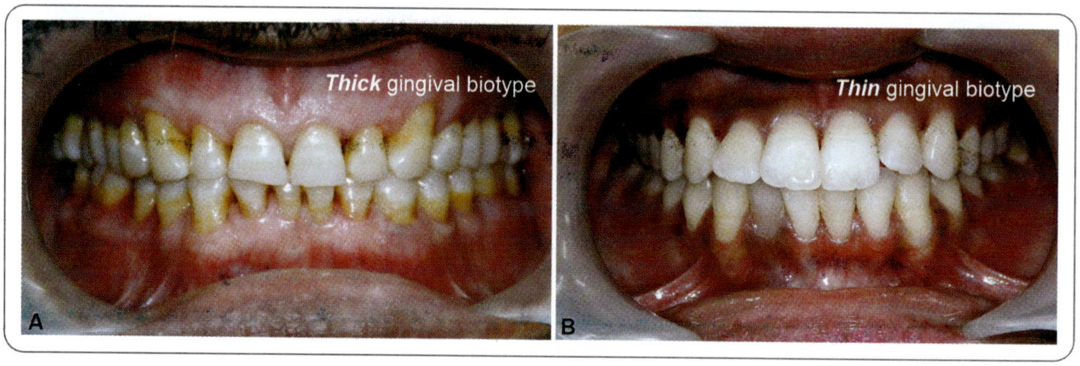

Fig. 2.22: Thick and thin gingival biotypes

VII. Shape of Normal Interdental Gingiva/Papilla

As discussed in preceding text, the shape of the interdental papilla is dependent on shape of the inter-proximal embrasure (*see preceding section and Fig. 2.11*).

Review Questions

1. Why is knowledge of normal periodontium essential for diagnosing periodontal disease?
2. What are the types of oral mucosa? What is gingiva?
3. What are supporting structures of teeth collectively called? Name tissues referred to by the term periodontium.
4. What is masticatory mucosa? Does it help in mastication?
5. Name clinical parts of gingiva.
6. Why is marginal gingiva also called free gingiva?
7. What is the anatomical boundary between free and attached gingivae called?

8. What is the width of free gingival groove?
9. What is gingival sulcus? Name its boundaries.
10. How wide is gingival sulcus? OR Is gingival sulcus easily accessible?
11. What is the relation between free gingival groove and base of gingival sulcus? How is free gingival groove formed?
12. What is the depth of gingival sulcus? How is depth of gingival sulcus measured?
13. How can average depth of 1.8–2.0 mm of normal sulcus be explained?
14. What is the difference between histological and clinical pocket depths?
15. Name the factors that cause deepening of sulcus.
16. Where would you expect sulcus depth of 0 mm?
17. What are the contents of gingival sulcus?
18. What is GCF? How can we measure rate of flow of gingival fluid?
19. What are the constituents of GCF? What are the functions of GCF?
20. Name boundaries of attached gingiva. What is the width of attached gingiva?
21. What kind of epithelium covers the attached gingiva?
22. Which areas of gingiva are keratinized?
23. What is the function of attached gingiva?
24. How is adequacy of attached gingiva known?
25. Where is interdental papilla located?
26. What is interdental col? What is its clinical importance?
27. What type of epithelium lines the interdental col area? Why is knowledge of type of epithelium lining interdental col important?
28. Name the types of epithelium covering various parts of gingiva.
29. Define keratinization. What is the function/purpose of keratinization?
30. Name the cell layers of the keratinized and non-keratinized epithelium.
31. What are parakeratinization and orthokeratinization?
32. What is a keratinocyte? Are keratinocytes found in oral epithelium?
33. What are melanocytes? Where are melanocytes found in epithelium?
34. What are melanosomes, premelanosomes, melanophages and melanophores?
35. Name different kinds of cells found in gingival epithelium.
36. Are mitotic rates in different areas of gingival epithelium same? Do other areas of oral epithelium exhibit similar mitotic rates as seen in the gingival epithelium?
37. Do mitotic rates of cells of gingiva vary during the day?
38. Is presence of inflammatory cells in gingival connective tissue considered to be normal or abnormal?
39. How is the epithelium joined to underlying connective tissue?
40. Describe the basal lamina of the gingiva.
41. Describe gingival connective tissue and gingival connective tissue fibers.
42. What is the other name of dento-periosteal group of fibers?
43. What is the difference between semicircular and circular group fibers?
44. What is the difference between transgingival and transseptal fibers?
45. What is junctional epithelium? What is the turnover rate of cells of JE?
46. Describe the DG junction.
47. Describe attachment epithelium or junctional epithelium.
48. What does dento-gingival unit mean?
49. What is the difference between dentogingival junction and dentogingival unit?
50. Name sources of blood supply of gingiva.
51. No vessels enter the epithelium, how do cells of epithelium receive their nutritional supply?
52. Discuss the innervation of the gingiva.
53. Name features of gingiva assessed while diagnosing the condition of the gingiva.
54. What is the normal color of free gingiva, attached gingiva and alveolar mucosa?
55. What is a coral pink color? Describe the racial variations in color of gingiva.
56. What are the features on which the color of gingiva depends? How do the above features modify color?

57. Describe contour of gingiva.
58. What does term scalloped or arcuate contour mean?
59. What does knife-edge deflecting contour mean?
60. What is normal consistency of gingiva? What is resiliency?
61. What is the surface texture of gingiva?
62. Why should the gingiva be dried before viewing stippling and deciding on its surface texture?
63. What is the size of pits present on a stippled gingiva?
64. What is the difference between pitting on pressure and pitted (*stippled*) surface?
65. Which parts of gingiva are stippled? Why is gingival surface stippled?
66. On which parts of gingiva is the test 'pitting on pressure' performed?
67. Is degree of keratinization related to coarseness, prominence and degree of stippling?
68. Where is the gingiva normally attached on the tooth?
69. What is reduced periodontium?
70. While diagnosing condition of gingiva as normal vs. abnormal, which is more important—the position of crest of free gingiva, base of sulcus or depth of sulcus?
71. What is the size of normal gingiva?
72. What is the shape of normal gingiva (*interdental papilla*)?

Chapter

3

Periodontal Ligament, Cementum and Alveolar Bone

The periodontium attaches teeth to the jaw bone and supports teeth during function. Of the four periodontal tissues, three, i.e. periodontal ligament, cementum and alveolar bone provide direct physical support to teeth whereas gingiva serves as a cover and provides protection to the other three.

PERIODONTAL LIGAMENT (*PDL*)

The periodontal ligament is a soft, fibrous specialized connective tissue that anchors and suspends the tooth within its bony socket. It covers roots of teeth and is present between cementum and the tooth-socket wall. PDL is also called periodontal membrane, pericementum, circular dental ligament, etc.

◂ *Which other periodontal tissues are present on the sides of PDL?*

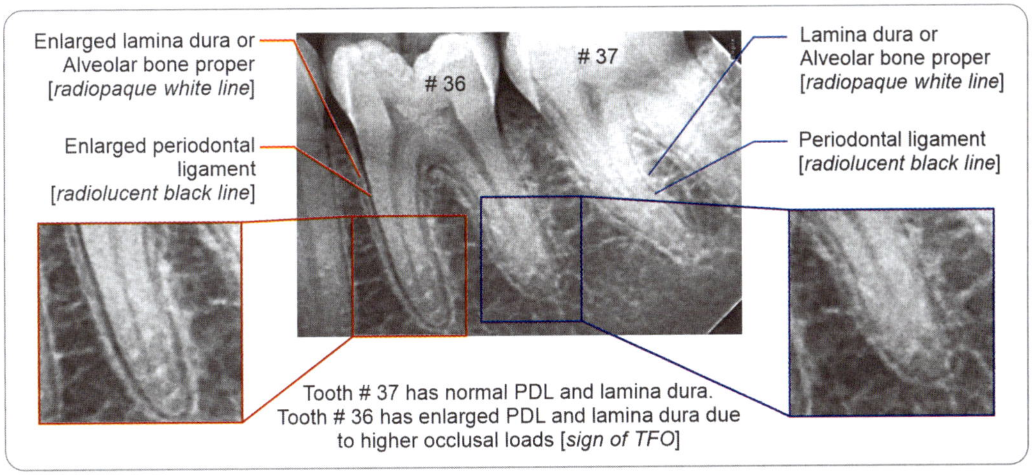

Fig. 3.1: Periodontal ligament is seen as a black (*radiolucent*) line surrounding roots of teeth

Shape and Width of PDL

- In a radiograph, the PDL appears like a ***black line*** surrounding the root of a tooth (*radiolucent*) and is shaped like an '***hourglass***' (Fig. 3.2). It is narrow in the middle and wider at its coronal 1/3rd and apical 1/3rd. The width of a normal PDL ***ranges from 0.15–0.38 mm***.
- The PDL ***widens*** (*hypertrophies*) when occlusal load on the tooth ***increases***. This is accompanied by an increase in number and thickening of collagen fiber bundles of PDL. The vice-versa is also true.

◂ *What is the normal width of PDL? How does it appear on a radiograph?*

◂ *What does widening of PDL indicate?*

CLINICAL UTILITY AND SHORT ANSWER

Does the width of the PDL increase or decrease with age?

The width of the PDL ***decreases*** with age.

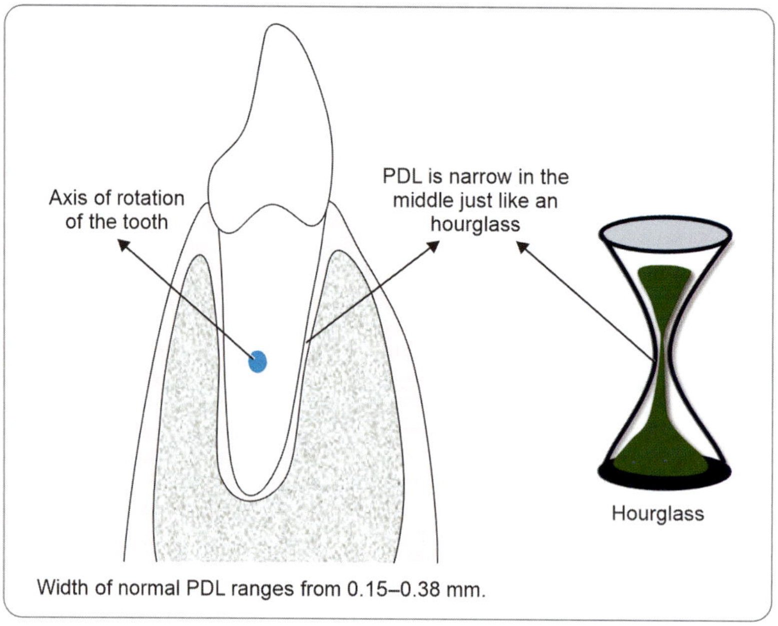

Fig. 3.2: Periodontal ligament is hourglass shaped

CLINICAL UTILITY AND SHORT ANSWER

What will happen when occlusal forces exceed load bearing capacity of PDL?

If excessive occlusal forces are put on the tooth (*traumatic occlusion*), PDL will get injured. This injury is called trauma form occlusion (*TFO*). A tooth with TFO will have wider PDL **(Figs 3.1 and 9.3)** and the socket may show widening at its opening **(*Fig. 9.4*)** (*funneling of the socket*).

Cellular and Extracellular Constituents of PDL

Name the cells found in the PDL. ▸

1. Cellular constituents of PDL include:
   i. **Synthetic cells** (*osteoblasts, fibroblasts and cementoblasts*).
   ii. **Resorptive cells** [*osteoclasts, fibroblasts* (*there are no fibroclasts; fibroblasts perform resorptive functions*) *and cementoclasts*].
   iii. **Progenitor cells** (*undifferentiated mesenchymal cells*).
   iv. Epithelial cell-rests of Malassez.
2. Extracellular constituents include collagen and oxytalan fibers, ground substance, nerves and vessels.

CLINICAL UTILITY AND SHORT ANSWER

Which pathological lesion can arise from epithelial cell rests of Malassez? ▸

What are epithelial cell rests of Malassez?

These are remnants of the Hertwig's root sheath in PDL. After formation of root of tooth, Hertwig's root sheath breaks into small islands of cells called epithelial cell rests of Malassez. The epithelial cell rests of Malassez can proliferate and lead to formation of periapical and lateral **cysts**.

Principal (*Collagen*) Fiber Groups of PDL

How much volume of the PDL do collagen fibers of the PDL collectively occupy? ▸

- Fibers of PDL are arranged in a complex ***three-dimensional*** network and they collectively comprise 2/3rd of total volume of PDL (*the other 1/3rd is occupied by ground substance, tissue fluid and neuro-vascular elements*).

Are PDL fibers straight or wavy? ▸

- When in a state of rest individual fibers are wavy, fibers show branching and union with other fibers. Fibers of PDL are made of type I and type III collagen and are arranged in groups called principal fiber groups. Nerves and blood vessels run between fiber bundles.

What are Sharpey's fibers? ▸

- Terminal-ends of individual fibers are embedded into cementum on one side and into alveolar bone on the other. ***Embedded terminal-ends*** of PDL fibers are called ***Sharpey's fibers*** **(Fig. 3.3)**.

The principal fiber groups of the PDL (Fig. 3.3) are:

1. **Alveolar crest group:** They run in an oblique direction, from crest of alveolar bone to the tooth's cementum just apical to the junctional epithelium (*JE*). The cemental attachment of the fibers is ***coronal*** to their attachment to alveolar bone.
2. **Horizontal group fibers:** They are located apical to alveolar crest group and run at right angles to long axis of tooth just apical to mouth of the socket.
3. **Oblique group:** These run obliquely from bone to cementum. The cemental attachment of these fibers is ***apical*** to their alveolar bone attachment.
4. **Apical group:** Fibers of this group run from apical cementum to surrounding alveolar bone forming fundus of the socket. These fibers form only ***after*** completion of root formation.
5. **Inter-radicular group:** These fiber bundles are found only in ***multirooted*** teeth. They run from crest of the inter-radicular bone to furcation of a multirooted tooth.
6. **Transseptal group:** They run from inter-proximal surface of one tooth to that of the adjoining tooth. These fibers occasionally pass-through crest of the alveolar bone (*interdental bone*) and continue as transseptal fibers of the adjoining tooth. Transseptal group fibers are classified both under gingival (*Chapter 2, Fig. 2.13*) and periodontal fibers groups. Transseptal fibers running between upper central incisors form only after growth in the central fissure stops.

◂ Name the fiber groups of PDL.

◂ What is the orientation of the alveolar group fibers of PDL?

◂ What is the orientation of the oblique group fibers of PDL?

◂ In which teeth are inter-radicular fibers of PDL present?

◂ Which group of PDL fibers is also classified as gingival group fibers?

◂ When do transseptal group fibers running between upper central incisors develop?

ALERT!

What is the difference between alveolar crest and oblique group fibers?

- Both alveolar crest fibers and oblique group fibers run in an ***oblique*** fashion.
- Cemental attachment of alveolar crest fibers is ***coronal*** to their attachment to alveolar bone.
- Cemental attachment ***of*** oblique fibers, is ***apical*** to their attachment to alveolar bone (Fig. 3.3).

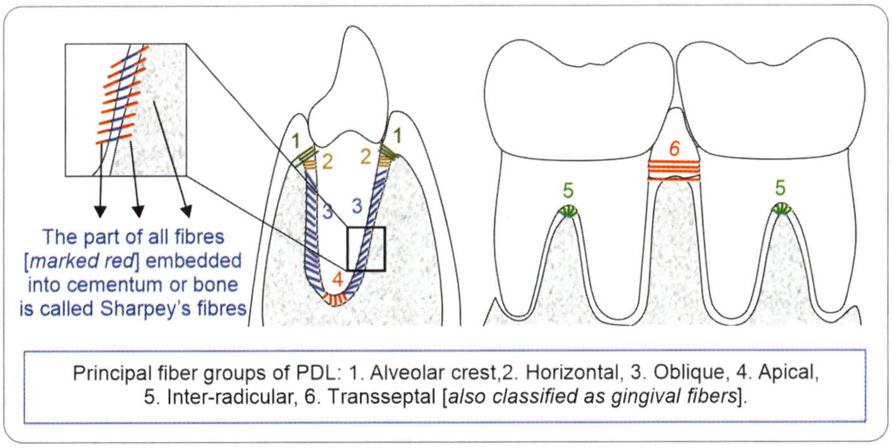

Fig. 3.3: Principal fiber groups of periodontal ligament and Sharpey's fibers (*embedded portion of fibers into cementum and bone are called Sharpey's fibers*).

CLINICAL UTILITY AND SHORT ANSWER

1. **Which fiber group out of all the gingival and periodontal ligament fiber groups develops first?**
   Dentogingival fibres of the gingival group develop first of all.
2. **What is the diameter of individual fibril of the PDL?**
   They have an average diameter of ***55 nm.***
3. **Which PDL fiber bundle group has the maximum number of constituent fibers?**
   Oblique group. They are the main attachment of tooth.
4. **Which group of PDL fibers is not found in teeth whose root formation is still continuing?**
   Apical group. They form only after root completion.
5. **What is the circular ligament?**
   Alveolar crest and ***horizontal groups*** are ***collectively*** called circular ligament.
6. **Which fibers rupture first during extraction of a tooth?**
   The fibers of the alveolar crest and horizontal group are the ***first to rupture during tooth extraction.***

◂ Which is the largest fiber group of PDL?

◂ When do apical group fibers form?

◂ What is circular ligament?

Functions of Individual Fiber Groups of PDL

The fiber bundles support the tooth in function and transfer the occlusal loads from tooth to bone. These fiber bundles perform the following functions:

How do alveolar crest fibers support the tooth?

- **Alveolar crest group:** They resist extrusion (*pulling out of tooth from its socket*), tilting and rotational forces on teeth. Fibers of one side resist lateral forces originating from same side.
- **Horizontal group:** Function is similar to that of alveolar group fibers.
- **Oblique group:** The oblique fibers suspend the tooth in the socket like a hammock (*hammock is a suspended bed of cloth or netting that is suspended by ropes between two firm anchor points, e.g. trees or posts and is used for swinging or resting*).

Which fibers (groups) bear most of the forces of occlusion (mastication)?

  a. These fibers take up bulk of occlusal load and transfer it to alveolar bone.
  b. Oblique fibers resist the horizontal and tilting forces. If a horizontal force is applied from direction A, the oblique group fibers coronal to the axis of rotation of side A will resist this force. The oblique group located apical to the axis of rotation on the opposite side (*side B*) will also resist force from side A.
     Oblique group fibers are also assisted by alveolar crest fibers and horizontal group fibers of side A in resisting force originating from side A.

Which fibers (groups) provide cushioning to the periapical tissues during intrusion of a tooth?

  c. They ***prevent*** injury to periapical tissues by preventing root apex from hitting against fundus of the socket.
- **Apical group:** They cushion impacts of root apex on periapical tissues during intrusion and resist extrusive and rotational forces on a tooth.
- **Inter-radicular group:** They prevent extrusion, tilting and cushion impacts of furcation of tooth on interdental bone.
- **Transseptal group:** They help maintain spatial relationships between adjoining teeth.

Other Fibers Found in the PDL

Which fibers other than collagen fibers are found in the PDL?

Two other types of fibers are found in the PDL. They are:
1. Oxytalan fibers
2. Eluanin fibers.

What is the function of oxytalan fibers?

Oxytalan and eluanin are immature forms of ***Elastin***. These are produced by fibroblasts. Oxytalan fibers are oriented vertically, i.e. parallel to root. They attach blood vessels to cementum and support them by preventing these from collapsing under pressure (*during loading of tooth*).

Ground Substance of PDL

Ground substance is amorphous (*has no definite shape*) both under light and the electron microscopes and is composed of hyaluronic acid, glycoprotein, proteoglycans, etc. It is produced by fibroblasts and is gel like with high water content (70%). Blood vessels, lymphatics, cementicles and nerves are present in it.

Blood Vessels of PDL

PDL has a very ***rich*** blood supply **(Fig. 3.4)**. This is required to maintain the high metabolic requirement of the PDL.

Which teeth have more blood supply?

- Blood supply of posterior teeth is more than anterior teeth and blood supply of maxillary teeth is more than that of mandibular teeth.

From where does the PDL receive its blood supply?

- Most of the blood supply to PDL comes from vessels running horizontally into the PDL from alveolar bone.
- Coronal most areas of PDL are also supplied by branches of gingival vessels.
- Vessels entering pulp through apical foramen also supply adjoining PDL.
- Blood vessels run parallel to long axis of tooth and between collagen fiber bundles. They form a flat basket like network of capillaries that surround root of the tooth. Glomeruli like capillaries are found in coronal 1/3rd of PDL.
- Veins run in an axial direction and drain into basket-like network in apical region of PDL or into larger veins located in septi of alveolar bone.
- Blood vessels play an important role in absorbing occlusal loads put on the PDL.

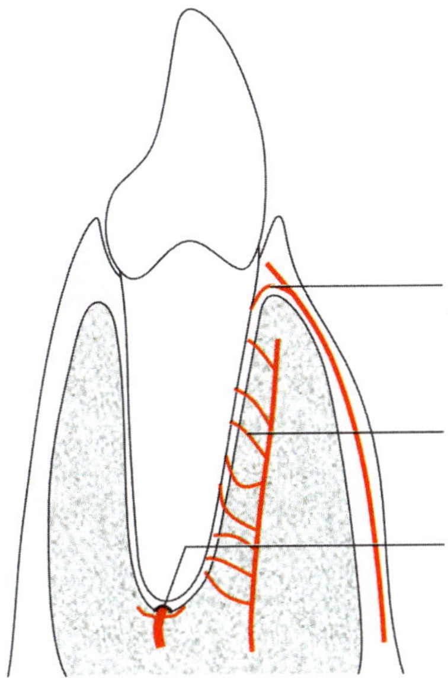

Fig. 3.4: Blood supply of PDL

Lymphatic Drainage of PDL

It is similar to that of gingiva (*see Chapter 2*).

Innervation of PDL

- Nerve supply of PDL originates from inferior alveolar nerve for mandibular teeth and superior alveolar nerves for maxillary teeth.
- Nerve fibers enter from apical region and lateral socket walls.
- Apical region of the PDL contains ***more*** nerve endings than middle and coronal regions.

◂ *Which area of PDL has more innervation?*

Function of Innervation of PDL

1. Nerves of PDL help in judgment of hardness, size, shape and texture of food or objects placed in the mouth.
2. Nerve receptors in PDL have directional sensitivity, they help in recognition of direction of force being applied on teeth. Directional sensitivity is different in different teeth, e.g. canines respond mainly to mesially or distally directed forces, whereas the incisors respond primarily to incisal or labially directed forces. This way, nerves of PDL help in ***adjusting*** occlusal forces according to need.
3. Nerve receptors in PDL ***limit*** maximum amount of force put on teeth during occlusal contact. This way they protect dentition and muscles (*gnathostomatic system*) from damage, e.g. if we bite onto a hard object and occlusal force widely exceeds load bearing capacity, an immediate paralysis of muscles of mastication is caused by ***reflex arcs***.

◂ *Do nerves of PDL enable recognition of direction of force being applied on a tooth?*

◂ *How does PDL prevent damage to the periodontium if excessive occlusal forces are suddenly exerted on a tooth?*

Different types of nerve endings are found in PDL:

1. Free nerve endings (*maximum in number, spread evenly along the root*)
2. Spindle-like nerve endings (*least in number, more in apical region*)
3. Ruffini corpuscle-like nerve endings (*more in apical region*).

◂ *Which type of nerve endings are found in the PDL?*

CLINICAL UTILITY AND SHORT ANSWER

What is the minimum amount of force that can be detected by a healthy PDL of a human tooth?

- Periodontal innervation in the ***incisors*** helps detect forces as little as ***0.01N.***
- The innervation of the PDLs of molars is less sensitive and ***molars*** can only detect forces of ***0.1 N*** or above.
- Force discrimination in PDL is better at lower occlusal loads levels than at higher occlusal loads.

Functions of PDL

What are the functions of PDL? ▶

1. Supportive (*physical*)
2. Formative
3. Sensory
4. Homeostatic
5. Nutritional

Supportive function of PDL

PDL helps bear occlusal loads by transmitting occlusal loads from tooth to bone.

How a tooth bears occlusal loads

Although occlusal-load bearing mechanisms are not fully known, two most widely accepted theories of how teeth bear occlusal loads are:

1. **Tensional theory:** According to this theory, principal fibers of PDL transmit occlusal forces from tooth to alveolar bone which further transfers these to facial skeleton. When occlusal load is applied on the tooth, the wavy fiber bundles get straightened and stretched and these then transfer occlusal force put on the tooth to the wall of tooth socket. The load is then further transferred onto the basal bone of the jaws as tension.

How does a tooth bear occlusal load? ▶

2. **Visco-elastic system theory:** According to this theory, a tooth bears occlusal forces in two phases. In the 1st phase, occlusal pressure forces free fluid of PDL to move out of PDL through holes in the wall of alveolar socket into marrow spaces of the alveolar bone. This mechanism functions like a hydraulic shock absorber to absorb occlusal forces.

   In the second phase, fibers of PDL get stretched and tightened and transmit the remaining occlusal force to the wall of the tooth socket. Stretching and tightening of the fibers also causes narrowing of vessels of PDL. This results in arterial back pressure and ballooning of vessels. Arterial back pressure forces blood fluids to come out of the vessels into the PDL. This fluid replenishes the PDL's lost fluids.

   Viscoelastic system theory is more ***accepted*** of the two theories.

ALERT!

How much occlusal force can a tooth bear?

1. Maximum occlusal forces in humans can range from 100–250 N (*Newton*) (*10–25 kg*) in the incisor region to 1000 N (*100 kg*) in the molar region.
2. However, ***actual*** average occlusal forces of mastication are only about ***150 N or 15 kg;*** these are much lesser than the maximum generatable forces.
3. When an occlusal force is put on a tooth, it gets divided into ***two*** vectors—horizontal and axial. The horizontal vector is much smaller than the axial vector. Horizontal vector of occlusal force pushes the tooth in the ***mesial*** direction. It thus produces ***mesial drift*** of teeth. Mesial drifting of teeth causes maintenance of tight inter-proximal contacts between adjacent teeth.

What causes mesial drifting of teeth? ▶

Formative and homeostatic functions of PDL

How do formative and homeostatic functions of PDL help? ▶

- These maintain function, integrity and functional relationship of PDL's constituents by formation and resorption of individual components of PDL.
- Formative and resorptive cells of PDL bring about healing and regeneration of periodontal tissues, i.e. cementum, alveolar bone and fibers of PDL.

Which cells of periodontium are required for periodontal regeneration? ▶

- This fact is used clinically for periodontal regeneration of lost periodontal tissues (*due to periodontitis*). For this, after periodontal surgery, only cells of PDL are allowed to populate the healing periodontal wound site. This type of regenerative surgery is called GTR (*guided tissue regeneration*) (*see Chapter 18 and Fig. 18.8*).

CLINICAL UTILITY AND SHORT ANSWER

What is homeostasis?

Maintenance of a state of equilibrium in the living body or tissue with respect to its various functions is called homeostasis.

Sensory function of the PDL

See section on nerve supply of the PDL.

CEMENTUM

Cementum covers anatomic roots of teeth. Unlike alveolar bone, cementum is ***avascular*** (*does not have blood and nerve supply*). Its main function is to provide attachment to principal fiber groups of PDL to tooth root.

◄ *Does cementum have blood supply?*

◄ *What is the main function of cementum?*

CLINICAL UTILITY AND SHORT ANSWER

Why cementum is a periodontal tissue despite it being anatomically a part of the tooth?

Classification of cementum as a periodontal tissue is based upon its use and purpose. Cementum provides anchorage to tooth by allowing insertion of the periodontal ligament's fibers within it. Therefore, cementum is classified as a periodontal tissue even though it is part of the tooth.

Thickness of Cementum

- Thickness of cementum varies from ***20–200 µm***.
- Cementum is deposited ***continuously*** over the root surface covered by PDL; thickness of cementum ***therefore increases with age***.
- Cementum is thinner (*20–50 µm*) on coronal 1/3rd of root and thicker (*150–200 µm*) on the apical 2/3rd of the root and in furcation regions of multirooted teeth.

◄ *What is the thickness of cementum?*

◄ *Why does thickness of cementum increase with age?*

Physical Characteristics of Cementum

1. Color of cementum is light yellow (*similar to that of dentin*).
2. As cementum is softer than dentin (*cementum is only 45–50% calcified*), it can be ***easily*** removed during scaling and root planing. If cementum is completely removed, dentin gets exposed, this leads to dentinal hypersensitivity.
3. Cementum is more ***permeable*** than other hard dental tissues.
4. As it does not have blood supply, cementum is more resistant to resorption than bone; this makes orthodontic movement of teeth possible.
5. PDL normally lies between cementum alveolar bone, however sometimes, the bone and cementum unite; this is called ankylosis (Fig. 3.7).
6. Cementum has ***high fluoride*** content (*highest amongst all dental tissues*). This makes roots more resistant to initial caries, but once caries starts and reaches dentin, root caries proceeds very fast (*as dentin is only half as calcified as enamel*).
7. Cementum on area of root covered by PDL ***always*** has a layer of uncalcified premature cementum called ***cementoid tissue*** over it.

◄ *Why does dentinal hypersensitivity occur after scaling?*

◄ *Why is cementum more resistant to resorption than alveolar bone?*

◄ *Why is cementum more resistant to caries than dentin?*

◄ *What is cementoid tissue?*

How PDL Fibers get Attached to Cementum

- The PDL fibers get inserted and attached to cementoid tissue (*uncalcified matrix of cementum*) before it gets calcified to become cementum.
- The embedded ends of PDL fibers then get calcified along with cementum that is undergoing calcification (*embedded ends are called Sharpey's fibers, see Fig. 3.3*).
- Cementoid tissue (*uncalcified cementum*) is always present on calcified cementum to allow attachment of newly formed PDL fibers.

◄ *How do PDL fibers that are soft get inserted into hard cementum for attachment?*

Types of Cementum

Based on the presence or absence of cells within its matrix and time of its formation, cementum is classified into ***two*** categories (Fig. 3.5):

1. Acellular cementum
2. Cellular cementum.

◄ *How many types of cementum are there?*

Which type of cementum forms first? ▶

Which type of cementum is more calcified? ▶

Table 3.1: Differences between acellular and cellular cementum from clinical point of view	
Acellular cementum	***Cellular cementum***
1. Forms first and till the time the tooth does not reach the occlusal plane.	1. Forms later and ***after*** the tooth has reached occlusal plane.
2. No cells and therefore no empty lacunae are seen within the calcified matrix.	2. Cementocytes are seen within the lacunae in the calcified matrix. In deeper layers cementocytes die, lacunae are therefore empty.
3. Slow rate of deposition	3. Faster rate of deposition
4. More perfectly calcified. Has higher degree of calcification.	4. Relatively imperfectly calcified. Has lesser degree of calcification.
5. Present over coronal 2/3rd of roots of all teeth.	5. Present on apical 1/3rd of roots of all teeth and inter-radicular regions of premolar and molar teeth.
6. It is present on roots of all teeth.	6. It may be absent in single rooted teeth.

Types of Cemento-enamel (CE) Junctions

There are three types of CE junctions (Fig. 3.6):

Type I: 60%; ***cementum overlaps*** enamel for a small distance.

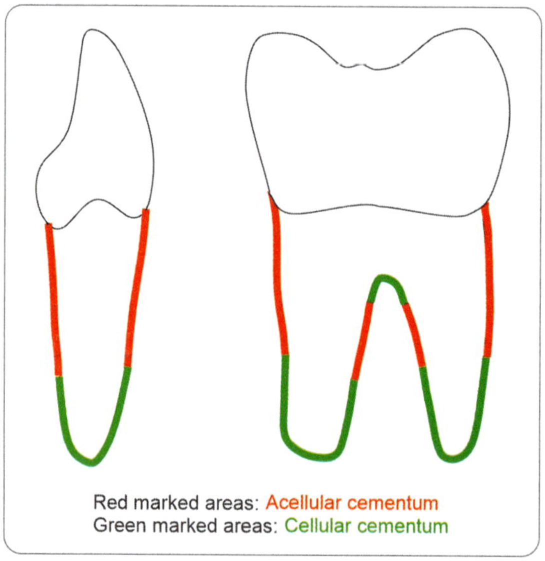

Fig. 3.5: Distribution of acellular and cellular cementum on roots of anterior and posterior teeth

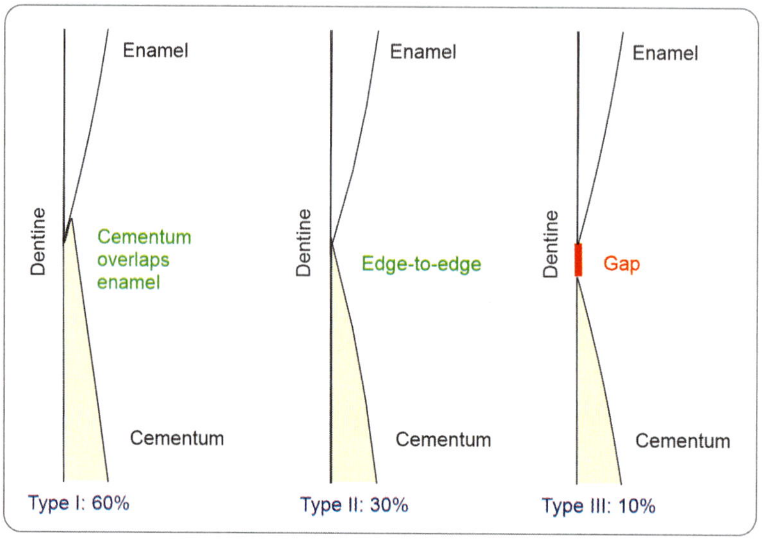

Fig. 3.6: Types of CE junctions. Teeth with type III (*gap junctions*) are more prone to dentinal hypersensitivity

Type II: 30%; cementum and enamel meet ***end-to-end***.

Type III: 10%; a small gap is present between enamel and cementum. This type of junction is also known as ***gap junction***. As dentin is exposed in this gap area, such teeth are prone to develop dentinal hypersensitivity.

◂ *What is the clinical importance of gap junction?*

CLINICAL UTILITY AND SHORT ANSWER

What is coronal cementum?

In some human teeth, small deposits of cementum called ***coronal cementum,*** are found on enamel. This occurs due to local disturbances at the time of tooth development. Coronal cementum, if present, is usually found in occlusal fissures of normal unerupted teeth of children and embedded teeth.

◂ *Where is coronal cementum usually present?*

CLINICAL UTILITY AND SHORT ANSWER

What is hypercementosis?

Hypercementosis is ***thickening*** of cementum. Hypercementosis maybe localized or diffused. It may involve one region of a root, single tooth or it may be seen in roots of all teeth. Hypercementosis is of two types:

1. ***Cemental hypertrophy:*** When hypercementosis improves function of cementum.
2. ***Cemental hyperplasia:*** When hypercementosis does not improve function of cementum.

It is often ***difficult*** to distinguish between these two types.

◂ *What is the difference between cemental hypertrophy and cemental hyperplasia?*

ALERT!

Cementicles

Cementicles are small (*less than **0.2 mm***) calcified bodies in PDL that are made of ***cementum-like tissue*** or ***cementum.*** They form due to ***calcification of dead cell rests of Malassez*** (*remnants of the Hertwig's root sheath*). They can be of two types:

1. **Attached cementicles:** Ones that are attached to root.
2. **Free cementicles:** Ones that are not attached and lie free within the PDL.

Adjacent cementicles may fuse to form a larger mass that may then fuse with the tooth root, this then causes ***hypercementosis***.

◂ *How do cementicles form?*

◂ *What is hypercementosis?*

Cementum Resorption and Repair

Cementum responds to stimuli not only by deposition but also by resorption. Resorption areas vary in size from small unidentifiable resorption bays to large areas easily detectable in radiographs. Cementum may resorb due to:

1. Trauma from occlusion (*TFO*), e.g. excessive occlusal or orthodontic force exerted over a long period of time, etc.
2. Periodontal or periapical disease.
3. Pressure on root from unerupted or embedded teeth or tumors.
4. Transplantation or re-implantation of teeth, etc.

◂ *What are the reasons for cementum resorption?*

Cementum resorption and repair can occur both in nonvital and vital teeth. After resorption, repair occurs by formation of cellular cementum. If repair activity re-establishes original outline of root surface, repair is called ***anatomic repair***. After repair, normal width of PDL is re-established by a matching indentation or projection of bone wall (*lamina dura*) opposite the root's cementum defect area.

◂ *Can cementum resorption and repair occur in non-vital teeth?*

◂ *What type of cementum forms after cementum repair?*

◂ *Does normal width of PDL get re-established after cementum repair?*

Ankylosis

Periodontal ligament is normally present between a tooth's root and the alveolar bone proper, i.e. the wall of the socket. Sometimes, a section of tooth root does not have PDL over it and in this area the tooth root is fused with alveolar bone, this is called ***ankylosis*** (**Fig. 3.7**). Ankylosis commonly occurs after cemental resorption. Ankylosis may be seen in:

1. Trauma from occlusion (*TFO*)
2. Chronic periapical inflammation.
3. In transplanted or re-implanted teeth (*because of death of cells of PDL due to drying of tooth when tooth remains out of tooth socket for more than thirty minutes*), etc.

◂ *What is ankylosis?*

◂ *What causes ankylosis?*

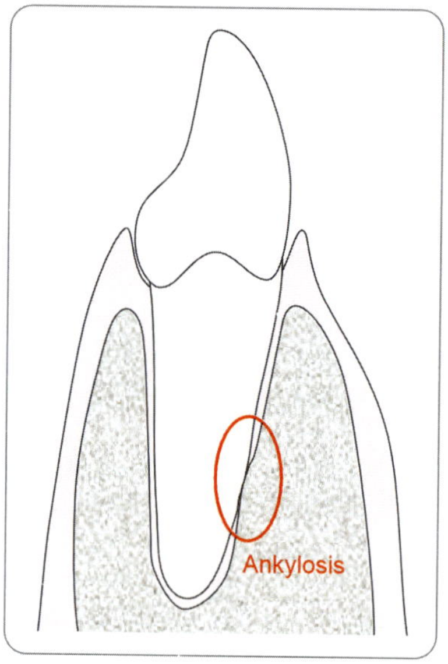

Fig. 3.7: Ankylosis

ALERT!

Osseointegration seen in implants is similar to ankylosis.

Osseointegration is a direct structural and functional connection between living bone and surface of a dental implant. Osseointegration is very similar to ankylosis as bone forms directly on the implant surface without any intervening connective tissue.

Cemental Tears

What causes cemental tear?

When teeth are subjected to severe physical trauma, fragments of cementum can get partially or completely detached from tooth root, these fragments of cementum are called cemental tears. Such cemental tears in the PDL may then get completely or incompletely resorbed or get reunited to the root surface by new cementum formation.

ALERT!

Cementomas and necrotic cementum

What is the radiographic picture of a cementoma?

Cementomas are cemental outgrowths on tooth roots of both vital or non-vital teeth. As they are ***radiolucent*** in their early stages, these if present at the root apex, look like periapical abscesses in a radiograph; however lamina dura in such cases is intact (Fig. 3.10). Cementomas become radiopaque in later stages.

If cementum gets denuded due to periodontitis, plaque and calculus form its surface. Bacterial toxins also get absorbed into cementum and these leach out into surrounding periodontal tissues to cause periodontitis. Such diseased cementum is called ***necrotic cementum.***

ALVEOLAR BONE

Alveolar bone forms sockets of teeth. It is an extension of body of mandible and maxilla.

What happens to alveolar bone after a tooth is extracted?

- It is similar to other bones of the body but has a relatively richer blood supply.
- It forms when teeth erupt and gradually resorbs after a tooth is extracted/lost. If teeth do not develop (***anodontia***), the alveolar process also does ***not*** develop despite normal development of facial skeleton.

Parts of Alveolar Bone

Alveolar bone has ***two*** parts:

What is the difference between alveolar bone proper and supporting alveolar bone?

1. **Alveolar bone proper** (*lamina dura or cribriform plate*): It is the thin plate of ***compact bone*** that lines sockets of teeth. Principal fibers of PDL attach into it (Fig. 3.8, *green line*).
2. **Supporting alveolar bone:** Bone that surrounds alveolar bone proper is called supporting alveolar bone. It is further of two types:

a. **Cortical plates:**
   i. They form outer and inner plates (*walls*) of alveolar processes **(Figs 3.8, red line and 3.9)** and are made of ***compact bone***.
   ii. Cortical plates of alveolar processes are continuous with cortical plates of maxilla and mandible.
   iii. They are thicker in the mandible; more so in the premolar region.

b. **Spongy or Cancellous or Trabecular bone:**
   i. It is the bone present between alveolar bone proper (*tooth socket wall*) and cortical plates **(Figs 3.8 and 3.9)**.
   ii. This bone has trabeculae that form a three-dimensional framework (*trabeculae are small supporting tissue elements*).
   iii. It is relatively less dense, less stiff, i.e. softer and weaker than compact bone.
   iv. Spongy bone is more vascular than compact bone and contains red bone marrow.
   v. In mandibular ***anterior*** region cortical plates are fused with alveolar bone proper, i.e. there is ***no*** intervening spongy bone.

◂ *What is the difference between cortical bone and spongy bone?*

◂ *In which area are the cortical plates thickest?*

◂ *Which of the two: Cortical or spongy bone has more blood supply?*

◂ *In which region of the mandible no spongy bone is present?*

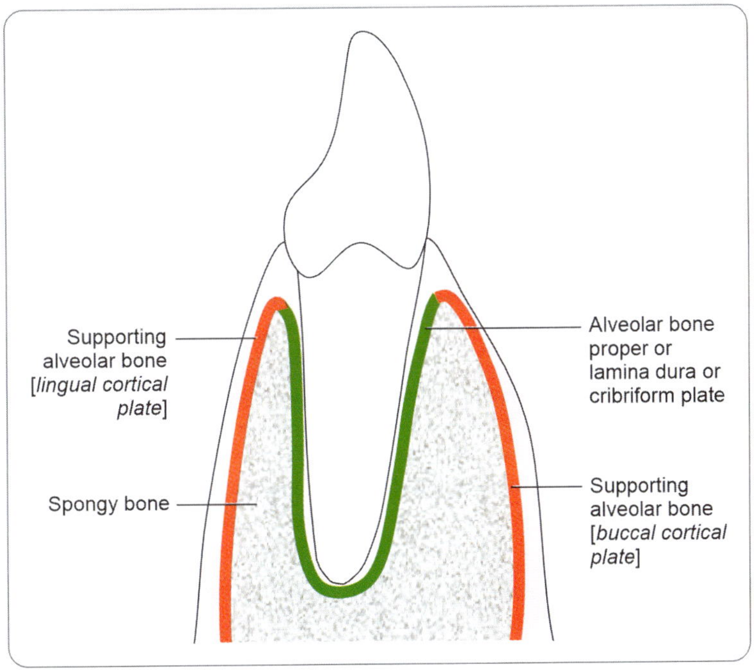

Fig. 3.8: Parts of alveolar bone

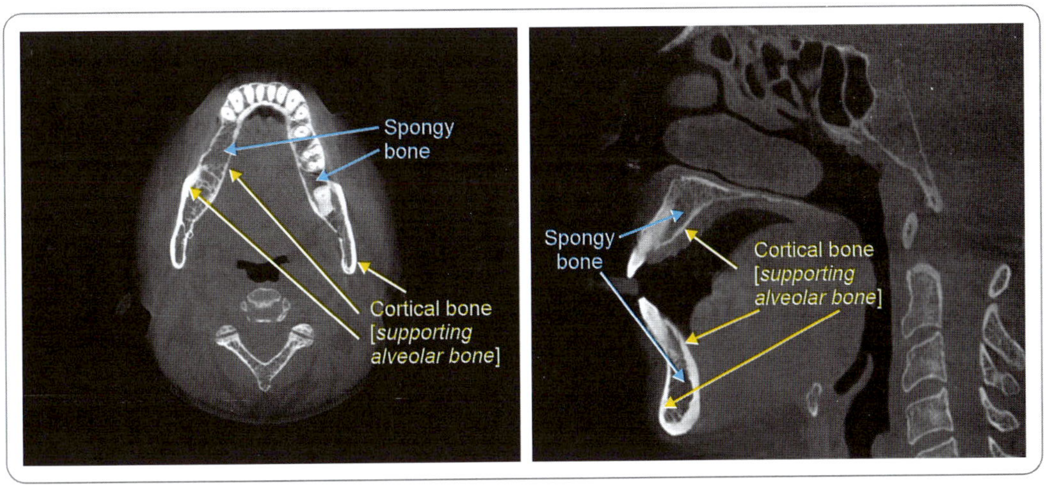

Fig. 3.9: Cortical and spongy bone seen in a CBCT radiograph

Lamina Dura

What is lamina dura? ▸

- Lamina dura is a ***radiographic entity***, i.e. it is the name given to alveolar bone proper when seen in a radiograph (Fig. 3.10).

How does lamina dura appear in a radiograph? ▸

- It is ***more calcified*** than surrounding supporting (*spongy*) bone, therefore lamina dura appears as a ***radiopaque*** (*white*) ***linear shadow*** (*line-like shadow*) surrounding root of the tooth on a radiograph.

What is the black line between lamina dura and tooth root? ▸

- A thin radiolucent shadow (*black line*) of PDL is present between root of the tooth and lamina dura (Fig. 3.10).

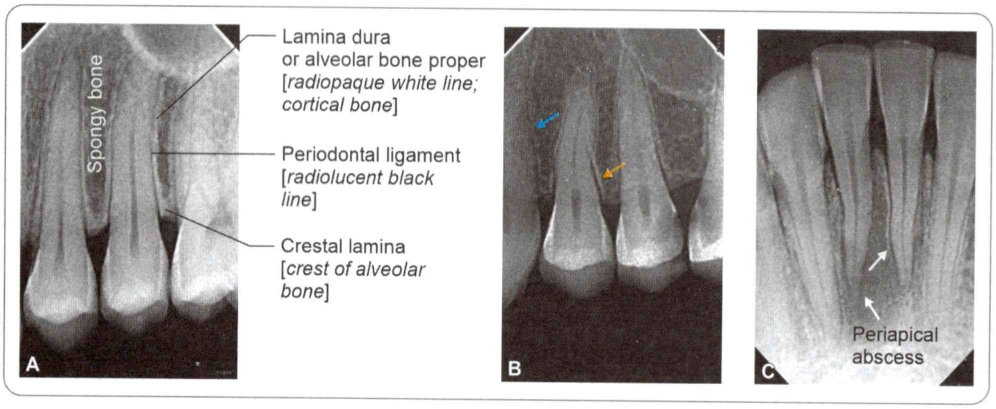

Fig. 3.10: Lamina dura (*alveolar bone proper*), crestal lamina and spongy bone as seen in a IOPA radiograph. Break in continuity of lamina dura is suggestive of pulpal pathology (*diag. C*).

ALERT!

Lamina dura has huge diagnostic value.

What does thickening of lamina dura suggest? ▸

1. If lamina dura is thicker than usual (*hypertrophy*), it suggests that the tooth has been subjected to high occlusal forces for a long time. This is a sign of trauma from occlusion (*TFO*) (Fig. 3.10, diag. B, *orange arrow*) (*see Chapter 9, 'Trauma from Occlusion, Bone Loss and Pathologic migration*).
2. Thin lamina dura (*atrophy*) suggests reduced or no occlusal load.

What does break in continuity of lamina dura suggest? ▸

3. Chronic periapical abscess resulting from an infected pulp causes periapical bone loss. In such cases, lamina dura is broken and a radiolucent (*black area*) is seen around the root apex (Fig. 13.10, diag. C, *white arrow*).
4. If lamina dura is intact and has no break in its continuity, especially around the root apex, this usually rules out possibility of chronic pulp pathology (*periapical abscess or granuloma*) (Fig. 13.10, diag. B).

Crestal Lamina

What is crestal lamina? ▸

- It is the radiographic image of the crest of the alveolar bone (Fig. 3.10, diag. A). It appears as a horizontal radiopaque line at the crest of the interdental bone or at the crest of the edentulous alveolar process.

Is crestal lamina continuous with lamina dura of teeth? ▸

- Crestal lamina is continuous with lamina dura of adjoining teeth.

When is crestal lamina not present? ▸

- Crestal lamina is absent in ongoing periodontitis (*bone loss*).
- Loss of crestal lamina is usually the first sign of start of bone loss in periodontitis (*incipient periodontitis*).

Location of alveolar bone crest in relation to base of sulcus, mucogingival junction and CE junction

Where is the crest of alveolar bone located in relation to the base of sulcus? ▸

1. **Location of bone crest in relation to base of sulcus:**
   - Bone crest is about 2–3 mm apical to base of sulcus (Fig. 3.11, X).
   - The distance between base of sulcus and crest of bone is called ***'biologic width'***. This is maintained even when bone loss occurs in periodontitis.

Where is the crest of alveolar bone located in relation to the mucogingival junction? ▸

2. **Location of bone crest to mucogingival junction:**
   - If teeth are in their ***normal position*** in the arch and there is ***no alveolar bone loss***:
     i. Crest of alveolar bone is located ***3 mm coronal*** to mucogingival junction on the ***buccal and lingual*** sides (Fig. 3.11, Y).
     ii. In the ***interdental region***, alveolar bone crest is located ***5 mm coronal*** to the mucogingival junction (Fig. 3.11, Z).

3. Location of bone crest in relation to CE junction:

- Interdental bone crest is normally located about ***2 mm apical*** and ***parallel*** to an ***imaginary line joining*** the two adjacent ***CE junctions*** of adjoining teeth (*range is 0.75 mm–2.81 mm*) (Figs 3.12 and 3.13).

Where is the crest of interdental bone located in relation to the CE junction?

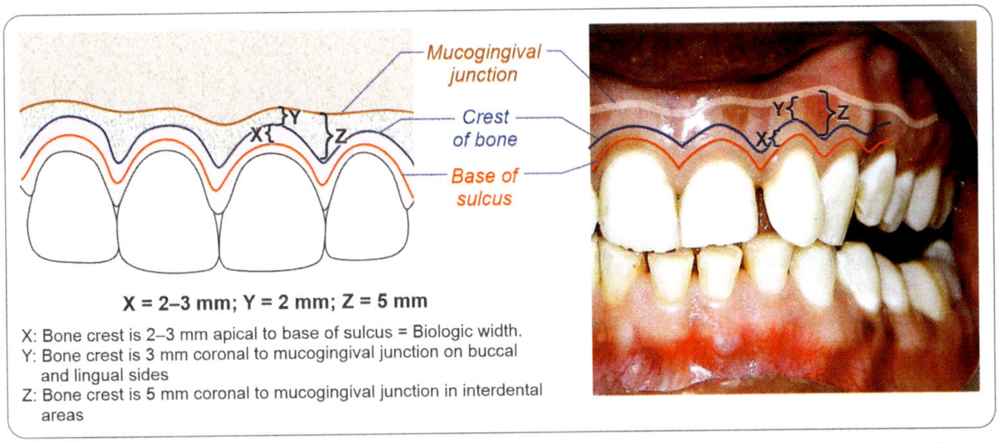

Fig. 3.11: Distance of alveolar bone crest from base of sulcus and mucogingival junction

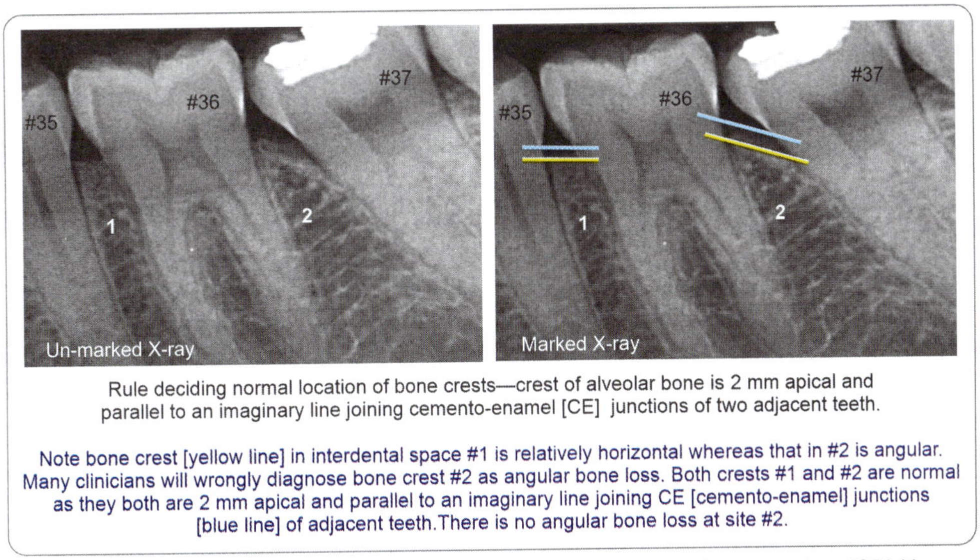

Fig. 3.12: Normal position of alveolar bone crest (*crestal lamina*) as seen in a IOPA X-ray

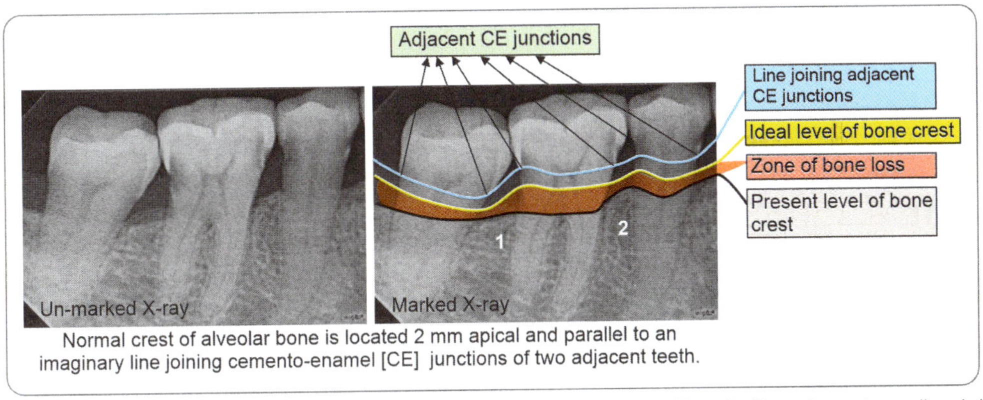

Fig. 3.13: How to know amount of bone loss in an IOPA radiograph. Step 1: Draw imaginary line joining adjacent CE junctions of adjoining teeth (*blue line*). Step 2: Draw an imaginary line parallel and 2 mm apical to line joining adjacent CE junctions (*blue line*) to know ideal location of normal alveolar bone crest in each interdental space, i.e. where bone crest should normally be in these interdental spaces (*yellow line*). Step 3. Draw imaginary line tracing the present alveolar crest (*black line*). The area between yellow and black line depicts the approximate bone loss (*red zone*).

ALERT!

How to know if there is interdental bone loss

Amount of interdental bone loss can be easily measured on a IOPA radiograph. As already discussed, interdental bone crest is located approximately 2 mm apical and ***parallel*** to an ***imaginary line joining*** the two adjacent ***CE junctions*** of adjoining teeth (*range is 0.75 mm–2.81 mm*) (Fig. 3.13, *yellow line*). Any increase in distance between CE junction and bone crest beyond 2 mm denotes bone loss (Fig. 3.13, *red marked area*).

However, it is important to remember the following points in this regard:

- In cases of healthy but reduced periodontium (*tooth out of arch, crown lengthening, previously treated periodontitis, etc.; 2018 classification*), alveolar crest is normally located ***more*** than 2 mm apical to the CE junction.

What causes crestal bone loss? ▶

- In both intact and reduced healthy periodontium, alveolar bone loss usually occurs only as result of periodontitis.

Interdental Septum

What is the interdental septum? ▶

- Alveolar bone between roots of two adjacent teeth is called interdental septum.
- It is composed of a core of cancellous bone that has a border of compact bone on all sides.
- In anterior teeth, interproximal space is small, therefore mesio-distal width of the alveolar crest is small and interdental septum is thin and conical (Fig. 3.14, *diag. A, white arrow*).
- In posterior teeth, interdental space is large, therefore, interdental septum is wider and flat (Fig. 3.14, *diag. B, white arrow*).
- When diastema is present between anterior teeth, alveolar crest is flat and rounded.

In which cases interdental septum is composed of compact bone only? ▶

- If interdental space is narrow, cancellous bone in interdental bone is thin or missing. In such cases, interdental septum is composed of compact bone only.
- In a thin interdental sptum, there may be a window-like opening connecting PDLs of the two adjacent teeth.

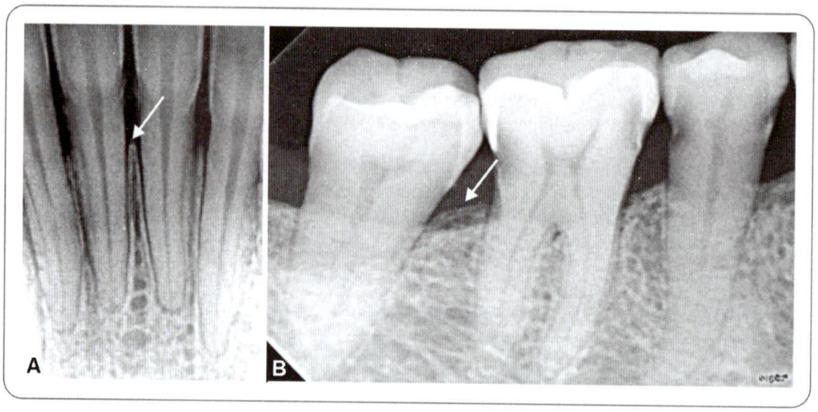

Fig. 3.14: Interdental septum. It is thin and conical in anterior teeth (*diag. B, white arrow*) and wide and flat in posterior teeth (*diag. B white arrow*)

ALERT!

Bone is remodeled continuously.

Does alveolar bone remain the same always? ▶

- The alveolar bone is ***constantly*** remodeled.
- Of all the four periodontal tissues (gingiva, alveolar bone, PDL and cementum), alveolar bone is the ***least stable***.
- Bone mass is maintained by a sensitive balance between bone resorption and formation.
- Any adverse change in the local and/or systemic conditions will result in immediate decrease in bone mass by bone resorption.
- Increase in bone mass due to increase in occlusal forces is called bone ***hypertrophy***.
- ***Disuse atrophy*** of bone occurs due to decrease in occlusal forces; this is characterized by decrease in bone mass.

What is disuse atrophy of alveolar bone? ▶

- Bone is resorbed in areas of pressure and formed in areas of tension.

ALERT!

- During healing of extraction sockets and bone defects, immature bone forms first. Such immature bone is ***radiolucent***. This bone due to its rich fibrillar and cell content, makes ***ideal bone graft*** material.
- After extraction/loss of teeth, alveolar process becomes thin due to bone atrophy. Such atrophied areas not only look unaesthetic but also cause dentures to become loose fitting and makes implant placement complicated or even impossible.
- As alveolar bone is richly supplied by blood, chances of osteomyelitis occurring after extraction of a tooth or surgical denudation of alveolar bone during periodontal surgery are usually negligible.
- When controlled orthodontic forces are applied, alveolar bone resorbs under pressure and forms in areas of tension (*pull*). As cementum is avascular, it remains unaffected by such forces. This makes orthodontic tooth movement possible.

◂ *Why does bone infection usually not occur when alveolar bone is exposed after periodontal surgery or extraction?*

External Contour of the Alveolar Bone

- External contour of alveolar bone is variable.
- In teeth with healthy periodontium, it is dependent on prominence and position of their roots in the dental arch.
- If a tooth is within curve of the dental arch and its root is not prominent, crest of alveolar bone is placed up to 2 mm apical to the CE junction (Figs 3.12 and 3.13).
- If a root is very prominent, the alveolar bone margin is located more ***apically*** and is thinner. The vice-versa is also true (Fig. 3.15).
- If ***excessive occlusal loads*** are being put on a tooth, its bone margins are thicker.

◂ *Where is the alveolar bone margin located on prominent surface of a tooth's root?*

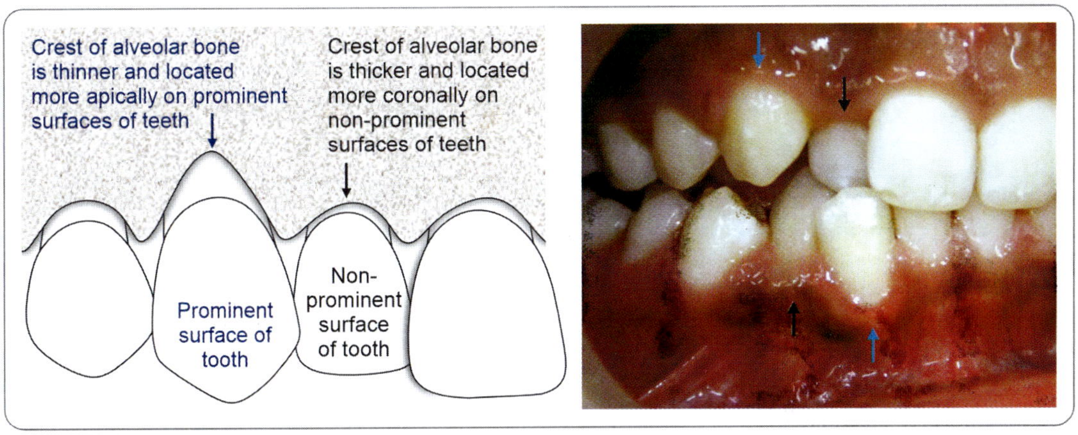

Fig. 3.15: Alveolar bone crest is normally located more apically on prominent surface of teeth (*blue arrow*). It is located more coronally on non-prominent surfaces of teeth (*black arrows*)

CLINICAL UTILITY AND SHORT ANSWER

What changes are seen in lamina dura, bone and PDL when teeth are subjected to increased occlusal loads over a long period of time?

If increased occlusal loads are put on teeth, it causes:

1. Thickening of lamina dura (*Figs 9.2 and 9.8*)
2. Thickening of spongy bone trabeculae (*Fig. 9.8*).
3. Enlarged PDL space (*Figs 9.2 and 9.8*).
4. Strengthening of cortical and spongy alveolar bone is called buttressing bone formation.
   a. Buttressing bone formation in cortical plates of the alveolar process (*in which teeth are present* is called peripheral buttressing bone formation.
   b. Buttressing bone formation within the body of maxilla or mandible is called central buttressing bone formation.
5. Peripheral buttressing bone formation may result in a bulging alveolar bone crest (*Fig. 9.5*). This is called lipping.

◂ *What do thick lamina dura, thick bone trabeculae and enlarged PDL space in a radiograph suggest?*

Fenestrations and Dehiscences in Alveolar Bone

What is the difference between fenestrations and dehiscences?

Are fenestrations and dehiscences in alveolar bone common?

Where are fenestrations and dehiscences usually seen?

- These are non-pathologic variations in bone.
- Fenestrations are ***window***-like defects on the surface of alveolar bone through which roots of teeth are exposed, i.e. these areas on the root ***do not*** have covering bone **(Fig. 3.16)**.
- If such alveolar bone defects extend through the margin of alveolar bone, they are called dehiscence (i.e. *dehiscence has bone on three sides only*) **(Fig. 3.16)**.
- Fenestrations and dehiscences on roots of teeth are covered only by periosteum and overlying gingiva.
- Both these defects can only be identified after reflection of a full thickness periodontal flap (*comprising gingiva and periosteum*).
- These defects are present in ***20% of teeth*** and are usually ***bilateral.***
- They are commonly seen on ***facial*** bone of ***prominent*** roots.
- ***No*** clinical features are associated with these defects.

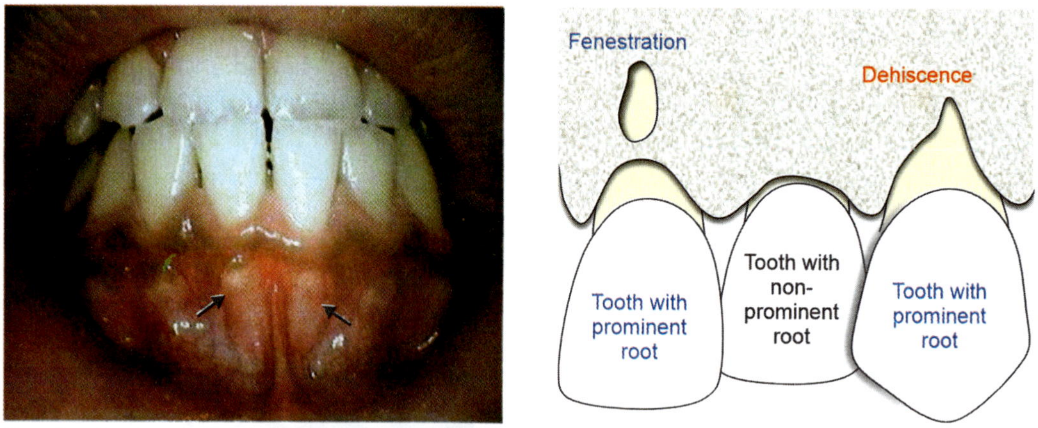

Prominent surfaces of roots [black arrows] are more likely to have fenestration and dehiscence bone defects

Fig. 3.16: Fenestration and dehiscence of alveolar bone

CLINICAL UTILITY AND SHORT ANSWER

Do teeth with dehiscences show increased or decreased mobility?

Do teeth with dehiscences show increased or decreased recession after flap surgery?

What are the clinical consequences of dehiscences?

- They usually do not affect health and function of teeth and periodontium.
- Teeth with large dehiscences can show increased mobility on the side where the dehiscence is present (*usually facial side*).
- After flap surgery ***more post-operative gingival*** recession is seen in areas of dehiscences.

Root Proximity

If roots of a tooth or teeth are placed very close to each other, this is called root proximity **(Fig. 3.16)**.

What are the clinical implications of closely placed roots?

- Root proximity can result because of position of teeth in the arch or closely formed roots of multirooted teeth.
- If roots are closely placed in their coronal-half, such tooth surfaces are more difficult to treat as instrument assess is not easy **(Fig. 3.17, red circle)**.
- Such areas are also difficult to clean **(Fig. 3.17, red circle)** and are therefore more prone to gingivitis and periodontitis.

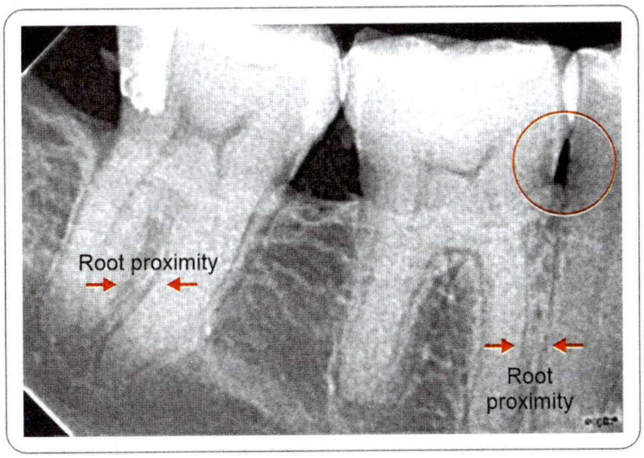

Fig. 3.17: Root proximity

Review Questions

1. What are different kinds of fibers found in PDL? Describe principal groups of fibers of PDL. Of all PDL fiber bundle groups, which group has maximum number of fibers?
2. Describe functions of individual fiber groups of PDL.
3. How does the tooth bear occlusal loads?
4. Write on importance of formative and homeostatic functions of PDL.
5. Name principal cells and extracellular constituents of PDL.
6. Write a short note on blood supply of PDL.
7. Write a short note on nerve endings found in PDL.
8. Write on the various functions of PDL.
9. Name clinically important characteristics of cementum.
10. Why is cellular cementum deposited continuously? Why is a layer of cementoid tissue always present on the root? How does cementum provide attachment to PDL fibers?
11. Why is new fiber insertion into cementum required?
12. Classify cementum. Write differences between cellular and acellular cementum.
13. Name different types of CE junctions. What is the importance of gap junction?
14. What are cementicles?
15. Write a short note on cementum resorption and repair.
16. What is ankylosis?
17. What are cemental tears?
18. Name parts of alveolar bone.
19. What is lamina dura? Lamina dura has immense diagnostic value, explain.
20. What is crestal lamina? Where is crestal lamina or alveolar crest ideally located?
21. Write a short note on external contour of alveolar bone in normal and reduced periodontium.
22. What is buttressing bone formation? What is lipping?
23. What are fenestrations and dehiscences in the alveolar bone? How are they important clinically?
24. Write a note on interdental septum.

Chapter

4

Classification and Epidemiological Assessment of Periodontal Disease

What is classification? ▸ Classification is a systematic arrangement of diseases in groups that possess common characteristics. In recent times, classifications of periodontal disease have been based on infection-host response paradigm (*etiology, pathology and host response*). The most recent classification of periodontal disease is the 2018 classification that has been ***jointly*** published by ***American Academy of Periodontology*** and the ***European Federation of Periodontology***. The earlier classification that was in wide use prior to the 2018 classification was the American Association of Periodontology's 1999 classification.

Uses of Classification

What are the uses of classification? ▸

1. Classification helps in diagnosis and assessment of relationship between members of the same disease group and between different groups.
2. It also helps in diagnosis and makes treatment of periodontal disease more systematic and convenient.
3. Classifying disease helps in accurate communication between professionals, determine prognosis, formulation of treatment plan and integrate resources to provide better health care.

2018 CLASSIFICATION OF PERIODONTAL AND PERI-IMPLANT DISEASES AND CONDITIONS

I. Periodontal Diseases and Conditions

A. Periodontal Health, Gingival Diseases and Conditions

1. Periodontal health and gingival health

a. Clinical gingival health on an intact periodontium
b. Clinical gingival health on a reduced periodontium
   i. Stable periodontitis patient
   ii. Non-periodontitis patient.

2. Gingivitis: Dental biofilm-induced

a. Associated with dental biofilm (*plaque*) alone
b. Mediated by systemic or local risk factors
c. Drug-influenced gingival enlargement.

3. Gingival Diseases: Non-dental biofilm (*plaque*)-induced

a. Genetic/developmental disorders
b. Specific infections
c. Inflammatory and immune disorders
d. Reactive processes
e. Neoplasms
f. Endocrine, nutritional and metabolic diseases

g. Traumatic lesions
h. Gingival pigmentation.

B. Periodontitis

1. Necrotizing periodontal diseases

a. Necrotizing gingivitis
b. Necrotizing periodontitis
c. Necrotizing stomatitis.

2. Periodontitis as a manifestation of systemic diseases

3. Periodontitis

a. **Stages:** Based on severity and complexity of management
   i. **Stage I:** Initial periodontitis
   ii. **Stage II:** Moderate periodontitis
   iii. **Stage III:** Severe periodontitis with potential for additional tooth loss
   iv. **Stage IV:** Severe periodontitis with potential for loss of dentition.
b. **Extent and distribution:** Localized; generalized; molar-incisor distribution.
c. **Grades:** Based on evidence of risk of rapid progression and anticipated treatment response
   i. **Grade A:** Slow rate of progression
   ii. **Grade B:** Moderate rate of progression
   iii. **Grade C:** Rapid rate of progression.

C. Other Conditions Affecting the Periodontium

1. **Systemic diseases or conditions affecting periodontal supporting tissues**
2. **Periodontal abscesses and endodontic-periodontal lesions**
3. **Mucogingival deformities and conditions**
   a. Gingival phenotype
   b. Gingival/soft tissue recession
   c. Lack of gingiva
   d. Decreased vestibular depth
   e. Aberrant frenum/muscle position
   f. Gingival excess
   g. Abnormal colour
   h. Condition of exposed root surface.
4. **Traumatic occlusal forces**
   a. Primary occlusal trauma
   b. Secondary occlusal trauma
   c. Orthodontic forces.
5. **Tooth and Prosthesis-related factors that modify or predispose to plaque-induced gingival diseases/periodontitis**
   a. Localized tooth-related factors
   b. Localized prostheses-related factors.

II. Peri-implant Diseases and Conditions

1. Peri-implant health
2. Peri-implant mucositis
3. Peri-implantitis
4. Peri-implant soft and hard tissue deficiencies.

Staging of Periodontitis

Severity of periodontitis is decided by staging it. Staging is done after diagnosis of periodontitis. Initial stage should be determined using clinical attachment loss (*CAL*). If CAL is not available, radiographic bone loss (*RBL*) is used.

◄ *Why is staging of periodontitis done?*

Table 4.1: Staging of Periodontitis

	Periodontitis	*Stage 1*	*Stage 2*	*Stage 3*	*Stage 4*
Severity	Interdental CAL (*at the site of greatest loss*)	1–2 mm	3–4 mm	≥5 mm	≥5 mm
	RBL	Coronal third (<15%)	Coronal third (15%–33%)	Extending to middle third of root and beyond	Extending to middle third of root and beyond
	Tooth loss (*due to periodontitis*)	No tooth loss	No tooth loss	≤4 teeth	≥5 teeth
Complexity	Local	• Max. probing depth ≤4 mm • Mostly horizontal bone loss	• Max. probing depth ≤5 mm • Mostly horizontal bone loss	In addition to Stage II complexity: • Probing depths ≥6 mm • Vertical bone loss ≥3 mm • Furcation involvement class II or class III • Moderate ridge defects	In addition to Stage III complexity: • Need for complex rehabilitation due to: – Masticatory dysfunction – Secondary occlusal trauma (*tooth mobility degree ≥2*) – Severe ridge defects – Bite collapse, drifting, flaring – <20 remaining teeth (*10 opposing pairs*)
Extent and distribution	Add to stage as descriptor	For each stage, describe extent as: Localized (*<30% of teeth involved*); Generalized or Molar/incisor pattern			

CLINICAL UTILITY AND SHORT ANSWER

How is stage of periodontitis determined?

For staging periodontitis, the following sequence is followed:

Staging of periodontitis is done based on which findings? ▸

1. Periodontal loss is evaluated in the entire mouth by determining CAL (*clinical attachment loss*) or RBL (*radiographic bone loss*).
2. Stage (*initial*) is then established according to the above table. It is based on the ***maximum*** CAL or RBL found at any site.
3. Now look for ***complexity*** factors that complicate periodontitis and establish ***final*** stage periodontitis according to the above table. The complexity factors that force upward revision of initially established stage (*point # 2 above*) are:
   a. Horizontal or vertical bone loss
   b. Furcation involvement
   c. Number of teeth lost to periodontitis
   d. TFO (*trauma from occlusion*)
   e. Drifting of teeth (*pathologic migration*)
   f. Flaring of teeth
   g. Need for complex treatment, etc.
4. If no complexity factors are present, the initially established stage (*point # 2 above*) becomes the final stage.

Grading of Periodontitis

Why is grading of periodontitis done? ▸

After establishing severity of periodontitis, we grade periodontitis to determine the rate at which periodontitis is likely to progress. Grading is also done to know the expected response of periodontitis to periodontal treatment and the potential effect of periodontitis on the patient's systemic health.

Table 4.2: Grading of periodontitis

	Progression		*Grade A: Slow rate*	*Grade B: Moderate rate*	*Grade C: Rapid rate*
Primary criteria	Direct evidence of progression	Radiographic bone loss or CAL	No loss over 5 years	<2 mm over 5 years	≥2 mm over 5 years
	Indirect evidence of progression	% bone loss/age	<0.25	0.25 to 1.0	≥1
Whenever available, direct evidence should be used.		Case phenotype	Heavy biofilm deposits with low levels of destruction	Destruction commensurate with biofilm deposits	Destruction exceeds expectations given biofilm deposits; specific clinical patterns suggestive of periods of rapid progression and/or early onset disease
Grade modifiers	Risk factors	Smoking	Non-smoker	<10 cigarettes/day	≥10 cigarettes/day
		Diabetes	Normoglycemic/no diagnosis of diabetes	HbA1c <7.0% in patients with diabetes	HbA1c ≥7.0% in patients with diabetes

ALERT!

- Grade A indicates slowly progressing periodontitis and low risk of progression of periodontitis in future.
- Grade B indicates periodontitis is progressing at a moderate speed and there is moderate risk of progression in future.
- Grade C denotes very fast progressing periodontitis and high risk of its very fast progression in the future.

◂ What do grade A, B and C periodontitis denote?

ALERT!

Salient features and important changes in the 2018 classification (*compared to the 1999 AAP classification*)

- ***Chronic periodontitis and Aggressive periodontitis*** are now ***no longer*** two separate diseases. They are now grouped under a ***single category–periodontitis***.
- Bleeding on probing (*BOP*) is now the ***main*** parameter for identification and classification of gingivitis.
- The classification accepts that site level health can be different from case level health. Site level health is used to decide case level diagnosis.
- A multi-dimensional staging and grading system for periodontitis has been made. This provides a structure for periodontal treatment planning, monitoring patient's response to therapy and assessing risk of future periodontal disease progression.
- Periodontal health and gingival inflammation in a reduced periodontium after completion of treatment of periodontitis have been characterized.

◂ What are the important features of 2018 classification?

EPIDEMIOLOGICAL ASSESSMENT OF PERIODONTAL DISEASES

Epidemiology is the study of distribution, causes and effects of health and disease in demarcated populations. It helps us to understand patterns of distribution and measure the amount of disease present at community and individual's oral cavity level.

◂ What is the definition and benefit of epidemiology?

CLINICAL UTILITY AND SHORT ANSWER

What are the benefits of studying epidemiology?

Epidemiological data can help to:

1. Determine etiological factors, risk factors, modes of transmission and amount and pattern of distribution of disease in a particular population group.
2. Monitor progress and control disease by surveillance.
3. Know effectiveness of treatment methods by clinical trials.
4. Develop strategies for research and preventive oral health care.

CLINICAL UTILITY AND SHORT ANSWER

How does data from epidemiological studies help in case management?

How does epidemiological data help in case management?

We can know the following from data generated by epidemiological studies:

1. How rare or common is a particular disease or condition. From this we can know the probability of a patient having that disease or condition.
2. Signs and symptoms of a disease and stage of that disease in a particular patient.
3. Natural history of events likely to occur during course of a disease or condition.
4. The right stage and time to treat a disease or condition.
5. Prognosis of a disease or condition.

Commonly used Epidemiological Terms

What is the difference between prevalence and incidence?

Prevalence: It is the total number of cases of a disease in a given population at a ***particular time***.

Prevalence tells us degree of ***commonness*** of something and the likelihood of finding something in a particular group at a ***particular time***.

Incidence: It is a measure of the probability of occurrence of a given disease in a population group during a specified ***period of time***.

Incidence tells us the number of new cases of a disease occurring in a span of time, e.g. in a month, year, etc.

Risk: It is the probability of a person getting a disease during a specific duration of time.

Risk factors: Factors that place individuals at higher risk of getting a particular disease or condition.

Prognosis: It is the prediction of course or outcome of a disease (*likelihood of successful treatment especially related to tooth loss, recurrent disease, loss of function, complete/partial recovery, etc.*).

Assessment of Gingival and Periodontal Disease

What is an index?

Gingivitis and periodontitis are assessed and measured (*quantified*) using indices. An ***index*** is a standard method of rating a disease on a graduated numerical scale. Numeric values of an index correspond to specific criteria. Indices can be used to:

1. Gauge disease status in individuals
2. Know prevalence and incidence of diseases in a population group
3. Know disease status in a particular patient.

Some commonly used indices for quantifying gingivitis and periodontitis are described hereunder.

Assessing and Measuring Gingivitis (*Quantifying Gingivitis*)

Gingival indices gauge inflammation and assign numbers to gingival characteristics like colour, gingival bleeding, etc. according to their intensity.

Commonly used Indices for Scoring Inflammatory Gingival Disease

Gingival inflammation is assessed around which teeth for GI?

How is BOP assessed for GI?

I. Gingival Index (*GI*) (*Loe, H. and Silness, J. 1963*): It assesses severity of gingival inflammation by assessing changes in ***colour, consistency*** and ***bleeding on probing*** in relation to ***facial, mesial, distal, and lingual gingiva*** around teeth **# 16, 11, 24, 36, 31, 44** (*FDI system*). Bleeding on probing is assessed by ***lightly running*** a periodontal probe along the soft tissue wall of gingival sulcus (*sulcular epithelium*) all around the selected teeth.

Score	*Scoring criteria of Gingival Index (GI)*
0	Normal gingiva, i.e. no clinically identifiable inflammation or bleeding on probing.
1	Mild inflammation, i.e. slight change in colour, slight edema and no bleeding on probing.
2	Moderate inflammation, i.e. redness, edema, shining surface of gingiva and bleeding on probing.
3	Severe inflammation, i.e. marked redness, edema, ulceration and tendency to spontaneous bleeding.

Scoring for GI

1. Scores of gingival units around a particular tooth are totaled and divided by four to attain a tooth score (*for a single tooth*).
2. Tooth scores are added and divided by the total number of teeth examined to get GI score for that patient.

◂ *How is scoring done for GI?*

Interpretation of GI Scores

Scores between

1. 0.1–1.0 indicate mild inflammation in the gingiva
2. 1.1–2.0 indicate moderate inflammation
3. 2.1–3.0 are indicative of severe inflammation.

II. Sulcus Bleeding Index (*SBI*) (*Muhlemann, H and Son, S; 1971*): This index scores bleeding after sulcular probing, change in gingival contour and color.

i. Assessment is done at ***four*** gingival units per tooth, i.e. labial and lingual marginal gingiva (*two M units*) and mesial and distal papillary gingiva (*two P units*) under good illumination and after drying gingiva.
ii. To score the 'M unit' a periodontal probe is held parallel to long axis of tooth and gingival sulcus is probed lightly.
iii. For scoring the 'P units', probe is inserted interproximally and directed towards center of the interdental space, i.e. interdental col area.
iv. After probing, scoring of bleeding is done ***after*** 30 seconds according to under-mentioned criteria:

◂ *How is scoring done for sulcus bleeding index?*

Score	*Scoring criteria of Sulcus Bleeding Index (SBI)*
0	Healthy looking papillary and marginal gingiva. No bleeding after probing of sulcus.
1	Healthy looking gingiva with no colour or contour changes but bleeding on probing is present.
2	Colour of gingiva is changed from light pink (*normal*) to dark pink, red or bluish red. There is ***no*** edema in marginal or papillary gingiva (*no change in contour*) and bleeding on probing is present.
3	Same as '2' but ***slight*** edema (*change in contour*) is seen in marginal and papillary gingiva.
4	Same as '2' but **marked** edema (*change in contour*) is seen in the marginal and papillary gingiva.
5	Same as '2' but **very severe** edema (*change in contour*) is seen in the marginal and papillary gingiva. ***Spontaneous bleeding*** on probing is seen.

Scores for four units are added and divided by four to obtain the SBI score for a tooth. SBI scores for all scored teeth are totaled and divided by the number of teeth giving the overall SBI score.

ALERT!

Bleeding indices can measure bleeding on probing in both gingivitis and periodontitis.

Assessing and Measuring Periodontitis (*Quantifying Periodontitis*)

Plaque-induced periodontitis is an extension of gingivitis into deeper periodontal tissues. Periodontal indices are used to assess status of health or disease of the periodontium and record changes in these over a period of time.

Commonly used Indices for Scoring Inflammatory Periodontal Disease

I. Periodontal Index (*PI*) (*Russell, AL; 1956*): This index measures both reversible and irreversible aspects of periodontal disease in relation to all teeth present in the mouth. Scores of 0, 1, 2, 6 or 8 are allotted after assessment of periodontal disease.

Russell's rule: Assign lower score "when in doubt".

◂ *What is Russell's rule?*

Score	*Scoring criteria of Periodontal Index (PI)*
0	No obvious inflammation or loss of function due to destruction of supporting tissues.
1	Mild gingivitis; i.e. an area of inflammation is present in the free gingiva but this area of gingival inflammation does not go around the tooth.
2	Gingivitis, i.e. free gingiva all around the tooth shows inflammation but there is no break in epithelial attachment (*no CAL, i.e. no periodontal attachment loss*).
6	Gingivitis with pocket formation, i.e. epithelial attachment has been broken (*CAL is present, i.e. periodontal attachment loss has occurred*) and there is true pocket formation. Masticatory function is normal and tooth is firm and has not drifted.
8	Advanced periodontal destruction with loss of masticatory function, i.e. tooth may be loose, may have drifted (*pathological migration*), may sound dull on percussion and may be depressible in its socket (*grade III mobile*).

How is an individual's and population PI score got? ▶

A patient's (*individual's*) total score can be obtained by adding all the tooth scores and dividing by number of examined teeth. Population score can be obtained by adding all individual scores and dividing this number by number of subjects that were examined.

Interpretation of scores of Periodontal Index (PI)	
0.0–0.2	Clinically normal tissue
0.3–0.9	Gingivitis
1.0–1.9	Start of destructive periodontal disease (*periodontitis*)
2.0–4.9	Established destructive periodontal disease (*periodontitis*)
5.0–8.0	Terminal disease (*periodontitis*)

II. Periodontal Disease Index (*PDI*) (*Ramfjord; 1957*): The periodontal disease index is a modification of periodontal index (*PI*) given by Russell. The PDI has the ability to measure periodontal attachment loss (*CAL*) by relating it to a fixed landmark: CE junction (*cementoenamel junction*) of teeth.

Which six teeth are called Ramfjord teeth? ▶

The PDI collects data of ***six*** pre-selected teeth. These teeth are called ***Ramfjord teeth.*** They are: Maxillary right first molar, left central incisor, left first premolar and mandibular left first molar, right central incisor and right first premolar (*i.e. teeth no. 16, 21, 24, 36, 41 and 44 FDI system*). PDI has ***three*** components:

i. Plaque component
ii. Calculus component
iii. Gingival and periodontal component.

Plaque component of PDI

How many surfaces of Ramfjord teeth are scored for scoring plaque component of PDI? ▶

i. ***Four surfaces***, i.e. facial, lingual, mesial and distal of six Ramfjord teeth are scored.
ii. For this, mouth mirror and dental explorer are used. To score dental plaque, two cotton pellets are soaked in Bismarck Brown solution (*plaque disclosing solution*) and are used to stain plaque over all surfaces of teeth including the occlusal surface.
iii. Plaque scoring is then done after thoroughly rinsing twice. Scoring criteria:

How is plaque scored using PDI? ▶

Score	*Scoring criteria of plaque component of periodontal disease index (PDI)*
0	No plaque.
1	Plaque is present on some but not all interproximal, buccal and lingual surfaces of tooth.
2	Plaque is present on all interproximal, buccal and lingual surfaces but covers less than half of these surfaces.
3	Plaque extends over all interproximal, buccal and lingual surfaces and covers more than half of these surfaces.

Individual plaque score is got by adding all tooth scores and then dividing this by the number of teeth examined.

Calculus Component of PDI: Calculus component of PDI assesses presence and extent of calculus deposits only on ***two***, i.e. buccal and lingual surfaces of six Ramfjord teeth. A mouth mirror and dental explorer is used for this. Scoring criteria:

◂ How many surfaces of Ramfjord teeth are scored for scoring calculus component of PDI?

Score	*Scoring criteria of calculus component of Periodontal Disease Index (PDI)*
0	No calculus.
1	Supra gingival calculus extending not more than 1 mm coronal to free gingival margin.
2	Moderate amount of supra and sub-gingival calculus or presence of only sub-gingival calculus.
3	Plenty of supra and sub-gingival calculus.

Calculus score of an individual is got by adding calculus scores of teeth and dividing this by the number of teeth that were examined.

Gingival and Periodontal Component of PDI

i. Gingival component of PDI is obtained by examining gingiva to note changes in colour, form, consistency and for any evidence of ulceration or bleeding.
ii. After this, sulcus depth is noted by relating it to the CE (*cemento-enamel*) junction. To obtain sulcus depth, university of Michigan number 0 probe (*markings at 3, 6 and 8 mm*) held in a light grasp and inserted into the gingival sulcus/pocket under light pressure while maintaining tooth contact, is used.
iii. Sulcus depth measurements are taken on four surfaces, i.e. facial, lingual, mesial and distal of six Ramfjord teeth.

◂ On how many surfaces of Ramfjord teeth is sulcus depth taken for PDI?

Score	*Scoring criteria of gingival and periodontal component of Periodontal Disease Index (PDI)*
0	No inflammation.
1	Mild-to-moderate gingival inflammation not extending around the tooth
2	Mild-to-moderately severe gingivitis extending all around tooth
3	Severe gingivitis characterized by marked redness, swelling, tendency to bleed, and ulceration
4	Gingival sulcus in any of the four measured areas (*mesial, distal, buccal, lingual*) extends apical to CE junction but not more than 3 mm
5	Gingival sulcus in any of four measured areas extends 3–6 mm apical to the cemento-enamel junction
6	Gingival sulcus in any of four measured areas extends more than 6 mm apical to CE junction.

Calculation of scores: PDI score for an individual is got by adding scores of all Ramfjord teeth that were examined and then dividing this by the number of examined teeth.

◂ How is final PDI score obtained?

Commonly used Indices to Score Dental Plaque

I. Shick & Ash (*1961*) modification of plaque criteria of PDI (*Ramfjord's 1957 Periodontal Disease Index*): Shick and Ash suggested scoring gingival half of crowns of six Ramfjord index teeth on both the facial and lingual surfaces (*instead of interdental areas for plaque deposits as done in Ramfjord's PDI*).

◂ What is the difference between recording plaque scores in PDI and Schick and Ash plaque index?

Scoring criteria:

Score	*Scoring criteria of Shick and Ash modification of plaque criteria of PDI*
0	No plaque
1	Plaque only at gingival margin covering less than 1/3rd of the gingival half of facial or lingual surfaces of crown of a tooth
2	Plaque covering more than 1/3rd but less than 2/3rd of gingival half of facial or lingual surface of crown of a tooth
3	Plaque covering 2/3rd or more of facial or lingual surface of crown of a tooth

Only fully erupted teeth are scored; missing teeth are not substituted, i.e.; no score is allotted for missing teeth.

II. Plaque index (*Silness and Löe; 1964*) (*PI*): This index records soft debris or plaque deposits on buccal, lingual, mesial and distal surfaces of teeth # 16, 12, 24, 36, 32 and 44 (*FDI system*). Missing teeth are not substituted.

Scoring criteria:

Score	Scoring criteria of plaque index (Silness and Löe; 1964) (PI)
0	No plaque
1	Plaque adhering to free gingival margin and adjacent area of teeth. Plaque is seen only after application of disclosing solution or by using a probe on a tooth's surface
2	Moderate accumulation of soft deposits within gingival sulcus or at the tooth-gingival margin which can be seen with naked eye
3	Abundance of soft matter within gingival sulcus and the tooth-gingival margin

How is PI score for a tooth and for an individual got?

Calculation of scores: PI score for a tooth is got by totaling scores of all four areas of the tooth and then dividing this by 4 to get plaque index score for that tooth. PI scores for an individual is got by totaling scores of individual teeth and dividing this by number of teeth examined.

Commonly used Indices to Score Calculus Deposits and Oral Debris

I. Simplified oral hygiene index (*Greene and Jack R. Vermillon 1964*) (*OHI-S*)

This is a widely used index used to score and quantify ***both*** calculus and oral debris.

i. Presence of oral debris or other soft deposit on a tooth's surface is known by running side of an probe/explorer over surface of a tooth (*six index teeth*).
ii. Different surfaces of six index teeth (*FDI system*) are examined:
   a. Buccal surface of tooth #16,
   b. Buccal surface of tooth #11,
   c. Buccal surface of tooth #26,
   d. Lingual surface of tooth #36,
   e. Buccal surface of tooth #31,
   f. Lingual surface of tooth #46.

Which surfaces of which six teeth are scored for OHI-S?

Scoring oral debris component of simplified oral hygiene index (*DI-S*)
Scoring criteria

How is oral debris component of OHI-S scored?

Score	Scoring criteria of oral debris component of Simplified oral hygiene index
0	No debris or stain
1	Soft debris covering not more than 1/3rd of tooth surface or presence of extrinsic stain without other debris regardless of surface area covered
2	Soft debris covering more than 1/3rd but not more than 2/3rd of exposed tooth surface
3	Soft debris covering more than 2/3rd of exposed tooth surface

Interpretation of scores of DI-S	
0.0–0.6	Good
0.7–1.8	Fair
1.9–3.04	Poor

Scoring calculus component of simplified oral hygiene index (*CI–S*)
Scoring criteria

Score	Scoring criteria of calculus component of simplified oral hygiene index
0	No calculus
1	Supragingival calculus covering not more than 1/3rd of exposed tooth surface
2	Supragingival calculus covering more than 1/3rd but not more than 2/3rd of exposed tooth surface or presence of individual flecks of sub-gingival calculus around cervical portion of tooth or both
3	Supra-gingival calculus covering more than 2/3rd of exposed tooth surface or a continuous heavy band of sub-gingival calculus around cervical portion of tooth or both

Interpretation of scores of CI-S	
0.0–0.6	Good
0.7–1.8	Fair
1.9–3.04	Poor

The scores of debris component are added and divided by number of (*tooth*) surfaces examined. Scores of calculus are also similarly added and divided by number of tooth surfaces examined. These two total scores are then added together to get OHI-S score for an individual.

◂ *How is OHI-S score for an individual obtained?*

Interpretation of OHI-S (got after adding DI–S and CI-S scores)	
0.0–1.2	Good
1.3–3.0	Fair
3.1–6.0	Poor

Review Questions

1. What is the need for classification of periodontal diseases?
2. Which classification of periodontal disease is the most accepted and in use today?
3. What are the important changes in 2018 classification as compared to 1989 AAP classification?
4. What is epidemiology?
5. What basic purposes do the study and the data of epidemiology serve?
6. Define prevalence and incidence. What is the difference between these two?
7. Write on risk and risk factors.
8. Why are indices important?
9. Write short note on gingival index.
10. Name some commonly used indices to score periodontal disease.
11. Write a short note on periodontal index or periodontal disease index.
12. Describe some commonly used indices for scoring plaque.
13. Write a short note on Shick & Ash modification of plaque criteria of PDI.
14. Describe commonly used indices to score calculus deposits and oral debris.
15. Write a short note on simplified-oral hygiene index.

Chapter

5 Basic and Applied Concepts of Immunology and Inflammation Related to Periodontology

IMMUNE SYSTEM AND IMMUNITY

What is the difference between immunity and immune system? ▸

The defense system of our body that provides us protection from microbial infections, disease and physical insults is called immune system. Protection provided by the immune system is called immunity. The immune system not only neutralizes infection causing microorganisms that have somehow entered our body but also kills pathologically altered cells, e.g. cancer cells, etc.

Types of Immunity (*Immune Responses*)

There are two types of immune responses:

What is the difference between innate and adaptive immunity? ▸

1. **Innate or natural immunity** (*it is non-specific in nature*): This includes barrier systems of our body and systems and cells that identify and eliminate all pathogens ***irrespective*** of their antigenic specificity.
2. **Adaptive immunity** (*individual components of this immunity are directed against specific microorganisms and cells*): Components of the adaptive immune system identify and adapt themselves to each new pathogen and disease that they come across in the body and generate a ***pathogen specific*** or ***disease specific*** immunity.

I. *Innate Immunity* (Non-specific Immunity)

Name some mechanisms of innate immunity. ▸

Innate immunity is the name given to ***natural*** disease preventing and fighting ability that a person is born with. Some such innate immunity mechanisms are:

1. Epithelium of skin and mucous membrane prevent entry of microbes and protect from physical damage.
2. Rapid shedding of cells of epithelium (*desquamation*); due to this microorganisms that have entered the layers of epithelium are also shed off along with the cells of the epithelium.
3. Sweat, tears, etc. have compounds that kill microorganisms, etc.

Chief features of innate immunity or non-specific immunity

1. It is naturally present in everybody regardless of presence of or previous exposure to microorganisms.

What are characteristics of innate immunity? ▸

2. It is always functional, ready and ***does not need activation***.
3. Response of the innate immune system does ***not*** change (*increase*) in strength if re-exposure to the same infectious agent occurs.

II. *Acquired Immunity* (Specific or Adaptive Immunity)

Acquired immunity is acquired disease fighting capability of our body. It is highly specialized and specific and acts through humoral (*mediated by secreted antibodies present in plasma that are produced by B-lymphocytes*) and cell mediated immunity (*involves T-lymphocytes*).

Chief features of acquired immunity

1. It eliminates microorganisms (*antigens*) by production or activation of a ***specific*** immune response that works against that particular microorganism only.
2. This specific response of acquired immunity develops only after an earlier exposure of the acquired immune system to that particular microorganism (*antigen*).
3. Acquired immune system creates a ***'memory'*** of a particular microorganism (*antigen*) after its first exposure to it. This is a special feature of this system.
4. After first exposure to a microorganism (*antigen*) subsequent exposure to it produces a faster and improved response than the initial (*first*) response.
5. The acquired immune system is finely tuned and controlled by other elements of the immune system.

◂ *How is adaptive immunity different from innate immunity?*

◂ *How does acquired immune system tackle secondary infections by the same microorganism?*

Basics of Immunology

Antigen

- An antigen is any molecule that is identified as foreign (*'non-self'*) by the immune system.
- Antigen is recognized and specifically bound by ***one*** specific antibody and specific lymphocytes.
- All antigens may not be recognized as foreign and are thus not immunogenic (*against whom antibodies are produced*).
- Antigenicity of an antigen depends on its chemical nature, molecular size (*large molecules are stronger antigens*), foreignness (*relative to host*), chemical complexity (*increases antigenicity of antigens*) and accessibility of its antigenic sites (*greater accessibility leads to more antigenicity*).

◂ *What is an antigen?*

◂ *What are the factors on which antigenicity of an antigen depends?*

Antibody

- Antibodies are also known as immunoglobulins (*Ig*).
- They are produced by ***plasma cells*** (*fully differentiated B-lymphocytes*).
- Antibodies are ***antigen specific***, i.e. they are produced in response to and only after exposure (*of immune system*) to particular antigens.
- They bind to microorganisms, infected cells etc. (*opsonization*) and make these identifiable by other components of immune system.
- ***Nine*** types of antibodies (*immunoglobulins*) are found in ***humans***, they are: IgM, IgD, IgG1, IgG2, IgG3, IgG4, IgA1, IgA2 and IgE.
- Antibodies occur in ***two*** physical forms:
  1. **Soluble form:**
     a. They are secreted by ***plasma cells*** (*fully differentiated B-lymphocytes*) and are released into blood, tissue fluids and secretions.
     b. They circulate in the body and continuously survey their environment for antigens (*e.g. invading microorganisms, etc.*).
  2. **Membrane bound form:**
     a. These are antibodies attached to surface of B-lymphocytes.
     b. They are also referred to as the B cell receptors (*BCR*).
     c. The BCR enables activation of B-lymphocytes and causes them to further differentiate into:
        i. **Plasma cells** (*antibody producing B-lymphocytes*).
        ii. **Memory B cells** B-lymphocytes that survive and maintain memory of a particular antigen (*after first exposure to it*). In future, if the same antigen invades the body again, B-lymphocytes recognize it faster and mount a stronger and faster response against it.

◂ *What is an antibody?*

◂ *Which cells produce antibodies?*

◂ *Does a universal antibody against all microorganisms exist?*

◂ *How many types of antibodies are present?*

◂ *What are plasma and memory cells?*

ALERT!

75% of serum antibodies (*immunoglobulins*) in humans are of ***IgG*** type making it the ***most abundant*** antibody found in the circulation.

◂ *Which type of antibody is found in the maximum quantity?*

Basic structure of antibodies (*Immunoglobulins*)

What is the structure of an immunoglobulin molecule? ▸

All immunoglobulins have the same basic structure:

1. Antibody molecule is 'Y' shaped (Fig. 5.1).
2. Each immunoglobulin has two identical heavy chains. The heavy chain isotope (γ, μ, α, δ or ε) determines biologic properties of that immunoglobulin class.
3. The two arms of the Y-shaped Ig molecule are Fab fragments (*fraction antigen binding*) and the base of Y is Fc (*fraction crystallizable*) fragment.
4. The Fab fragments have antigen binding sites. This region of Ig molecule is composed of a variable region and hyper-variable sub-region.

Importance of variable and the hyper-variable regions on Fab fragment of an antibody

To how many antigens can an antibody bind to? ▸

- Though the overall structure of all antibodies is almost similar, antigen binding sites at tips of the Fab fragments are different in different antibodies (Fig. 5.2). These regions allow binding of a particular antigen only.

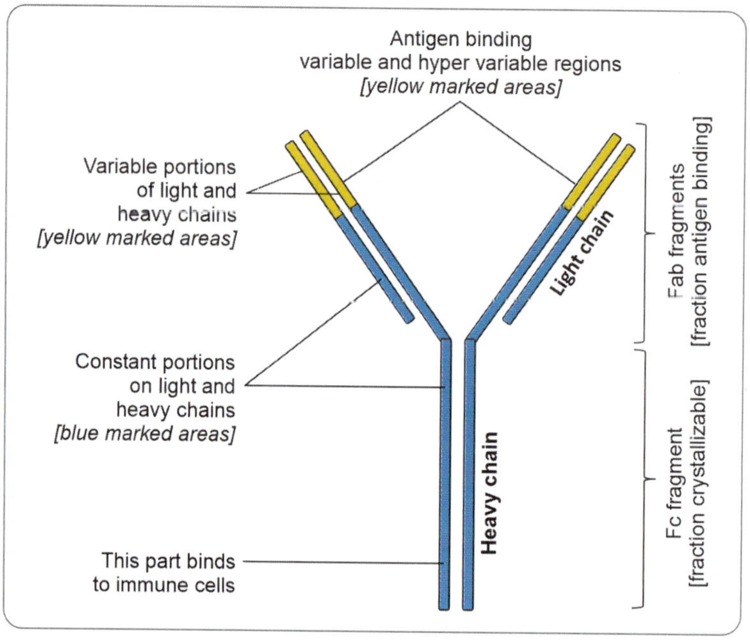

Fig. 5.1: Two-dimensional structure of antibody (*immunoglobulin*)

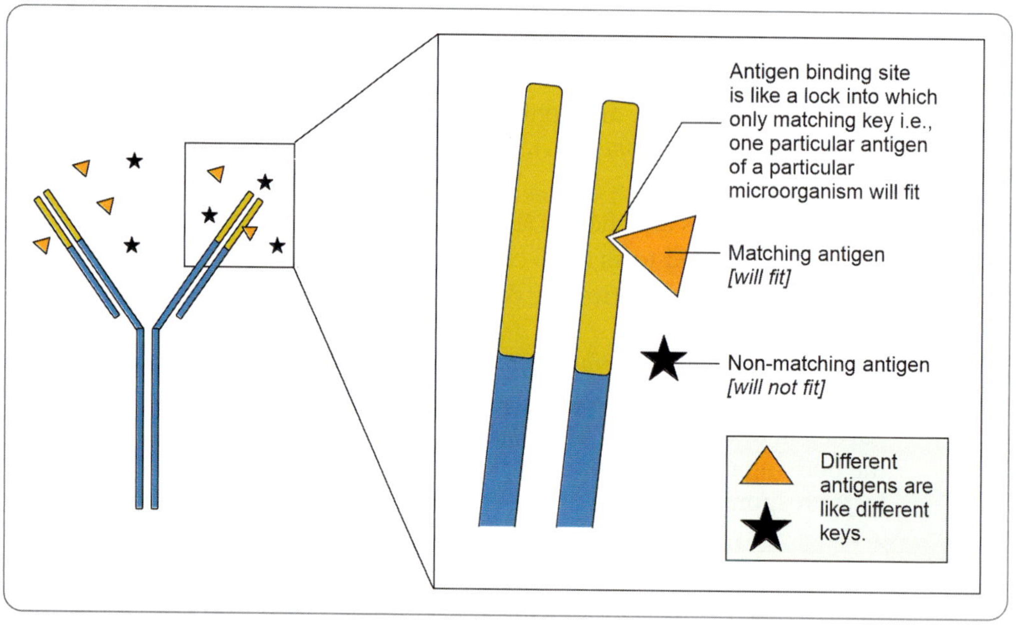

Fig. 5.2: Antibodies can bind only to specific antigens

- Antibody specificity to a particular antigen is because of a lock-key mechanism that exists between variable and hyper-variable regions and that specific antigen (Fig. 5.2).
- Because antigens can be of different types and a specific antibody will only bind to particular antigen, variability in antigen binding sites ensures specific response to a wide variety of antigens.
- Presence of a lock and key mechanism for antigen binding to antibodies allows maintaining of antigen specificity of antibodies.

◂ *Why is variability of antigen binding sites of an antibody important?*

◂ *How does an antibody allow binding of a particular antigen only?*

Opsonin and opsonization

- An ***opsonin*** is a marking molecule that binds to the microorganism's cell wall to 'mark' it and make the microorganism recognizable for ingestion and killing by a phagocyte.
- Examples of opsonins are antibodies IgG and IgA, components of the complement system e.g. C3b, C4b, etc.
- The process of binding of an opsonin to a receptor is called opsonization.

◂ *What is opsonin?*

◂ *What is opsonization?*

ALERT!

IgG and C3b are the ***most effective*** and important opsonins.

The Complement System

After antibodies bind to an antigen (*antigen-antibody reaction*) and label it as foreign (*opsonization*), complement system recognizes and destroys such labelled antigens (*microorganisms, etc.*). Complement system is a part of the ***innate immune system*** and it therefore shows similar response against all antigens. Complement system is also used by the adaptive immune system. Some important features of the complement system are:

1. It comprises of about ***30*** different proteins; there are ***no*** cells in the complement system.
2. When components of complement system come across a trigger, e.g. an opsonized microorganism's cell wall, the system's components are activated. This leads to a sequence of events that ends in destruction of the microorganism.

◂ *Complement system is a part of innate or adaptive immunity?*

◂ *Are there cells in the complement system?*

The complement system can be triggered by ***three*** pathways (Fig. 5.3): **Classical, alternate and lectin pathways.** All these eventually produce similar variants of C3 convertase, a ***key enzyme***, in the complement system.

◂ *How many pathways are there in the complement system?*

Functions of complement system

- Complement factors attract phagocytes to infection site by chemotaxis (Fig. 5.5).
- Complement factors also opsonize the microorganisms; this enables phagocytes to identify and ingest microbes and kill them.
- One of the end products of the activated complement pathways, the membrane attack complex (Fig 5.3, *yellow circle*) breaks the cell wall of cells of microorganisms leading to their death.
- Complement system's components bind to cells of immune system and trigger inflammation, immune mechanisms and regulatory molecules for the immune system.

◂ *What are the basic functions of complement system?*

CLINICAL UTILITY AND SHORT ANSWER

What happens if functioning of complement system is defective?

A malfunctioning or deficient complement system predisposes an individual to recurrent and severe infections. Unregulated or deficient complement system can cause many auto-immune diseases, e.g. arthritis, asthma, systemic lupus erythematosus, etc.

◂ *What will happen if complement system does not function properly?*

Toll Like Receptors (*TLRs*)

TLRs are a part of the innate immune system. 13 TLRs have been identified in humans.

- TLRs are ***pattern recognizing receptors*** present on ***surfaces*** of different immune competent cells like the ***macrophages, mast cells, monocytes, dendritic cells***, etc.

◂ *Is TLR a part of innate or adaptive immunity?*

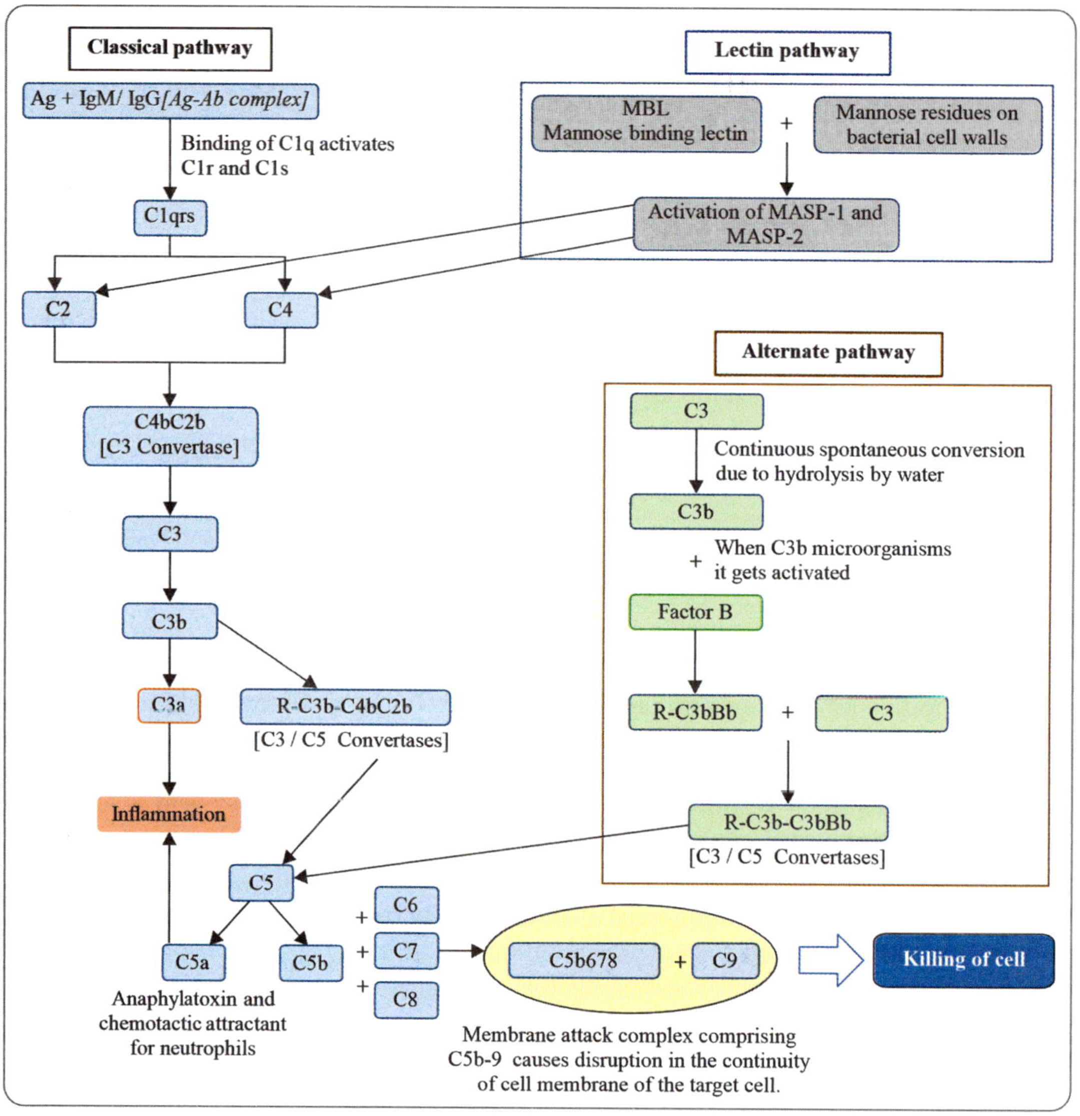

Fig. 5.3: The complement system

- TLRs do not recognize specific microorganisms but recognize their race in general, e.g. they will recognize bacteria but will not recognize particular species of bacteria. They do this by identifying molecular patterns common to cell walls of all bacteria.
- After microorganisms penetrate skin and mucosa, defense cells of innate immune system kill them using TLRs.

When do TLRs provide immunity during infection? ▸

- TLRs on defense cells provide protection against microorganisms in ***early stages*** of infection. Later, when invading pathogen is precisely identified, a more specific and stronger defense is mounted by the acquired immune system.

ALERT!

Why are TLRs critical to our body's defense?

TLRs and similar components of the innate immunity are very important for fighting infections.

Why are components of innate system very important although they are not as specialized as components of the adaptive immunity? ▸

- Adaptive immunity takes at least 4–7 days to get activated.
- If innate immunity components like the TLRs are not present, the body would remain defenseless in these initial 4–7 days of infection. This would cause severe infection that will then be very difficult to control by the adaptive immunity.
- TLRs recognize the most critical and unchangeable (*in which no mutations occur*) components of microorganisms, e.g. bacterial cell-surface constituents like lipopolysaccharides, etc. Therefore, TLRs help host immune system to recognize even those microorganisms that have undergone mutation.

Host Factors Influencing Ability and Response of Immune System

1. **Health and nutritional status of host.**
2. **Dose of antigen**. A minimum concentration of antigen is required to produce an immune response.
3. **Elapsed time after earlier exposure.** If repeated exposures to a particular microorganism keep occurring, the memory of that particular microorganism remains 'fresh' in the host's immune system. As a result, the host's immune system can then react quickly and strongly to that microorganism after repeat exposure to it.
4. **Foreignness** of the antigen relative to the responding host.
5. **Genetic background** of responding host, etc.

◄ *Which factors affect immunity of an individual?*

INFLAMMATION

Definition: Inflammation is a ***non-specific*** and ***local*** protective response of ***living*** and ***vascular tissue*** to infection and injury (*physical, thermal or chemical*).

◄ *What is inflammation?*

ALERT!

- Inflammation is the ***first step*** in healing. Wounds would not heal and infections would not resolve if inflammation is not present.
- However, excess and uncontrolled inflammation can negatively affect outcome of many diseases.
- Uncontrolled and excessive inflammation can also cause severe tissue damage leading to inflammatory disease, e.g. rheumatoid arthritis.

◄ *Is inflammation required for healing?*

Inflammation is of Two Types

1. **Acute inflammation**
2. **Chronic inflammation.**

◄ *How many types of inflammation are there?*

The ***initial*** inflammatory response is called acute inflammation. During this phase, increased outward movement of blood plasma and leukocytes occurs from blood vessels into affected tissues. Several biochemical events involving local vascular, cellular elements and the immune system occur during acute inflammation.

In due course of time, acute inflammation gives way to chronic inflammation. Shift from acute to chronic inflammation is characterized by a progressive shift in type of inflammatory cells present at the site of inflammation. Chronic inflammation is also characterized by ***start of healing***.

There are five basic signs of inflammation:

1. **Redness (*rubor*):** Because of increased blood flow.
2. **Swelling (*tumor*):** Due to collection of inflammatory fluid called exudate.
3. **Heat (*calor*):** This is also due to increased blood flow.
4. **Pain (*dolor*):** Caused by release of compounds like bradykinin which increase sensitivity of pain sensing nerve endings.
5. **Loss of function (*functio laesa*):** This occurs due to pain and collection of exudate in the tissue, etc.

◄ *What are the signs of inflammation?*

ALERT!

All signs of inflammation may not be seen in ***chronic inflammation***.

CLINICAL UTILITY AND SHORT ANSWER

What is exudate and purulent exudate?

Inflammatory fluid is called exudate. It is composed of water, WBCs, platelets etc. and contains high concentrations of plasma proteins (e.g. *fibrin, etc.*).

If exudate contains pus, it is called purulent exudate or suppurative exudate or pus. It contains plasma, active and dead neutrophils, fibrinogen and necrotic tissue components.

◄ *What is exudate?*

Outcomes of Inflammation

What are the possible outcomes of inflammation? ▶

Inflammation could result in the following outcomes:

1. **Resolution:** Complete restoration of inflamed tissue to normal. If inflammation is short lived, this is the most common outcome.
2. **Fibrosis:** If large amount of tissue destruction has occurred and tissues are unable to regenerate completely, healing then occurs by formation of fibrous tissue (*scar tissue*) (*repair*). Functional impairment is seen in tissues in which fibrosis has occurred. *What is fibrosis?* ▶
3. **Abscess formation:** Localized collection of pus can occur; pus will have to be drained out of the abscess for resolution of inflammation.
4. **Chronic inflammation:** Chronic inflammation results if cause of acute inflammation cannot be completely removed or persists for a long time. Body's own tissues are also damaged and destroyed in chronic inflammation.

Cells Playing Important Roles in Inflammation and Immunity

Mast cells, PMNs (*neutrophils*), macrophages, lymphocytes, etc. are actively involved in inflammation.

Mast Cells

Where are mast cells located in maximum numbers? ▶

- Mast cells are resident cells of several tissues.
- They are present near blood vessels and borders between outer and internal body environment, e.g. skin and mucosa of lung, mouth and nose.

What do chemicals produced in mast cells cause? ▶

- When inflammation occurs, mast cells release histamine, heparin (*an anticoagulant*), prostaglandins, cytokines, etc. into surrounding tissues. These bioactive chemicals cause increased permeability of blood vessels. This results in swelling, increased mucus production, etc.
- Mast cells have the ability of responding to ***specific antigens*** of particular micro-organisms.

Neutrophils (PMNs)

- Neutrophils comprise 50–70% of the WBCs found in blood.

What is chemotaxis? ▶

- Neutrophils leave blood vessels and migrate to the site of inflammation by ***chemotaxis***, i.e. moving along increasing chemical gradient of chemicals released at the site of inflammation. Neutrophils can detect increasing chemical gradients of interleukins, interferons and complement factor C5a.

What is the main function of neutrophils? ▶

- They have a short life and their main function is phagocytosis (*eating of infection causing microbes*). When neutrophils ingest microbes, they release superoxide and proteins from their cytoplasmic granules. The superoxide converts to hypochlorous acid that kills ingested bacteria. Neutrophils die after this.
- Neutrophils can kill ***all*** microbes. They ***do not need to differentiate*** amongst different microbes to phagocytose a particular microbe for killing it.

Why are neutrophils best suited to kill microbes in a periodontal pocket? ▶

- Because neutrophils derive most of their energy from glycolysis (*a cellular energy producing process that does not need oxygen for energy production*) they can ***function quickly*** and ***efficiently*** in ***anaerobic environments*** like the periodontal ***pocket***.

Which cells are present in the maximum quantity in pus? ▶

- Neutrophils form majority of cells in pus. Pus is white due to neutrophils in it.

Macrophages

- Macrophages are large phagocytosing cells (*'big eaters'*); they originate from monocytes and mature in local tissues.

What is the main function of macrophages? ▶

- After phagocytosis and digestion of microorganisms, they present the microorganism's antigens on their cell membranes to the lymphocytes and other immune cells.
- Macrophages also secrete powerful chemical substances that play a crucial role in inflammation and immunity, e.g. enzymes, regulatory factors like interleukin-1, etc.

Dendritic Cells

- Dendritic cells are named because of their surface projections that make them look like neurons; otherwise, they are ***not*** related to neurons in any way.
- They are antigen presenting cells and are present in all tissues that are in contact with the external environment, e.g. skin and mucosa of mouth, nose, lungs, etc.

◂ *Dendritic cells look like neurons, are they related to them?*

◂ *What is the main function of dendritic cells?*

Lymphocytes

- Lymphocytes are primary cellular components of acquired immune response.
- They are of three types: ***B lymphocytes***, ***T lymphocytes*** (*B cells, i.e. bursa-derived cells; T cells i.e. thymus cells*) and ***natural killer lymphocytes*** (Fig. 5.4).
- After an antigen has been killed and neutralized, B and T lymphocytes leave behind ***memory cells*** that maintain a lasting memory pool of antigens they had encountered.
- Memory cells thus help control any future infections by the same microorganism in a faster and more effective way.
- When a microbe (*antigen*) is found, ***B lymphocytes*** differentiate into dedicated antibody producing factories called ***plasma cells.*** Antigen (*microbe*) specific soluble antibodies are secreted into the body's fluids where they interact with antigens. ***B lymphocytes*** are therefore active components of ***humoral immunity***.
- ***T lymphocytes*** are responsible for ***cell-mediated immunity.*** They interact directly with their targeted cells, e.g. they directly attack body cells that have been infected by viruses or have become malignant.

◂ *What are the types of lymphocytes?*

◂ *What are memory lymphocytes?*

◂ *What is the main function of B lymphocytes?*

◂ *What is the main function of T lymphocytes?*

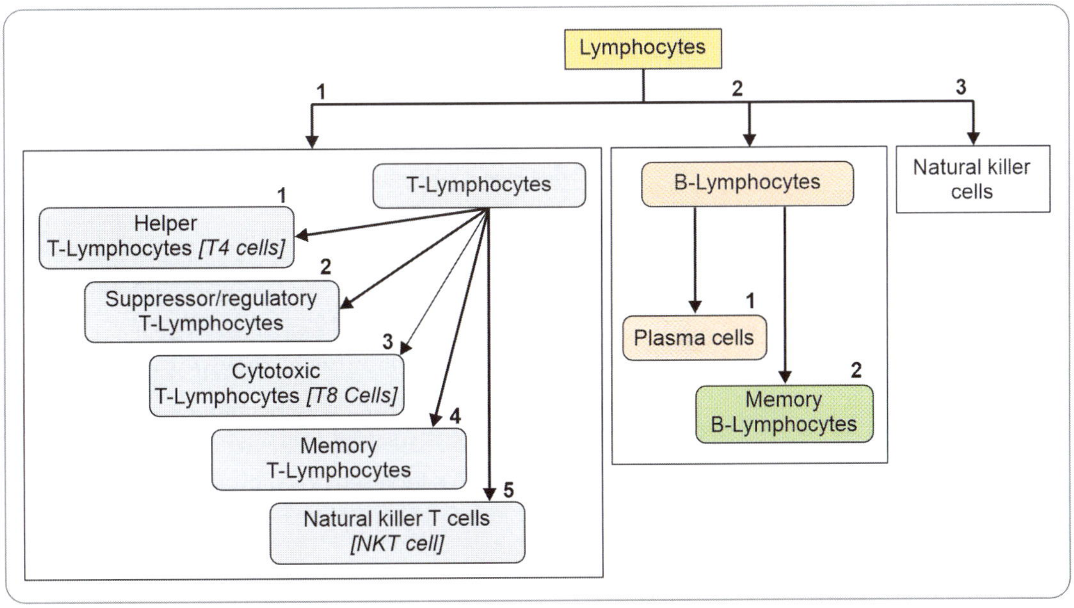

Fig. 5.4: Types of lymphocytes

WHAT HAPPENS WHEN AN INFECTION OR INJURY OCCURS

When injury or infection occurs, an inflammatory response is triggered. A complex series of events occurs that helps WBCs reach site of infection or injury. These are:

Step I: Trans-endothelial Migration of Leucocytes

1. *Rolling and Rolling Adhesion*

i. In a blood vessel with normal blood flow, WBCs normally roll slowly along endothelial cells of walls of blood vessels.

ii. While doing this, WBCs constantly but ***temporarily*** 'stick' to blood vessel walls and ***scan*** endothelial cells of the blood vessel wall to 'sense' molecules that are signals for further action. This process is called ***rolling***.

◂ *What is rolling?*

iii. When inflammation occurs, signaling molecules of inflammation, e.g. histamine, etc. reach the blood vessel walls and make the endothelial cells express chemical molecules called selectins on their luminal cell membranes.

iv. Selectins act as binding agents for rolling leucocytes.

What is rolling adhesion? ▸

v. Under the effect of selectins, leucocytes start to slow down and begin sticking along the inner surface of the vessel wall. This is called ***rolling adhesion*** of leukocytes.

What is rolling arrest? ▸

2. *Rolling Arrest or Tight Adhesion*

After rolling adhesion occurs, WBCs bind (*get attached*) to endothelial cells of the blood vessel walls.

How do leucocytes migrate out of walls of blood vessels? ▸

What is trans-endothelial migration? ▸

3. *Trans-endothelial Migration*

The leucocytes attached to the blood vessel wall ***flatten*** by rearranging their cytoskeletons and ***migrate out*** of the blood vessel through the endothelial cell junctions.

Step II: Chemotaxis

What is chemotaxis? ▸

After WBCs come out of the blood vessel, they start to migrate towards site of injury or infection by moving towards increasing concentration of inflammatory chemical molecules (*chemokines,* e.g. *TNF, interleukins, etc.*) released by local cells at the site of inflammation or injury. This movement towards an increasing chemical gradient is called chemotaxis **(Fig. 5.5)**.

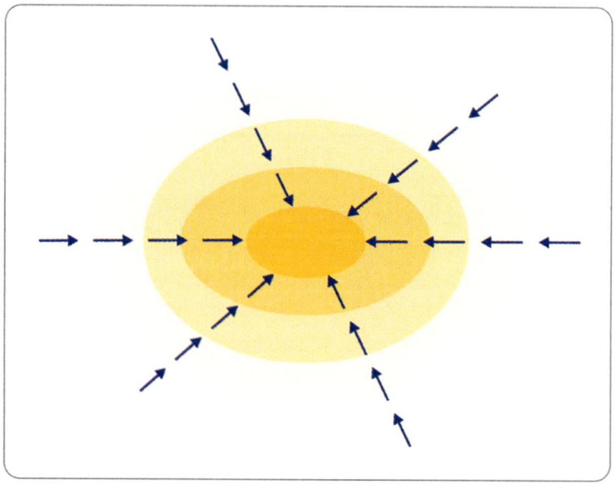

Fig. 5.5: Chemotaxis. Increasing chemical concentration is represented by circles of darker colour

Step III: Killing of Microorganisms by WBCs

Before arrival of WBCs at site of infection or injury, components of complement system, etc. label (*opsonize*) the invading microorganisms for identification by the arriving WBCs. The WBCs then kill microorganisms and control infection in four stages:

What is phagocytosis? ▸

1. *Phagocytosis*

- Phagocytosis is a cellular process that involves engulfing and ingestion of solid particles by phagocytes (*PMNs, monocytes and macrophages*).
- After reaching the site of inflammation (*injured or infected site*), phagocytes kill and eat (*phagocytose*) microorganisms to manage infection.

2. *Killing of Ingested Microorganism (After Phagocytosis)*

The microorganism is killed in two ways within the phagocyte after phagocytosis:

i. Non-oxidative killing:

What is non-oxidative killing? ▸

- Non-oxidative killing does ***not*** require presence of oxygen, therefore, this mechanism is effective even in ***deficiency*** of ***oxygen***.

- As oxygen concentration in periodontal pockets is low (*anaerobic environment*), non-oxidative killing plays a very important role in eliminating microorganisms from the pockets.
- After phagocytosis, a phagosome is formed within cytoplasm of the phagocyte.
- Lysosomes of the phagocyte then fuse with the phagosome and form a phagolysosome.
- Phagocytes have two types of granules called specific and azurophil granules within their cytoplasm. After a phagolysosome forms, specific granules release lysozyme, lactoferrin, etc. and azurophil granules release elastase, cathepsin, lysozyme, etc. into the phagolysosome to kill the phagocytosed microorganism.

◂ *Why is non-oxidative killing important from the periodontal point of view?*

◂ *Name the two types of granules present in the cytoplasm of phagocytes.*

◂ *Which chemical compounds do the granules of phagocytes contain?*

ii. Oxidative killing:

- Oxidative killing uses oxygen to kill the microorganisms. Oxidative mechanism therefore works only in presence of ***abundant oxygen***.
- In this mechanism, a superoxide anion O_2- and hydrogen peroxide are produced within the phagocyte. This is followed by formation of myeloperoxidase. Hydrogen peroxide and myeloperoxidase activate a halogenating system that results in formation of hypochlorous acid (*HOCl*) which kills phagocytosed microorganisms.

◂ *What is oxidative killing?*

3. *Antigen Processing and Presentation*

Antigen processing and presentation breaks antigens of microorganisms into small fragments and presents these to T-lymphocyte.

◂ *What is antigen processing and presentation?*

4. *Co-stimulation*

- After recognition of an antigen that is presented on surface of an antigen presenting cell, T lymphocytes bind to it.
- To activate T-lymphocytes into action, a second signal from the antigen presenting cell is given to them. This is called co-stimulation.
- If antigen binding T-lymphocytes do not receive the second signal they self-destruct.
- Co-stimulation is also required by B-lymphocytes to proliferate further after recognition and binding to the antigen.

◂ *What is co-stimulation?*

HOW MICROORGANISMS ESCAPE HOST DEFENCES AND PRODUCE INFECTION DESPITE AN ACTIVE IMMUNE SYSTEM

Microorganisms possess certain features that allow them to escape host defences and produce infection and disease (*also see* Fig. 6.18). Some of these are:

1. Cell membranes of some pathogenic bacteria like G –ve bacteria cannot be penetrated by lysozymes, etc.
2. Preventing inflammatory response against infection. Without inflammatory response the host is unable to activate its phagocytic defenses.
3. Inhibition of chemotaxis of phagocytes. Several microorganisms produce compounds that suppresses neutrophil chemotaxis even in very low concentrations, e.g. streptococcal streptolysin.
4. Inhibiting engulfing by phagocytes. Some pathogens have special features on their cell walls, e.g. fimbriae, capsules, etc. that prevent phagocyte's contact with microorganisms for phagocytosis.
5. Some pathogens can survive within the phagocyte after phagocytosis. This is due to their resistance to lysosomal constituents of phagocytes.
6. Killing of phagocytes before and after phagocytosis.

◂ *How do microorganisms evade host defences to produce infection and disease?*

APPLICATION OF CONCEPTS OF INFLAMMATION AND IMMUNOLOGY TO PERIODONTICS

Although etiology of periodontitis is microbial (*primarily bacterial*), but the disease itself is produced by harmful products of microorganisms and actions of host's inflammation and immunity that responds to the infection:

- The first response to the microbial infection is inflammation.

◂ *Does damage to periodontal tissues in periodontitis occur due to infection or host response to the infection or both?*

- Presence of bacteria in periodontal tissues stimulates host defense mechanisms of innate and specific immunity which then eliminate microorganisms that are present in periodontal tissues.
- However, these host defense mechanisms also cause simultaneous host tissue damage while tackling infection. This causes periodontal loss and damage seen in periodontitis.

Stages in Production of Periodontitis

Which stages are seen in production of periodontitis? ▸

Page and Schroeder in 1970 induced experimental periodontitis in dogs and described ***four*** stages of periodontitis that are applicable to humans also. These stages are:

1. *Initial Lesion*

How many days does the initial lesion of periodontitis last? ▸

i. It is seen within 2–4 days after stopping oral hygiene measures and thereafter lasts for 2–4 days before shifting to the next stage.
ii. This is characterized by presence of a few PMNs within the junctional epithelium, that are in the process of moving into the gingival sulcus.
iii. A small number of macrophages and lymphocytes (*mostly T-lymphocytes*) are seen in adjoining connective tissue.

2. *Early Lesion*

How many days does the early lesion of periodontitis last? ▸

Which cells are predominantly present in the infiltrate collected in the early lesion? ▸

i. This stage develops after 4–7 days of start of initial lesion and continues for up to 14–21 days.
ii. During this phase, increase in PMNs is seen in periodontal pocket till the 12th day.
iii. A marked increase in lymphocytes (*predominantly T-cells and few B-cells*), comprising up to ***75% of the infiltrate*** is also noticed in connective tissue adjoining the periodontal pocket.

3. *Established Lesion*

Which stage in history of production of periodontitis is the most prevalent and most commonly clinically seen stage? ▸

i. After about 14–21 days from start of initial lesion, ***intense*** PMN infiltration in junctional epithelium and pocket is seen.
ii. B-lymphocytes are now increased and they can be seen converting to plasma cells (*for antibody production*).
iii. Monocytes are seen to covert to macrophages.
iv. This phase is the ***most common clinically*** seen stage and is also the most ***prevalent***.
v. It lasts for an ***indefinite*** period.

4. *Advanced Lesion*

In which stage of periodontitis is destruction of alveolar bone seen? ▸

In which stage does apical shift of junctional epithelium occur? ▸

i. The periodontal lesion is considered advanced when ***destruction*** of ***alveolar bone*** is seen.
ii. Pocket epithelium is ulcerated and ***apical shift of junctional epithelium is seen.***
iii. Plasma cells now dominate in the connective tissue, whereas neutrophils dominate the junctional epithelium and gingival sulcus.
iv. This phase also lasts for an ***indefinite*** period.

What is the leukocyte wall? ▸

In which area of periodontal tissues are maximum number of leukocytes present? ▸

Which leucocytes are present in maximum and minimum numbers in the periodontal tissues? ▸

How many PMNs are present in junctional epithelium and GCF? ▸

ALERT!

Distribution of leukocytes in periodontal tissues is not uniform.

- Neutrophils (PMNs) readily infiltrate into gingival sulcus and form a '***leukocyte wall***' between plaque and junctional and sulcular epithelium.
- ***50%*** of leukocytes in ***junctional epithelium*** are PMNs.
- ***90%*** of leukocytes in ***GCF*** (gingival crevicular fluid) are PMNs.
- Neutrophils are the first WBCs to arrive at the site of periodontitis.
- On the other hand, lymphocytes and other mononuclear cells usually infiltrate into junctional epithelium only in small numbers and generally remain confined within the connective tissue.

HOW HOST PREVENTS AND MANAGES PERIODONTAL INFECTIONS (*PERIODONTITIS*)

In the beginning, components of innate immunity control infection and present antigens of invading microorganisms to cells of acquired immunity. Later acquired immune responses become active. Events that prevent periodontal infection and resulting periodontitis are:

1. The first line of defense against plaque induced periodontitis is innate immunity which includes the following:
   - **Intact layer of epithelium:** This acts like a physical barrier and prevents entrance of most of the microorganisms.
   - **Continuous shedding of epithelial cells:** Shedding of top layers of epithelium continuously ensures that microorganisms that had somehow gained entry into epithelium are also shed off and these therefore cannot enter into gingival connective tissue where they can cause infection.
   - **Gingival crevicular fluid (*GCF*):** As GCF flows ***outward*** from the sulcus into the oral cavity, it physically flushes out microorganisms out of the sulcus. Microbicidal substances like lysozyme, etc. in GCF also kill microorganisms.
   - **Neutrophils in the sulcus:** They kill microorganisms that are present in the sulcus.
2. Despite the above, some microorganisms still manage to break the epithelial barrier and gain assess into the underlying connective tissue. In the connective tissue such microorganisms are recognized and eliminated by the humoral (*serum*) components of innate immunity, e.g. complement system, lysozyme, etc. and some components of specific immune system.
3. Inflammation: After microorganisms have gained entry into connective tissue, they trigger inflammation at that site. Mast cells release histamine, prostaglandins, cytokines, interleukins etc. into the surrounding tissues. These chemical mediators of inflammation produce local responses like increased permeability of blood vessels. Acute inflammation also causes release of chemical substances that make more neutrophils come to the infected/inflamed area by chemotaxis.
4. Neutrophils and other phagocytes phagocytose and kill infection causing microorganisms to control infection.
5. Lymphocytes then enter the scene. This marks the start of the phase of ***chronic inflammation***.
   - T helper lymphocytes 'learn' about the infection after interaction with antigen presenting cells that exhibit the infecting microorganisms' antigens on their surfaces. A particular line of T helper cells recognizes only one specific microorganism.
   - T helper lymphocytes then increase in numbers by clonal expansion and activate other immune cells for attacking the invading pathogen.
   - T-lymphocytes also activate B-lymphocytes to produce antibodies against that microorganism. These antibodies opsonize, i.e. tag the infecting microorganisms by sticking onto microorganisms to mark them out for phagocytes to phagocytose them.
   - Microorganisms are also memorized by lymphocytes. This enables faster and stronger response against that particular microorganism in future.
6. Cytokines (*signaling chemicals*) released by lymphocytes, monocytes and other resident cells present in the infected tissue cause differentiation and activation of immune cells. They also result in connective tissue remodeling that may be destructive in nature.
7. When the infection has been controlled, inflammatory activity is brought down by release of chemical signals by the resident cells of infected-inflamed tissue. Tissue remodeling then starts and results in healing (*constructive activity*).

◄ *How do components of innate immunity protect entry of microorganisms into periodontal tissues?*

◄ *How does continuous exfoliation of epithelium prevent periodontal infection?*

◄ *How does GCF help in maintaining periodontal health?*

◄ *How are microorganisms controlled in the initial stages of infection?*

◄ *When does phase of chronic inflammation start?*

◄ *Is response of T lymphocytes microorganism specific or not?*

HOW PERIODONTITIS (*INFECTION*) OCCURS DESPITE PRESENCE OF AN ACTIVE IMMUNE SYSTEM

Microorganisms can evade several layers of host defenses and can cause periodontitis even in healthy people with a 'normally' functioning immune system.

- Usually infection by plaque microorganisms (*periodontitis*) is kept under control by body defenses (*immune system*); this is clinical health.

◄ *How do microorganisms evade host defenses?*

When does clinically recognizable disease result? ▸

- When disease produced by the infection surpasses disease controlling capacity of the immune system, tissue destruction increases and clinically apparent disease results.
- Additionally, if host has a deficiency in its immune components, e.g. neutropenia (*reduced number of PMNs*) or if phagocytes are defective in their functioning, disease occurs easily and is more severe.

Give examples of how bacteria produce periodontitis. ▸

- Microorganisms that cause periodontitis are known to possess several factors that help them survive within periodontal tissues despite a healthy and robust immune system. These factors also increase their periodontitis causing ability. Two of the most studied periodontitis causing bacteria are *P. gingivalis* and *A. actinomycetemcomitans*. Bacterial factors of these bacteria that help them cause periodontitis are:

What is the etiological importance of lipopolysaccharides in periodontitis? ▸

  - Lipopolysaccharides in cell wall of bacteria provide protection against phagocytosis and are strongly antigenic.
  - Lipopolysaccharides induce a very strong defensive inflammatory reaction by the host. This inflammatory reaction causes more periodontal destruction in periodontitis than the overall beneficial and protective effects of inflammation caused by Lipopolysaccharides.
  - Adhesins and Fimbriae of bacteria not only help them stick to host cells but also to other bacteria to form a bio-film. This helps in invasion and colonization of periodontal tissues.
  - Bacteria produce:
    - Invasins to help penetrate into cells.

Name some chemical compounds that help bacteria evade host defences and produce periodontitis. ▸

    - Enzymes like collagenase, fibrinolysin, etc. that help them degrade connective tissue and thus allow easy entry into tissues.
    - Cytotoxins to hinder PMN chemotaxis, phagocytosis and intracellular killing and inhibit proliferation and functioning of fibroblasts.
    - Leukotoxin to inhibit PMN activity, immunoglobulins and complement activation. It is one of the most potent toxins produced by bacteria against the human body defenses.
    - Endotoxins to induce inflammation and bone resorption.

DESTRUCTION OF PERIODONTAL TISSUES IN PERIODONTITIS IS ALSO CAUSED BY HOST'S IMMUNE MECHANISMS AND INFLAMMATION

Periodontitis is not only caused by destruction of periodontal tissue by microorganisms but also by components of the host defense systems that destroy periodontal tissues in their effort to control periodontitis. For example:

How do host defences damage host tissues during periodontitis? ▸

a. In the process of killing pathogens, PMNs and macrophages cause host tissue damage due to spilling of their enzymes (*e.g. proteolytic enzymes of the PMNs*) into the surrounding periodontal tissues. These enzymes destroy periodontal tissues.
b. Lipopolysaccharide are components of bacterial cell walls. When host defenses kill bacteria, their cell wall breaks down and lipopolysaccharides are released into the surrounding tissues.
c. As lipopolysaccharides are strongly antigenic they induce a strong inflammatory reaction that leads to production of arachidonic acid metabolites like prostaglandin E2 (*PGE2*), etc.

What are MMPs? ▸

d. PGE2 and several such compounds cause release of matrix metalloproteinases (*MMPs*) in host tissues. MMPs are potent molecules that cause destruction of periodontal tissues.

How do cytokines and other chemical regulators of inflammation help in production of periodontitis? ▸

e. Cytokines like interleukin 1 (*IL-1*) are released from periodontal tissue cells during periodontitis. Cytokines are important regulators of inflammatory and immune responses. In addition to their beneficial role, cytokines also inhibit new bone formation (*reduce healing*) and increase bone loss in periodontitis.

Review Questions

1. What is immunity? Why is the immune system needed?
2. What is an antigen?
3. What is an antibody? Name types of antibodies.
4. Write a note on complement system.
5. What is the basic structure of an immunoglobulin?
6. In the presence of so many types of antigens, how do antibodies manage to react to each one of them in a very specific manner?
7. Why is inflammation needed? What are the 'cardinal signs' of inflammation?
8. How do leucocytes reach the area of infection? How do leucocytes eliminate pathogens after they reach the infected site?
9. What are chemotaxis and phagocytosis?
10. What are toll like receptors (*TLRs*)?
11. Describe the stages in production of periodontitis and emphasize on the changes with respect to the immune system.
12. Is the distribution of leukocytes within the periodontal tissues uniform?
13. Which of the two cell types, neutrophils and lymphocytes, are more abundantly seen in the diseased periodontal tissues?
14. How can an infection occur in the periodontal tissues despite the presence of an active immune system?
15. How does the host defense tackle a periodontal infection?
16. Name the host mechanisms and molecules that cause destruction and healing in periodontal disease.
17. Write on bacterial factors causing tissue destruction.

Chapter

6

Dental Plaque (Oral Biofilm)

The human oral cavity has ***no*** microorganisms at time of birth (*sterile*). Later, more than 500 species of bacteria can be found in the oral cavity. Large proportion of these microorganisms is normal commensals (*non-disease causing and beneficial*) and they live in a symbiotic relationship with us.

Define plaque? ▸

Definition: Dental plaque is a soft white/light-yellow adherent substance that accumulates on all surfaces of the oral cavity including teeth, restorations, prostheses, soft tissues and in sulci and pockets (Figs 6.1 and 6.2).

Do bacteria in plaque live in a random unorganized fashion? ▸

Plaque has a highly ***organized*** structure and is composed of diverse microbial communities embedded and living together in a matrix of polymers of microbial and salivary origin.

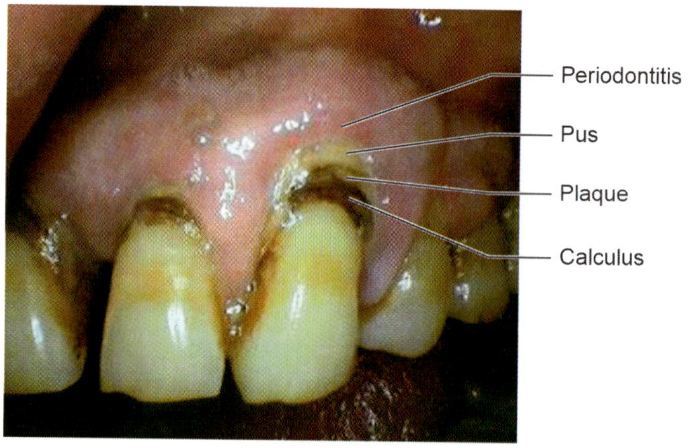

Fig. 6.1: Dental plaque and calculus cause gingivitis and periodontitis and complicate clinical features of other diseases and conditions affecting periodontium

DENTAL PLAQUE HAS BEEN RE-NAMED AS ORAL BIOFILM

Biofilm—What is it?

What is a biofilm? ▸

Definition: A biofilm is a complex collection of different species of ***cooperating*** micro-organisms that live in an excreted protective adhesive matrix.

What are planktonic microorganisms? ▸

Are bacteria living as planktonic microbes different from those living in biofilms? ▸

- Bacteria live in the oral cavity either in colonies as ***biofilms*** or as solitary cells floating in the saliva as ***planktonic*** microbes.
- Because living in a biofilm requires establishing complex relationships with other microorganisms, therefore, bacteria in biofilms, have different characteristics than the same bacteria living as solitary cells (*planktonic microbes*).
- Biofilms are usually attached to a surface (*substrate*).

- Living together in biofilms provides microorganisms several benefits, these include:
  - Physical security. Bacteria in biofilms resist physical forces better than solitary cells of the same bacterial species that are collected and clumped together.
  - Protection against chemical antimicrobials. Bacteria in plaque (*oral biofilm*) are many more times ***resistant*** to antiseptic mouthwashes.
- As dental plaque possesses all characteristics of a biofilm, it has been renamed plaque biofilm or oral biofilm.
- This change in name represents a significant shift in our understanding of the power and ability of a very powerful biological entity—plaque, that affects all of us. It also forces us to shed our casualness and to re-look at plaque as a more formidable enemy than we earlier thought.
- ***In common usage though, because of habit and tradition, the term 'dental plaque' or simply 'plaque' is used more commonly and accepted.***

◂ *How do bacteria benefit from staying together in a biofilm?*

◂ *What are the new names of plaque?*

◂ *Why is the term plaque used more commonly than oral biofilm?*

Materia Alba

Materia alba (Fig. 6.2) is an unorganized collection of food debris, bacteria and tissue cells that loosely sticks to the oral surfaces.

- Materia alba is very ***similar*** to plaque as it has practically the same constituents, color and consistency.
- The difference between materia alba and plaque is in their internal structure. While plaque is ***highly organized***, i.e. bacteria in plaque live together in an organized manner in colonies that firmly stick onto oral surfaces, no such organization and adherence is seen in materia alba.

◂ *What is materia alba?*

◂ *What is the difference between dental plaque and materia alba?*

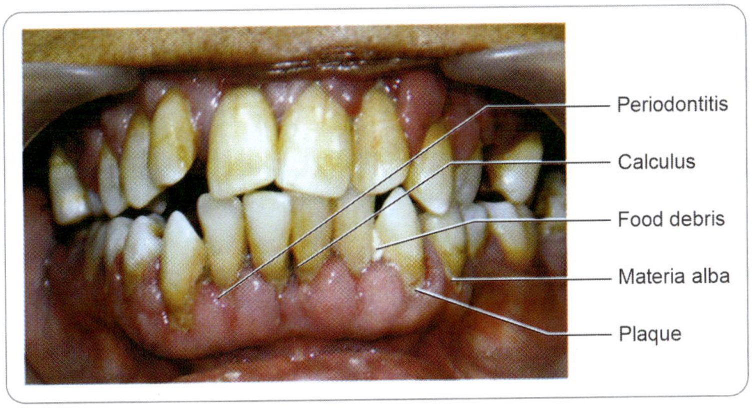

Fig. 6.2: Dental plaque, calculus, materia alba and food debris in a patient suffering from periodontitis

Areas Where Dental Plaque (*Oral Biofilm*) Deposits are Found

- Plaque regularly forms on surfaces of teeth, restorations, oral prostheses, sulci and pockets and oral soft tissue (*areas and surfaces that remain wet with saliva or GCF*).
- Occlusal surfaces of teeth and restorations and soft tissue surfaces that get cleaned during mastication of food or by tooth brushing, etc. do not show plaque.
  Plaque may form on these surfaces if a patient is not eating on that side (*unilateral mastication*) or in case the patient is tooth brushing properly (Fig. 6.6).

◂ *Where is plaque usually seen?*

◂ *Where is plaque usually not seen?*

◂ *When does plaque form on oral hard and soft tissue surfaces where it not usually seen?*

How Can Dental Plaque (*Oral Biofilm*) Be Seen and Identified?

Because dental plaque is white/light-yellow in colour, it ***cannot*** be easily seen if it is present over surface of teeth or tooth-coloured restorations. Presence of plaque can be known by:

1. **Direct viewing** (Figs 6.1 and 6.2).
2. **Scrapping the tooth surface:** If a dental instrument, e.g. probe etc. is moved over a tooth surface, plaque if present, will collect on tip and blade of the instrument.

◂ *What is the colour of plaque?*

What are plaque disclosing solutions?

What is the best way to identify plaque?

3. **Staining plaque with plaque disclosing solutions:** Plaque disclosing solutions stain plaque to make it readily identifiable. This is the most accurate way of knowing presence and extent of plaque **(Fig. 6.3)**.
   a. They contain dyes, e.g. basic fuchsin, erythrosin (*FDC Red No. 3*), etc.
   b. Two tone staining solutions containing FDC red no. 3 and FDC green no. 3. are also available. Such solutions stain old and new plaque in two different colours.
4. **Visualizing plaque on surfaces of teeth with intra-oral cameras using fluorescence technology:** This is the simplest and digital method of plaque identification. When teeth are illuminated with a special light at specific wavelengths, plaque that was not visible under normal daylight, shows fluorescence and can be easily seen on a computer screen **(Fig. 6.4)**.

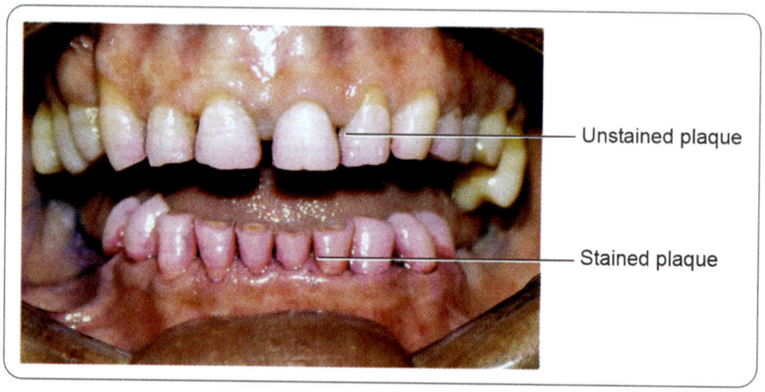

Fig. 6.3: Dental plaque (*oral biofilm*) seen in daylight and after disclosing with two tone disclosing solution. Older plaque deposits stain bluish red while more recent plaque stains pink

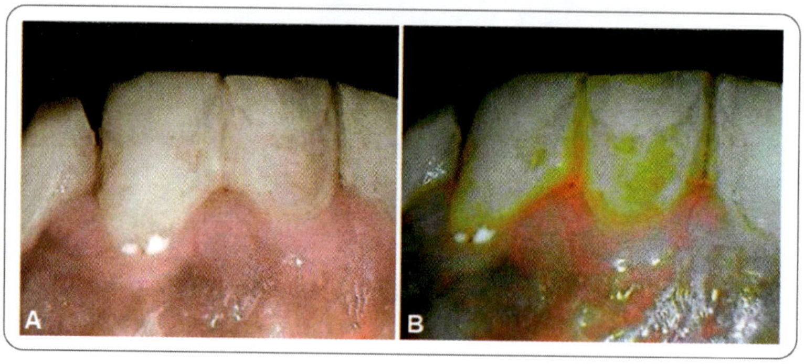

Fig. 6.4: Special intra oral cameras are available which can take pictures both in daylight (*diag. A*) and after illuminating teeth with light that causes plaque to show fluorescence (*diag. B*). Note fluorescence of plaque in picture B taken under special light. Such pictures serve as an excellent educational and motivational tool for plaque control

ALERT!

Some terms used to describe type of bacteria found in oral cavity.

Aerobic: Oxygen loving microorganisms.

What is the difference between facultative aerobes and facultative anaerobes?

1. **Obligate aerobes:** Can survive only in oxygen rich atmosphere.
2. **Facultative aerobes:** Use oxygen, but also have anaerobic methods of energy production.

Anaerobic: Carbondioxide loving microorganisms.

1. **Obligate anaerobes:** Microorganisms that live in absence of oxygen and will die when exposed to oxygen.
2. **Facultative anaerobes:** Prefer carbondioxide but can use oxygen when it is present.

Which type of microorganisms, aerobic or anaerobic are present in a pocket in maximum numbers?

Microaerophiles: Microorganisms that use oxygen only at low concentrations (*normal concentrations of oxygen will inhibit their growth*).

The periodontal ***pocket,*** especially if it is more than 3–4 mm deep has an ***anaerobic*** environment.

Types (*Classification*) of Dental Plaque (*Oral Biofilm*)

Based on anatomical location of plaque with respect to gingival margin, plaque can be classified as (Fig. 6.5):

What are the different types of plaque?

1. Supra-gingival plaque.
2. Sub-gingival plaque.
   a. Tooth attached/associated (*most disease causing*).
   b. Epithelium associated.
   c. Unattached (*suspended in GCF within the sulci/pocket*) (*most disease causing*).
3. Peri-implant plaque.

Which type of plaque has the maximum capacity to produce periodontitis?

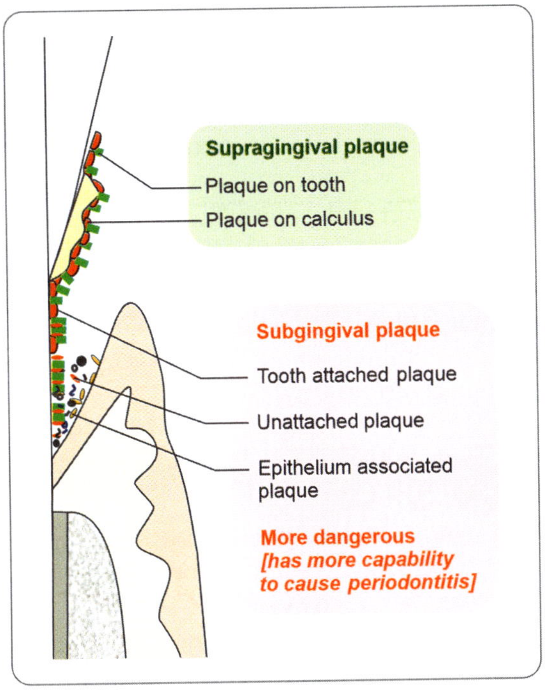

Fig. 6.5: Types of plaque/oral biofilm

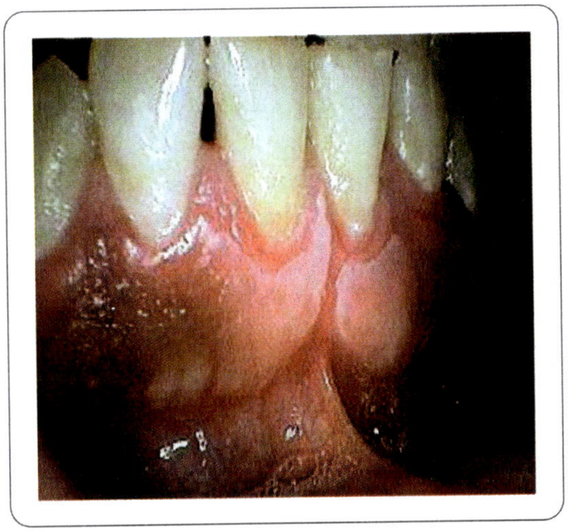

Fig. 6.6: Plaque can also form on oral soft tissue surfaces, e.g. gingiva and tongue (*oral mucous membrane*). In this diag. plaque has formed on gingiva of a sick patient who is only on liquid diet and is not brushing his teeth

CLINICAL UTILITY AND SHORT ANSWER

What are the differences between supragingival and subgingival plaque?

	Supragingival	*Subgingival*
1. Location and distribution	Coronal to crest of free gingiva	Apical to crest of free gingiva
2. Retention	Adheres to supra-gingival rough tooth surfaces, restorations, calculus, etc.	Adheres to sub-gingival tooth and calculus surfaces; epithelium attached plaque adheres to the sulcular/pocket epithelium; unattached plaque microorganisms remain suspended in sulcus/pocket.
3. Source of nutrients	Saliva and ingested food	Gingival crevicular fluid (*GCF*)
4. Type of microorganisms	Primarily aerobic	Primarily anaerobic
5. Type of calculus that forms after calcification of plaque	Forms supragingival calculus that is soft in consistency and is light in colour.	Forms subgingival calculus that is hard in consistency and is dark green or black in colour.

Physical Features of Dental Plaque (*Oral Biofilm*)

- It is white/light-yellow in color and soft in consistency.
- Each 1 mg. wet weight of dental plaque can contain 10^8–10^{11} bacteria and many species of microorganisms.
- An individual pocket around the tooth can be populated by more than 150 species.

What is the colour of plaque?

How many species of microorganisms can be present within a pocket?

- Inter-microbial matrix of plaque (*substance in which cells of plaque microorganisms are embedded*) makes almost 25% of its total volume.

Clinically Important Characteristics of Dental Plaque (*Oral Biofilm*)

1. Quality of plaque (*types of microorganisms in plaque*) is different at different sites of the oral cavity.

How soon does plaque start to form after complete removal? ▸

2. Plaque formation starts within few minutes of complete removal of all disclosable plaque. Rate of formation of plaque is increased in gingivitis and periodontitis.
3. Plaque formation starts as small colonies. These spread out and mass of plaque increases in quantity for about a week or so. After one week, only quality of plaque changes with time, increase in quantity is not seen.
4. G +ve bacteria are the first bacteria to be seen in supra-gingival plaque. Later G –ve cocci and G +ve and G –ve rods and filaments colonize developing plaque.

Does the number of plaque microorganisms increase as depth of pocket increases? ▸

5. The number of anaerobic microorganisms in sub-gingival plaque increase as depth of sulci/pockets increases.

How do plaque micro-organisms enter gingival connective tissue? ▸

6. Bacteria enter gingiva through temporary tunnels left in the epithelium by migrating PMNs as they migrate from gingival connective tissue into gingival sulcus.
7. Epithelial attachment weakened by inflammation allows colonization of plaque bacteria in the space between junctional epithelium and tooth.
8. Spread of plaque microorganisms and resultant gingivitis and periodontitis can be easily reduced by controlling plaque by tooth brushing, etc.

In which areas is plaque control difficult? ▸

9. Plaque control is difficult on rough surfaces of calculus, fissures, carious lesions and hard to reach areas like furcations, crowded teeth, under overhanging restoration margins, etc.

Plaque calcifies to form what? ▸

10. Supra-gingival plaque calcifies to form light-coloured, lightly adherent and supra-gingival calculus. Sub-gingival plaque calcifies to form dark coloured, strongly adherent and harder sub-gingival calculus.
11. Plaque and calculus contain a large quantity of bacterial endotoxins. These cause inflammation in periodontal tissues.

Formation of Dental Plaque (*Oral Biofilm*)

How does plaque form? ▸

Name the three stages in which plaque forms. ▸

There are basically three stages in development of plaque:

1. Adhesion to a surface (*substrate*)
2. Maturation
3. Dispersion.

1. Adhesion to a surface (*substrate*)

a. Formation of acquired pellicle

- As soon as any surface of the oral cavity is thoroughly cleaned or a new surface of new restoration or prosthesis becomes available in the oral cavity, a ***sticky*** layer called acquired pellicle, begins to form on that surface.

What is acquired pellicle? ▸

- The acquired pellicle is made up of macromolecules derived from ***saliva***, e.g. mucin, proteins, etc.
- This starts plaque formation.

b. Microbial adhesion to acquired pellicle

Free-floating (*planktonic*) microorganisms start to stick on the sticky acquired pellicle by:

- **Reversible attachment:** Initially microorganisms stick on acquired pellicle using weak ***Van der Wall*** forces of attraction.
- **Irreversible attachment:** If initial colonizing microorganisms remain on acquired pellicle surface for some time, they get attached to the pellicle more firmly.

2. Maturation

- Colonies of microorganisms start to grow on the pellicle. New microorganisms join the ones already present. An extracellular matrix that is secreted by these microorganisms holds colonies together.
- As time passes, more microorganisms (*of different species*) attach to the growing plaque mass. Each new microorganism provides a surface to other new microorganisms for adhesion. Plaque mass now starts to grow fast due to rapid cell divisions of microorganisms and new cell adhesions to the biofilm.
- As plaque mass is a relatively thinner in the initial few hours after start of plaque formation, oxygen is abundantly available to microorganisms. Therefore, the initial colonizers of plaque biofilm are aerobic and G +ve microorganisms. Later rods and filaments and other G –ve microorganisms join them.
- As thickness of plaque mass gradually increases with time, oxygen availability reduces in deeper layers of plaque and anaerobic conditions develop. As a result, aerobic species are eliminated and are replaced by anaerobic species in the deeper layers of plaque mass.
- A few hours after plaque started to develop, its constituent microbial cells start to communicate amongst themselves. This marks the beginning of establishment of the biofilm.

◂ *What type of microorganisms are found in initial and matured plaque?*

◂ *Deeper layers of a thick plaque deposit will contain which type of microorganisms?*

3. Dispersion

- After plaque matures, physical forces of food and saliva dislodge bacteria from its surface into saliva. These microorganisms are then spread to other sites in the oral cavity.
- This allows bacteria to colonize new sites in the oral cavity.

◂ *Why do bacteria disperse from surface of established plaque?*

CLINICAL UTILITY AND SHORT ANSWER

Time zones in formation of dental plaque (*oral biofilm*)

- Acquired pellicle starts to form on oral surfaces (*teeth, restoration, prostheses, etc.*) within ***minutes*** of thorough removal.
- Plaque grows steadily during the first 24 hours of initiation of plaque formation and if left undisturbed, grows rapidly during the next 2–3 days.
- Undisturbed plaque reaches its maximum physical bulk by the ***4th day***.
- Further increase in bulk of the dental plaque oral/biofilm is restricted by natural cleaning mechanisms of oral cavity and shearing forces of food (*during mastication*).
- As plaque matures, its quality changes. Early G +ve aerobic/facultative anaerobic bacteria are replaced by G –ve anaerobic bacteria.
- Very high morphological diversity is seen in dental plaque (oral biofilm) from 7 to 14 days. Many cocci and rods and filament shaped bacteria are seen. Later, filamentous organisms dominate over other types.

◂ *How soon does acquired pellicle start to form on freshly cleaned oral surfaces?*

◂ *After how many days plaque reaches its maximum bulk after start of plaque formation?*

ALERT!

Microbial complexes in subgingival plaque (*Socransky 1998*)

Collection pf bacterial species in dental plaque is not by chance but happens in a coordinated way. Socransky *et al* in 1998 identified and labelled groups of subgingival bacterial species closely associated with health and disease with colours: red, orange, green, yellow and purple (Fig. 6.7). These groups facilitate aggregation of compatible species in plaque.

- The purple and yellow group bacteria are early colonizers, followed by green complex.
- The red complex bacteria are capable of producing periodontal tissue destruction (*periodontitis*) and are also called ***marker*** bacteria for periodontitis. They are associated with deep pockets and bleeding on probing.
- After treatment, red complex bacteria are reduced in plaque samples.
- Red complex species are generally found in association with orange complex bacteria.

◂ *What are marker bacteria?*

◂ *Bacteria of which group are associated with deep pockets and bleeding on probing?*

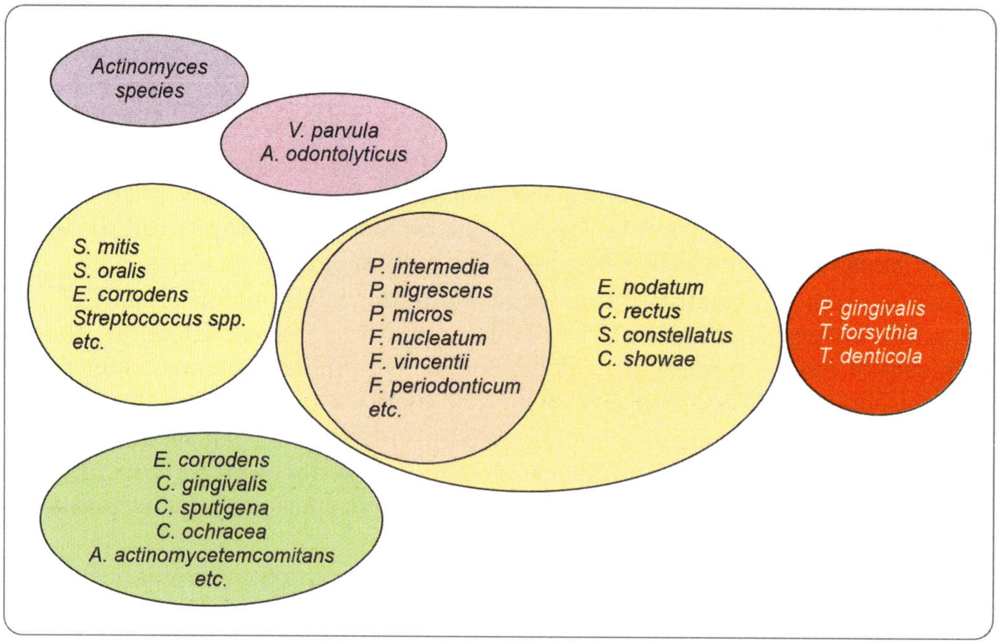

Fig. 6.7: Microbial complexes in subgingival plaque (*Socransky 1998*)

CLINICAL UTILITY AND SHORT ANSWER

Which areas of the mouth are more prone to plaque formation and maturation?

Plaque formation can start on any surface of the oral cavity but plaque bulk will increase and mature ***only*** in areas where plaque remains undisturbed (*by forces of saliva, tongue, cheeks and food being masticated*). After initiation of plaque formation, plaque extend sideways and coronally. It seen more in:

- Fissures, cracks, deformities, enamel imperfections, etc. on tooth surfaces.
- Tooth surface area just coronal to the gingival margin.
- Rough surfaces of restorations and prostheses.
- Beneath overhanging restorations (Fig. 6.8).
- On surface of calculus.
- Interdental areas.

ALERT!

Calculus always has a layer of uncalcified plaque over its surface.

Where is plaque present in relation to calculus?

- Calculus forms after calcification of plaque.
- Calculus has a rough surface that enables formation and retention of plaque over it (Fig. 6.1).
- If plaque covering the surface of calculus is not removed, it will calcify and add another layer to bulk of the calculus.
- Calculus and the layer of plaque over it cause gingivitis and periodontitis.

ALERT!

Dental restorations, appliances and prostheses increase plaque formation and retention

All dental restorations, appliances and prostheses increase plaque accumulation. This is true even if these are well made and polished well. If restoration margins are defective, rough or are placed sub-gingivally, more plaque formation is seen (Fig. 6.8).

Factors on Which Rate of Formation and Amount of Plaque Depends

Rate of plaque formation varies from person to person and at different sites in the same oral cavity. It is dependent on:

Which factors increase plaque?

1. Oral hygiene measures, i.e. physical and chemical plaque control measures used by an individual. If these measures are inadequate, more plaque will form (Figs 6.6, 6.9 and 6.13).

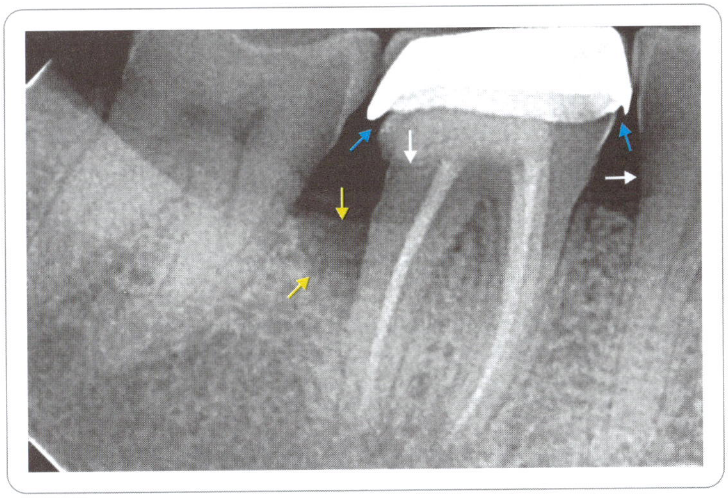

Fig. 6.8: Defective restorations, e.g. overhanging restorations of crowns are ideal places for plaque collection and maturation. Note that plaque under overhanging crown margins (*blue arrows*) has led to bone loss (*yellow arrows*) and caries (*white arrows*).

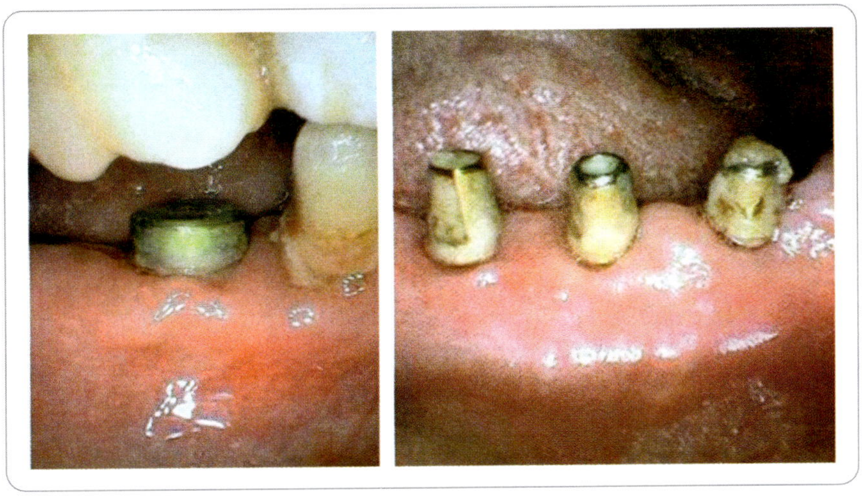

Fig. 6.9: Plaque forms even on well-polished oral surfaces like implant components. More plaque will form if oral hygiene measures are not followed properly.

2. Ease of assess of oral hygiene measures to a particular site. More the access lesser the plaque accumulation **(Fig. 6.10)**. Prominent surfaces of teeth are more likely to be cleaned better than non-prominent surfaces **(Fig. 6.11)**.
3. Over-crowding of teeth. More the crowding, more will be the accumulation of plaque. More plaque is seen in furcation areas of multirooted teeth.
4. Degree of roughness of oral surfaces. Rough surface of teeth, caries, unpolished restorations and prostheses, incomplete removal of calculus from tooth surface during scaling, skipping polishing of teeth after scaling, etc. show more plaque formation. More the crowding and roughness, more will be the accumulation of plaque.
5. Type of diet. Rough and coarse food cleans oral surfaces; such surfaces are relatively plaque free.
6. Unilateral mastication (*eating on one side only*). More plaque formation is seen on the lesser used or unused side. Patients do not eat on a particular side if there is pain or there are missing teeth on that side **(Fig. 6.13)**.
7. Rate of formation of plaque is more if there is preexisting gingivitis and periodontitis **(Fig. 6.12)**.
8. Sick patients who are on a soft diet and are not tooth brushing their teeth also show more plaque deposits.

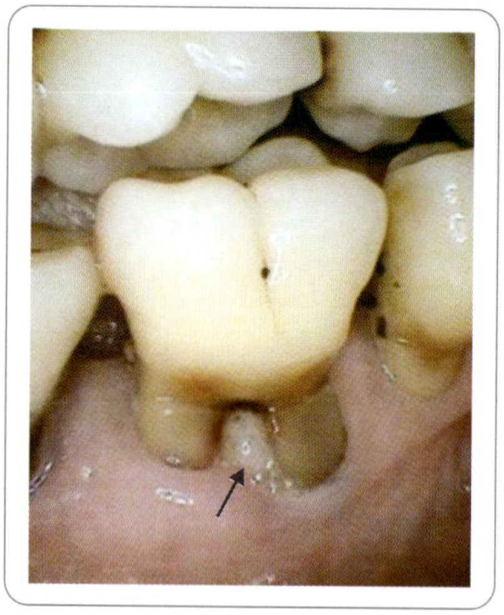

Fig. 6.10: Increased plaque is seen on relatively inaccessible areas of teeth. In this picture plaque is seen in inaccessible furcation area of a mandibular molar whereas other surfaces of teeth are relatively clean.

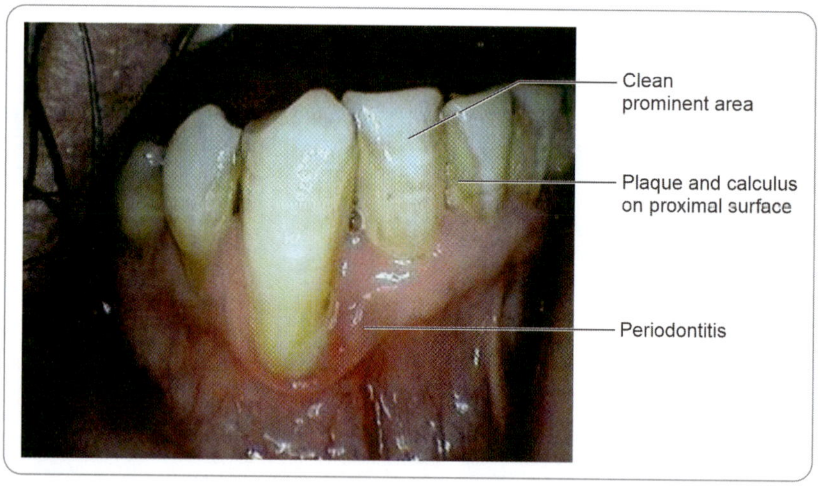

Fig. 6.11: Prominent areas of teeth are cleaned better by natural and instituted mechanisms and vice-versa. In this picture, note that prominent areas of teeth are cleaner while less prominent, receded and less accessible areas, e.g. proximal surfaces of teeth have more plaque, stains and calculus.

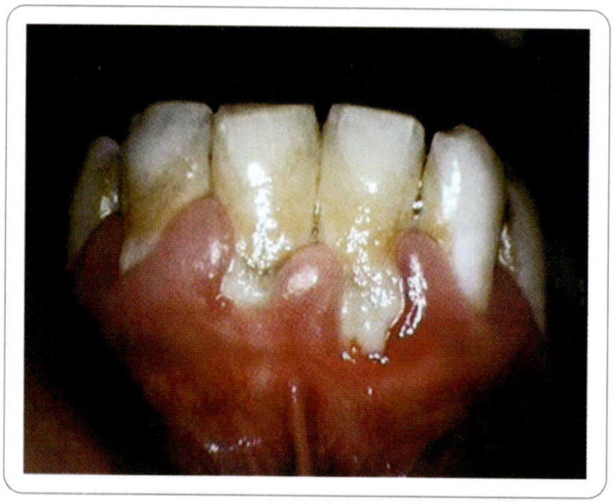

Fig. 6.12: More plaque is seen if there is preexisting gingivitis and periodontitis. This is so because, in such cases, rate of formation of plaque increases (*due to increased nutrition from GCF*), plaque now has more physical protection (*from enlarged gingiva*) and patient with ongoing gingivitis or periodontitis starts to restrict oral hygiene measures due to fear of gingival bleeding after tooth brushing, flossing, etc.

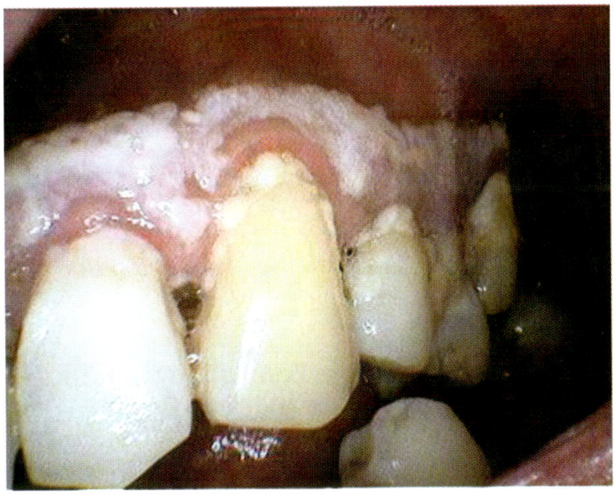

Fig. 6.13: Plaque deposits on gingiva in a 65-year-old male patient who does not brush his teeth due to untreated trigeminal neuralgia (*brushing triggers unbearable severe flashes of pain in this patient*).

Role of Saliva in Formation of Plaque

Saliva plays a role in both formation and reduction of plaque. On the whole, saliva's role in plaque formation and maturation is more of protective nature. Plaque forms in greater quantity and higher speed in patients with relatively less saliva (*xerostomia*) (**Fig. 6.14**).

Saliva *helps* in formation of plaque by:

◂ *How does saliva increase plaque formation?*

◂ *How does saliva help plaque formation at other sites?*

1. Causing formation of acquired pellicle, which is the first step in formation of plaque.
2. Acting like as a reservoir of microorganisms. Solitary (*planktonic microbes*) are suspended in saliva which scatters them to other oral sites and thus helps plaque formation at new sites.
3. Salivary constituents act as food and nutrients for plaque bacteria.
4. Bacteria clump together using salivary proteins, this helps bacteria survive their dispersion to other sites.
5. Serving as a circulatory medium. Saliva flows in and out of plaque mass via channels within plaque. This crude circulatory system of plaque helps in plaque growth by enabling nutritional and metabolic exchanges, intra and inter-species communication, etc.

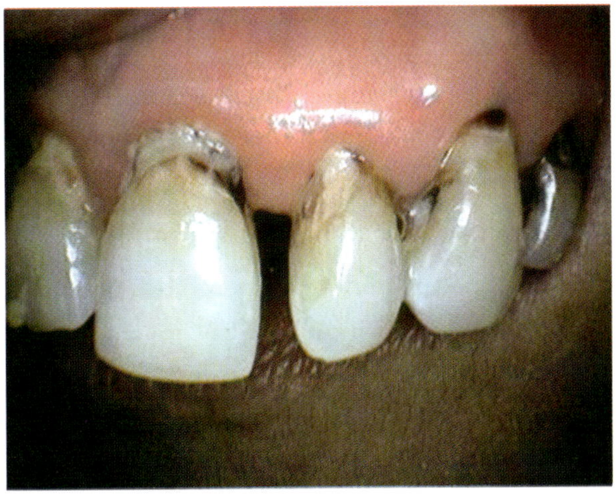

Fig. 6.14: Increased caries and periodontitis (*plaque induced diseases*), in a patient with dry mouth (*xerostomia—less saliva*)

How does saliva reduce plaque formation? ▸

Saliva *reduces* formation of plaque in the following ways:

1. Physically removing bacteria from the mouth. Saliva when swallowed or spitted out reduces bacterial numbers in the mouth.
2. Antibacterial factors found in saliva kill oral bacteria (*e.g. lysozyme, salivary peroxidase, IgA, etc.*).
3. Salivary proteins that cause bacteria to clump together and survive also make swallowing of bacteria easier thereby reducing bacteria numbers in the mouth.
4. Flushing out food debris (*that acts like a source of nutrition for plaque bacteria*) from the mouth. This reduces plaque growth rate.

Role of GCF (*Gingival Crevicular Fluid*) in Formation of Dental Plaque (*Oral Biofilm*)

What is the role of GCF in plaque formation? ▸

GCF is an inflammatory fluid (*exudate*). It is present in gingival sulcus and pockets. It has a ***similar*** role as saliva in formation of plaque (*see chapter 2 'Gingiva'*).

CLINICAL UTILITY AND SHORT ANSWER

Is rate of plaque formation proportional to salivary flow? ▸

Does rate of growth of plaque increase or decrease at night (*during sleep*)?

Saliva serves as an important nutritive medium for plaque growth. On the other hand, as discussed above, it also reduces rate of plaque growth. Quirynen and Steenberghe (*1989*) have shown that plaque formation ***reduces*** with reduction in salivary flow and that at night plaque growth rate decreases by up to 50%.

CLINICAL UTILITY AND SHORT ANSWER

Is rate of plaque formation proportional to consumption of dietary sugar? ▸

What is the role of *sugar* (*sucrose*) in formation of plaque?

Sugar ***increases*** rate of growth and maturation of plaque. Therefore, patients who eat sugar many times a day have more plaque formation.

NON-SPECIFIC, SPECIFIC AND ECOLOGICAL PLAQUE HYPOTHESES

How does plaque cause periodontitis? ▸

These are theories that explain role of plaque bacteria in causing gingivitis and periodontitis. As our knowledge of plaque changed with time, different hypotheses were proposed. Management of plaque induced gingivitis and periodontitis and other periodontal diseases have accordingly changed over time.

Nonspecific Plaque Hypothesis

This hypothesis was put forth many decades ago when we had very little knowledge of plaque. This hypothesis proposes:

- Plaque is a homogenous mass.
- All microorganisms in plaque have similar disease-causing potential.
- As plaque mass increases, severity of gingivitis and periodontitis also increase proportionally.

Specific Plaque Hypothesis

The specific plaque hypothesis became popular after middle of the last century, especially after 1960s when our knowledge of plaque microbiology increased. The specific plaque hypothesis suggests:

- Bacterial species in plaque change as plaque matures.

Why quality of plaque is more important than quantity of plaque? ▸

- Particular bacterial species are found in high numbers at diseased sites; such bacteria may be absent or present in low numbers at healthy sites. This means that only these particular bacterial species cause gingivitis and periodontitis.
- Therefore, it was proposed that quantity of plaque is not as important as quality of plaque (*composition*).

Ecological Plaque Hypothesis (*Marsh 1994*)

The ecological plaque hypothesis merges key elements of specific plaque and non-specific plaque hypotheses. According to this hypothesis:

- An ***everchanging*** (*dynamic*) relationship exists between environment, composition of plaque and periodontal health or disease of a host.
- Plaque-mediated oral diseases are a consequence of relative increase in numbers of disease-causing microorganisms in plaque.
- Disease causing potential of plaque increases due to physical and chemical changes in habitat of plaque. Such changes favour overgrowth of disease producing bacteria (*periodontopathogens*).

Non-specific plaque hypothesis	• All bacteria are disease causing • More plaque = more gingivitis and periodontitis
Specific plaque hypothesis	• Only some plaque bacteria cause gingivitis and periodontitis • Quality of plaque [bacteria species in plaque] is more important than quantity [number of bacteria in plaque]
Ecological plaque hypothesis	• Dynamic relationship between environment, plaque composition and periodontal health • Gingivitis and periodontitis occur due to relative increase in disease causing bacteria • Increase in disease causing bacteria occurs due to physical and chemical changes in environment of plaque

Fig. 6.15: Non-specific, specific and ecological plaque hypotheses

ALERT!

Prevention of gingivitis and periodontitis by regular plaque control and SRP is based on nonspecific plaque hypothesis.

Though we have moved away from the nonspecific plaque hypothesis, the prevention and treatment of gingivitis and periodontitis by regular plaque control (*tooth brushing, etc.*) and scaling and root planing (*SRP*) is based on it. This is helpful because:

- Plaque control measures cause reduction of both disease-causing and non-disease-causing bacteria (*normal commensals*) from the mouth.
- Reduction of overall bacterial load of the mouth is helpful in preventing initiation and worsening of gingivitis, periodontitis and caries.

Treatment of periodontitis by local or systemic antibiotics is based on specific plaque hypothesis

It is now known that periodontitis is caused largely by anaerobic bacteria therefore, antibiotics against these bacteria are helpful in controlling periodontitis, e.g. metronidazole, an antibiotic against anaerobic bacteria, is used in treatment of periodontitis in some cases.

CLINICAL UTILITY AND SHORT ANSWER

Why severe periodontitis occurs only in some individuals?

Clinicians frequently find that despite presence of ***similar*** amount of plaque, severe periodontitis will only occur in some individuals. This is so because mere presence of microorganisms in the mouth ***alone cannot*** cause severe periodontitis (Figs 6.16 and 6.17). To produce severe periodontitis, the following conditions have to be fulfilled:

◂ Can oral microorganisms cause severe periodontitis on their own?

1. An individual must also have some defect in his/her immune system, i.e. must be susceptible to disease (***a susceptible host***).
2. Environment of the mouth must also be suitable for disease causing microorganisms to survive and produce disease.

Hence:

1. Adequate plaque control is essential to prevent and treat periodontitis in immunocompromised individuals just as it is in healthy individuals.

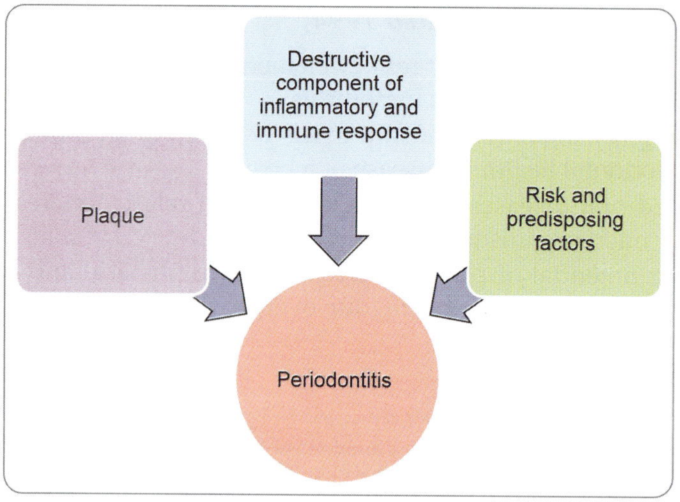

Fig. 6.16: Periodontitis and gingivitis are produced by combined actions of risk and predisposing factors, plaque and destructive component of host inflammatory and immune response

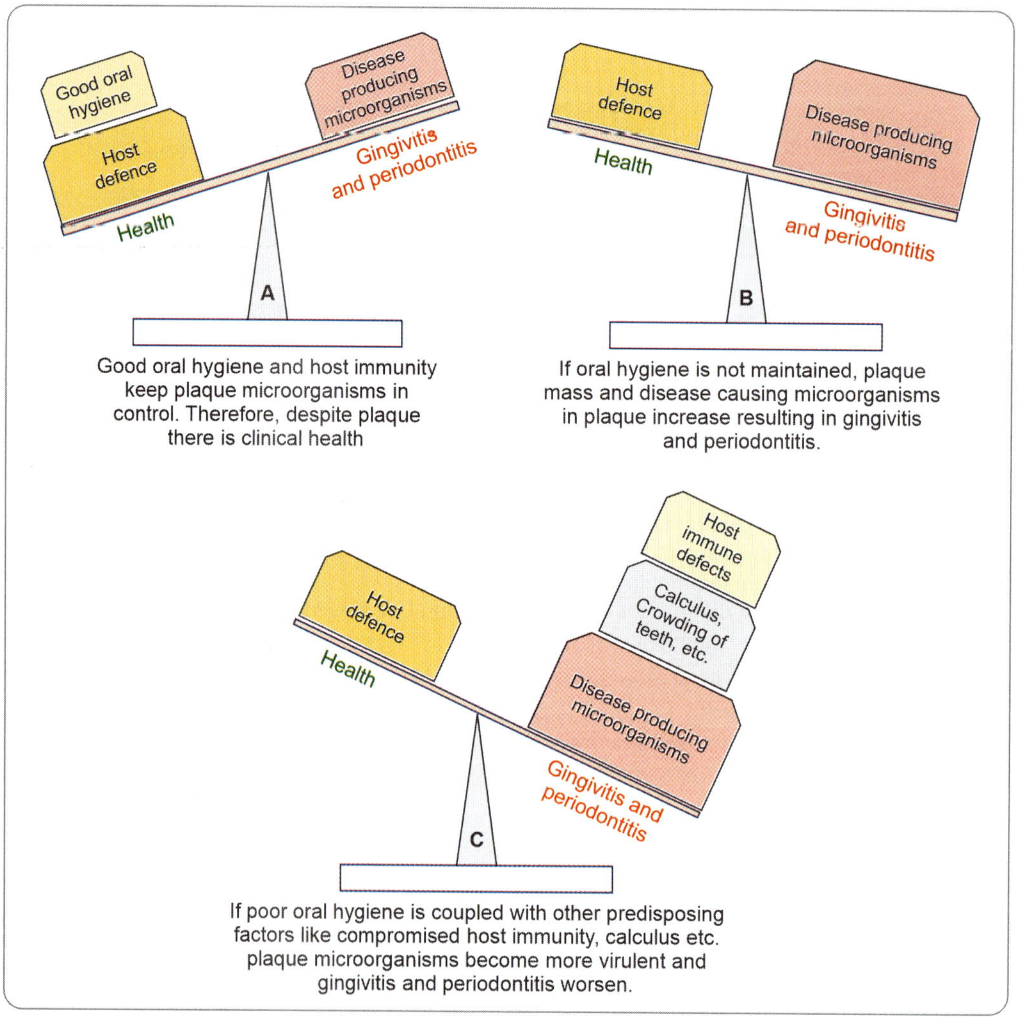

Fig. 6.17: Role of balance between host defenses, disease causing microorganisms and oral hygiene in periodontal health and disease. Diag. A: When host defense, i.e. immunity is good and patient is maintaining good oral hygiene, disease causing microorganisms in plaque cannot produce disease and clinical health is seen. Diag. B: When patient does not maintain good oral hygiene, plaque deposits increase and plaque matures and disease causing microorganisms in plaque increase in proportion. This results in gingivitis and periodontitis. Diag. C: When a patient has immune deficiencies, predisposing factors that increase plaque retention and factors that increase plaque formation, severe gingivitis and periodontitis will result.

ALERT!

Bacteria cause gingivitis and periodontitis only after they combine resources and come together to form pathogenic complexes.

Bacteria cause gingivitis and periodontitis when they collect in large numbers and work ***in*** close collaboration. They are known to collectively produce factors and conditions that allow establishment of 'red-complex' bacteria (*P. gingivalis, T. forsythensis* and *T. denticola*) in plaque biofilm (Fig. 6.7).

To prevent bacteria from collecting in large numbers and causing disease, plaque bacteria must be physically removed by tooth brusing, etc. When plaque is removed and its growth is disturbed by tooth brushing, etc. we actually ***stop*** plaque from maturing, i.e. plaque bacteria from organizing themselves into dangerous periodontitis producing complexes amongst themselves.

◂ *Do microorganisms cooperate with each other to produce periodontitis?*

A. actinomycetemcomitans causes severe periodontitis

Establishes itself and survives killing by:
- Resistance to killing by complement factors
- Inhibits PMN chemotaxis,
- Evades killing by PMNs and monocytes,
- Stops multiplication of immune cells,
- Produces proteases that destroy IgG, etc.
- Producing cytolethal toxin

Causes periodontal destruction by:
- Adhering firmly to epithelial and tooth surfaces due to micro-vesicles and fimbria.
- Stops multiplication of fibroblasts.
- Inhibits healing of connective tissue by fibroblasts
- Causes bone resorption
- Induces release of cytokines that cause tissue destruction.
- Resistant to antibiotics

P. Gingivalis collaborates with other bacteria to cause severe periodontitis

Establishes itself and survives killing by:
- Destabilizing complement pathway
- Modifying immune response by impairing signaling and destroying antibodies.
- Destroys cytokines that recruit PMNs to infection site thus allows uncontrolled colonization of healthy periodontal sites by bacteria.

Coordinates resources and multiplies virulence of other microbes to cause periodontal destruction
- Fimbriae aid in its adhesion with bacterial and host cells and surfaces improving invasion and colonization.
- Coordinates integrity of plaque biofilm
- Increases the virulence of other bacteria in plaque
- Causes direct destruction of periodontal tissues and slows tissue healing and contributes to inflammation.
- Provides nutrients to bacteria by degrading hcst tissue.

Fig. 6.18: Defensive and virulence factors of two of the most implicated marker bacteria in periodontitis: *P. gingivalis* and *A. actinomycetemcomitans*

ALL BACTERIA FOUND IN PLAQUE/ORAL BIOFILM DO NOT CAUSE GINGIVITIS AND PERIODONTITIS

We at present, have little knowledge of only about 10% of the more than 500 species of microorganisms found in plaque. This means, contrary to our present-day knowledge, bacteria presently believed to be causing gingivitis and periodontitis may actually be secondary inhabitants at the disease site and may have no or little role in causing gingivitis or periodontitis. In this context is important to remember:

Are all bacteria in plaque capable of producing gingivitis and periodontitis? ▶

- Most bacterial species in the oral cavity are believed to be normal commensals. These microorganisms normally do not cause disease but if conditions of the oral cavity or host change, these can cause opportunistic infections.
- It may be possible that these bacteria cause gingivitis and periodontitis only when working in combination with some presently unknown microorganisms.

MICROBIOLOGY OF PERIODONTALLY HEALTHY AND DISEASED SITES WITH GINGIVITIS AND PERIODONTITIS

Different microorganisms are present in healthy and diseased sites (Fig. 6.19).

What are the basic types of bacteria found at sites with periodontitis? ▶

- Diseased sites contain more than ***double*** the number of bacteria as compared to healthy sites.
- 70–75% of bacteria at healthy sites are G +ve facultative cocci and rods; whereas only 10–15% of bacteria at severely diseased sites are of G +ve facultative cocci and rods.
- The opposite is true for anaerobic bacteria which increase from 13% at healthy sites to about 70–75 % in severely diseased sites.

Name some bacteria present in healthy and diseased periodontal sites. ▶

1. **Healthy** periodontal sites have:
   a. Primarily G +ve facultative species, e.g. *S. sanguis, A. viscosus, A. naeslundii*, etc.
   b. A smaller number of G –ve species are also found, e.g. *Capnocytophaga, F. nucleatum, P. intermedia*, etc.
   c. A few spirochetes and motile rods are present.
2. **Gingivitis** sites (*plaque induced*) have:
   a. G +ve species, e.g. *S. sanguis, A. viscosus, A. naeslundii, P. micros*, etc.
   b. G –ve species, e.g. *Capnocytophaga, F. nucleatum, P. intermedia, V. parvula, Campylobaeter*, etc.
3. **Periodontitis** sites (*all stages and grades*) have:
   a. *Up to 90%* anaerobic and G –ve bacteria, e.g. *P. gingivalis, A. actinomycetemcomitans, P intermedia, P micros, C. rectus, E. corrodens, F. nucleatum, Treponema* species, etc.
   b. ***Viruses***, e.g. ***EBV-1*** (*especially in grade C periodontitis*).

CLINICAL UTILITY AND SHORT ANSWER

Plaque is present in all individuals at all times, why then do we not see gingivitis and periodontitis in all individuals all the time?

As plaque is always present, gingivitis and periodontitis are always a constant possibility. Clinical condition of gingiva at a particular time is the result of balance between host defense on one side and plaque + predisposing factors on the other (Fig. 6.17).

Factors that increase plaque deposition and retention, favour gingivitis and periodontitis. If such factors increase, gingivitis and periodontitis results. On the other hand, factors that increase host's defense capability and decrease plaque favor establishment of clinical gingival health.

Simply put:

1. Normal host defenses can manage normal microbial challenge from plaque bacteria if good oral hygiene is maintained. This results in clinical gingival health (*no BOP or features of gingival inflammation and PD less than 3 mm; 2018 classification*) (Fig. 6.17 diag. A).
2. Reduced or defective host defenses (*immune compromised state, e.g. uncontrolled diabetes, etc.*) cannot control normal microbial challenge from plaque bacteria. This is especially true if good oral hygiene is not maintained. This leads to moderate periodontal disease (*mild to moderate gingivitis or grade A or B periodontitis; 2018 classification*) (Fig. 6.17 diag. B).
3. Reduced or defective host defenses (*immune compromised state, e.g. uncontrolled diabetes, etc.*) + ***increased*** microbial challenge, totally overwhelms host defenses. Severe and fast progressing periodontal disease results in such cases (*moderate to severe gingivitis or grade B or C periodontitis; 2018 classification*) (Fig. 6.17 diag. C).

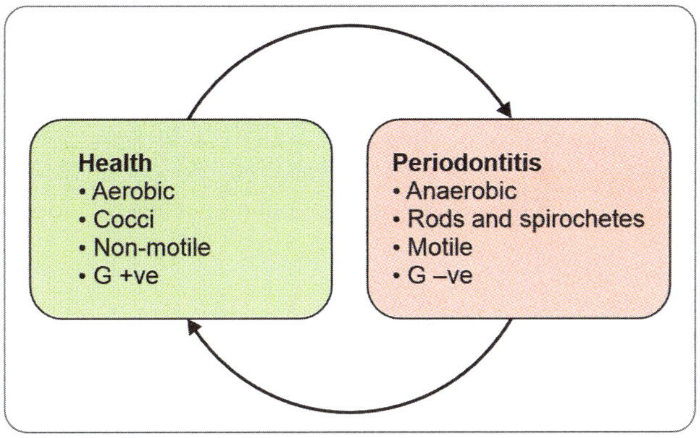

Fig. 6.19: Basic differences between plaque in health and periodontitis

ALERT!

- As natural vulnerability of an individual to periodontitis (*host's immunity*) ***cannot*** be changed, periodontal treatment is primarily focused on ***reduction*** in depth of the pocket and decreasing periodontal disease-causing microorganisms (*periodontopathogens*) within the pocket.
- According to the 2018 classification's criteria of health for a treated case of periodontitis, probing pocket depth (*PD*) must be maintained at less than 4 mm for it remain healthy (*also see Chapter 10A, 'Making clinical diagnosis of gingivitis and periodontitis using the 2018 classification' and Figs 10A.6 and 10A.7*).
- A PD of less than 4 mm reduces anaerobic conditions in the sulcus and facilitates establishment of aerobic microorganisms that are helpful in maintenance of periodontal health in that sulcus.

MICROBIOLOGICAL METHODS USED TO IDENTIFY BACTERIA

◂ *Name some tests used for identification of plaque bacteria.*

Several techniques can be used to identify bacteria in plaque. These include microscopy, bacterial culture, ELISA (*enzyme-linked immunosorbent assay—species specific*), PCR (*polymerase chain reaction*), Checkerboard DNA–DNA hybridisation (*this allows quantitative analysis of microbial species*), 16S rDNA amplification cloning (*this allows bacterial identification to species level*), etc.

◂ *Can tests used for identification of plaque bacteria be commonly used for periodontal case management?*

The above techniques are time consuming, expensive, are not 100% efficient and can identify only a limited number of microorganisms for which specific probes (*tests*) have been developed. In other words, these tests are not a fool-proof way to identify disease producing microorganisms in particular patient with a particular disease.

CLINICAL UTILITY AND SHORT ANSWER

◂ *Can periodontitis be diagnosed on the basis of tests alone?*

Why we cannot make a diagnosis of periodontal health or periodontitis based only on microbial analysis of plaque composition.

This is so because:

1. Our knowledge of plaque microorganisms is very limited. We only know 'something' about very small percentage of plaque bacteria; the rest are unknown. These unknown microorganisms (*bacteria*) maybe playing a crucial role in pathogenesis of periodontitis.
2. Microbial species found in diseased sites are also found in plaque samples collected from healthy periodontal sites and vice versa.

The presence or absence of particular microbes therefore cannot be used to differentiate between different forms of infectious periodontal diseases.

ALERT!

Some bacteria in plaque are protective in nature and prevent gingivitis and periodontitis!

Examples of such bacteria include: *S. sanguis*, *C. ochraceus*, *Veillonella parvula*, etc. Such protective species of bacteria are found in high numbers and proportions at healthy sites and in low numbers and proportions at diseased sites. These protective species of bacteria control gingivitis and periodontitis by:

1. Physically occupying available space within the sulcus that would otherwise be taken up by disease causing bacteria (*periodontopathogens*).

2. Not allowing the periodontopathogens to stick onto gingival and oral surfaces by pre-occupying available sites or by making sticking mechanisms of periodontopathogens ineffective by direct interference with them.
3. Killing periodontopathogens, e.g. *S. sanguis* produces hydrogen peroxide (H_2O_2) that kills *A. actinomycetemcomitans (a dangerous bacteria that causes periodontitis)*, etc.
4. Interfering with production of virulence factors of periodontopathogens and their degradation.

Review Questions

1. What is dental plaque (*oral biofilm*)? How can it be visualized?
2. What are the stages in formation of dental plaque (*oral biofilm*)?
3. What are the types and physical characteristics of dental plaque (*oral biofilm*)?
4. What is the difference between supragingival and subgingival dental plaque (*oral biofilm*)?
5. Why are initial colonizing bacteria of plaque biofilm aerobes and facultative anaerobes while mature plaque biofilm is primarily anaerobic?
6. In what areas/sites of the oral cavity is plaque more likely to form and mature?
7. What is the role of saliva in the formation of dental plaque (*oral biofilm*)?
8. Do all bacteria found in dental plaque (*oral biofilm*) cause periodontal disease? Name some periodontopathogens.
9. What are the implications of the fact that our knowledge of periodontopathogenecity of plaque microorganisms is limited?
10. Describe the concept of microbial specificity. Compare specific, non-specific plaque hypothesis and ecological plaque hypothesis.
11. Write a note on factors that increase susceptibility of the host to periodontitis.
12. Name specific bacteria associated with major periodontal infections.

Chapter

7

Dental Calculus and Other Factors Contributing to Periodontal Disease

Plaque calcifies to form calculus. Because of its rough surface, calculus provides an ideal surface for plaque accumulation. While plaque can be easily removed by tooth brushing, etc. calculus cannot be removed this way; it can only be removed by scaling.

Several other etiologic factors, e.g. impacted food, iatrogenic factors, injuries inflicted during dental treatment, etc. also play important roles in periodontal health and disease. Acting in combination with dental plaque, they contribute and predispose to gingivitis and periodontitis.

DENTAL CALCULUS

Definition: Calculus is mineralized dental plaque. Plaque starts to mineralize into calculus between the ***1st*** and ***14th*** day of plaque formation.

◂ *What is calculus? When does plaque start to mineralize to form calculus?*

Calculus can therefore form on all surfaces on which plaque accumulates, e.g. surfaces of natural teeth, restorations and dental prostheses.

◂ *Can calculus form on surface of a prosthesis?*

Classification

Depending on its ***location*** in relation to ***margin of free gingiva***, calculus is classified as:

◂ *Name the types of calculus.*

1. Supragingival calculus
2. Subgingival calculus.

Supragingival Calculus

Portion of calculus that is ***coronal*** to the gingival margin is called supragingival calculus (Fig. 7.1). Important characteristics of supragingival calculus are:

◂ *What is supragingival calculus?*

1. It is visible in the oral cavity (*subgingival calculus is hidden under the gingiva*) and is usually cream or light yellow in color. If stained with tea or coffee, tobacco or pigments from pigment producing bacteria, etc. it may be dark coloured.

◂ *What is the colour of supragingival calculus?*

2. If calculus has large bulk, it may be seen in radiographs. ***Interdental calculus*** is more ***readily*** identified in radiographs (Fig. 7.2).

◂ *Can calculus be seen in a radiograph?*

3. It has dried clay-like consistency and is softer than sub-gingival calculus.

◂ *How hard is supra-gingival calculus?*

4. It can be easily removed (*by scaling*).
5. With time, as its bulk increases, it may form a 'bridge' like mass over teeth (Fig. 7.3, diag. B).
6. It may even form on occlusal surfaces of teeth if the patient is not eating on the same side for a long time (*unilateral mastication*).

◂ *If calculus is present on occlusal surface of teeth what does it suggest?*

7. Maximum deposition of supragingival calculus is seen on lingual surfaces of mandibular incisors and buccal surfaces of maxillary 1st and 2nd molars (Fig. 7.3).

◂ *Where does maximum calculus deposition occur?*

8. It usually ***re-forms*** rapidly at the same sites after removal. (*that is why scaling is required repeatedly every 3–6 months*).

Subgingival Calculus

What is subgingival calculus?

Portion of calculus located ***apical*** to the gingival margin is called sub-gingival calculus (Fig. 7.4).

1. As it is located under the free gingiva:
   a. It is not visible.
   b. It may be seen after gently pulling the marginal gingiva outwards with a probe.
   c. Its presence can be felt by light exploration of surfaces of teeth with an explorer or periodontal probe (*though an explorer is better suited*).
   d. ***Only 60–70%*** of the entire subgingival calculus can be clinically identified and located. This is done by exploration using hand instruments without elevation of a periodontal flap.

Can the entire supra-gingival calculus be felt with an instrument without raising a flap?

What is the colour of subgingival calculus?

2. It is dark brown or greenish black in colour.
3. Large mass of sub-gingival calculus can sometimes be seen in dental radiographs. Interdental calculus is more readily identified in radiographs (Fig. 7.2).
4. It is harder than supragingival calculus.
5. It more firmly attached and more difficult to remove than supra-gingival calculus.
6. Its re-formation after removal is ***slower*** than that of supragingival calculus.

Which of the two supra-gingival or subgingival calculus re-forms faster after removal?

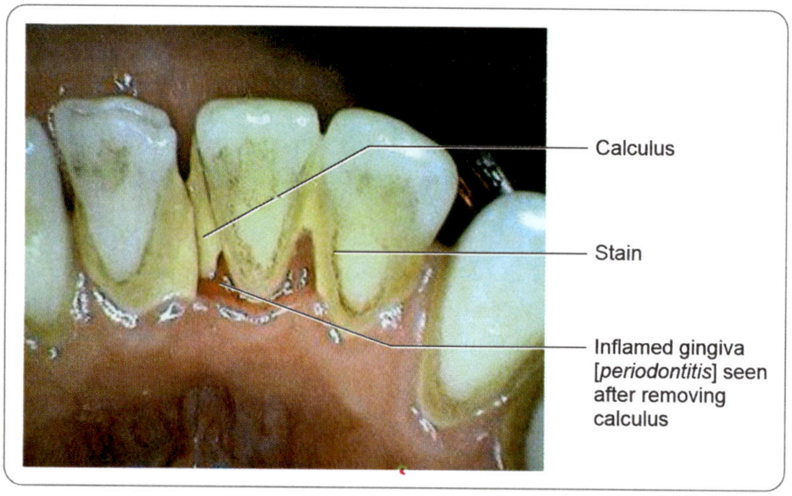

Fig. 7.1: Supra-gingival calculus. It is cream or light-yellow in colour but stained at some places. Note gingiva is red under it (*inflammatory changes—periodontitis*).

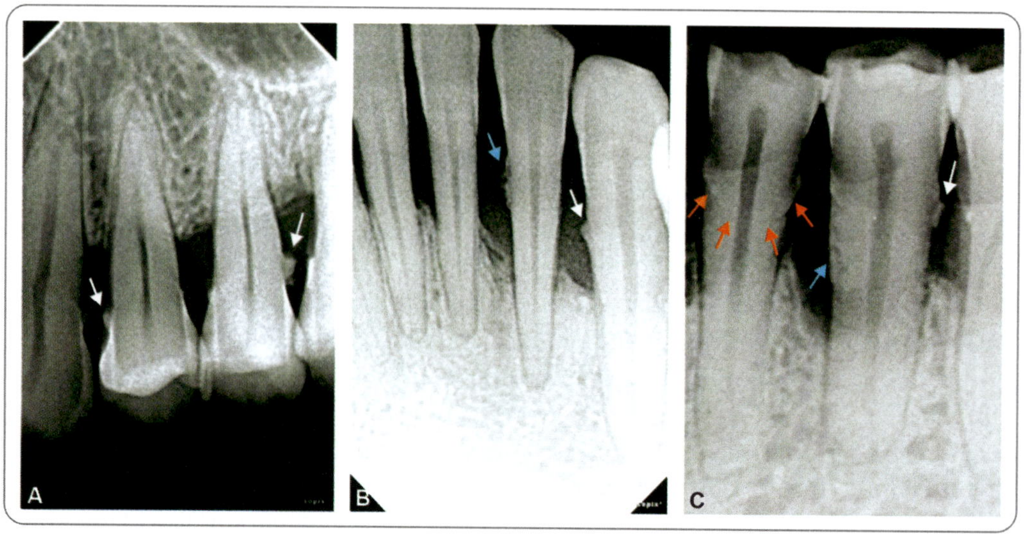

Fig. 7.2: Appearance of calculus in a radiograph. Calculus is seen as radiopaque projections or spurs (*white arrows*), crusts (*blue arrows*) protruding into the interdental space or as ledges extending as a ring around a tooth (*red arrows*).

CLINICAL UTILITY AND SHORT ANSWER

Why does maximum calculus deposition occur on lingual surfaces of mandibular incisors and buccal surfaces of maxillary molars?

This is because of increased salivary flow over these areas.

- ***Stensen's duct*** discharges saliva from parotid gland on facial surfaces of maxillary 1st and 2nd molars (Fig. 7.3, diag. A).
- ***Wharton's*** and ***Bartholin's ducts*** discharge saliva from submandibular and sublingual glands respectively on lingual surfaces of mandibular incisors (Fig. 7.3, diag. B).
- As surfaces of these teeth receive more saliva and remain continuously coated with salivary mucins (*that increase plaque formation during initial stages*) more calculus formation is seen over these surfaces.

◂ *Why does maximum calculus formation occur on lingual surfaces of mandibular incisors and buccal surfaces of maxillary molars?*

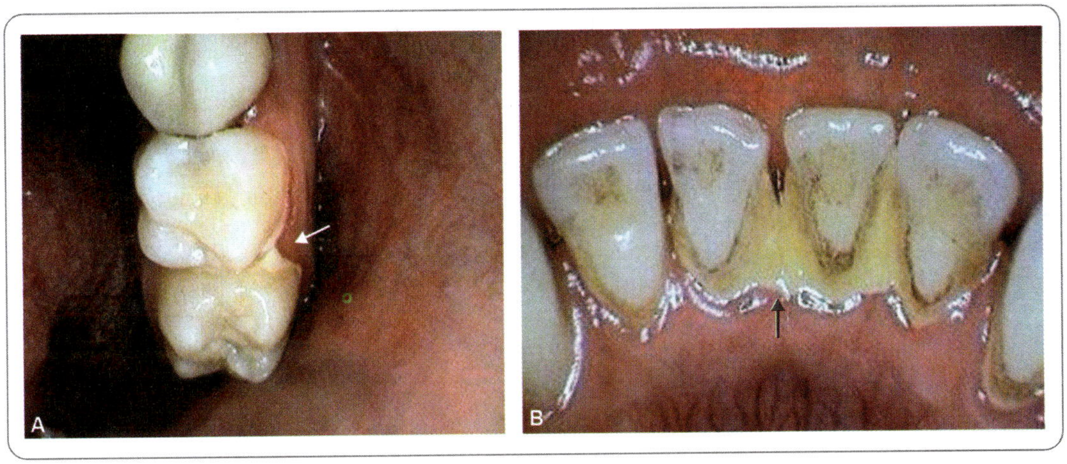

Fig. 7.3: Maximum calculus deposits are seen on buccal surfaces of maxillary 1st and 2nd molars (*opposite opening of duct of parotid salivary gland—Stensen's duct, diag. A*) and lingual surfaces of mandibular incisors (*opposite opening of ducts of submandibular—Wharton's duct and sublingual glands—Bartholin's duct, diag. B*).

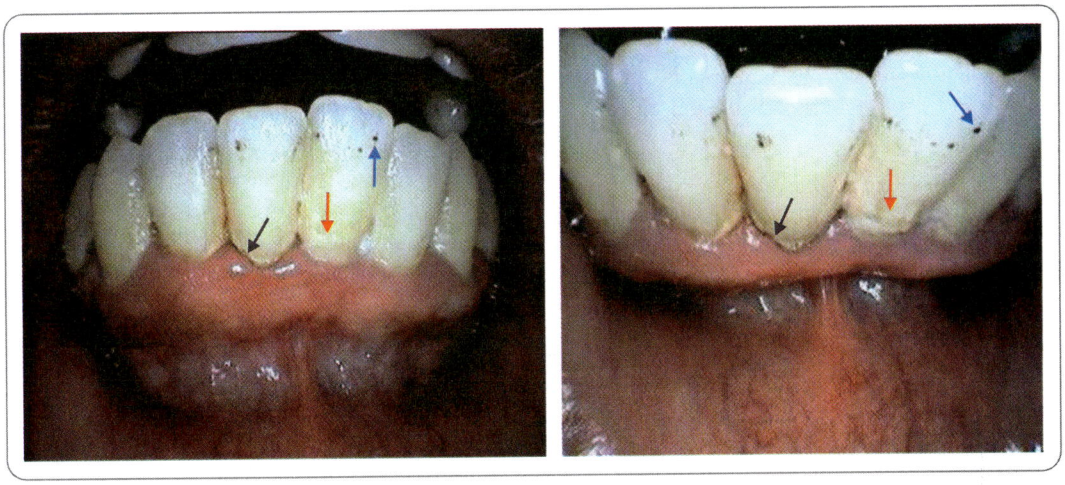

Fig. 7.4: Subgingival calculus located just under the crest of free gingiva may be visible if free gingiva is gaping or if it is pulled outwards (*black arrows*). Supragingival calculus is covered by plaque (*red arrows*). Also note presence of extrinsic stains on teeth (*blue arrows*).

ALERT!

- Supragingival and subgingival calculus usually occur together but one may be present without the other.
- Apical margin of subgingival calculus ends 500 to 800 μ coronal to base of the pocket (*junctional epithelium*).
- Attached and un-attached plaque is present between apical end of calculus and junctional epithelium.
- That calculus deposits lead to gingivitis and periodontitis is proved by the fact that gingival inflammation and probing depth reduce (*gain in clinical attachment*) after removal of calculus.

◂ *How far is margin of supragingival calculus from junctional epithelium?*

Table 7.1: Differences between supragingival and subgingival calculus

	Supragingival calculus	*Subgingival calculus*
Location	Coronal to gingival margin.	In the pocket, apical to gingival margin.
Distribution	On all teeth but more on lingual surfaces of mandibular incisors and buccal surfaces of maxillary 1st and 2nd molars.	Can occur at all sites. More in deeper pockets and hard to reach areas (*inaccessible areas*).
Colour	Cream or light yellow in colour	Dark brown, green or black in colour
Consistency	Soft and clay like. Easier to remove.	Hard and tenacious. Difficult to remove.
Rate of formation	Relatively faster. In some individuals, it re-forms within days after complete removal.	Slower
Morphology	• Can be of variable size and shape. • Morphology is influenced and limited by available dimensions of space between teeth and oral soft tissues.	• Present in smaller masses than supragingival variety. • Usually present as crusts, spines, nodules or ledges that may be extending as a ring around the tooth.
Detection	• Can be seen with naked eye. Extent can be known with explorer. • Calculus present in interdental areas can be seen in radiographs.	• Can be identified using tactile sensation with an explorer or a probe during probing. • Subgingival calculus present near gingival margin can be seen by gently pulling out free gingiva. • Small dark smooth protuberance on the free gingva can at hint the possibility of subgingival calculus present under it. • Subgingival calculus present in interdental areas can be seen in radiographs. • If gingival recession occurs, subgingival calculus can become supragingival and is then easily visible.
Composition	• Inorganic content 70–80%: calcium, phosphate, magnesium, sodium, carbonate and fluoride. • Organic matrix is 15–20% of dry weight.	• More mineral content than supragingival calculus.
Mineral content and source	• Relatively less mineralized. • Minerals derived from saliva.	• Relatively more mineralized. • Minerals derived from GCF.
Crystal type	• Octacalcium phosphate • Hydroxyapatite • Whitlockite • Brushite	• Octacalcium phosphate • Hydroxyapatite • Whitlockite

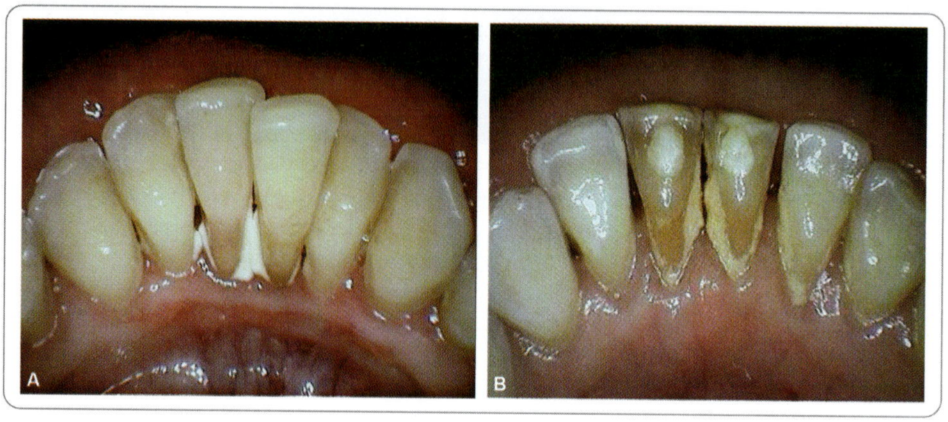

Fig. 7.5: Calculus can re-form very soon after removal. In these pictures of two individuals, calculus has formed to sizeable amount within four (*diag. A*) and six weeks (*diag. B*) after scaling. Note that calculus has a 'fresh' unstained look and surfaces of teeth are still relatively clean and stain free due to scaling done earlier.

ALERT!

- Portions of sub-gingival calculus often becomes visible and exposed to the environment due to recession of gingiva following incomplete periodontal therapy. It can also become visible due to antibiotic induced shrinkage of inflamed gingiva (*temporary*). Such calculus although placed supra-gingivally will still have characteristics of sub-gingival calculus (Fig. 7.6).
- Portions of supra-gingival calculus can also often become sub-gingival because of coronal shift of crest of gingiva due to gingival enlargement. Such calculus although placed sub-gingivally will still retain characteristics of supra-gingival calculus.

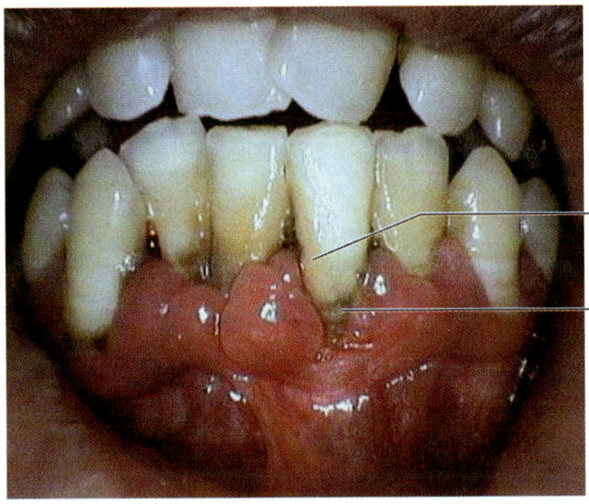

Fig. 7.6: If gingival recession occurs, subgingival calculus can become supragingival and is then easily visible.

How Calculus Attaches to Surfaces of Teeth

Differences in the way in which calculus is attached to the tooth surface affects its tenacity (*grip on underlying surface*) and is responsible for the relative ease or difficulty with which it can be removed during scaling.

◄ How does calculus attach to underlying surfaces?

1. Calculus attaches physically to surfaces of teeth, restorations and oral prostheses. This physical attachment occurs due to close adaptation of calculus over gentle elevations, depressions and micro-surface irregularities on surfaces of teeth (*C-E junction of teeth, perikymata, fissures or hypocalcified areas on surfaces of teeth, rough surfaces of restorations, prostheses, etc.*).
2. The attachment is strengthened by organic pellicle and calcified 'bodies' of plaque bacteria that have penetrated into the underlying surface over which calculus has formed.

Etiologic Significance of Calculus

Calculus causes gingivitis and periodontitis and it does that in the following ways:

◄ How does calculus cause gingivitis and periodontitis?

◄ How does calculus increase gingivitis and periodontitis potential of plaque?

1. Calculus has a rough surface, therefore it provides increased and firm attachment to plaque. This makes plaque removal (*by tooth brushing, etc.*) more difficult.
2. A layer of plaque is thus ***always*** present on surface of calculus. This way calculus maintains a layer of plaque close to sulcular and junctional epithelia of gingiva. This increases gingivitis and periodontitis producing potential of plaque (Fig. 7.7).
3. Calculus also has ***living bacteria*** within it.
4. As bulk of calculus increases, it lowers effectivity of plaque control measures in that area. This compromises oral hygiene and further increases plaque deposition (Fig. 7.8).
5. When subgingival calculus is present, sulcular epithelium gets injured as it rubs over underlying calculus during mastication of food. This causes ulcerations in the sulcular epithelium thus allowing easy access of bacteria into gingiva (*break in continuity of epithelium is called an ulcer*).
6. Calculus has endotoxins (*components of bacterial cell walls that are released after the death and disruption of bacterial cells*). These seep out from the calculus into the surrounding gingival tissues and worsen inflammation in gingivitis and periodontitis (Fig. 7.8, diag. B, black arrows).

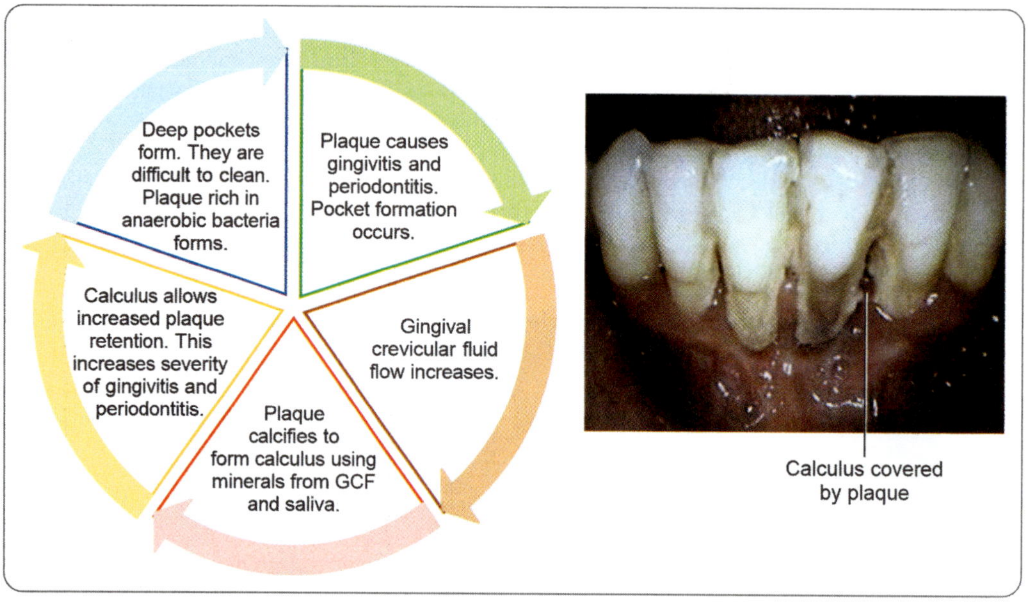

Fig. 7.7: Calculus is an important factor in etiology of gingivitis and periodontitis as it allows increased plaque retention and maintains a layer of plaque close to gingiva.

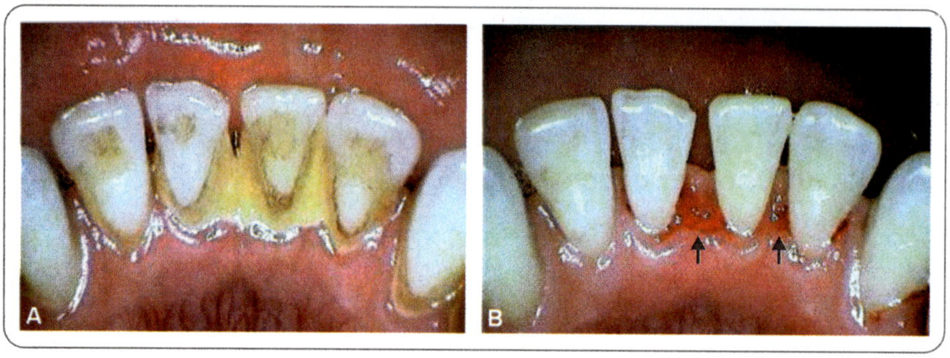

Fig. 7.8: Blocking of interdental spaces by calculus prevents interdental cleaning (*diag. A.*). Note the gingival inflammation seen after removal of calculus by scaling (*diag. B, black arrows*).

CLINICAL UTILITY AND SHORT ANSWER

What is calculocementum?

- Calculus embedded deep into cementum of root of a tooth is called ***calculocementum***.
- It is morphologically ***similar*** to cementum.
- Just like calculus, calculocementum can also lead to gingivitis and periodontitis.
- Calculocementum must therefore be carefully identified and removed (*by root planing*) to produce a smooth and healthy root surface.

Why must calculocementum be removed? ▸

How Calculus Forms

Calculus is formed by mineralization of plaque. However, all plaque does ***not*** calcify to form calculus.

- Plaque contains a small amount of inorganic material that increases as plaque mineralizes into calculus. If calculus formation does not take place, inorganic content of plaque reaches maximum level in approximately two days.
- Mineralization of plaque to form calculus usually starts between ***1st–14th*** day of plaque formation. Mineralization of plaque to form calculus and its rate of formation ***varies*** at different sites, times and from person to person.
- Bulk of the mineralization (*50%*), occurs within the ***1st two days*** of initiation of mineralization.

When does plaque start to convert to calculus? ▸

When does majority of mineralization of plaque occur during calculus formation? ▸

- Mineralization begins in the central areas of plaque, i.e. areas nearest to tooth surface.
  - Intercellular matrix of plaque gets crystallized first.
  - This is followed by crystallization of bacteria.
  - Small foci of mineralization that form initially, increase in size and subsequently unite to form larger chunks of calculus.
- Calculus is formed in layers. After one layer of plaque mineralizes to form calculus, plaque present over it then mineralizes to form another layer of calculus.
- ***Supragingival*** plaque derives minerals for mineralization primarily from ***saliva***, and a small component from gingival crevicular fluid (*for plaque located near the gingival crest*). ***Subgingival*** plaque derives its major component of mineralization from ***gingival crevicular fluid*** and a small component from saliva (*for plaque near the gingival crest*).
- Calcification starts by binding of calcium to the carbohydrate–protein complexes of the organic matrix of plaque. This is followed by precipitation of calcium salts. Some individuals have relatively higher phosphorus content in their un-calcified plaque, this is the reason for repeated heavy calculus deposition in these individuals.
- Calculus may reach its ***maximum*** physical bulk between ***two–six months*** beyond which increase in size does not occur. This is so because, increasing size of calculus makes it vulnerable to fracture due to mechanical forces generated in the oral cavity (*food being masticated, movement of lips, cheek tongue, tooth brushing, etc.*).

◂ *Does all of plaque mineralize to calculus at the same time?*

◂ *Where does the mineral for calcification of plaque come from?*

◂ *How much time does it take for calculus to reach its maximum bulk?*

How Mineralization of Calculus Occurs

1st theory: Increase in local concentration of calcium and phosphate ions causes mineralization of plaque to calculus.

2nd theory: Epitactic concept: Carbohydrate-protein complexes in plaque take up calcium from saliva and form small foci of calcification. These small foci then act like seeding agents for further calcification of plaque to form a larger calcified mass—calculus.

◂ *How does calculus mineralize?*

EXTRINSIC DENTAL STAINS (*PIGMENTED DEPOSITS*)

Extrinsic dental stains are ***not*** implicated in etiology of periodontal disease. However, as they are unaesthetic, their removal is one of the chief objectives of scaling.

- Chromogenic materials (*colour pigment containing materials*), e.g. tobacco products, food pigments, medicinal syrups containing iron, etc. beverages like tea, coffee, etc. anti-plaque mouth-wash, e.g. chlorhexidine, etc. can cause staining of dental pellicle and produce extrinsic dental stains on surfaces of teeth, oral appliances and prostheses (Fig. 7.9).
- Chromogenic microorganisms can also cause external stains.
- Mechanisms of formation of extrinsic stains are different for each causative agent.

◂ *What are extrinsic dental stains?*

Removal of extrinsic stains

- External dental stains are largely an aesthetic problem.
- They can usually be removed by scaling and polishing.

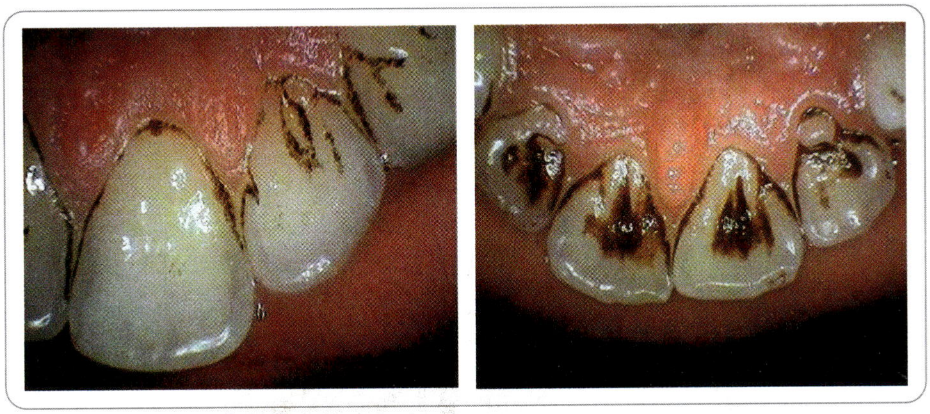

Fig. 7.9: Extrinsic dental stains

What are intrinsic dental stains?

ALERT!

Intrinsic dental stains

- These are formed within the tooth structure and are produced because of developmental anomalies, hematological causes, tetracycline, degradation of hemoglobin after pulp death, etc.
- They cannot be removed by treatments meant for removing extrinsic stains. Bleaching and veneering (*covering with restorative material*) of affected area of teeth are done to treat internal stains.

IATROGENIC FACTORS CONTRIBUTING TO PERIODONTAL DISEASE

What are iatrogenic factors?

How do iatrogenic factors cause periodontal disease and caries?

Disease caused by treatment is called iatrogenic disease. Dental restorations, prostheses, etc. can act as contributing factors for periodontal disease.

- They act by favoring retention of plaque and causing increased occlusal loads on the periodontium.
- If a restoration is over or under contoured or if its margins do not flush with those of the tooth (*e.g. overhanging margins*), food debris and plaque will accumulate at margins of such restorations. This will lead to gingivitis and periodontitis.
- Additionally, as accumulated food starts to decay, it will produce foul taste and bad breath (*halitosis*) and caries in the long-term.

CHARACTERISTICS OF DENTAL RESTORATIONS THAT ACT AS PREDISPOSING FACTORS FOR PERIODONTAL DISEASE AND CARIES

How can restorations and crowns predispose to periodontitis?

Which is the safest location for a restorative margin in relation to gingival crest?

The features of dental restorations and prostheses that can contribute to and cause periodontal disease and caries are:

1. Location of gingival margin of restoration in relation to the crest of gingiva:
   a. Gingival margin of restoration is ***coronal*** to crest of gingiva. As the area of the tooth with the prepared margin of the restoration can be cleaned easily, this placement is the ***safest*** and is least likely to lead to gingivitis, periodontitis or caries **(Fig. 7.10, diag. A)**.
   b. Gingival margin of restoration is at ***same*** level as crest of gingiva. This is considered almost as safe as the first option described above point (a) **(Fig. 7.10, diag. B)**.
   c. Gingival margin of restoration is ***apical*** to crest of gingiva but not ingressing into biologic width (*gingival margin is within gingival sulcus*). In this case, as tooth area with prepared margin of the restoration is not visible and not easily reachable, it cannot be cleaned properly. Therefore, there is a constant risk of periodontitis and caries in this region **(Fig. 7.10, diag. C and 7.12)**.

   Why are restoration margins ingressing into biologic width considered unsafe?

   d. Gingival margin of restoration is ***apical*** to crest of gingiva and ingressing into biologic width. In addition to risk mentioned in point c, this will always cause persistent inflammation in gingiva which will eventually lead to periodontitis **(Fig. 7.10, diag. D and 21.1)**.

Why is presence of space between restoration margin and prepared tooth structure likely to lead to periodontitis and caries?

2. Presence of space between margin of restoration and margin of the prepared tooth surface. Because plaque will form and food debris will get stuck in this space, it will certainly lead to periodontitis and caries **(Fig. 7.11)**.

How does an overhanging restoration contribute to periodontitis and caries?

3. Degree of overhang in relation to class II, III, IV or V restorations. Plaque is always present under the overhanging margin. Also as this area is very difficult to clean, therefore, larger the overhang, more are the chances of periodontitis and caries in the tooth structure immediately under the overhanging restoration margin **(Fig. 7.11)**.

What is the importance of tooth contours for periodontal health?

4. Cracked or broken or underfilled restorations. These will encourage plaque formation.

Why more plaque and food debris accumulate apical to an over contoured restoration?

5. Faulty contours of restoration. During mastication of food, over contoured restorations deflect food far away from surface of gingiva and prevent the gingiva from getting cleaned by passage of food over it. On the other hand, under contoured restorations allow food to hit and injure gingival margin during mastication. If restorations

with faulty contours also have defective embrasures; this will encourage plaque accumulation in the interdental area which will lead to gingivitis and periodontitis.

6. Type of occlusion attained with a restoration:
   a. Hyper-occlusion. This causes acute TFO (*Trauma from occlusion*) in short term, if it is not corrected, chronic TFO results.
   b. Less than normal or no occlusal contact. This decreases masticatory efficiency.
7. Open interdental contacts in relation to class II, III or IV restorations or crowns **(Fig. 7.13)**. Open interdental contacts will lead to interdental vertical food impaction **(Fig. 7.14, diag. A)** that will result in periodontitis and caries.
8. Physical and chemical properties of materials used for the restorations. Restorative materials may chemically irritate oral soft tissues, e.g. acrylic resins.
9. Degree of roughness of the restoration's surface. If restorative material is not polishable it will encourage plaque deposition on its surface, e.g. glass ionomer. This will lead to periodontitis and caries in nearby tooth structure and gingiva.
10. Degree of injury produced in periodontal tissues during placement of the restoration.

◂ *How are under contoured restorations likely to cause periodontal disease?*

◂ *Why must restorations have tight interdental contacts?*

◂ *Why must restoration be smooth and polished?*

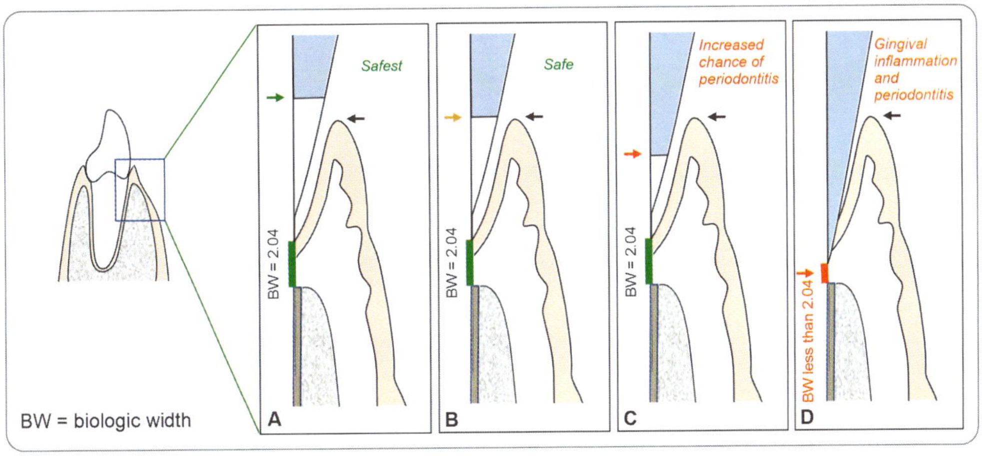

Fig. 7.10: Margins of crowns and restorations (*blue shaded area*) can be placed at three locations in relation to crest of gingiva: coronal to the gingival crest (*green arrow, diag. A*), at level of gingival crest (*orange arrow, diag. B*) and apical to gingival crest (*red arrows, diag. C and D*). To allow maintenance of biologic width (*BW*) of 2.04 mm, restoration margins must be placed at least 3–4 mm coronal to crest of alveolar bone (*green lines, diag. A, B and C*). If restoration or crown margins crosses into biologic width and distance between crest of alveolar bone and restoration or margin of crown is less than biologic width (*red line, diag. D*), gingival inflammation and periodontitis will occur in that area.

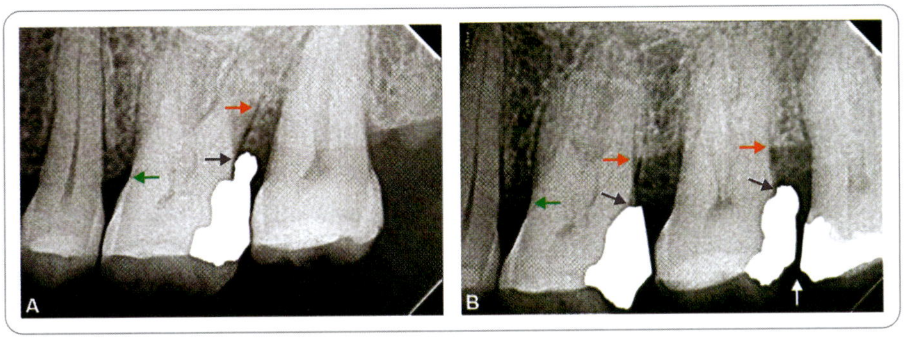

Fig. 7.11: Iatrogenic factors contributing to periodontal disease. In both diags A and B, overhanging margins of the restorations (*black arrows*) encourage plaque accumulation under them and have resulted in bone loss (*periodontitis*) (*red arrows*). Note that contact of restoration in diag. B is open (*white arrow*), this causes food impaction which also has led to periodontitis and bone loss. Compare normal level of bone crest in relation to mesial surfaces of first molars (*restored teeth*) (*diags A and B, green arrows*) with the apically placed bone crest on distal surfaces of same teeth (*diags A and B, red arrows*) thus proving the role of overhanging restorations in causing periodontal loss in the area.

CLINICAL UTILITY AND SHORT ANSWER

What is biologic width? What is its clinical importance?

Biologic width is a ***2.04 mm*** (*average*) normal space between crest of alveolar bone and base of gingival sulcus in which supra-alveolar gingival connective tissue, fibers, etc. are located **(Fig. 7.12)**. This space includes junctional epithelium (*average 0.97 mm*) and gingival supra-alveolar connective tissue attachment (*connective tissue and gingival fibers; average 1.07 mm.*).

Why must margins of restorations end 3–4 mm coronal to crest of bone?

- Prevention of breach of biologic width is of utmost clinical importance.
- To prevent breach of biologic width, a minimum distance of at least ***3–4 mm*** must be maintained between restoration margins and the alveolar crest **(Fig. 7.10 A, B and C)**.
- This will accommodate a normal gingival sulcus of around 1 mm and biologic width of 2.04 mm.
- If the minimum biologic width distance is not maintained when restoration or crown is placed, ***untreatable*** gingival inflammation leading to periodontitis will occur **(Fig. 7.10 D)**.
- Such gingiva will bleed and also look unaesthetic.
- If biologic width is violated, bone loss will eventually occur in the area causing the alveolar crest to move apically till biologic width is re-attained.
- If 3–4 mm height of crown is not available coronal to bone crest, it must be created by crown lengthening (*Chapter 21, 'Interdisciplinary Interrelationships and Supportive Periodontal Therapy'* and *diag. 21.6*).

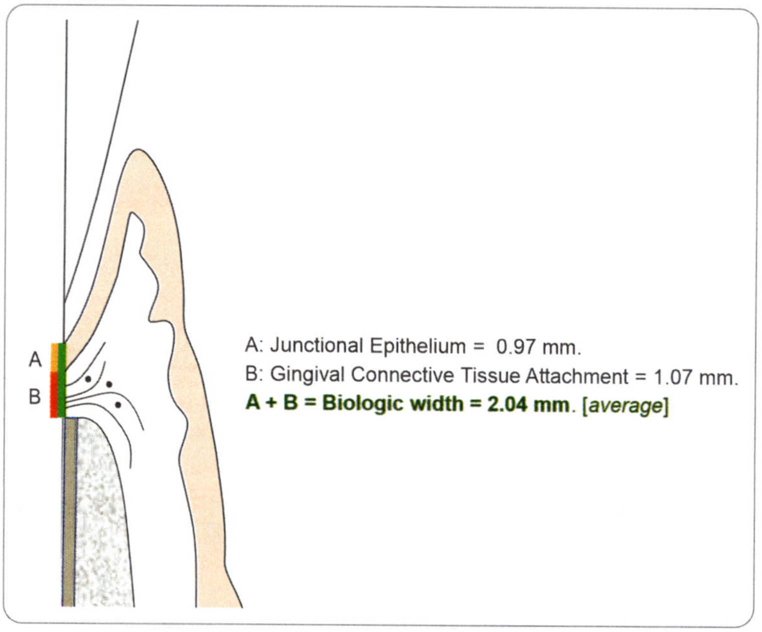

Fig. 7.12: Biologic width

Why Tooth Contours should be Made Properly

See section on 'characteristics of dental restorations that act as predisposing factors for periodontal disease and caries', in the preceding text.

OPEN PROXIMAL TOOTH CONTACTS

How do open tooth contacts predispose to periodontal disease?

A tight proximal contact between two adjacent teeth and proper location of proximal contacts and embrasures are essential for preventing interproximal food impaction. Even a slightly open interproximal tooth contact will result in food impaction in the interproximal region **(Figs 7.11 and 7.13)**. This is harmful for the health of the periodontium as explained in the preceding text.

INJURIES INFLICTED TO PERIODONTAL TISSUES DURING DENTAL TREATMENT

Dental treatments can cause chemical and physical injuries to periodontal tissues. These injuries may be small traumatic injuries, like cuts, penetrations or abrasions that occur during cavity preparation, matrix band and retainer placement, crown preparation, scaling, etc. Occasionally,

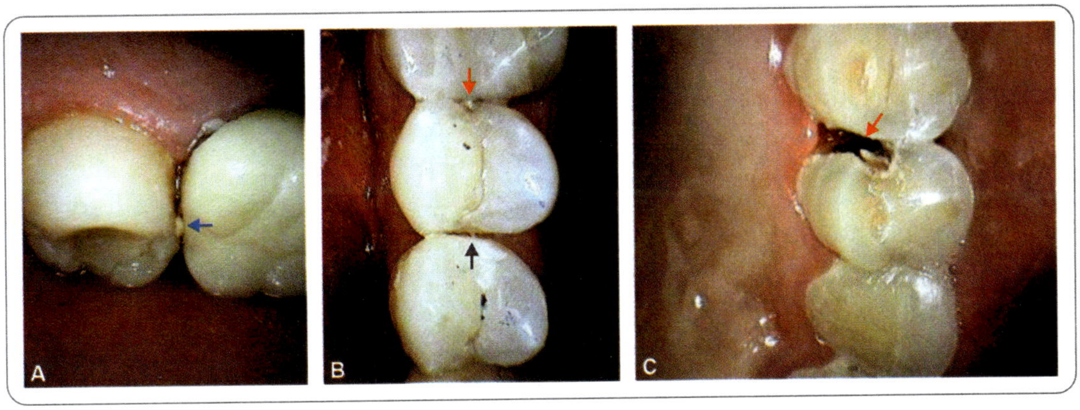

Fig. 7.13: Open contacts due to faulty crowns (*pic. A, blue arrow*), restorations (*pic. B, black arrow*), caries (*pic. B and C, red arrows*), etc. cause food impaction and predispose to periodontitis.

injuries may be more severe, e.g. severe trauma to periodontium during elevation of an adjoining tooth during extraction, excessive orthodontic force resulting in (*TFO*), etc.

- In most cases till such injuries heal completely, they continue to cause discomfort to the patient. As a result, patients may not be able to eat on the same side and clean such areas properly.
- Forceful impaction of restorative material into periodontal tissues during dental treatments may also lead to a foreign body reaction and resultant gingival/periodontal abscess formation. Chemical injury (*burns*) in gingiva may result from application of medications during dental treatments, e.g. use of sodium hypochlorite during RCTs, application of pH 1 citric acid for root preparation, etc.

MATERIA ALBA

Definition: Materia alba is a soft and sticky cheese like material comprising microorganisms, food debris, desquamated epithelial and blood cells that is deposited on and around the teeth and other surfaces of the oral cavity.

◂ *What is materia alba?*

- Although contents of materia alba are same as those of plaque; yet materia alba is different from plaque as it does not have the internal organized structure of plaque.
- It is also not as firmly adherent to the underlying surface as plaque.
- It is usually yellowish or grayish white in colour. It may be also be of the colour of food that was recently consumed. At first look, it appears to be plaque.
- The etiologic significance of materia alba is because of its nutritive value for oral bacteria. Bacteria get ***nutrition*** from materia alba and then flourish to cause gingivitis and periodontitis.
- Such bacteria also metabolize carbohydrates in materia alba and produce organic acids (*lactic acid*, etc.). These organic acids then cause caries.
- Untreated carious lesions, especially those that are near the gingiva encourage plaque formation, food impaction, etc. and cause gingivitis and periodontitis.

◂ *What is the difference between materia alba and plaque?*

◂ *How does materia alba cause oral disease?*

FOOD IMPACTION

Definition: Forceful wedging of food into interdental space or gingival sulcus or pocket is called food impaction (**Fig. 7.14**).

◂ *What is food impaction?*

It is of Two Types

Vertical and Horizontal (*lateral*).

Vertical Food Impaction

◂ *What is the difference between vertical and horizontal food impaction?*

When food impaction occurs into interdental spaces due to vertical occlusal forces (*during mastication of food*) (**Fig. 7.14, diag. A, red arrow**).

Lateral Food Impaction

When food impaction occurs into and around embrasures and interdental spaces of teeth due to lateral pressure of tongue, lips or cheeks (Fig. 7.14, diag. B, black arrow).

What causes worsening of food impaction?

Increased food impaction is seen in the following situations:

1. Loss of proximal contact: This is the commonest cause of food impaction. Proximal contacts may be lost due to:
   a. Pathologic migration of teeth (*e.g. in severe stage III and IV periodontitis, TFO, etc.*).
   b. Migration of teeth due to non-replacement of lost or missing teeth.
      1. Mesial or distal migration of teeth towards edentulous space in the same arch (Fig.7.15, diag. B).
      2. Supra-eruption of teeth into edentulous space in the opposite arch.
   c. Proximal caries (Fig. 7.13, diag. C)
   d. Attrition of proximal surfaces of teeth that is not compensated by mesial migration.
2. Faulty restorations, e.g. those with open interproximal contacts, improper form and embrasure reconstruction (Fig. 7.13, diag. B), etc.
3. Occlusal wear, attrition of teeth may result in a tooth form that does not allow normal deflection of food away from proximal areas but instead encourages food impaction. Attrition may also lead to formation of 'plunger cusps' that typically force food into interdental spaces of opposing teeth.
4. Abnormal biting habits.
5. Crowding of teeth (Fig. 7.15, diag. A).
6. Congenital morphologic abnormalities of teeth.

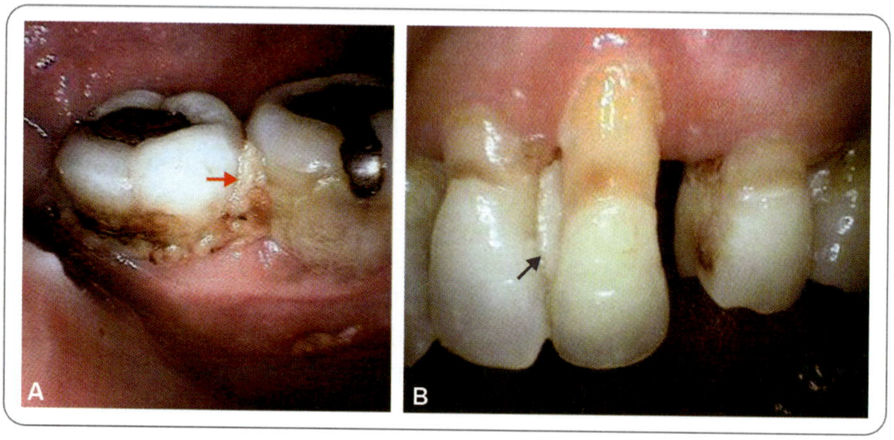

Fig. 7.14: Food impaction. Vertical food impaction (*diag. A, red arrow*) and horizontal food impaction (*diag. B, black arrow*).

Clinical features of chronic food impaction

What are the chief complaints of a patient with food impaction?

1. Feeling of pressure and vague pain between teeth and urge to dig impacted material from these interdental spaces (*especially after meals*).
2. Occasional deep radiating pain (*into jaw*).
3. Tendency to suck out impacted food from interdental spaces (*that may have a foul taste and smell*).
4. Gingival inflammation and bleeding (*from such interdental spaces*).
5. Tenderness in adjoining teeth.
6. Deep impaction of food into periodontal tissues may result in formation of an abscess.
7. If food impaction is chronic, it can also cause:
   i. Local alveolar bone loss
   ii. Gingival recession
   iii. Root caries.

CLINICAL UTILITY AND SHORT ANSWER

What are plunger cusps?

Definition: Plunger cusps are those cusps of teeth that are so shaped and positioned that they force (*wedge*) food into interproximal spaces of antagonist teeth (*opposite teeth in the opposite arch*) during mastication.

◄ *How do plunger cusps affect periodontal health?*

- Plunger cusps form due to abnormal attrition of occlusal surface of a tooth that wears down most of the occlusal surface but selectively leaves out a particular cusp relatively intact (*plunger cusp*).
- This cusp is ***protruding*** and ***fits*** relatively well against contours of the opposite teeth. This way plunger cusps forces food into interdental spaces and worsens food impaction.
- Repeated food impaction into such interdental spaces can cause gingival inflammation, bone loss and even abscess formation in such interdental spaces.

FOOD DEBRIS AND IMPACTED FOOD

Food debris: Remnants of food (*debris*) left back in the mouth after swallowing is called food debris.

◄ *What is food debris and impacted food?*

Impacted food: During mastication, food can be forcefully impacted in interdental areas (*between teeth*) or into sulci or pockets. This is impacted food.

Etiologic significance of food debris and impacted food is primarily because of its ability to sustain plaque bacteria which cause dental diseases.

◄ *How do food debris and impacted food cause oral disease?*

- If food debris or impacted food remain in the mouth for a very long time, it starts to get digested in the mouth (*by action of salivary enzymes and bacteria*). This digested (*'and liquefied'*) food debris is then cleared from the oral cavity by swallowing or spitting.
- Food debris and impacted food can however remain stuck at a site for many hours or days. This food, then, over a period of time, decays (*due to bacteria*) and produces foul mouth taste and odour (*halitosis*).
- Food debris and impacted food serves as a source of nutrition for plaque bacteria and it thus causes:
  - Caries
  - Contributes to gingivitis and periodontitis.
- When food is being chewed it can cause direct physical or thermal injury to gingiva and other periodontal tissues especially if food is very hard or very hot or very cold.

CLINICAL UTILITY AND SHORT ANSWER

How long does it take for food debris to be cleared from the mouth?

◄ *What is the rate of clearance of food?*

- Food debris stays in the mouth for an average time of 15 minutes. This is called ***'rate of clearance of food'***; it varies with kind of food and from person to person.
- Liquids and non-sticky foods are usually cleared in about ***15 minutes*** or so, whereas sticky foods may remain for more than ***one hour***.
- If food is impacted, i.e. forcibly stuck between two teeth, it can remain stuck there for many hours until it decays or is physically removed (*by a tooth pick, etc.*).

ROLE OF MALOCCLUSION, ANATOMICAL FACTORS AND CARIES IN PERIODONTAL DISEASE

Anatomical factors can cause and contribute to gingivitis and periodontitis. Such anatomical factors include: Radicular (*root*) grooves seen on palatal aspect of upper lateral incisors, narrow furcations, high frenal attachments, malocclusion, etc.

- Anatomical abnormalities increase plaque accumulation and thus act as predisposing factors for gingivitis and periodontitis.
- High frenal attachments not only restrict oral hygiene measures (*especially tooth brushing*) but are also associated with narrow zone of attached gingiva which predisposes to gingival recession and mucogingival complications.

Does malocclusion always cause gingivitis and periodontitis? ▸

- Malocclusion only acts as a ***predisposing*** or ***contributing*** **factor** for gingivitis and periodontitis by facilitating more food impaction, plaque accumulation and making plaque control more difficult (Fig. 7.15). If an individual performs adequate plaque control and maintains teeth surfaces in a relatively 'plaque free' state constantly, malocclusion stops being a contributing or predisposing factor.
- Malocclusion resulting in lingual/palatal or buccal version of teeth may be accompanied by more apical placement of the crest of the free gingiva (*'recession'*) and alveolar bone on such prominent root surfaces. According to the 2018 classification of periodontal diseases, such receded gingiva is called 'reduced periodontium'. Teeth with reduced periodontium may have gingival health or gingivitis or periodontitis.

How do malplaced teeth predispose to gingivitis and periodontitis? ▸

- Malplaced teeth and supra erupted teeth also disturb normal pattern of force dissipation in the periodontium and movement masticated food in the mouth. These factors, thus favour food impaction, plaque formation and retention and may also result in trauma from occlusion (*TFO*). The possibility of formation of plunger cusps also increases manifold in malocclusion.

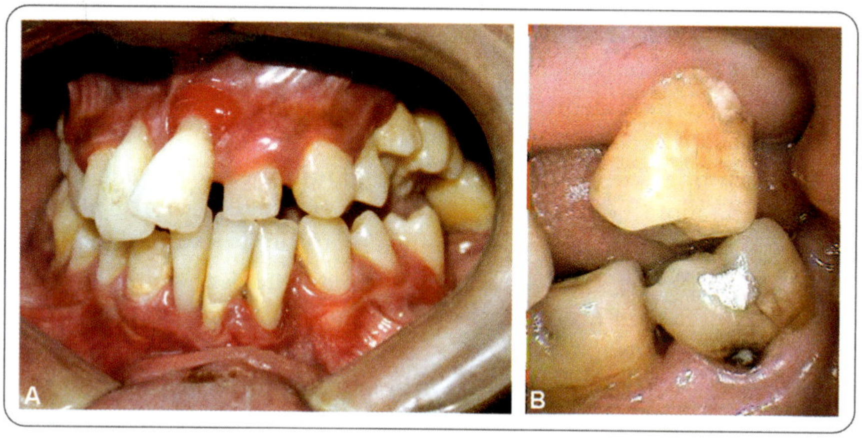

Fig. 7.15: Malocclusion and pathologic migration seen in periodontitis (*diag. A*) and due to un-replaced missing teeth (*diag. B*). Such cases present with more plaque and calculus formation and food impaction. As plaque control is more difficult in such cases, malocclusion and pathologic migration act as predisposing and contributing factors for gingivitis, periodontitis and caries.

HABITS AND SELF-INFLICTED INJURIES AFFECTING THE HEALTH OF THE PERIODONTIUM

How are some habits detrimental to periodontal health? ▸

- Habits like prolonged and forceful tooth brushing (*done every day and over a very long period of time*) may cause gingival trauma and abrasion and may also produce gingival recession.
- People in the habit of smoking, consuming strong alcohol or keeping snuff or chewing tobacco in their buccal or lingual vestibules, also have a risk of developing hyperkeratosis in the gingiva. Such hyperkeratotic lesions may transform to malignancy.
- Some individiuals may place medicines, e.g. aspirin or strong chemicals, e.g. battery acid, clove oil, nail paint, nail paint remover, etc. by the side a tooth to relieve tooth pain. Such chemicals can cause chemical burns in the gingiva. Hot foods can cause thermal burns, e.g. hot potatoes, cheese, etc.
- Oral jewelry (*piercing jewelry*) may also physically or chemically (*by its corrosion products*) harm oral tissues and gingiva. This may result in recession and loss of height of alveolar bone.

Review Questions

1. What is dental calculus? Classify it.
2. Describe the supra-gingival and sub-gingival calculus and enumerate differences between these two.
3. Write on etiologic significance of calculus.
4. Why is maximum deposition of calculus seen on lingual surfaces of mandibular incisors and buccal surfaces of maxillary 1st and 2nd molars?
5. How does calculus attach to oral surfaces?
6. How does calculus form?
7. What is calculocementum?
8. What is materia alba? How is it different from food debris?
9. What is the rate of clearance of food products from the mouth?
10. Write a note on extrinsic dental stains.
11. How do overhanging and under-filled restorations cause gingivitis and periodontitis?
12. Why is it important to restore a tooth to its original form and shape with a restoration?
13. Write on role of iatrogenic factors, like dental restorations, restoration margins and their design in causing gingivitis and periodontitis.
14. What is biologic width? How is invasion of biologic width by restorations related to inflammation of gingiva?
15. What is food impaction? Differentiate between vertical and horizontal/lateral food impaction.
16. What are the clinical features of chronic food impaction?
17. What are plunger cusps? How do they contribute to food impaction and periodontal disease?
18. How do open proximal contacts of teeth contribute to periodontal disease?
19. Write on role of malocclusion and anatomical factors in causing gingivitis and periodontitis.
20. What is the role of habits in causing gingivitis and periodontitis?

Chapter

8

Systemic and Periodontal Interrelationships

It is commonly found that despite having comparable etiological factors, periodontal damage in periodontitis is more severe in some individuals. This increased periodontal damage is because of an individual's decreased immunity. On the other hand, some individuals show a very high degree of immune response against periodontopathogens; this too is harmful and increases tissue damage in periodontitis. A defective immune response is often associated with some systemic illnesses. Individuals with defective immunity or systemic illnesses that cause defective immunity are called individuals with a '***systemic background***'.

What is implied by the term individual with a systemic background? ▶

Just as the systemic health affects periodontal health, periodontitis can also harmfully affect an individual's systemic health. Periodontal infections (*gingivitis and periodontitis*) affect and act like predisposing, contributing and aggravating factors for many serious systemic diseases and conditions like coronary heart disease (*that causes heart attacks*), diabetes, pneumonia, preterm labor, low birth weight babies, etc.

The interrelationship between periodontitis and systemic health is very complex. It is briefly discussed in two sections:

SECTION 1: Systemic disorders contributing to and aggravating periodontal disease

SECTION 2: Periodontal (*oral*) diseases contributing to and aggravating systemic diseases and conditions (*Periodontal medicine*)

SECTION 1: SYSTEMIC DISORDERS CONTRIBUTING TO AND AGGRAVATING PERIODONTAL DISEASE

Several systemic factors that include psychological, environmental and physical factors, can affect periodontitis. These factors ***cannot initiate*** but can only ***predispose*** to periodontitis. When present, they accelerate and increase severity of periodontitis.

Systemic diseases and conditions that affect periodontal health and disease

1. Endocrine disorders (*hormonal imbalances*) related to:
    a. Pancreas—diabetes mellitus
    b. Sex hormones
    c. Adrenal hormones
    d. Thyroid hormones
    e. Parathyroid hormones
    f. Pituitary hormones
2. Chronic liver disease
3. Blood (*haematological*) disorders
4. Psychological stress
5. Nutritional imbalances
6. Acquired immune deficiency syndrome (*AIDS*), etc.

1. Endocrine Disorders (*Hormonal Imbalances*) Affecting Periodontium

Endocrine disorders like hormonal fluctuations during pregnancy or puberty, diabetes, etc. are excellent examples of harmful influences of body's hormones on periodontal health. Some common endocrinal diseases affecting periodontium are discussed below:

1a. *Effect of Diabetes Mellitus (DM) on Periodontium*

Diabetes is a metabolic disease characterized by chronic ***hyperglycemia*** (*raised blood glucose*). In normal individuals, blood glucose levels after eight hours of fasting are less than 100 mg/dL; post prandial (after eating a meal) blood glucose levels two hours after a normal meal, are less than 140 mg/dL. Normal HbA1c range to between 4–5.6%.

◂ *What is diabetes mellitus?*

◂ *What are normal blood glucose levels?*

CLINICAL UTILITY AND SHORT ANSWER

What is HbA1c blood test?

HbA1c is a blood test to know an individual's average plasma glucose concentration (*blood levels of **glycated** hemoglobin*) over the ***past 2 to 3 months***. Consistently high blood glucose levels lead to a corresponding increase value of HbA1c. Reference values for HbA1c are:

- 4–5.6% = Normal range, no diabetes
- 5.7% and 6.4% = Pre-diabetic state or increased risk of diabetes
- Higher than 6.5% = Diabetes

The HbA1c test serves as a very good indicator of diabetic control in diabetic patients.

Insulin

- It is a hormone produced by pancreas.
- It regulates and maintains blood glucose levels and is released in response to several stimuli that include increased blood levels of glucose, eating protein and carbohydrates, etc.
- Insulin is needed by cells for absorption of glucose from blood.
- Diabetes mellitus (*DM*) is caused either by decreased production or impaired action of insulin. Therefore, any imbalance in production or action of insulin causes high blood glucose.
- Chronic high blood glucose damages tissues and organs.

◂ *What does insulin do?*

Diabetes is primarily of two types: Type I and Type II

Type I DM is relatively ***uncommon*** (*5–10% cases*). It results due to destruction of insulin producing β-cells of the islets of Langerhans of pancreas.

◂ *Which type of diabetes is more common?*

Type II DM is far ***more common*** than type I DM. It is caused by decreased or impaired insulin secretion, peripheral resistance to insulin action and/or increased glucose production of glucose in liver.

Systemic clinical features of diabetes:

- High blood glucose levels
- ***Polyphagia*** (*excessive hunger*), ***polydipsia*** (*excessive thirst*), ***polyuria*** (*excessive urination*).
- Such individuals also have:
  - ***Increased*** tendency to infections,
  - Poor wound healing,
  - Nephropathy, retinopathy, neuropathy, etc.

◂ *What are the common clinical features of diabetes mellitus?*

ALERT!

- Type I DM usually occurs in thin (*non–obese*) individuals whereas, type II DM usually occurs in obese (*fat*) individuals.
- Type I DM is more difficult to control than type II DM. To control type I DM regular insulin injections are needed. Type II DM can be controlled by oral hypoglycaemics, diet control, exercise and weight reduction.
- Ketosis and coma (*complications of diabetes*) occur far more commonly in patients with Type I DM.
- Diabetes can also occur due to other causes, e.g. gestational diabetes (*occurs in 2–5% of pregnant women*), after surgical removal of pancreas, in patients of cushing's syndrome, etc.

◂ *Which individuals are more prone to type I diabetes?*

◂ *Which type of diabetes cannot be controlled only by oral hypoglycaemics?*

Oral manifestations of poorly controlled diabetes mellitus (*DM*)

What are the oral clinical features of diabetes mellitus? ▸

Patients of poorly controlled DM can show many clinical changes in their oral health. DM itself does ***not*** cause these diseases and conditions, but only serves as a ***predisposing*** and ***aggravating*** factor. These changes may not be present in all cases and when present may show great degree of variation in patients. Common oral manifestations of ***poorly controlled*** DM include:

What are the specific features of periodontitis complicated by diabetes? ▸

1. Severe periodontitis ***not*** relatable to amount of identifiable local factors:
   a. Moderate-to-severe periodontitis that is fast progressing (*grade B or C periodontitis*) (*deep periodontal pockets, increased tooth mobility*)
   b. Multiple recurrent chronic periodontal abscesses that are difficult to treat (Fig. 8.1).
2. Reduced flow of saliva (*dry mouth—xerostomia*).
3. Angular cheilitis (*painful cuts in angles of mouth that ooze exudate and bleed when stretched; caused by fungal infection*).
4. Burning mouth.

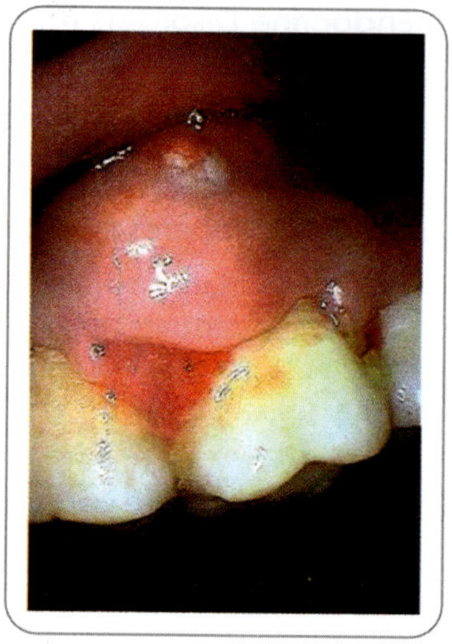

Fig. 8.1: Recurrent multiple chronic periodontal abscess in a patient with uncontrolled diabetes and stage III grade C periodontitis.

CLINICAL UTILITY AND SHORT ANSWER

Why do poorly controlled diabetics show increased tendency to severe periodontal infections?

Increased chances of severe infections in ***poorly controlled*** diabetic patients are due to reduced immunity. This is due to:

Why are diabetic patients more prone to severe periodontitis? ▸

1. PMN defects, that cause defective:
   a. Chemotaxis (*of PMNs to site of infection*)
   b. Adherence (*of PMNs to invading microorganisms*)
   c. Phagocytosis (*engulfing of microorganisms by PMNs*)
2. Functional defects of monocytes and macrophages resulting in impaired killing of invading microorganisms.

Poorly controlled diabetics also show increased rate of periodontal loss due to:

1. Impaired collagen metabolism that reduces collagen synthesis and maturation (*in extracellular connective tissue*).
2. Increased collagen destruction.
3. Defective collagen repair due to presence of larger amount of 'accumulated glycation end products' (*AGEs*). These AGE products cause cross linking of collagen making collagen less soluble and therefore less likely to be repaired or replaced in the normal way.

Diabetes and periodontitis have a *two-way* relationship.

Does treatment of DM and periodontitis have a beneficial effect on the control of these two diseases individually? ▸

- Poorly controlled DM increases severity of periodontitis and untreated periodontitis causes ***worsening*** of DM and makes its management difficult.
- Treatment of periodontitis improves a diabetic patient's control of blood sugar with existing medications and diet control; similarly, improvement in diabetes leads to improvement in periodontal health of a diabetic patient.

1b. *Effect of Sex Hormones on Periodontium*

Do changes in an individual's sex hormones affect periodontal tissues? ▸

Fluctuations in sex hormones in the human body can have ***significant*** effects on gingiva. Fluctuating hormone levels do not by themselves cause gingival disease but they act only as initiating or complicating factors and condition the gingiva to produce an ***exaggerated*** response to the already present local factors. Such conditioning causes puberty gingivitis, pregnancy gingivitis, menopausal gingivostomatitis, etc.

Pregnancy and puberty gingivitis or periodontitis

These are discussed in Chapter 11, 'Plaque Associated Periodontal Disease and Gingival Enlargements'.

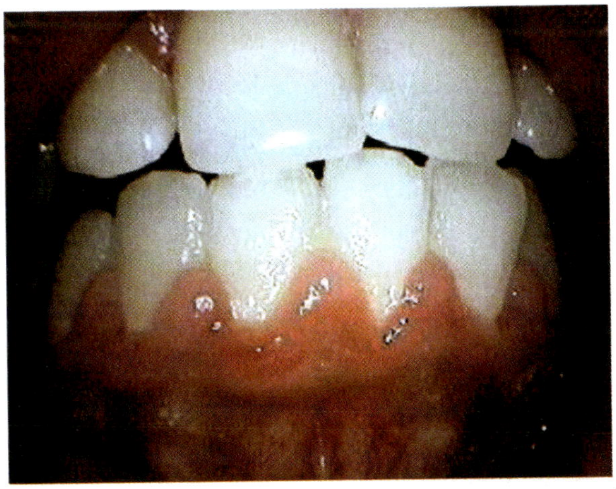

Fig. 8.1a: Pregnancy gingivitis (*or pregnancy periodontitis if base of pocket is apical to CE junction*)

Gingival changes associated with menstrual cycle

Menstrual cycle is usually ***not*** accompanied by any clinically noticeable changes in the gingiva in most females. However, gingiva may show some increase in severity of:

◂ *Does menstrual cycle affect gingival health?*

- Gingivitis and gingival bleeding
- Swelling and slight increase in GCF flow.

After menopause, due to change in concentration and proportion of a female's sex hormones, ***Menopausal gingivostomatitis*** (*senile atrophic gingivitis*) may occur. Clinical features of menopausal gingivostomatitis are similar to those of chronic desquamative gingivitis. These include:

◂ *Enumerate the changes in gingiva related to menopause.*

- Thinning and ulceration of gingiva and oral mucosa (*atrophy of epithelium, mildly red colour of gingiva, etc.*)
- Dry mouth with burning sensation and changes in taste, etc.

Gingival changes associated with use of oral contraceptives

If oral contraceptives are consumed continuously by females for many months, they can cause gingival changes that are similar to ones seen in pregnancy gingivitis.

◂ *Do oral contraceptives affect gingival health?*

1c. *Effect of Adrenal Gland Hormones on Periodontium*

Adrenal glands are endocrine glands located on kidneys. They produce ***corticosteroids*** (*mineralocorticoids for regulation of blood pressure and electrolyte balance, glucocorticoids for regulation of glycogen and lipid metabolism and immune system suppression and androgens* (*they are converted to sex hormones*) and ***catecholamines*** (*adrenaline and noradrenaline*).

Excessive blood levels of corticosteroid hormones can cause:

◂ *What are the ill affects of excessive corticosteroid levels in blood?*

- Suppression of immune system resulting in recurrent and severe infections
- Bone resorption and reduced bone formation
- Osteoporosis
- Reduction in collagen and reduced number of collagen fibers in PDL (periodontal ligament) and increased destruction of periodontal tissues in periodontitis.

Corticosteroids levels in blood ***increase*** in ***stress***. If an individual remains under continuous psychological stress for very long, high corticosteroid levels in the blood will reduce the individual's natural immunity against infection. This will lead to recurrent infection and also increase severity of pre-existing infections including periodontitis.

◂ *How does stress affect corticosteroid levels in blood?*

1d. *Effect of Thyroid Hormones on Periodontium*

No specific clinical changes in gingiva are seen in hypothyroidism or hyperthyroidism.

1e. *Effect of Parathyroid Hormones on Periodontium*

Parathyroid glands secrete parathyroid hormone which controls and maintains calcium and phosphate levels in blood and bones.

What are normal calcium levels in blood? ▸
What happens when calcium levels in blood drop below normal? ▸
What is the effect of hyperparathyroidism on bone health? ▸

- Parathyroid hormone increases blood calcium levels by causing bone resorption (*calcium from resorbed bone moves into blood stream*).
- The ***normal*** levels of the ***calcium*** in blood are ***9.0–10.5 mg/dL***. Decrease in calcium blood levels produces ***Tetany***.
- **Hyperparathyroidism** causes ***osteoporosis*** (*increased bone resorption causing generalized demineralization of the bones of body including alveolar bone*). Lamina dura may be thinned but remains intact despite osteoporosis.
- Such patients complain of vague pain and tenderness in bones, jaws and teeth.

ALERT!

Tetany is a sign of severe hypocalcemia (*low blood calcium level*) (*normal blood calcium level is 9.0–**10.5** mg/dl*) and is characterized by involuntary contraction of muscles. Tetany is confirmed by ***Chvostek sign*** (*tapping just anterior to the ear, where facial nerve emerges, results in twitching of nose and/or lips*).

CLINICAL UTILITY AND SHORT ANSWER

Can calcium content of bone be known by blood test? ▸

Can calcium deficiency in an individual be assessed by blood calcium level?

Calcium content of bones and severity of osteoporosis ***cannot*** be gauged by blood calcium levels! This is so because blood calcium levels are always maintained between 9.0 and 10.5 mg/dL (*if levels of calcium fall below normal, tetany will occur*). When blood levels of calcium start to fall below normal, calcium is removed from bones and moved into blood to maintain normal blood calcium levels. This happens even in cases of severe osteoporosis and chronic severe dietary deficiency of calcium.

To gauge osteoporosis and level of calcification of bones (*bone density*), ***DEXA scan*** (*dual energy X-ray absorptiometry*) is done. A good estimate of decrease in bone density can also be had by assessing CBCT. In IOPA radiographs, osteoporotic bones with low density present a rarefied look.

2. Effect of Chronic Liver Disease on Periodontium

How does liver disease affect periodontal health? ▸

Liver plays a major role in metabolism, glycogen storage, decomposition of RBCs, protein synthesis, etc. Chronic liver disease therefore results in impaired glucose metabolism and poor blood glucose level control.

- Chronic liver disease complicates pre-existing diabetes and periodontitis, making periodontitis more severe and difficult to treat.
- The liver also makes many coagulation factors that play a major role in blood clotting. Patients with periodontitis and chronic liver disease often present with increased gingival bleeding that may be difficult to control.

3. Blood Disorders Affecting Periodontium

Blood (*haematological*) disorders can be broadly grouped into WBC, RBC and haemostatic disorders. Of these, WBC disorders (*leukocyte disorders*) constitute a major proportion of blood disorders that affect the periodontium.

3a. *Leukemia*

It is a disease characterized by very high numbers of WBCs in blood. Leukemia may be of acute or chronic types.

Why do patients with leukemia have frequent unexplained gingival bleeding? ▸

- Anemia and thrombocytopenia (*deficiency of platelets*) are present in patients with all types of leukemias. Leukemic patients therefore often complain of frequent unexplained bleeding from their gingivae, formation of petechiae and ecchymosis in the palate (*despite absence of severe periodontitis*).
- Such patients also have deficient immune and inflammatory responses.

- Leukemic patients frequently have gingival enlargement, bleeding from gingiva, oral ulcerations and recurrent infections. Gingival enlargement is caused by leukemic cell infiltration in gingiva; it starts in interdental papilla.
- As gingiva enlarges due to leukemic infiltrate, it causes pocket formation. Marginal gingiva and interdental papillae then become inflamed, enlarged and of bluish-red color. Enlarged gingiva subsequently partially covers crowns of teeth. Leukemic enlargement also increases severity of periodontitis (*if already present*) resulting in rapid periodontal loss.

◂ *Why do patients with leukemia have gingival enlargement?*

3b. *Neutropenia*

Deficiency of mature neutrophils (*PMNs*) in circulation is called neutropenia. It may be chronic or cyclic, severe or benign. Neutropenia increases severity of periodontitis and leads to increased destruction of periodontal tissues (*PMNs play a critical role in maintenance of periodontal health as they are the first line of defense against infection—innate immunity*).

◂ *Why are patients with neutropenia more likely to have severe periodontitis?*

- Neutropenia may be caused by many systemic diseases and conditions that may be drug induced, genetic, resulting from a viral infection or as an after effect of chemotherapy for cancer.
- In many diseases and conditions, normal functioning of PMNs is affected, e.g. agranulocytosis, lazy leukocyte syndrome, down's syndrome, papillon-lefevre syndrome, inflammatory bowel disease, etc. Patients suffering from these diseases can have severe periodontitis.

3c. *Agranulocytosis* (Neutropenia is a Part of This)

It is reduction in number of circulating granulocytes (*PMNs, basophils and eosinophils*). Less severe forms of the disease are called neutropenia or granulocytopenia. Agranulocytosis is most commonly caused by adverse drug reactions (*sulfonamides, drugs containing arsenic, gold salts, etc.*). Agranulocytosis may be chronic or periodic with recurring neutropenic cycles (*e.g. cyclic neutropenia occurring every three weeks and lasting three to six days at a time*).

◂ *What are less severe forms of agranulocytosis?*

◂ *What is the difference between agranulocytosis and neutropenia?*

◂ *How does agranulocytosis affect oral health?*

- Agranulocytosis results in severe infections that include ulcerative and necrotizing lesions of oral mucosa, skin and gastrointestinal and genitourinary tracts.
- Such lesions ***do not*** show clinical signs of inflammation (*because normally functioning PMNs are required for inflammation*).
- Such cases have severe periodontal destruction but may present with little inflammatory changes in the gingiva. Gingival bleeding, necrosis, increased salivation and fetid odor (*features similar to NUG (necrotizing ulcerative gingivitis)*) may also be seen.
- Isolated sharply demarcated greyish-black necrotic patches may develop from such necrotizing lesions later.
- Agranulocytosis can be differentiated from NUG, NOMA/cancrum oris/necrotizing ulcerative stomatitis, etc. (*that present similar clinical features*) by assessing blood counts (*that will show pronounced leukopenia and almost complete absence of neutrophils*).

3d. *Anemia*

Iron deficiency and pernicious anemia (*caused by vitamin B_{12} deficiency*) are common types of anemias. In severe anemia:

- Tongue appears red, smooth and shiny due to atrophy of its papillae.
- Ulcerations of the oral mucosa and oropharynx may also be seen and these cause painful swallowing of food (*dysphagia*).
- Many cases of anaemia have concurrent neutropenia (*decrease in the number of PMNs*). This results in increased susceptibility to periodontal infections and severe periodontitis.

◂ *What are the oral changes seen in anaemia?*

3e. *Thrombocytopenia*

It is a condition in which there is a reduction in circulating platelets in blood. It may be idiopathic, due to decreased production of platelets in bone marrow in aplastic anaemia, leukemia, etc. or as a result of increased destruction of platelets in diseases like dengue or after intake of certain drugs etc.

◂ *What are the main causes of reduction of platelets in blood?*

- Thrombocytopenia is characterized by a increased bleeding time (*clotting time is normal or slightly increased*), spontaneous bleeding under the skin or mucous membranes (*purpura*), petechiae, ecchymosis and formation of hemorrhagic vesicles (*particularly in the palate, tonsillar pillars, and buccal mucosa*).

What are the oral features of reduction in platelet numbers?

- Gingiva is inflamed, soft, friable and bleeds on slightest injury or even spontaneously. Bleeding from gingivae is persistent and is difficult to control. Local plaque control measures like tooth brushing, flossing, etc. and scaling also cause increased bleeding.

CLINICAL UTILITY AND SHORT ANSWER

What are the typical normal blood counts in humans?

TLC: *4,000–11,000 per microliter of blood*

DLC: PMNs: *40–80%,* ***Eosinophils:*** *2–3%,* ***Basophils:*** *<2%,* ***Lymphocytes:*** *20–40%*

Monocytes: *5–6%*

Hb: Men: *13.8 to 18.0 g/dL;* Women: *12.1 to 15.1 g/dL of blood*

RBCs: *4 to 5 million per microliter of blood*

Platelets: *150,000–400,000 per microliter of blood*

Bleeding time (*Duke method*): *1–5 minutes.*

Clotting time (capillary tube *method*): *3–8 minutes*

Prothrombin time: *11–16 seconds* (interpret using laboratory's reference range)

Prothrombin ratio: *0.9–12* (interpret using laboratory's reference range).

CLINICAL UTILITY AND SHORT ANSWER

Common syndromes that complicate periodontitis

Lazy Leukocyte syndrome

- It is a disorder caused by defective leucocyte function and results in compromised immune and inflammatory response.
- Such individuals have increased susceptibility to ***recurrent severe neutropenia*** and microbial infections including grade C periodontitis (*aggressive periodontitis*) characterized by severe destruction of alveolar bone and early tooth loss.

Papillon-Lefevre syndrome

- It is a genetically inherited condition.
- It is characterized by ichthyosis (*dry, scaly or flaky skin*) of localized areas on palms, soles, knees and elbows, hyperkeratotic skin lesions, severe destruction of periodontium (Fig. 8.2).
- Skin and periodontal lesions appear by four years of age.
- Due to very fast rate of periodontal destruction, deciduous teeth are lost by 5 or 6 years of age and permanent teeth are usually lost in teenage or early adulthood.

Acquired immunodeficiency syndrome (*AIDS*)

AIDS is discussed in detail later in this chapter.

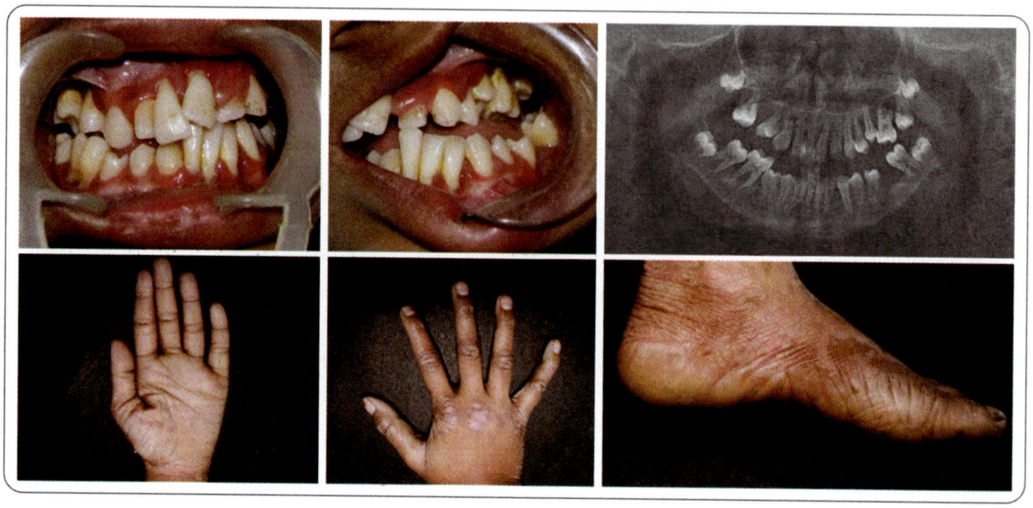

Fig. 8.2: Papillon-Lefevre Syndrome presents with stage III grade C periodontitis (*severe periodontitis in early age*). The syndrome is also characterized by dry, scaly or flaky skin (*ichthyosis*) on hands and feet, hyperkeratotic skin lesions.

4. Psychological Stress and its Effect on the Periodontium

Stress itself does not cause destructive periodontal disease but, it creates the right conditions for the pre-existing infection to become more virulent; thus, periodontitis becomes more severe.

- An individual's capacity to bear psychological stress determines the degree of worsening in severity of periodontitis caused by stress.
- Therefore, even when several individuals have similar degree of psychological stress, all of them will not develop psychological stress related destructive periodontal disease.

◂ *Does psychological stress affect severity and rate of progress of periodontitis in all patients?*

Psychological stress contributes to periodontal disease by:

1. Increasing production of corticosteroids which regulate blood pressure, glycogen and lipid metabolism and causes immune system suppression.
2. Individuals with psychological stress are known to have dry mouth (*low saliva production*), high blood pressure, high blood sugar levels, poor control of hypertension and diabetes and increased susceptibility to infections, osteoporosis, cancers, etc.
3. Chronically psychologically stressed individuals usually do not bother to maintain adequate oral hygiene and tend to consume a diet that consists of soft foods with high sugar content. This results in poor oral health and nutritional status.
4. Individuals under chronic psychological stress may develop a tendency to inflict injuries in their gingivae and develop para-functional habits like bruxism and bruxomania, nail biting, biting onto hard objects, etc. which damage teeth and periodontium. Self-inflicted injuries in the gingiva often result in gingival recession in that area.
5. Psychologically stressed individuals become 'frustrated' with life and have a tendency to live in 'denial' of their ill health. Such individuals are ***less likely*** to seek timely treatment. This complicates systemic and periodontal diseases further.

◂ *Why are individuals with psychological stress likely to have poor oral hygiene?*

5. Malnutrition and its Effect on Periodontium

A balanced diet contains adequate quantity and proportions of proteins, fats, carbohydrates, vitamins and minerals. Nutritional deficiencies affect body functions and slows down repair and regeneration of body tissues. Effect of some specific components of nutrition on oral and periodontal health is described below:

5a. *Vitamin A*

Deficiency of vitamin A causes delayed wound healing.

5b. *Vitamin B Complex*

i. Vitamin B complex deficiency causes glossitis (*inflammation of tongue*), glossodynia (*pain in tongue*), angular cheilitis and oral mucositis (*inflammation of entire oral mucosa*).
ii. Deficiency of riboflavin (*vitamin* B_2) is known to cause severe lesions in gingiva and oral mucosa and Noma (*necrotizing ulcerative stomatitis*).
iii. Deficiency of Niacin (*vitamin* B_3) and Folic acid (*vitamin* B_9) causes black tongue and increase in severity of gingivitis and periodontitis.

◂ *What are the oral signs and symptoms of vit. B complex deficiency?*

CLINICAL UTILITY AND SHORT ANSWER

What is Noma?

Noma (*necrotizing ulcerative stomatitis*) is a severe destructive disease of oral cavity produced by a rapidly progressing, polymicrobial and often gangrenous infection. It is caused by *F. necrophorum* and *P. intermedia;* these act along with other bacteria like *S. aureus, Streptococci, B. vincentii, P. gingivalis,* etc.

5c. *Vitamin C*

Vitamin C plays an important role in collagen metabolism. Its deficiency has a huge impact on periodontal health because connective tissue of the periodontium is primarily made of collagen. Vitamin C also controls immune pathways.

◂ *How does deficiency of vitamin C affect periodontal health?*

Deficiency of vitamin C causes ***scurvy*** and this produces a conditioned enlargement of the gingiva (*described in detail in Chapter 11*).

5d. *Vitamin D*

How does deficiency of vitamin D affect periodontal and systemic health? ▶

It is essential for absorption of calcium in GIT and helps in the regulation of calcium-phosphorus balance and bone density and strength (Fig. 8.3). Severe vitamin D deficiency results in weak bones (*osteoporosis*) and weak immunity. Osteoporosis results in ***loss of bone mass***; this can complicate periodontitis and cause implant failure.

ALERT!

Vitamin B complex and vitamin C being water soluble vitamins are not stored in the body. As a result, these have to consumed in recommended daily doses to prevent deficiency. If balanced nutritious diet is not consumed, deficiencies of these vitamins result easily.

On the other hand, fat soluble vitamins, A, D E and K are stored in our body fat. Therefore, if a balanced diet containing RDA of these vitamins is consumed regularly, chances of deficicncy of these vitamins is less.

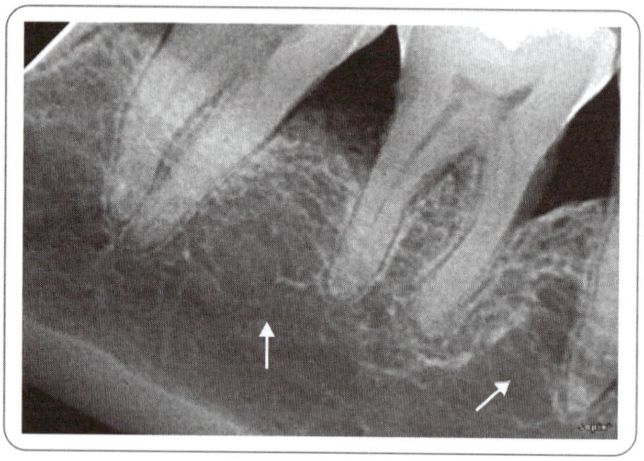

Fig. 8.3: Rarefaction (*osteoporosis*) of alveolar bone caused by vitamin D deficiency. Note that spongy alveolar bone has fewer and widely spaced trabeculae (*white arrow*).

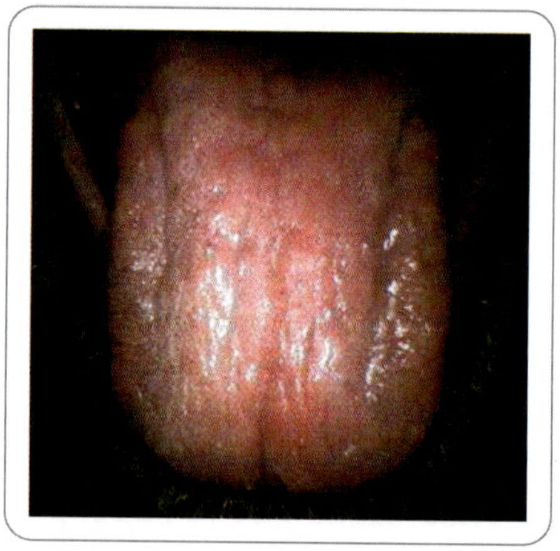

Fig. 8.4: Bald tongue and glossitis. It is usually caused by deficiency of iron and vitamin B_{12}.

5e. *Antioxidants*

Their role in prevention and treatment of periodontal disease is unclear. Antioxidants like vitamin C, E, selenium, etc. are used to treat oral leukoplakia and other pre-cancerous lesions like oral sub-mucus fibrosis, lichen planus, etc.

5f. *Proteins*

How does deficiency of protein affect an individual's health? ▶

Deficiency of proteins leads to loss of tissue mass, delayed wound healing defective and insufficient immunity, etc. making the individual liable to disease. Severe protein deficiency causes glossitis, increased gingival inflammation and alveolar bone loss in plaque induced periodontitis.

5g. *Iron*

Iron deficiency causes iron deficiency anaemia. It can result from chronic blood loss and/or decreased iron in diet. It affects women more often than men (*due to loss of blood during menstruation*). Effects of anaemia on periodontium have already been described earlier in this chapter.

5h. *Metal Intoxication*

Increased levels of mercury, lead, arsenic and bismuth is harmful for general health (*metal intoxication*) and produces pigmentation (*discoloration*) of gingiva.

- Bismuth sulphide produces a ***bluish-black*** discoloration of ***gingival margin*** in areas with pre-existing gingivitis.

What is Burtonian line? ▶

- Lead intoxication produces a grey-coloured linear discolouration (*line like*) called ***Burtonian line***.

CLINICAL UTILITY AND SHORT ANSWER

What is the effect of tooth loss on diet and nutrition of an individual?

If a permanent tooth is lost and is not replaced with a prosthesis, it can have huge impact on an individual's dietary habits:

- With loss of a tooth (*especially a posterior tooth*) an individual is forced to eat on the opposite side. This reduces masticatory efficiency and increases occlusal loads on the remaining teeth.
- Increased occlusal loads can cause TFO (*trauma from occlusion*) in these teeth and can also produce injury in temporomandibular joints.
- Individuals with reduced number of teeth (*or with teeth that are mobile due to periodontitis, mutilated with caries, etc.*) develop a preference for softer diets and may have increased refined sugar consumption.
- Soft diets are often not as nutritious as normal diets and they fail to physically clean teeth and oral soft tissues during mastication of food (*as would a firm normal diet*).
- This predisposes an individual's dentition to several diseases including periodontitis and caries.
- Such individuals have poor nutritional status and are therefore prone to several systemic diseases.

◂ *How does loss of tooth/teeth affect an individual's health?*

6. Acquired Immune Deficiency Syndrome (*AIDS*) and its Effects on Periodontium

Acquired immunodeficiency syndrome (*AIDS*) results in severe immune deficiency and is caused by infection by human immunodeficiency virus (*HIV*). An individual with HIV infection has greater chances of getting opportunistic infections (*by fungi, bacteria and viruses*) and malignancy.

◂ *What is AIDS?*

- HIV infection occurs most commonly after unprotected sexual contact, sharing of hypodermic needles with an HIV infected individual, transfusion of HIV infected blood, etc. HIV is usually not found in saliva, but HIV from blood can find its way into saliva if bleeding occurs in the oral cavity (*from the inflamed gingiva or mucosal injury*).
- HIV infection remains hidden (*latent*) for several weeks to months. Later the individual seroconverts (*develops detectable antibodies against the HIV in the blood*) and clinical features of the disease start appearing.
- Usually, first signs of HIV infection appear in the oral cavity and therefore can be recognized by a dental surgeon during a routine dental visit. Early detection enables better treatment and increased life expectancy of the patient. It also prevents further transmission of infection to other individuals.

◂ *How does AIDS occur?*

◂ *How soon after HIV infection does AIDS occur?*

There are many oral manifestations of AIDS:

a. **Linear Gingival Erythema** (*LGE*) (*HIV gingivitis*) is seen in some HIV +ve patients.
   - It is a refractory (*not responding to treatment*) linear (*line like*) or semilunar patch of gingivitis that may bleed easily. This gingivitis does not improve with scaling or other periodontal treatment. This is one of the chief differentiating features of LGE from plaque induced gingivitis (*which is easily treatable with treatment*).
   - LGE may only involve marginal gingiva or it may extend into attached gingiva and alveolar mucosa in a punctate or diffuse manner.
   - It may be localized or generalized and may worsen to necrotizing ulcerative periodontitis (*NUP*).
   - LGE is thought to be caused by a fungal infection (*candida*). Although LGE may show improvement with anti-fungal therapy, it can also be non-responsive to all treatment (*refractory*).
   - LGE may also undergo spontaneous remission due to unknown reasons.

◂ *What are the oral manifestations of AIDS?*

◂ *What is linear gingival erythema/HIV gingivitis?*

◂ *What is the difference between linear gingival erythema and plaque induced gingivitis?*

b. **Necrotizing Ulcerative Gingivitis** (*NUG*) was called Acute Necrotizing Ulcerative Gingivitis (*ANUG*) few years ago. It is a rare disease that is more likely to occur in patients with severe immune deficiency, e.g. AIDS patients or patients under extreme psychological stress. When NUG is diagnosed, testing for AIDS must always be done as a precautionary measure.

   The reader is referred to Chapter 12, 'Desquamative Gingivitis and Acute Gingival Infections' for a more detailed section on NUG.

◂ *What is NUG? What was its earlier name?*

◂ *Why must AIDS be ruled out if NUG/NUP have been diagnosed?*

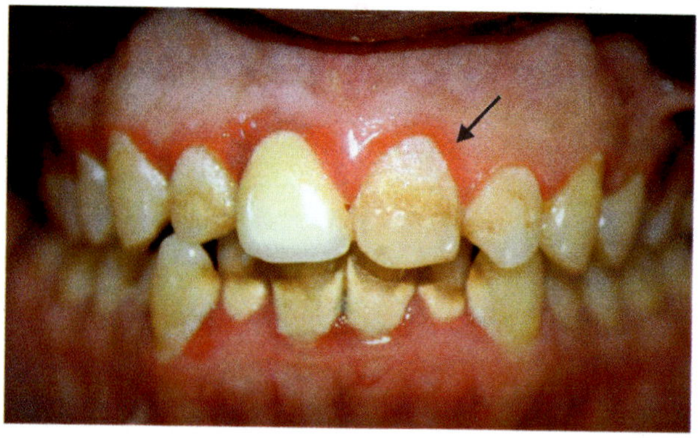

Fig. 8.5: Linear gingival erythema (*HIV gingivitis*)

What is NUP? ▶

c. **Necrotizing Ulcerative Periodontitis** (*NUP*) is a necrotizing, ulcerative, rapidly progressing and destructive type of periodontitis.
   - It is rarely seen in the normal individuals but is frequently seen in patients in advanced stage of AIDS (*with severe immune deficiency* and *very low CD4 T-lymphocyte counts*). NUP may arise from worsening of NUG.
   - It is characterized by extremely painful lesions, rapid destruction and sequestration of alveolar bone and gingival necrosis.

   NUP is treated by scaling and root planing, local irrigation using antimicrobial agents, e.g. chlorhexidine and povidone-iodine followed by oral hygiene maintenance. Healed NUP lesions usually leave behind deep interproximal craters in gingiva.

What is NUS? ▶

d. **Necrotizing Ulcerative Stomatitis** (*NUS*) is a rare destructive disease of oral and peri-oral tissues that causes painful lesions that affect large areas that may also involve underlying alveolar bone. It is generally reported in individuals with either severe immune deficiency or severe chronic malnutrition, e.g. patients of AIDS having very low CD4 T-lymphocyte counts. NUS may lead to NUP. Management of NUS is similar to that of NUP.

e. **Severe and complicated periodontitis** is common in individuals with AIDS. It can worsen to NUP. As long as clinical and systemic condition (*immunity*) of an HIV infected individual remains normal, periodontal health can be easily maintained with routine oral hygiene measures and periodontal treatment. Such an individual can also receive dental implants.

What is Kaposi's sarcoma? ▶
What is the clinical implication of oral Kaposi's sarcoma? ▶

f. **Kaposi's sarcoma** is a ***rare*** tumor of blood vessels of skin. It, if present, in the oral cavity is pathognomonic of AIDS (*its presence means that patient has AIDS*). Kaposi's sarcoma usually occurs on the palate or gingiva. In its early stages, oral Kaposi's sarcoma appears as painless, reddish-purple macules. Later, the lesions become nodular. Patients suffering from AIDS also have chance of developing other oral malignancies, like oral squamous cell carcinoma.

When does oral candidiasis occur? ▶
How many types of oral candidiasis lesions are there? ▶

g. **Candidiasis** is caused by *Candida albicans* and is an ***opportunistic*** fungal infection. Candidiasis can occur if an individual is taking ***broad spectrum antibacterial*** (*antibiotic*) for a long time. It can also occur if an individual's immunity is lowered, e.g. after taking ***immune suppressants*** (*steroids and anti-graft rejection medications*). When oral candidiasis appears without these causes, a clinician should explore the possibility of ***HIV infection.*** Oral candidiasis may be present in any of its four clinical types: pseudomembranous, erythematous, hyperplastic candidiasis or angular cheilitis.

What causes oral hairy leukoplakia and where does it cccur? ▶

h. **Oral hairy leukoplakia** is caused by Epstein-Barr virus. It usually occurs bilaterally on lateral borders of ***tongue***. It appears as a poorly demarcated keratotic (*white*) area that does not rub off and has a corrugated appearance. When dried, these lesions look 'hairy', due vertical striations in them.

7. COVID-19 and its Effect on Oral Tissues and Periodontium

Coronavirus disease (*COVID-19*) is an infectious disease caused by the novel corona virus (*nCoV*). Most individuals infected with nCoV (*COVID-19*) experience only mild-to-moderate respiratory illness and recover without extensive treatment and hospitalization. Whereas old individuals and/or those with underlying systemic problems, like diabetes, cardiovascular disease, chronic respiratory disease, cancer, etc. may develop serious illness due to COVID-19.

◂ Which oral lesions are found in patients with COVID-19?

Although lungs are the primary site of involvement by COVID-19, oral lesions have also been reported in patients hospitalized patients with severe COVID-19. Oral manifestations include xerostomia, petechiae, candidiasis, geographic tongue, non-specific ulcerations, ***gingivostomatitis*** presenting as recurrent herpes simplex lesions on lips, multiple irregular ulcers with red-yellowish halo on palate and tongue, etc. As many patients are treated with high doses of systemic steroids, some such patients develop mucormycosis infection (*black fungus*) (*fungal infection of jawbones, sinuses, eyes, brain, etc.*). It is only treatable if it is diagnosed early and therefore results in death in a significant number of patients.

SECTION 2: PERIODONTAL (*ORAL*) DISEASES CONTRIBUTING TO AND AGGRAVATING SYSTEMIC DISEASES AND CONDITIONS (*PERIODONTAL MEDICINE*)

◂ How does the periodontium act like a focus of infection?

The periodontium, *especially gingiva, sulci and pockets* that may be healthy or clinically infected (*gingivitis, periodontitis or periodontal abscesses*) act like reservoirs of bacteria and their endotoxins. Chewing, massaging of gingiva, routine daily oral hygiene measures like tooth brushing and scaling and root planing causes bacteria and their toxins to be pushed from the pockets into the blood stream resulting in bacteremia and endotoxemia (*toxemia resulting from circulating endotoxins of bacteria*). The number of circulating bacteria and concentration of endotoxin in blood of individuals suffering from periodontitis is more than ***four*** times greater than in those with healthy periodontiums. Periodontium thus acts as a ***focus of infection***.

CLINICAL UTILITY AND SHORT ANSWER

What is a focus of infection?

Definition: A focus of infection is localized area of infection in an individual's body that is usually hidden and presents ***no*** apparent clinical features.

◂ How does a focus of infection cause disease at other sites of the body?

- Microorganisms and their toxins leak out of the focus of infection via blood stream and reach different tissues within the individual's own body and cause infection at these distant sites.
- Immune-inflammatory response against such infection results in tissue damage at these sites. This can lead to severe damage to body organs leading to their dysfunction.
- Arthritis, narrowing of arteries of the heart (atherosclerosis), pre-term labor, low birth weight babies, cancer, mental illness, etc. are believed to be caused in some part by such infections (*whose source is from foci of infection elsewhere in the body*).

Oral Foci of Infection can Cause Myocardial Infarctions, Cerebral Strokes and Atherosclerosis

Research has found that oral foci of infection including periodontitis (*especially untreated periodontitis deep pockets*) can act like etiological and predisposing factors for myocardial infarctions (*heart attacks*), ischaemic cerebral strokes (*brain attack*) and atherosclerosis (*obstructions in blood vessels of tissues and organs*). This can happen in the following ways:

1. **By causing formation of thrombus by platelets**

◂ What is a thrombus? How does it form?

   - Platelets bind to circulating oral bacteria (*e.g. S. sanguis, P. gingivalis, etc.*) in the blood stream and form a lump. If a big lump of aggregated platelets called thrombus forms, it can block blood vessels and thus obstruct blood flow to tissues supplied by that blood vessel.

◂ What is a thromboembolism?

   - If such a thrombus starts to circulate in the blood (*thromboembolism*) it can get stuck in a blood vessel of smaller diameter at a distant site from its place of origin. This

How are thrombus and thromboembolism harmful? ▶

causes reduction or stopping of blood supply to the area supplied by the vessel. Reduction or complete stopping of blood supply causes death of local tissue and organ damage (*ischaemic damage*).

- If this event happens in the heart, it causes heart attacks and if it happens in the brain, it causes ischaemic cerebral strokes.

How does bacteraemia increase viscosity of blood? How is it harmful? ▶

2. **By increasing viscosity of blood:** In response to bacteremia (*very high number of bacteria circulating blood*), leukocytosis occurs (*increase in number of circulating WBCs in the blood to counter this bacteremia*). This causes increased blood viscosity (*increased thickness of blood*). Increased viscosity of blood increases chances of thrombus formation and resultant vessel blockage.

How can oral infections increase chances of thrombus formation? ▶

3. **By increasing coagulability of blood:** Bacteremia originating from oral foci of infections can lead to increase in fibrinogen and other blood coagulation factors in blood. This increases coagulability of blood and chances of thrombus formation.

How can oral infections lead to formation of atherosclerotic plaques? ▶

4. **By formation of atherosclerotic plaques:** Atherosclerotic plaques cause narrowing of blood vessels and thickening of vessel walls leading to reduction in blood supply to the areas these vessely supply. Several factors related to oral microorganisms that are circulating in the blood can cause atherosclerosis [e.g. *bacterial lipopolysaccharides, prostaglandins, tumor necrosis factor alpha (TNF-α), interleukin-l (IL-l), etc.*].

ALERT!

What are cerebral strokes?

Cerebral strokes (*cerebro-vascular accidents*) are caused by sudden death of a part of the brain due to an abrupt disruption of its blood supply that may occur due to a blocked artery (*ischaemic stroke*) or bursting of a blood vessel (*haemorrhagic stroke*).

- Ischaemic cerebral strokes are often preceded by systemic bacterial or viral infection about ***one week before*** the stroke. Recent infection is now considered a significant risk factor for cerebral ischaemic strokes.
- Periodontitis and infected periapical lesions are predisposing factors for cerebral strokes. They are believed to be as important risk factors for stroke as smoking.
- Such infections contribute to formation of atherosclerotic plaques by producing a mild but continuous bacteremia that can cause platelet aggregation in the vessels and produces an inflammatory response in the blood vessel walls (*as discussed above*).
- Treatment of periodontitis is very important for this reason also.

Untreated Gingivitis and Periodontitis Worsen Diabetes Mellitus

How does periodontitis complicate management of diabetes? ▶

As has been discussed in previous sections of this chapter, diabetes can predispose to and worsen periodontitis. It is now well-known that the reverse relation also exists between periodontitis and diabetes, i.e. ***periodontitis can worsen diabetes*** of a diabetic individual. This can happen due to:

- Systemic infection (*bacteremia*) arising from periodontitis is known to increase tissue resistance to insulin (*prevent uptake of glucose by body's cells*), **both** in individuals with and without diabetes leading to persistent high blood glucose levels.
- When systemic infections occur in individuals with type 2 diabetes (*who already have high tissue resistance to insulin*) an additional increase in insulin resistance occurs. This ***worsens*** an individual's glycemic control and blood glucose levels. Such patients require more medication and diet control to keep blood glucose levels in control.
- Treatment of periodontitis reduces bacterial load and systemic bacteremia. Periodontal treatment thus improves insulin sensitivity in diabetic individuals over time.

Untreated Gingivitis and Periodontitis can Lead to Pre-term Labor and Low Birth Weight Babies

As discussed above, any systemic infection either through bacteremia or circulating by-products of bacteria and other microorganisms has the capacity of damaging body tissues.

How does periodontitis affect outcome of pregnancy? ▶

- Periodontal infection caused bacteremia sends bacteria like *P. gingivalis* etc. into circulation.
- If these bacteria settle in a pregnant uterus, they induce release of pro-inflammatory molecules like *TNF-β, PGE2*, etc. in the uterus. This makes the uterine muscles very

sensitive. This can result in pre-mature cervical dilatation, rupture of membranes and uterine muscle contractions, all of which lead to pre-mature labor and pre-term births and low birth weight babies (*less than 2.5 kg*).

Untreated Gingivitis and Periodontitis can Cause Chronic Obstructive Respiratory Disease

Chronic obstructive respiratory disease, e.g. chronic bronchitis or emphysema causes obstruction in respiratory passages causing restricted airflow. This obstruction is caused by enlargement of bronchial mucous glands and chronic inflammation.

◄ *How does periodontitis cause bronchitis?*

- Chief causes of chronic inflammation in chronic obstructive respiratory disease are smoking, respiratory tract infections caused by periodontal (*oral*), nasal and pharyngeal microorganisms that are transported into the respiratory tract.
- Individuals with poor oral hygiene and severe periodontitis are at a higher risk of developing chronic obstructive respiratory disease.
- Medical literature suggests that patients of chronic obstructive respiratory disease benefit immensely when their periodontitis is treated.

Review Questions

1. Name systemic diseases and conditions that affect periodontal health.
2. Write oral manifestations of diabetes.
3. How does diabetes affect periodontitis? Why do poorly controlled diabetics have more susceptibility to infections?
4. How does periodontitis complicate diabetes?
5. How do sex hormones affect periodontium?
6. How do corticosteroid hormones affect the periodontium?
7. Can osteoporosis be diagnosed by blood levels of calcium?
8. What is the effect of chronic liver disease on periodontium?
9. How do blood disorders affect periodontitis? Describe gingival enlargement in leukaemic patients.
10. What is agranulocytosis? How does it affect periodontal health?
11. How does psychological stress and malnutrition affect periodontal health?
12. How does vitamin D deficiency affect the periodontium?
13. What is acquired immunodeficiency syndrome (*AIDS*)? Describe periodontal disease in patients of AIDS.
14. What is a focus of infection?
15. How does periodontitis complicate pregnancy?
16. Discuss the two-way relation between periodontitis and diabetes.
17. How does periodontitis cause and affect chronic obstructive respiratory disease?

Chapter

9

Trauma from Occlusion, Bone Loss and Pathologic Migration

How much load can human teeth withstand? ▶

What is the clinical diagnosis if enlarged PDL is seen in a radiograph? ▶

Human teeth can withstand very high occlusal forces that range from 100 N (*Newton*) (*10 kg*) in the incisor region to 1000 N (*100 kg*) in the molars. This maximum occlusal load is generated only for a very small-time during mastication. Actual average occlusal forces of mastication are only about 150 N or 15 kg. If an individual has higher occlusal forces, the periodontium hypertrophies, i.e. adapts itself by remodeling (*number of PDL fibers increase, lamina dura and PDL space widen*) to be able to bear high occlusal forces thereby preventing injury to the periodontium. The periodontium atrophies when overall occlusal forces decrease (*number of PDL fibers decrease, lamina dura and PDL space become narrower*).

TRAUMA FROM OCCLUSION (*TFO*)

What is TFO? ▶

Definition: If occlusal forces exceed load bearing capacity of the periodontium, it causes injury in the periodontium. This ***injury*** in the periodontium is called trauma from occlusion (*TFO*).

What is the difference between traumatic occlusion and TFO? ▶

Traumatic occlusion: The ***occlusion*** that produces TFO is called traumatic occlusion.

Classification of TFO

TFO can be classified in two ways:

1. **According to duration and severity of occlusal force**

What is acute TFO? ▶

   a. **Acute TFO:** When very high occlusal forces are ***suddenly*** put on teeth for a ***short duration***, e.g. biting over a very hard object, 'high' restorations and prostheses, orthodontic appliances that put excessively high force on teeth, etc.

What is chronic TFO? ▶ *What is the difference between acute and chronic TFO?* ▶ *Which is more common, acute or chronic TFO?* ▶

   b. **Chronic TFO:** When high occlusal forces are put on teeth for a ***long period*** of time, e.g. clenching, movement of teeth into unfavorable positions leading to higher occlusal forces on teeth (*orthodontic movement or pathologic migration*). Chronic TFO is ***more common*** than acute TFO.

2. **According to magnitude and direction of occlusal force in relation to condition of the periodontium**

   a. **Primary TFO:**

What is primary TFO? ▶

      - When TFO results from ***excessive*** occlusal forces exerted on normal periodontium, e.g. TFO resulting after a high restoration in a tooth with normal periodontium, orthodontic movement of teeth into positions resulting in excessive occlusal stresses on them, etc. **(Figs 9.1, 9.2, 9.3 and 9.8)**.

Is primary TFO acute or chronic? ▶

      - Primary TFO can be ***acute or chronic***.

   b. **Secondary:**

What is secondary TFO? ▶

      - When TFO results from ***reduced ability*** of the periodontium to withstand even 'normal' occlusal forces, e.g. teeth with ***periodontal* (bone) *loss*** (*due to periodontitis*) **(Figs 9.1, 9.2 and 9.8)**.

Is secondary TFO acute or chronic? ▶ *What is the difference between primary and secondary TFO?* ▶

      - ***Secondary TFO is usually chronic***, however acute TFO (*periodontal injury*) can occur if very high occlusal force is suddenly put on teeth with reduced periodontal support.

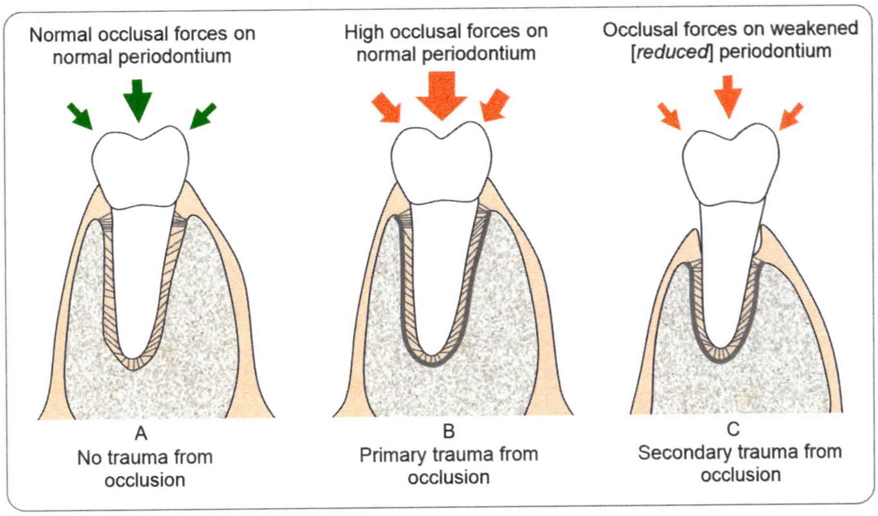

Fig. 9.1: Primary and secondary TFO

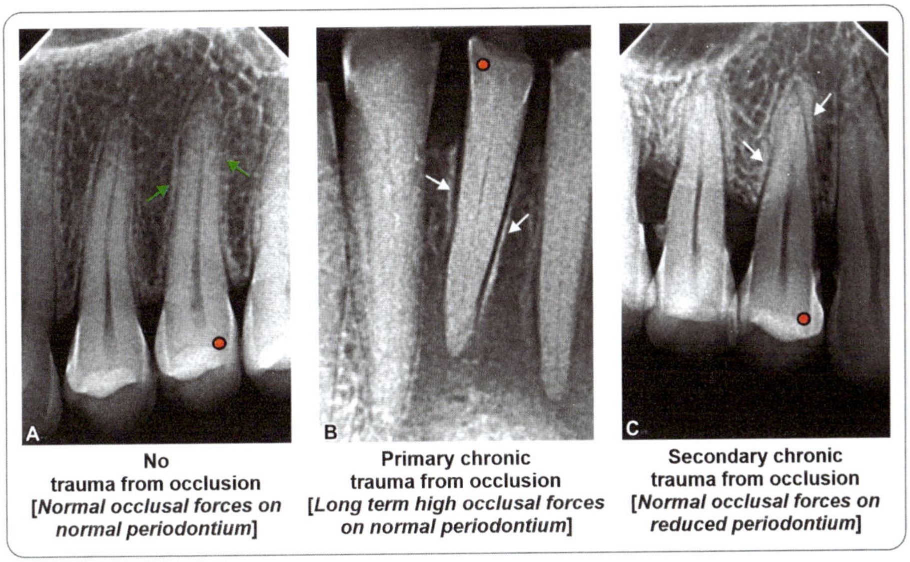

Fig. 9.2: Primary (*diag. B*) and secondary TFO (*diag. C*) in teeth marked with red dots. TFO is diagnosed by a wider periodontal ligament and thick lamina dura (*white arrows and white line diags B and C*). Normal periodontal ligament and lamina dura are relatively thinner (*green arrows, diag. A*).

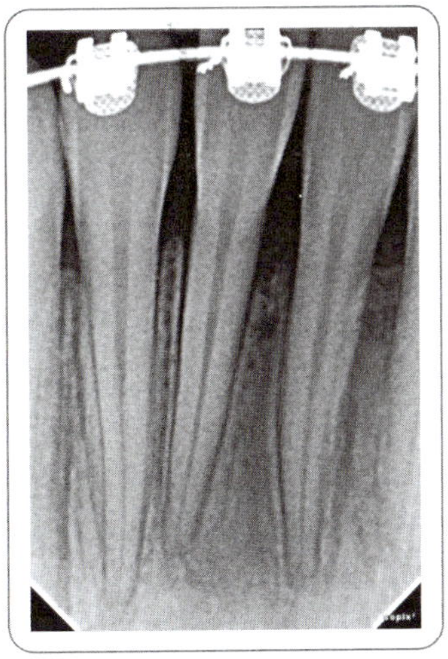

Fig. 9.3: Primary acute trauma from occlusion in a patient undergoing active orthodontic movement. Note enlarged PDL.

Clinical Features of TFO

Can features of TFO increase or decrease in severity? ▸

Clinical features of TFO can vary in different patients and in different teeth in the same patient. If occlusal forces are reduced, TFO will decrease and continue in a ***chronic*** (***milder***) form or may subside completely. The clinical features of TFO are:

What are the clinical features of TFO? ▸

1. ***Pain*** and ***tenderness*** in:
   a. Affected teeth (*due to inflammation in periodontal ligament*).
   b. Muscles of mastication (*especially in temple region and on sides of mandible*). This is commonly seen in cases where TFO is due to bruxism.
   c. Temporo-mandibular joints (*TM joints*).
2. ***Increased mobility*** in involved teeth.
3. ***Attrition*** (*excessive*) of incisal and occlusal surfaces of teeth (Fig. 9.5, diags B and C) and abfraction cavities (Figs 9.5. diag. D).

Why do teeth with TFO become hypersensitive and non-vital? ▸

4. ***Hypersensitivity*** to cold and hot foods in the affected teeth. This happens when inflammation extends from PDL into pulp (*via apical foramen or accessory canals*).
5. Teeth can become ***non-vital***. This happens if vessels supplying the pulp of the tooth get damaged due to very high occlusal forces.
6. Radiographic features:

What are the radiographic features of TFO? ▸

   a. ***Widening of periodontal ligament and lamina dura*** (Fig. 9.2, diags B and C).
   b. ***Funneling of tooth socket*** (Figs 9.4 and 9.8).
   c. Increased thickness and radiopacity of alveolar bone trabeculae.
   d. Change in direction and orientation of bone trabeculae.

What causes change in position of a tooth? ▸

7. ***Drifting*** or ***pathologic migration:*** If traumatic occlusal forces remain for a long period of time, it can lead to change in position of the tooth (*tooth shifts to a new position where occlusal forces are lesser*) (Fig. 9.16) (*pathologic migration is described in detail later in this Chapter*).
8. ***Acute*** TFO can cause:
   a. Cemental tears
   b. Necrosis in periodontal ligament.
   c. Abscess formation in periodontal ligament.

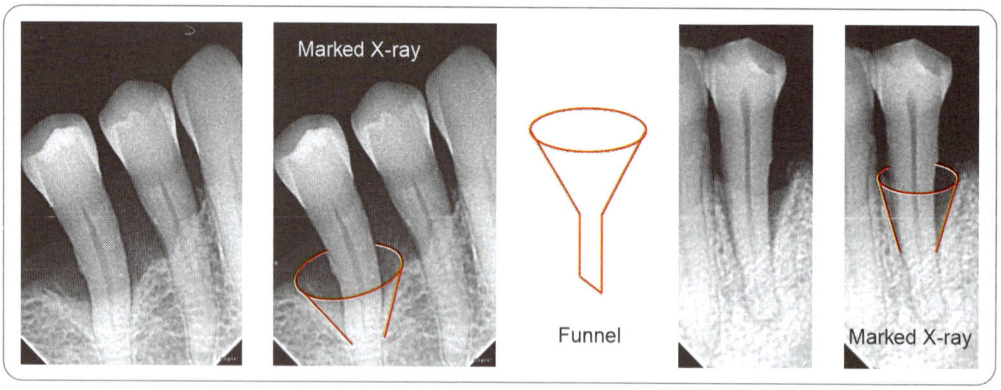

Fig. 9.4: Funneling of socket in TFO (*red marking*) is classical sign of chronic TFO

Stages of TFO

What are the stages of TFO? ▸

If high (*traumatic*) occlusal forces are put on teeth, the periodontium responds to them in ***three*** distinct stages:

Stage I: Injury; Stage II: Repair; Stage III: Adaptive remodeling.

What is the first stage of TFO? ▸

Stage I: Injury

Which periodontal tissue does not get affected by traumatic occlusal force? ▸

- Injury occurs because high occlusal forces exceed load bearing capacity of periodontium. Injury is seen in alveolar bone, PDL and cementum. ***Gingiva*** is ***not*** affected by traumatic occlusal force; it therefore shows no features of TFO.
- High occlusal force causes areas of increased ***pressure*** and ***tension*** within the periodontium.

- **Increased pressure** causes:
  - ***Resorption*** of alveolar bone. In extreme cases tooth resorption may also be seen.
  - Compression of blood vessels which results in reduced blood supply to periodontal tissues; this is the chief cause of injury due to TFO.
  - Elongation and compression of periodontal ligament fibers.
- **Excessive tension** (*stretching/pulling*) occurs as a result of high occlusal force. It causes stretching of PDL fibers. While normal tension results in formation, excessive tension results in:
  - ***Resorption*** of alveolar bone.
  - Pulling and tearing of walls of blood vessels leading to hemorrhage in PDL.
  - Tearing and breaking of PDL fibers.

◂ *What does increased pressure on the periodontal tissues result in?*

◂ *What effect does normal tension on periodontal fibers have on alveolar bone?*

◂ *What does increased tension on the periodontal fibers result in?*

CLINICAL UTILITY AND SHORT ANSWER

Which area of the periodontium/teeth is the most susceptible to injury by traumatic occlusal force?

Periodontium of furcation area of multi-rooted teeth is the most susceptible to injury by traumatic occlusal forces (*TFO*).

Stage II: Repair

- Repair activity in periodontium is significantly increased after injury (*TFO*).
- For this, resorptive cells of the periodontium, i.e. osteoclasts, cementoclasts and fibroblasts first remove damaged tissue.
- The formative cells, i.e. osteoblasts, cementoblasts, fibroblasts then lay down new periodontal tissue to increase load bearing capacity of alveolar bone, PDL and cementum. As ***gingiva*** is ***not*** affected by traumatic occlusal force; it shows no features of TFO.

◂ *What is the second stage of TFO?*

◂ *Which periodontal tissue does not show increased repair after injury by traumatic occlusal force?*

Stage III: Adaptive Remodeling

If TFO (*injury in the periodontium*) continues and the existing periodontal tissues are unable to bear higher occlusal forces, the periodontium then adapts itself by increasing its load bearing capacity to prevent further injury. This occurs by:

i. ***Widening*** of periodontal ligament (Fig. 9.2, diag. B and C white arrows)
ii. ***Thickening*** of lamina dura
iii. Thickening of cementum (*microscopic*).
iv. Formation of reinforcing new bone (*buttressing of alveolar bone*) to reinforce existing alveolar bone. If the reinforcing bone forms within the jaws, it is called ***central buttressing***. If reinforcing bone forms on facial and lingual/palatal alveolar cortical bone plates it is called ***peripheral buttressing***.
  Peripheral buttressing may produce a 'shelf' like enlargement of the alveolar bone margin called '***lipping***' (*more commonly seen on facial side*) (Fig. 9.5, diag. B).

After repair and adaptive remodeling, periodontium becomes stronger and can now bear increased occlusal forces better. Due to this, high occlusal forces now do not cause TFO (*injury in the periodontium*).

◂ *What is the third stage of TFO?*

◂ *What is adaptive remodeling?*

◂ *What are the features of adaptive remodeling?*

◂ *What is buttressing bone formation?*

◂ *What is central buttressing bone formation?*

◂ *What is peripheral buttressing bone formation?*

◂ *What is lipping?*

◂ *Can periodontium bear increased occlusal forces better after repair and adaptive remodeling?*

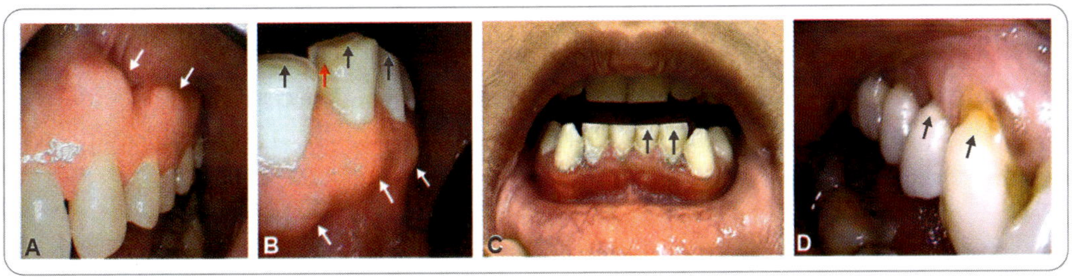

Fig. 9.5: Bone exostosis (*diag. A, white arrows*) and lipping (*peripheral buttressing*) of alveolar bone crest (*diag. B, white arrows*) in a patient of chronic TFO (*bruxism*). Presence of prominent wear facets, incisal and occlusal attrition (*diags B and C, black arrows*), tooth fracture (*diag. B, red arrow*), abfraction cavities (*diag. D, black arrows*) are other signs of TFO.

CLINICAL UTILITY AND SHORT ANSWER

Can we know stage of TFO clinically? ▸

Can the three stages of TFO (*injury, repair and remodeling*) be differentiated clinically?

The three stages of TFO are overlapping. Pain and tenderness may be present in the first stage (*injury*) of TFO, other than this, there is ***no*** fool proof way to differentiate these stages ***clinically***.

CLINICAL UTILITY AND SHORT ANSWER

What is the difference between torus and peripheral buttressing of alveolar bone?

What is a torus? ▸

Torus (*plural: tori*): It is a round bony outgrowth apical to crest of the alveolar bone. Tori is usually present on the lingual/palatal sides. Mandibular tori are more common than palatal tori.

Peripheral buttressing (*strengthening*) of alveolar bone strengthens the bone and causes lipping or formation of a distinct bulge in the contour of the alveolar bone crest. They are more commonly seen on the facial sides of both the jaws. Tori, Lipping and bulging of the crest of alveolar bone are caused by TFO.

TFO is Reversible

Is TFO reversible? ▸

TFO (*damage and injury in the periodontium*) is reversible. It can happen in two situations:

When can TFO reverse? ▸

1. If occlusal forces are reduced to 'normal' (*come within load bearing capacity of periodontium*).
2. If periodontal tissues (*alveolar bone, PDL and cementum*) are strengthened by adaptive remodeling (*hypertrophy*). This will enable periodontal tissues to easily bear high occlusal forces being put on the tooth without producing injury and damage (*i.e. without producing TFO*).

There is however a ***limit*** to such repair and adaptive remodeling of periodontal tissues by hypertrophy. If for some reason, high occlusal forces persist and the periodontium cannot further strengthen itself by continued reinforcement (*hypertrophy*), periodontal damage, i.e. TFO will worsen.

CLINICAL UTILITY AND SHORT ANSWER

What is the role of malocclusion in TFO? ▸

Does malocclusion always result in TFO?

No, malocclusion does ***not*** always cause TFO. Teeth in any dentition keep adjusting to occlusal forces over time. TFO results if occlusal forces increase suddenly or if periodontium of such misplaced teeth becomes weakened due to periodontal pathology, e.g. bone loss due to periodontitis.

Does crowding of teeth always cause TFO? ▸

From the ***periodontal point of view, any dentition that can be maintained in a reasonably clean and plaque free state and one which does not cause TFO is normal*** (*despite teeth being crowded, etc.*).

BONE LOSS IN PERIODONTITIS, FORMATION OF INFRABONY POCKETS AND ROLE OF TRAUMA FROM OCCLUSION IN THESE

How is mass and height of alveolar bone maintained? ▸

Balance between bone destruction (*resorption*) and formation of new bone maintains the height and density of alveolar bone. Amount of bone loss can be known by assessing the relative position of level of crest of interdental bone with respect to the CE junction of adjoining teeth (*interdental bone is easily visible in IOPA radiographs*). For knowing how to do this, the reader is referred to Chapter 3, 'Periodontal ligament, Cementum and Alveolar bone' (***Figs 3.12 and 3.13***).

What Causes Loss of Alveolar Bone during Periodontal Disease?

Alveolar bone loss can occur due to reduction of height of bone crest or loss of bone mass. ***Height*** of alveolar bone is reduced due to:

What are the reasons for loss of height of alveolar bone? ▸

1. Periodontitis
   - Conversion of gingivitis to periodontitis.
   - Worsening of ongoing periodontitis.
2. TFO
   - Loss of bone height occurs ***without*** increase in pocket depth (*progression of periodontitis*).
3. Combination of periodontitis and TFO.

Bone mass of alveolar bone can be lost due to:

1. Osteoporosis (*loss of bone mass*) can occur due to calcium deficiency, vit. D deficiency, systemic illnesses, long term steroid medication, etc. These diseases and conditions do not cause loss of height of bone; rather, in all such cases, ***loss of bone height*** will ***only*** occur as a result of ***periodontitis***.
2. Specific pathologies, e.g. abscess, tumors, etc.

◂ *What are the usual reasons for loss of bone mass?*

◂ *Can loss of alveolar bone height occur due to osteoporosis?*

ALERT!

- Bone loss seen in radiographs is indicative of ***past disease*** activity. Such loss of alveolar bone height does ***not*** automatically suggest ongoing periodontitis.
- On the other hand, ***changes in the gingiva, are indicative of the present-day*** health status of the periodontium.

◂ *What does height of bone as seen in a radiograph signify?*

Why and How Vertical (Angular) Bone Loss Occurs and Infrabony Pockets form (*Why Vertical Bone Loss Occurs at Some Sites While at Other Sites Horizontal Bone Loss Occurs*)

In periodontitis, bone loss (*loss of height of alveolar bone crest*) occurs in ***two*** patterns: ***horizontal*** and ***vertical***. In horizontal bone loss, alveolar bone crest is horizontal and suprabony pocket forms **(Fig. 9.12)**. In vertical bone loss, bone crest is angular and an infrabony pocket forms **(Fig. 9.11)**. *See section on Types of bone defects (bone loss patterns) seen in periodontal disease, presented later in this Chapter and Section on 'Pockets' in Chapter 10, page 138*).

◂ *Name the two patterns of loss of height of bone crest.*

In ***most*** cases, ***horizontal bone loss*** is seen whereas, vertical bone loss is seen at some sites only. To explain why some sites have horizontal while some other sites have vertical bone loss, ***three*** viewpoints have been popular. These are:

◂ *Which of the two, horizontal or vertical bone loss is more common?*

I. *Glickman's Concept*

- Glickman suggested that formation of horizontal and vertical (*angular*) interdental bone defects (*loss*) is dependent on the path taken by periodontitis induced inflammation to reach and ***enter*** the interdental bone crest.
- He believed that if inflammation travelling along blood vessels and transseptal fibers enters in the center of the interdental bone crest, horizontal bone loss occurs. If on the other hand, TFO causes change in the angulation of transseptal fibers, it leads to channeling of inflammation into the side of the interdental bone crest thus resulting in vertical (*angular*) bone loss in the interdental crest.

◂ *What is Glickman's concept of formation of angular bone loss?*

II. *Waerhaug's Concept*

- Waerhaug found ***no*** role of TFO in vertical (*angular*) interdental bone loss.
- Waerhaug however suggested two ***pre-requisites*** to explain formation of vertical defects:
  i. Presence of plaque micro-organisms at a more apical level
  ii. Presence of larger volume of, i.e. ***thicker*** alveolar bone.
- According to Waerhaug's concept, vertical (*angular*) bone loss occurs in the ***same way*** as horizontal bone loss; however, when alveolar bone septum is wide, plaque induced inflammation cannot destroy the entire width of the alveolar bone septum. This results in vertical (*angular*) bone defect/loss (*and infrabony pockets*).

◂ *What is Waerhaug's concept about reasons for vertical bone loss?*

◂ *What is the basic necessity for vertical bone loss according to Waerhaug's concept?*

ALERT!

Today it is clear that traumatic occlusion does ***not*** cause vertical (*angular*) interdental bone loss. In fact, it can also ***not*** cause deepening of pockets (*apical shift of junctional epithelium i.e. loss of connective tissue attachment*). It can however cause widening of mouth of the tooth's socket (*funneling*). This funneling can ***appear*** like angular bone loss in some radiographs **(Fig. 9.4)**.

III. *The Radius of Action Concept*

What is the radius of action concept? ▶

What is the bone resorptive range of action of plaque colonies? ▶

Why partial and angular destruction of alveolar bone septum is seen only if bone septum is more than 2.5 mm wide? ▶

How does radius of action concept explain formation of vertical bone defects? ▶

To explain why vertical (*angular*) bone loss and infrabony pockets occur only in a few cases (*of the so many individuals having periodontitis*), a very good explanation called 'Radius of action concept' has been given by Garant and Cho (*1979*) **(Fig. 9.6)**.

- According to this concept, plaque bacteria have a ***bone resorptive range of action*** of only ***1.5–2.5 mm*** from edge of the plaque colony (**Fig. 9.6** *red circles*), ***beyond this distance, bacterial colonies cannot cause bone destruction.***
- Therefore, bone tissue of the interdental septum that is up to 2.5 mm away from the edge of the plaque colony can get resorbed while, bone tissue of the same interdental septum that is more than 2.5 mm away from the edge of plaque colony will not show any resorption **(Fig. 9.6, diags B–D′)**.
- Consequently, we will see ***partial and angular (vertical) destruction*** of alveolar bone septum (*angular bone loss and infra bony pocket*) due to bone destroying effect of a plaque colony located on the same side as the angular bone loss ***only if an alveolar bone septum is more than 2.5 mm wide*** **(Fig. 9.6, diags B–D′)**.

  This is how angular destruction of bone septum results and vertical bone defects infrabony pockets form.

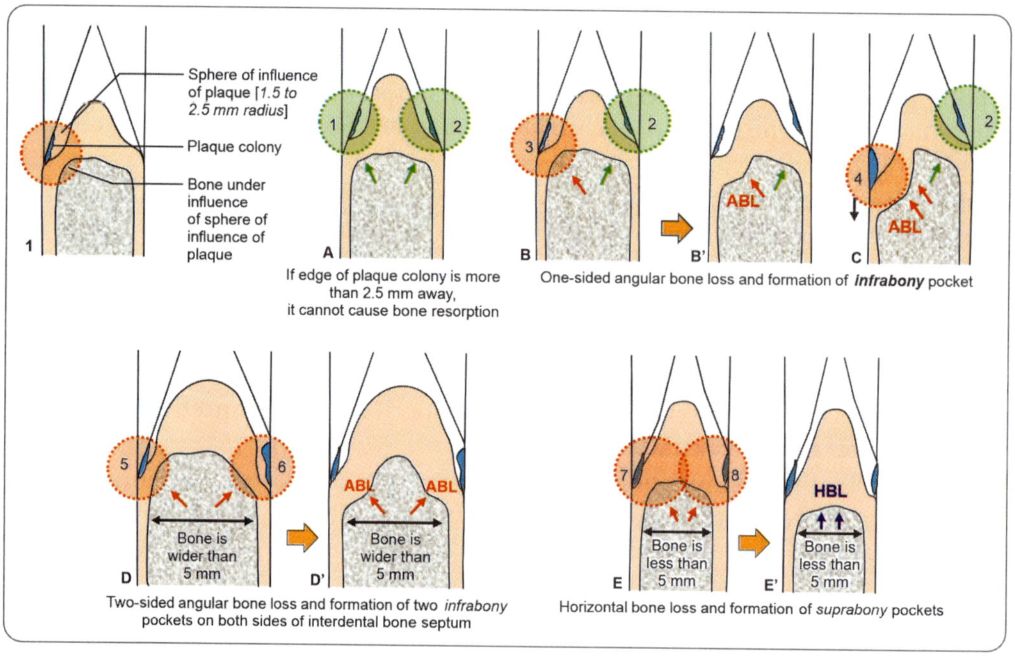

Fig. 9.6: The 'Radius of action' concept. A colony of plaque can cause bone resorption (*red circle*) only up to a distance of 1.5 to 2.5 mm from edge of the plaque colony (*diag. 1*). If plaque colony is more than 2.5 mm from crest of the alveolar bone (*green circles*), bone resorption will not occur (*green arrows*) (*diag. A, B and C*). Bone resorption occurs when plaque colony shifts apically and lies within 2.5 mm from bone crest (*red circles*) (*diag. B*).
Vertical (angular) bone loss and infrabony pocket formation is depicted in diagrams A, B, B′, C, D and D′. If a plaque colony is located only on one side and less than 2.5 mm from the interdental bone, resorptive influence of plaque will cause vertical (*angular*) bone loss (*ABL*) on the same side (*red circle 3 and red arrows, diag. B and B′*). As plaque colony shifts further apically (*red circle 4, diag. C*), vertical bone loss and depth of infrabony pocket increases (*red arrows, diag. C*). If two plaque colonies are present less than 2.5 mm from bone on both sides of an interdental septum that is ***more*** than 5 mm wide (*red circles 5 and 6, diag. D and D′*), they will cause two angular (*vertical*) bone loss defects and infrabony pocket formation on each side of the interdental septum (*red arrows, diag. D and D′*).
Horizontal bone loss and suprabony pocket formation is depicted in diagrams E and E′. If two plaque colonies are present on either side of interdental bone that is ***less*** than 5 mm wide and each of them is less than 2.5 mm from the bone (*red circles 7 and 8, diag. E*), they will exert overlapping spheres of influence and cause overlapping bone resorption on both sides of the interdental bone (*red arrows, diag. E and E′*). This will lead to horizontal bone loss (*HBL*) and formation of suprabony pockets on either side of the interdental septum (*blue arrows, diag. E′*).

- Formation of ***horizontal defects*** can also be explained by this concept easily. If a combined two-sided attack (*i.e. from both mesial and distal sides*) by plaque bacteria occurs in an interdental bone septum that is narrower than 2.5 mm, it will show bone loss on both mesial and distal sides. This will produce two bone loss defects on both sides. As the two get combined, a horizontal bone loss pattern and suprabony pocket results (Fig. 9.6, diags E and E').
- As interdental septum in anterior teeth is seldom wider than 2.5 mm, the entire bone crest gets resorbed this way and horizontal bone loss is usually seen. Angular (*vertical*) defects are therefore ***not*** seen in the anterior region (Fig. 9.6, diags E and E').

◄ *How does radius of action concept explain formation of horizontal bone defects?*

◄ *Why are vertical defects not seen in anterior teeth?*

Rate of Loss of Alveolar Bone

(*in active phase of periodontitis*)

Many factors, e.g. genetic, immunity, level of oral hygiene, systemic health, etc. affect the rate of loss of alveolar bone during ongoing periodontitis. As these factors can act singly or collectively, accurate assessment of the rate of bone loss due to periodontitis is very difficult.

- Loe *et al* (1986) found that ***0.2–0.3 mm*** height of alveolar bone is lost ***every year*** in ***untreated*** grade A and B periodontitis (*chronic periodontitis*).
- Rate of bone loss is more in complicated cases of periodontitis and in grade C periodontitis (*aggressive periodontitis*).

◄ *Which factors affect rate of bone loss*

◄ *How much loss of bone height occurs during periodontitis?*

CLINICAL UTILITY AND SHORT ANSWER

What is the rate of loss of attachment (*true pocket formation*) in periodontitis?

- Loss of attachment (*true pocket formation*) occurs ***6–8 months before*** alveolar bone resorption occurs.
- Rate of loss of attachment (*true pocket formation*) is ***similar*** to the rate of loss of alveolar bone, i.e. pocket depth increases by ***0.2–0.3 mm every year*** in untreated cases of periodontitis.
- Rate of loss of attachment (*true pocket formation*) has been estimated to be about ***1–3 µ/day*** in grade A and B periodontitis (*chronic periodontitis*).
- Rate of loss of attachment (*true pocket formation*) increases to ***3–5 µ/day*** in grade C periodontitis (*aggressive periodontitis*); which is ***3–5 times*** more than the rate of attachment loss in grade A and B periodontitis (*chronic periodontitis*).

◄ *Which occurs earlier, loss of attachment or bone loss?*

◄ *What is the rate of formation/deepening of true pockets in periodontitis?*

CLINICAL UTILITY AND SHORT ANSWER

Do systemic diseases and conditions affect resorption and density of alveolar bone?

- Just as in other bones of the body, systemic diseases and conditions (*stress, ageing, malnutrition, cancer, diabetes, hyperthyroidism, hyperparathyroidism, etc.*) can lead to loss of total mass alveolar bone but ***height of alveolar bone is not affected*** by them.
- Systemic diseases and conditions therefore only add on to rate of loss of bone occurring due to local periodontal disease activity.
- Loss of alveolar bone height primarily occurs due to local periodontitis or TFO (*TFO will however not cause pocket deepening*).

◄ *What is the role of systemic diseases and conditions in periodontal bone loss?*

Mechanisms by which Plaque Microorganisms Cause Bone Destruction in Periodontitis

Mechanisms of bone destruction are not fully clear. Plaque microorganisms cause bone resorption by:

1. Increasing number of osteoclasts (*thereby increase bone resorption*).
2. Inhibiting osteoblasts (*thereby reducing or stopping new bone formation to replace lost bone*).
3. Causing periodontal tissue destruction directly.
4. Producing inflammation and causing release of chemicals by inflammatory cells (e.g. *prostaglandins*) that cause bone resorption.

◄ *How is bone resorbed in periodontitis?*

How Bone is Resorbed

- The first step in bone resorption is formation and activation of osteoclasts.
  - Osteoclasts differentiate from monocytes or macrophages in the presence of macrophage colony-stimulating factor.

◄ *How is bone resorbed by osteoclasts?*

- Regulation of bone resorptive (*osteoclastic*) activity is done by osteoprotegerin (*OPG*) produced by osteoblasts.

- After activation, osteoclasts move to surface of bone by chemotaxis.

What are Howship's lacunae? ▶

- Osteoclasts make small resorption bays (*small cavities*) called ***Howship's lacunae*** to resorb underlying bone.
- Osteoclasts resorb bone at the molecular level by secreting acid and enzymes **(Fig. 9.7)**. To do this,
  - Cell membrane of the osteoclast that is opposite to the surface of bone develops a 'ruffled border'. This increases the cell surface area for secretion and uptake of resorption products.
  - An isolated area (*sealing zone*) is then produced under the ruffled border. Chemicals secreted by the osteoclast can be maintained in high concentration in this sealing zone.
  - After this, environment of the Howship's lacunae is made highly acidic by release hydrogen ions (H^+) by the osteoclast. This decalcifies the underlying bone surface by removing mineral (*calcium*) of the bone.
  - The osteoclast also releases enzymes like matrix metalloprotease (*MMP*), collagenase, etc. to cause degradation and dissolution of the organic matrix of bone.

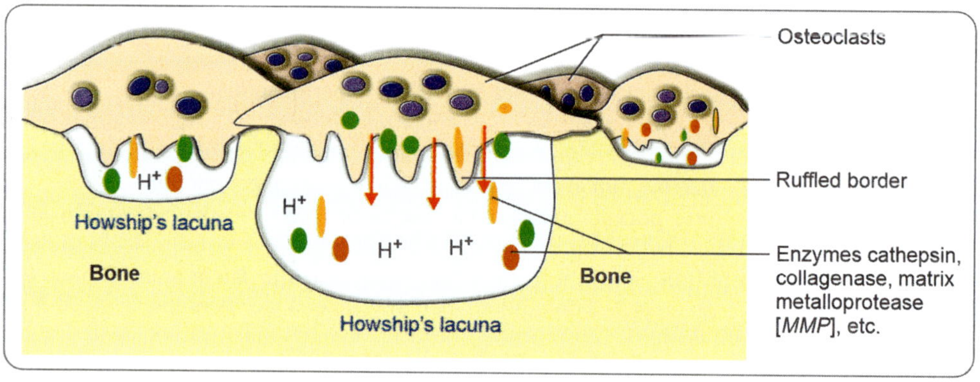

Fig. 9.7: Bone resorption by osteoclast

ALERT!

Bone formation also occurs along with bone resorption during periodontitis.

Does bone formation also occur during periodontitis? ▶

- New bone is formed during periodontitis in an attempt to compensate alveolar bone loss.
- As rate of bone formation is slower than rate of bone resorption in active periodontitis, there is net bone loss.
- New bone formation during ongoing periodontitis also occurs to reinforce the remaining bone to make it more resistant to resorption (*buttressing bone formation*).

Types of Bone Defects (*Bone Loss Patterns*) seen in Periodontal Disease

Two types of changes can be seen in alveolar bone in periodontal disease:

I. **Bone defects** (*bone loss patterns*)

II. **Bullous contours** (*thickening of contours of alveolar bone*).

I. *Bone Defects*

1. **Horizontal bone loss:**

What are horizontal bone defects? ▶

- Here the crest of resorbed bone is almost horizontal **(Fig. 9.12)**.
- Crest of interdental alveolar bone is normally placed about 2 mm apical and parallel to an imaginary line joining the CE junctions of two adjacent teeth (*see Chapter 3, Fig. 3.13*).

Which type of defect is commonly seen? ▶

- Horizontal bone loss is the ***commonest*** bone defect.

- Loss of horizontal height of bone is usually ***not uniform*** on all sides of a tooth.
- It is important to remember that, normal (*un-resorbed*) alveolar bone crests are usually located more apically on the more prominent root surface of teeth (*which may be facial or lingual*). This is called ***'reduced periodontium due to tooth position'*** in the 2018 classification of periodontal diseases and conditions (*see Chapter 10A and Fig. 10A.1, page 158*).
- In bitewing/IOPA radiographs, horizontal bone loss can be identified only in the interdental areas.

2. **Vertical or angular bone loss:**
   - In vertical bone loss, the crest of the resorbed alveolar bone is angular **(Fig. 9.11)**.
   - Vertical bone loss defects form 'within' the body of the alveolar bone, they are therefore also called ***intrabony*** or ***infrabony*** defects.
   - These are classified according to number of ***remaining*** walls of the defect **(Fig. 9.10)**.
3. **Osseous craters:** These are shallow craters (*concavities*) in the coronal most portion of the interdental septum bound by facial and lingual bony plates of almost equal heights.
4. **Reversed architecture:** When after resorption, crest of interdental bone septum is placed apical to the crest of the alveolar bone on the facial and/or lingual sides of the tooth (*normally crest of interdental bone is coronal to crest of bone on facial or lingual side*) (*see Chapter 18, Fig. 18.1, page 319*).
5. **Ledges:** When a thickened crest of alveolar bone undergoes resorption, it produces a ***plateau*** like flattened crest called a ledge (*this is different from lipping*).
6. **Combination of above defects.**

Is horizontal bone loss uniform on all sides of the same tooth/different teeth in the same mouth?

In an IOPA radiograph, where can bone loss be identified?

What are vertical bone defects?

How are vertical bone defects classified?

What are osseous craters?

What is reverse architecture of alveolar bone?

What are ledges?

II. *Bullous Contours*

Increased occlusal forces over a long period of time causes hypertrophy (*strengthening*) of alveolar bone that results in thickening of alveolar bone contours. Such contours are called bullous contours **(Fig. 9.5)**. They are of two types:

1. **Lipping (*peripheral buttressing of alveolar bone*): *Strengthening*** (*buttressing*) of alveolar bone that has been weakened by periodontitis induced resorption may produce a bulge in the alveolar crest; this is called lipping **(Fig. 9.5, diag. B)**. It is often seen after formation of osseous craters and vertical (*angular*) bone loss.
2. **Exostoses:** Outgrowths of alveolar bone are called exostoses. They form as adaptation to increased occlusal stresses (*traumatic occlusion*) and are of different sizes and shapes **(Fig. 9.5, diag. A)**.

What are bullous contours?

What is lipping?

How are ledges different from lipping?

What are bone exostosis?

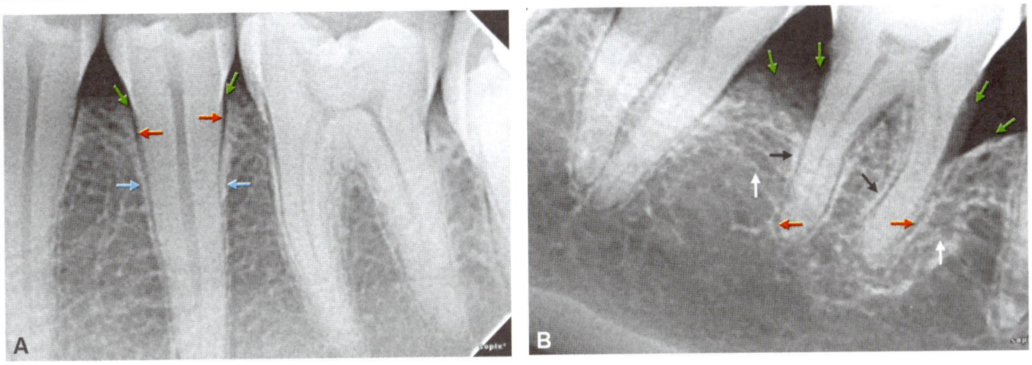

Chronic primary TFO
[*high occlusal force over normal height periodontium*]

Chronic secondary TFO
[*normal / high occlusal force over reduced height periodontium*]

Fig. 9.8: Changes seen in alveolar bone in early (*diag. A*) and late (*diag. B*) stages of TFO. Note in diag. A, slight funneling (*green arrows*) slightly thickened lamina dura (*blue arrows*), thickened PDL (*red arrows*) and normal trabecular pattern. In diag. B, note great amount of funneling (*double green arrows*), thick lamina dura (*black arrows*), thickened PDL (*red arrows*) and thick bone trabeculae (*white arrows*).

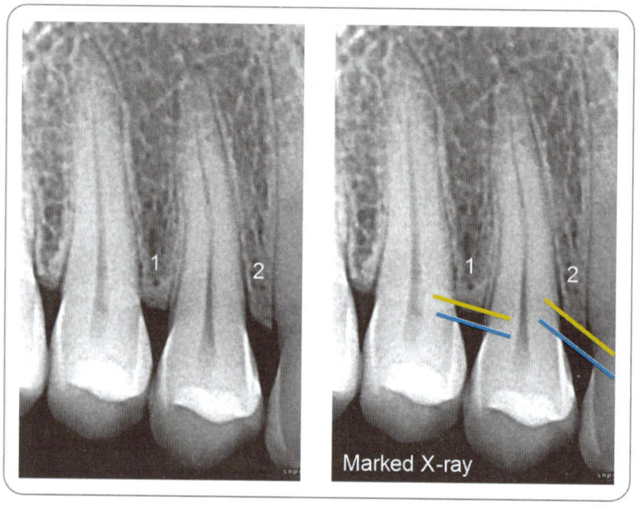

Fig. 9.9: All interdental bone crests that are angular do not have angular (*vertical*) bone loss. Although interdental bone crests marked 1 and 2 appear angular, both are *normal* as they are parallel and about 2 mm apical to an imaginary line connecting the two adjoining CEJs.

Factors that Affect and Modify Pattern of Bone Resorption in Periodontal Disease

Presence or absence of the following factors can change the type and amount of bone loss seen in periodontal disease. These are:

Which factors can modify bone loss? ▶

1. **Anatomical variations** (*of tooth and bone affecting type and amount of bone loss*).
   - Original angulation and thickness of crest of interdental septum and facial bone plates.
   - Presence of fenestrations and dehiscences.
   - Root and root furcation anatomy.
2. **Bone enlargements** (*lipping and exostoses*)
3. **Trauma from occlusion**
4. **Type of periodontal disease,** e.g. grade C periodontitis with molar-incisor distribution produces typical semilunar vertical bone loss patterns around 1st molars.
5. **Systemic diseases and conditions**
6. **Other complicating factors:**
   - Food impaction
   - Habits, e.g. bruxism, etc. may result in increased occlusal loads on the periodontium and may cause bone to hypertrophy thereby producing exostosis, lipping, buttressing bone formation, etc.
   - Smoking
7. **Iatrogenic factors**, e.g. overhanging restorations cause increased plaque accumulation under them resulting in more bone loss.

Vertical (*Angular*) Bone Defects

(*See section on TFO in this chapter and section on 'Classification of Pockets' in Chapter 10, page 141*).

Classification

Are vertical defects classified according to number lost or remaining bone walls of the bone defect? ▶

- Vertical (*angular or infrabony*) alveolar bone defects are classified according to number of ***remaining bone walls*** (*of the defect*) (Figs 9.10 and 9.11).

Is tooth surface and floor of the defect counted as a wall of the vertical bone defect? ▶

- Tooth surface and floor of the bone defect are ***not*** counted as a wall of the defect.

Classify vertical defects. ▶

1. **One-walled defect:** It has only one remaining bone wall; it is also called a ***hemi-septum***.
2. **Two-walled defect:** It has two remaining walls.
3. **Three-walled defect:** It has three remaining walls.
4. **Combined osseous defect:** If number of walls are more at the base (*apical end*) of the defect than at the top (*coronal end*) the bone defect is called a combined bone defect. Such defects are produced due to ***incomplete resorption*** of one of the walls of the defect.

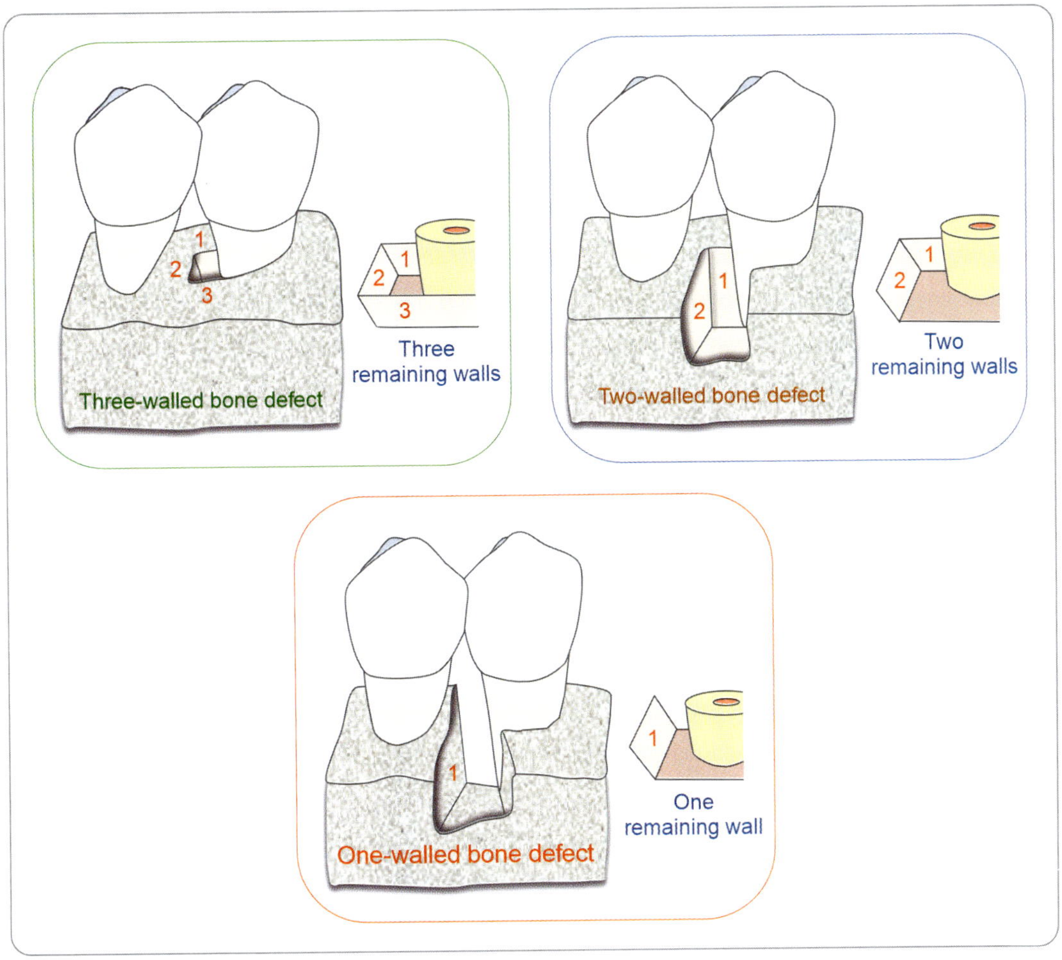

Fig. 9.10: Types of vertical (*angular*) bone defects. They are classified according to the number of *remaining bone walls*; tooth surface and floor are *not* countable as a wall of the defect.

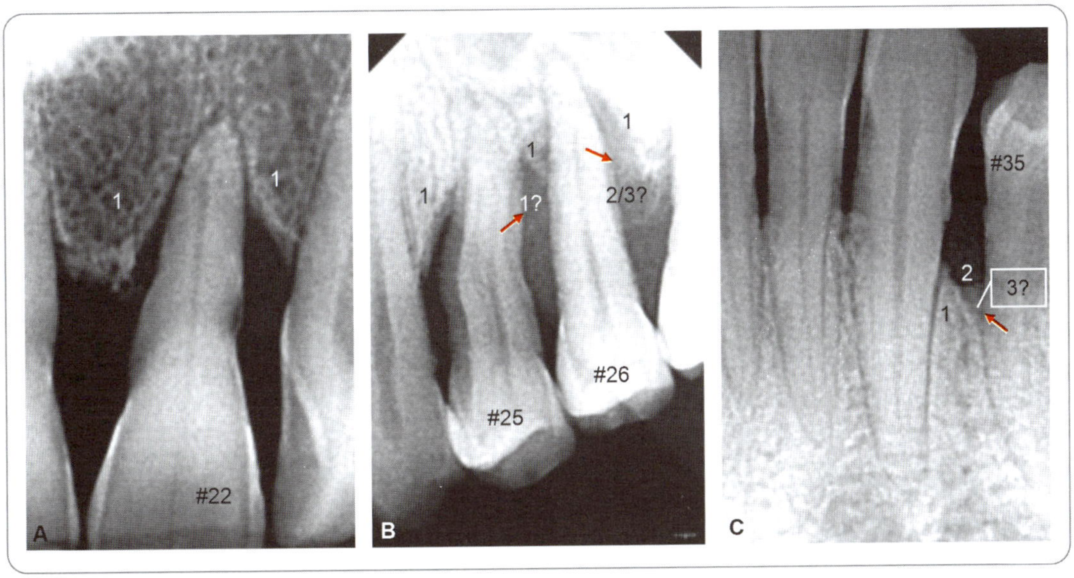

Fig. 9.11: Radiographic appearance of vertical (*angular*) bone defects (*number of walls marked on the defect*). One-walled defects are easily identified (*diag. A*). Two- and three-walled defects walled defects (*diag. B and C*) may not always be clear, but can be expected if a zone of fuzziness is seen in the bone adjacent to the root (*diags B and C, red arrows*). Light fuzziness suggests a one walled defect (*diag. B, red arrow*), whereas dark fuzziness can be due to a thick one walled circumferential defect, two or even three walled defects (*diags B and C, red arrows*).

CLINICAL UTILITY AND SHORT ANSWER

Which vertical defect has the best chance of bone regeneration?

Which vertical defect have the worst chance of bone regeneration?

Which type of vertical (*angular*) defect has the best and worst prognosis?

- ***Three-walled*** defects **(Figs 9.10 and 9.11)** have the ***best*** prognosis because, after treatment:
  - i. Healing of the bony defect occurs from three sides (*walls*).
  - ii. Healing tissues (*clot, granulation tissue, etc.*) and bone grafting material (*if used*) are better supported and protected.
  - iii. Blood supply to healing wound comes from all three sides.
- ***One-walled*** defects have the ***worst*** prognosis because blood supply, healing cells and support to the wound come only from one side (*compared to the same coming from three sides in a three-walled bone defect*).

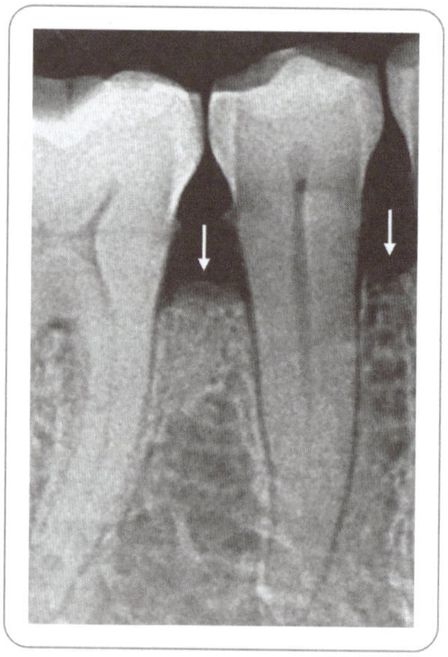

Fig. 9.12: Horizontal bone loss (*white arrows*) as seen in radiographs.

How Vertical (Angular) Osseous Defects are Identified

1. **Probing:** Probing of the pocket is done with a periodontal probe at multiple locations and at all these locations, probe is lightly moved outward buccally or lingually. If vertical bone defect is present, resistance will be felt.

What is bone sounding?

2. **Bone sounding:** This is an extension of periodontal probing. The site suspected to have a vertical bone defect is ***anaesthetized*** and probe is pushed down (*apically*) till bone crest is felt. Probe is moved lightly in all directions to assess the bone defect **(Fig. 9.13, diag. A)**.

What is transgingival probing?

3. **Transgingival probing:** After anaesthetizing gingiva, a periodontal probe is inserted ***horizontally*** from the buccal/lingual side into the gingiva till the tooth/bone is felt. Probe tip is then moved lightly in all directions to feel and map the bone topography **(Fig. 9.13, diag. B)**.
4. **Radiographs (*'X-rays'*):** Radiographs can give a good idea of type of bone defects in the ***interdental*** alveolar bone. They however, usually do not give us an accurate assessment of bone defects present on facial/lingual surfaces as the radiographic image of such bone defects is overlapped by images of facial and lingual bone plates and tooth **(Fig. 9.11)**.
5. **Direct viewing after surgical exposure:** Visual and tactile exploration of the defect after surgical exposure (*raising a full thickness flap*) is the only ***foolproof*** way of detection and classification of osseous defects.

Radiographic Diagnosis of Bone Defects

What are the radiographic features of interdental bone loss?

How interdental bone loss appears in an IOPA radiograph:

1. Fuzziness (*haziness*) or break in continuity of crestal lamina **(Fig. 9.12, white arrow)** and lamina dura **(Figs 9.11, 9.14 and 9.15)**.

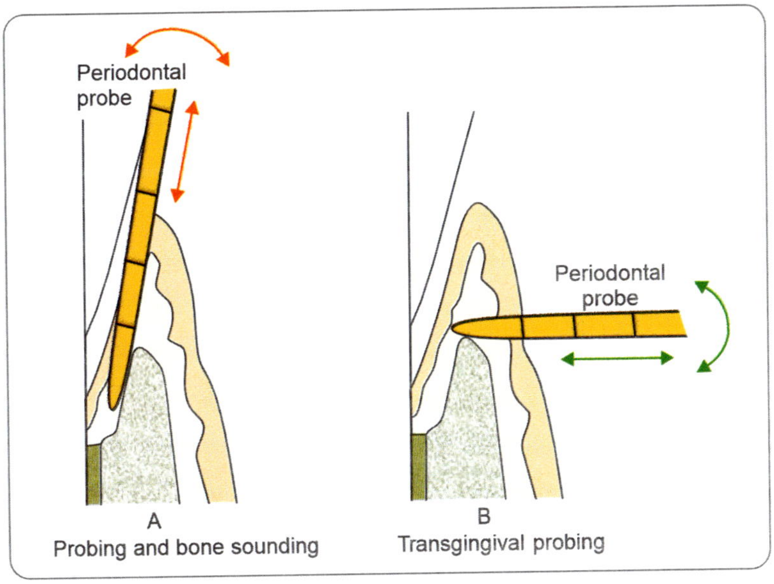

Fig. 9.13: Transgingival probing

3. Presence of craters or thin finger-like radiolucent projections in the interdental septum are suggestive of incipient periodontitis (*periodontitis that has just started; this is the only fully reversible stage of periodontitis*).
4. Presence of triangular wedge-shaped partially radiolucent areas at crest of alveolar bone (*appearing as grey triangles whose base is coronal and apex is apically pointed*) on the proximal aspects of tooth roots.
5. Loss of height of alveolar bone.

◂ *What is incipient periodontitis?*

Shortcomings of IOPA Radiographs When used for Diagnosis of Bone Defects

1. Defects on facial and lingual sides ***cannot*** be identified.
2. Grade I and II furcation defects ***do not appear clearly*** on radiographs due to overlapping of images of facial and lingual bone plates over image of the tooth.
3. Radiographs provide ***two-dimensional*** projections of three-dimensional alveolar bone and teeth.
4. Actual bone loss is usually about ***25% more*** than what appears in the radiograph.
5. Radiographic picture is representative of ***past*** changes (*does not tell the present health or disease status of periodontium; condition of gingiva tells present status*).

◂ *Which defects cannot be identified on IOPA radiographs?*

◂ *Do radiographs present accurate picture of the amount of bone loss?*

◂ *Radiographs present past or present condition of bone loss in periodontal disease?*

CLINICAL UTILITY AND SHORT ANSWER

Which radiographs are best suited for identification and assessment of periodontal bone defects?

Four radiographs are used for assessment of periodontal bone defects. These are:

1. **IOPA radiograph:** The 2018 classification necessitates bone loss assessment in relation to the length of the tooth's root to stage and grade periodontitis. Therefore, ***IOPA radiographs are best suited*** and most ***commonly*** used radiographs to identify and assess bone loss.
2. **Bite wing radiograph:** These must ***not*** be used for periodontal assessment of bone defects as bite wing radiographs provide images of only coronal half of opposing maxillary and mandibular teeth. Therefore alveolar bone defects that are beyond the physical range (*dimensions*) of bite wing radiographs cannot be assessed.
3. **OPG** (*orthopantomogram*): It is ***not*** preferred because it provides enlarged (*usually 25%*), blurred and at times distorted image of teeth and jaws. Overlapping teeth and superimposition of image of the back bone over images of anterior teeth make assessment of these areas impossible.
4. **CBCT** (*Cone Beam Computed Tomography*): This allows accurate three-dimensional imaging of bone defects. CBCT is however, ***rarely*** used for this purpose as it delivers many times ***more radiation*** than conventional dental X-rays. CBCT scans are also very ***costly***.

◂ *Which radiograph is the best suited for making a periodontal diagnosis?*

◂ *Which radiograph will you choose for periodontal diagnosis?*

◂ *Why OPG cannot be used for diagnosis of bone defects?*

ALERT!

What are the radiographic features of TFO.

Specific radiographic features suggestive of some ***specific*** periodontal diseases and conditions are:

- **TFO** (Figs 9.2, 9.4 and 9.8)
  - Funneling of periodontal ligament at the coronal end.
  - Increase in width of the periodontal ligament.
  - Increase in thickness (*radio-opacity*) of lamina dura.
  - Increase in thickness and change in angulation of the trabeculae of the alveolar bone.
- **Periodontal abscess**

Which radiographic finding is suggestive of periodontal abscess.

  - Radiolucency along lateral aspect of root that may or may not be in communication with the crestal lamina.
  - The abscess will appear in a radiograph only if the amount of bone loss is large enough to appear in a radiograph and also if the position of the abscess is such that it is not obliterated by superimposition of image of roots of the tooth.
- **Grade C periodontitis with molar-incisor distribution** (***localized aggressive periodontitis***) (Fig. 9.14)
  - Localization of alveolar bone loss (*either vertical or horizontal*) to **incisors** and **first molars** (*similar picture is present on the opposite side teeth also*)
  - Bone loss around first molars is ***cup-shaped*** (**semilunar**).
  - Despite severe bone loss around molars and incisors, other teeth usually do not have bone loss.
  - In advanced stages of the disease, more teeth get involved and a more generalized bone loss is seen.
- **Furcation involvement** (Fig. 9.15) (*see Chapter 20 for details*)

How does furcation involvement appear in a radiograph?

  Slightest radiolucency in the furcation especially so if there is loss in bone height along the adjoining roots may be an indication of furcation involvement.
  - **Grade I furcations:** Usually, no change is noticeable in grade I furcation. Initial stages of furcation involvement are ***most difficult*** to detect in a radiograph.
  - **Grade II furcation:** A slight radiolucency or fuzziness in the furcation area can be seen in grade II furcations.
  - **Grade III and IV furcations:** Frank radiolucency is seen in grade III and IV furcations. However, as images of furcations are often ***superimposed*** and obliterated by superimposition of tooth roots (*especially palatal root of maxillary teeth*), they can be difficult to detect radiographically. In case maxillary premolars have two roots, the buccal and palatal roots ***superimpose*** over the furcation's image. This makes it practically ***impossible*** to make a radiographic diagnosis of furcation involvement maxillary premolars.

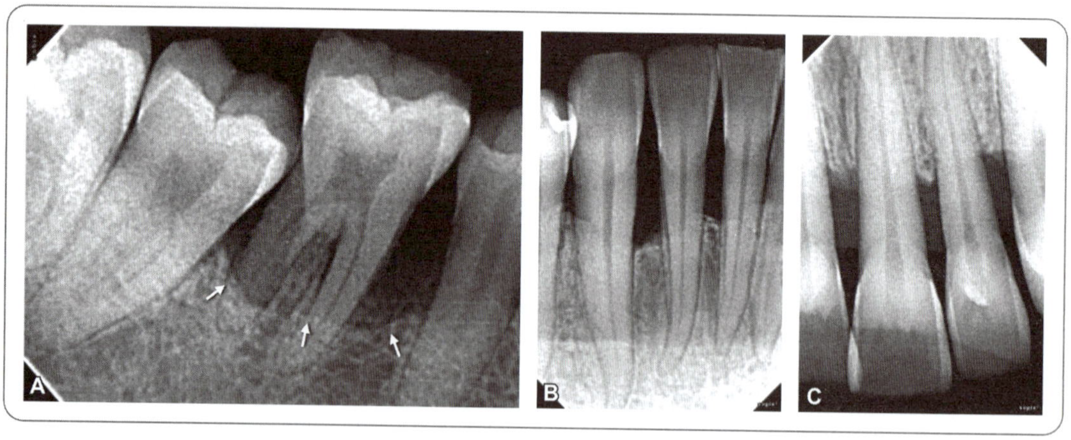

Fig. 9.14: Radiographic features of grade C periodontitis with molar–incisor distribution (*localized aggressive periodontitis*) include cup shaped or semi-lunar bone loss (*diag. A, white arrows*) in relation to first molars and severe bone loss in relation to all incisors (*Diag. B and C*). Other teeth may not show any bone loss or may only show minimal bone loss.

PATHOLOGIC MIGRATION

What is pathologic migration?

Where is pathologic migration seen more commonly?

Definition: Change in position of a tooth due to a disruption in the balance of forces that maintain it in its normal position is called pathologic migration.

- Pathologic migration is more commonly noticed in anterior teeth. Usually more than one tooth is involved.

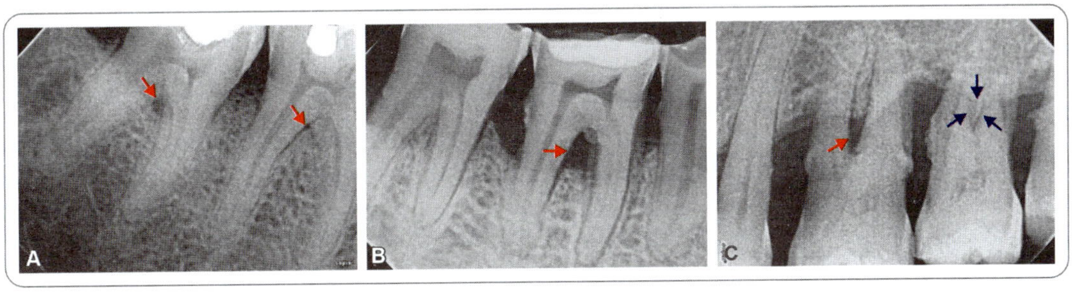

Fig. 9.15: Radiographic identification of furcation involvement. Slight radiolucency or fuzziness in furcation area is indicative of furcation involvement (*diag. A, red arrow*). Furcation involvement usually appears clearly in mandibular teeth (*diag. B, red arrows*). In maxillary teeth, furcation involvement is often difficult to identify as it is usually superimposed by image of palatal root (*diag. C, blue arrows*). If palatal root is placed to one side (*usually distal*), furcation involvement may then be clearly seen in a radiograph (*diag. C, red arrow*).

- Teeth undergoing pathologic migration may move in any direction, i.e. occlusal/incisal (*extrusion*), mesial or distal and buccal or lingual.
- Pathologically migrated teeth are often rotated and show increased mobility.
- Pathologic migration is usually a sign of periodontitis.

Factors Maintaining a Tooth in its Normal Position

There are many factors that maintain a tooth in its normal position; a change in the balance amongst these will lead to pathologic migration. These factors are:

◂ *Which factors maintain a tooth in its normal position?*

1. Health and normal height of the periodontium.
2. Counter balancing of inward pressure on a tooth by muscles of cheeks and lips by outward pressure of the tongue.
3. Forces of occlusion. Occlusal forces put on a tooth are split into two vectors, a smaller anterior vector and a larger vertical vector. The larger vertical vector is borne by the periodontium. The smaller ***anterior vector pushes all teeth anteriorly***; this is responsible for ***mesial migration*** and ***maintenance of proximal contacts*** (*by compensating for proximal attrition of the teeth*) **(Fig. 9.16)**.
4. Morphology of tooth, cuspal inclines, contact points and axial inclination.

◂ *How are proximal contacts of teeth maintained despite attrition?*

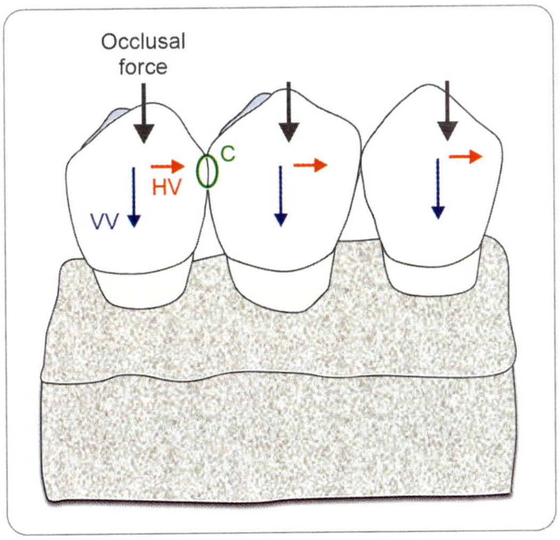

Fig. 9.16: Occlusal force (black arrow) splits into two vectors: a smaller horizontal vector (HV) that is directed anteriorly (mesially) (red arrow) and a larger apically directed vertical vector (VV) (blue arrow). The horizontal (mesial) vector puts a mesially directed force on teeth when teeth come in contact. This pushes teeth anteriorly and helps maintain tight contact (C) between adjacent teeth and compensates loss of proximal tooth structure due to proximal attrition. Tight proximal contacts help prevent food impaction and distribute occlusal forces along the entire arch (splinting effect) thus allowing bearing of high occlusal forces while preventing overloading of any particular tooth.

Factors that Cause Pathologic Migration

What causes pathologic migration? ▶

Pathologic migration may occur because of:

1. **Periodontitis:**

Why does a tooth with periodontitis show pathologic migration? ▶

   - A periodontally diseased tooth is unable to maintain its position in the arch and can move under the effect of occlusal and oral muscular forces. Such a tooth shifts its position till it gets to a more favourable position where the same forces become balanced and can be borne easily by the tooth.
   - Pressure from granulation tissue that is always present in periodontal pockets exerts a small but continuous force which over a period of time can force a tooth out of its normal position.

Why does a tooth with traumatic occlusion show pathologic migration? ▶

2. **Traumatic occlusion (*increased occlusal forces*):**
   - Teeth under the effect of higher and directional forces move to new positions where the same occlusal forces can be better tolerated.
   - Loss of teeth in the arch results in increased occlusal load on remaining teeth. This can cause teeth to change their position **(Fig. 9.17)**.
3. **Supra-eruption:** After a tooth is lost and is not replaced for a long time, the opposite tooth (*of opposite arch*) then supra erupts. This change in position of teeth results in changed occlusal forces on them.
4. **Habits:** Bruxism and bruxomania **(Fig. 9.5)**, tongue thrusting, thumb sucking, etc. all put excessive and directional pressure on teeth (*especially anterior ones*) resulting in pathologic migration.
5. **Loss of contact of a tooth with opposite teeth:** This results in changed direction of force put on such teeth by tongue, masticated food and swallowing leading to pathologic migration.

Management of Pathologic Migration

How is pathologic migration treated? ▶

Pathologic migration can be managed by:

- Identification of reasons behind pathologic migration
- Periodontal treatment to treat periodontitis
- Counseling for correction of oral habits
- Orthodontic correction of position of affected teeth
- Replacement of missing teeth, splinting, etc.

CLINICAL UTILITY AND SHORT ANSWER

What are bruxism and bruxomania?

- Bruxism and Bruxomania are para-functional habits.
- Periodic repetitive ***clenching*** and forceful ***grinding*** of teeth during ***sleep*** is called ***bruxism***.
- If this is done when a person is ***awake***, it is called ***bruxomania***.
- Causes of bruxism and bruxomania are: stress, anxiety, smoking, alcohol consumption, etc.

What is the difference between bruxism and bruxomania? ▶

What are the clinical features of bruxism? ▶

Clinical features:

- Loss of tooth substance (*attrition, abfraction cavities*) and tooth fracture **(Fig. 9.5)**.
- TFO (*bone resorption, mobility of teeth, etc.*)
- Vague or sharp pain (*unexplainable due to other reasons*) in head and neck region and ear either on one side or bilaterally.
- Stiffness and feeling of fatigue of muscles of mastication after waking up from sleep (*especially in the morning*).
- TMJ (*Temporo-mandibular joint*) disorders (*pain and tenderness due to inflammation, clicking, etc.*), etc.

ALERT!

Diastema formation is a sign of pathologic migration.

What are the important clinical considerations of diastema formation? ▶

- Pathologic migration is a sign of severe (*stage III or IV*) periodontitis.
- Anterior teeth generally show a tendency to extrude and migrate ***distolabially***.
- This distolabial migration of anterior teeth causes spaces between teeth (*diastema formation where none existed earlier*).
- Open proximal contacts invite food impaction that further leads to worsening of periodontitis.

ALERT!

Reactive positioning

After periodontal treatment, pathologically migrated teeth regain their periodontal health. Such teeth can then either ***move back*** to their ***original*** position or change their position further to move to a more stable position (*on their own*). This is called reactive positioning.

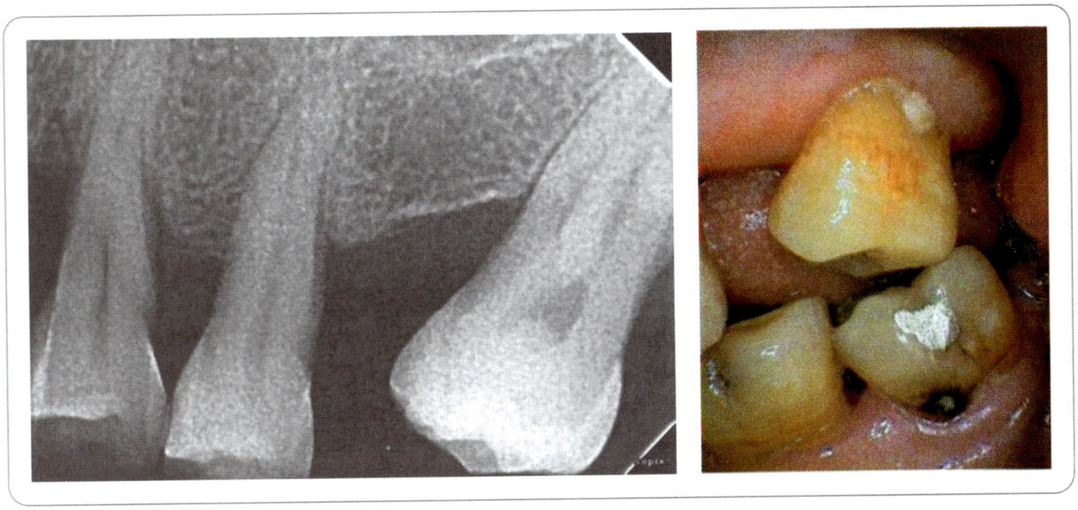

Fig. 9.17: Pathologic migration

Review Questions

1. What is trauma from occlusion (*TFO*) and traumatic occlusion? Does malocclusion always result in TFO? Do all malocclusions produce TFO?
2. Classify TFO. What are the clinical features of TFO? Write stages of TFO. Is TFO reversible?
3. Does periodontal bone loss occur only due to plaque induced periodontitis?
4. What is the 'radius of action' concept?
5. What is the rate of loss of alveolar bone in periodontitis? What is the rate of loss of periodontal attachment?
6. Does bone form during periodontal disease?
7. What are the differences between horizontal bone loss and vertical/angular bone loss?
8. What are osseous craters and ledges?
9. What is reversed architecture of crest of alveolar bone?
10. Classify vertical defects of alveolar bone. Which vertical defect type has the best and worst prognosis?
11. How can infrabony osseous defects be identified?
12. Which radiographs are best suited for identification and assessment of osseous defects?
13. What radiographic features are suggestive of occlusal trauma (*TFO*)?
14. Which radiographic features are suggestive of furcation involvement?
15. What is pathologic migration? What causes it? How can pathologic migration be managed?
16. What are bruxism and bruxomania?

Chapter 10

Plaque Induced Gingivitis and Periodontitis

Gingivitis and periodontitis are plaque induced inflammatory diseases of the periodontium (*'itis'—inflammation*). Periodontitis differs from gingivitis only in the extent of damage produced in the periodontal tissues. Otherwise, both gingivitis and periodontitis have the same causes and similar pathological processes.

For ease of understanding, the basic pathology of gingivitis and periodontitis will be discussed first. Specific points of these two diseases are discussed in subsequent sections of this Chapter.

ALERT!

By convention and unless specifically mentioned, both the terms gingivitis and periodontitis are used to refer only to plaque induced inflammatory disease of the periodontium *(gingiva, periodontal ligament and alveolar bone; cementum does not get inflamed as it does not have blood supply).*

If gingivitis and periodontitis caused by some other predominating causative and/or contributing factor have to be referred to, a definite mention of this is made specifically, e.g. pregnancy gingivitis, gingivitis caused by thermal injury, periapical periodontitis due to a non-vital pulp, etc.

CLINICAL UTILITY AND SHORT ANSWER

Terms used to describe clinical presentation of periodontal disease (*including gingivitis and periodontitis*)

Based on severity, rate of progress, inflammation type, response to treatment and duration, periodontal disease can be:

How is acute disease different from chronic?

1. **Acute:** This has short history and duration, is fast progressing and of high severity. Underlying inflammation is of acute type (*PMNs predominate*), e.g. acute gingivitis, acute periodontal abscess, etc.
2. **Chronic:** This has long history and duration, is slowly progressing and of low severity. Underlying inflammation is of chronic type (*plasma cells predominate*), e.g. chronic gingivitis, chronic periodontitis, etc.
3. **Sub-acute:** Disease with features that are in-between chronic and acute forms, e.g. sub-acute gingivitis, sub-acute periodontitis, etc.

What is the difference between recurrent and refractory disease?

4. **Recurrent:** Disease which recurs after complete treatment and elimination (*this is different from disease that recurs due to incomplete treatment*), e.g. recurrent gingivitis and periodontitis, etc.
5. **Refractory:** Disease which does not get treated with usual (*conventional*) treatment, e.g. refractory periodontitis (*cannot be treated with scaling and root planing—the usual treatment*), etc.
6. **Localized:** When less than 30% teeth or sites are involved with the disease, e.g. localized gingivitis, etc.
7. **Generalized:** When more than 30% teeth or sites are involved with the disease, e.g. generalized gingivitis, etc.
8. **Discrete:** When disease or condition is restricted to a specific area, e.g. localized tumor-like enlargement.
9. **Marginal:** When disease is identifiable only in marginal gingiva, i.e. other parts of the gingiva (*interdental papilla and attached gingiva*) are not affected by the disease, e.g. marginal gingivitis, etc.
10. **Papillary:** When disease is restricted to interdental papilla only, i.e. other parts of the gingiva (*marginal and attached gingiva*) are not affected by the disease, e.g. papillary gingivitis.

What is diffused disease? How is it different from generalized disease?

11. **Diffuse:** When all parts of the gingiva, i.e. interdental papilla, marginal and attached gingiva are involved by disease, e.g. diffuse gingivitis.

The above-mentioned terms are often used together to describe the disease and its presentation precisely, e.g. localized marginal gingivitis, generalized diffuse gingivitis, etc.

GINGIVITIS AND PERIODONTITIS

Gingivitis

- Gingivitis literally means inflammation of the gingiva (i.e. *the term refers to the pathologic process–inflammation of/in the gingiva*). ◂ *What is gingivitis?*
- However, in clinical use, the term gingivitis is used to refer ***only to plaque induced gingivitis*** (*inflammatory disease restricted to the gingiva caused by plaque microorganisms*).
- Plaque induced gingivitis is characterized by ***false*** pockets (*base of pocket is coronal to CE junction*) (Fig. 10.4, diag. 2). ◂ *What is chief distinguishing feature of gingivitis from periodontitis?*

Periodontitis

- Technically, any inflammation in deeper periodontal tissues will produce periodontitis (*inflammation of periodontium*). However, in clinical use, the term periodontitis is generally used to refer ***only to plaque induced periodontitis*** (*inflammatory disease of periodontium caused by plaque microorganisms*). ◂ *What is periodontitis?*
- Periodontitis is an ***extension*** of gingivitis and plaque induced gingivitis always ***precedes*** periodontitis but gingivitis does not always lead to periodontitis. ◂ *Is periodontitis related to gingivitis?*
- It is characterized by formation of ***true*** pockets, i.e. shifting of base of pocket apical to CE junction (*clinical attachment loss*) due to plaque induced inflammation (Fig. 10.4, diags 3 and 4). This differentiates periodontitis from gingivitis. ◂ *What is chief distinguishing feature of periodontitis from gingivitis?*

Pathogenesis of Gingivitis and Periodontitis (*Pocket*)

Briefly and simplified what happens is this: ◂ *How does gingivitis develop?*

1. Plaque deposits are always present near gingiva and within gingival sulcus.
2. If plaque deposits are small, body's defenses (*immune system*) can control the infection caused by plaque microorganisms and this does not allow plaque to produce clinically identifiable inflammation (*gingivitis*). If, however, body defense is unable to do this, clinical gingivitis (*clinically evident inflammation*) will result. ◂ *Does plaque always produce gingivitis?*
3. Gingivitis causes swelling and increase in size of gingiva. This results in increase in depth of the gingival sulcus (Figs 10.2 and 10.4).
4. Due to increased depth, anaerobic conditions develop in the sulcus and G –ve anaerobic bacteria now establish in it. ◂ *How does gingivitis cause increase in sulcus depth and how does this lead to clinical gingivitis?*
5. With time, bacterial numbers in the sulcus increase. This causes more gingival inflammation which then results in worsening of severity of clinical features of gingivitis and increase in sulcus depth (*coronal shift of crest of gingiva due to increase in swelling of gingiva*).
6. Gingival sulcus now becomes clinically diseased and deepened and is now called a gingival pocket. Bleeding from gingiva and other clinical features of gingivitis can now be seen.
7. As gingiva is swollen and depth of gingival sulcus has increased, oral hygiene measures become less effective. This results in even more plaque accumulation in the pocket which further leads to more gingival inflammation. Thus, a vicious cycle is established.
8. At this stage:
   - ***Sulcular epithelium*** and ***junctional epithelium*** start to show rete pegs (*finger-like projections of epithelium into underlying connective tissue*). ◂ *When do sulcular and junctional epithelia develop rete pegs?*
   - Junctional epithelium also lets out ***2–3 cell thick finger like projections*** into the gingival connective tissue along root of the tooth. The cells of these 'finger' like projections attach onto the root surface and become ***apical extension*** of the junctional epithelium. ◂ *How does junctional epithelium migrate apically?*
   - 2–3 layers of coronal most cells of the junctional epithelium (***cells forming the attachment epithelium***) are shed off and the junctional epithelium migrates apically causing deepening of the sulcus and loss of attachment.
9. Apical migration of junctional epithelium continues and ultimately ***junctional epithelium migrates apical*** to the CE junction. At this stage ***gingivitis converts to periodontitis***. Further progression of periodontitis occurs due to continued apical movement of junctional epithelium. ◂ *When does gingivitis convert to periodontitis?*

How does severity of periodontitis increase? ▶

10. Severity of periodontitis increases due to:
    - Increasing periodontal tissue loss (*breakdown*) at the already involved sites.
    - Involvement of newer sites around the same tooth.
    - Initiation and progression of periodontitis at new sites around other teeth of the mouth.

CLINICAL UTILITY AND SHORT ANSWER

At what stage does junctional epithelium shift apically during progression of periodontitis?

The junctional epithelium shifts apically when:

1. The PMN concentration within the junctional epithelium reaches 60% of the total volume of the junctional epithelium.
2. It starts to show rete-pegs and lets off 2–3 cell thick finger like projections into the gingival connective tissue.

Stages in Conversion of Clinically Healthy Gingiva to Periodontitis

Name the stages through which gingiva pass when gingival health converts to periodontitis? ▶

Conversion from clinical gingival health to periodontitis occurs in four stages:

1. **Normal or clinically healthy gingiva**
2. **Early gingivitis**
3. **Established gingivitis**
4. **Periodontitis**

1. *Normal or Clinically Healthy Gingiva*

What is normal gingiva? ▶

Clinically healthy gingiva has ***very little*** plaque in its vicinity and in the sulcus. Although the small amount of plaque produces inflammation in the gingiva at the histological level but this inflammation is so little that it does ***not*** show up in the gingiva clinically. Such gingiva that shows ***no*** features of inflammation clinically, is termed normal gingiva.

2. *Early Gingivitis*

Gingiva in this stage shows very mild clinical features of inflammation (*gingivitis*), e.g. slight bleeding on probing, slight change in color of marginal gingiva (*from light pink to red*), etc. Early gingivitis can revert to clinically healthy (*normal*) gingiva by scaling and good plaque control.

3. *Established Gingivitis*

At which stage is gingivitis easily diagnosable clinically? ▶

As the disease progresses, features of gingivitis increase in severity and are now ***easily*** recognized clinically. This is established gingivitis. Untreated established gingivitis lesions can:

a. ***Remain as such*** for an indefinite period of time.
b. If treated successfully, ***revert*** back to clinically healthy normal gingiva.
c. ***Progress*** to periodontitis.

4. *Periodontitis*

As gingivitis progresses further, base of the sulcus ***shifts apical*** to the CE junction on the root; this marks conversion of gingivitis to periodontitis. Loss of height of supporting alveolar bone and periodontal support are seen.

Histopathology of Different Stages during Conversion of Clinically Healthy Gingiva to Periodontitis

Histopathological features of each of these stages are ***overlapping*** and are carried over to the next stage.

Are inflammatory cells present in gingiva and sulcus in normal gingiva? ▶

Normal or Clinically Healthy Gingiva

Normal or clinically healthy gingiva shows few bacteria and very little inflammation (*characterized by very few PMNs in sulcular epithelium and sulcus*).

Early Gingivitis

- As early gingivitis sets in, more bacteria can be identified in gingival tissues and inflammatory changes become evident.
- PMNs and lymphocytes are predominant cell and these cells comprise 5–10% connective tissue volume.
- Very few plasma cells antibody producing B-lymphocytes are also seen.
- Capillaries in the neighborhood of junctional and sulcular epithelia appear dilated and many new capillaries are also seen.
- Sulcular and junctional epithelia are thickened and develop rete pegs (*rete pegs are not present in sulcular and junctional epithelia of normal gingiva*).

Established Gingivitis

- Inflammation becomes more severe. PMNs and plasma cells (*antibody producing B-lymphocytes*) now occupy almost 50% of total gingival tissue volume and are now prominent in sulcular epithelium which is loosely attached to tooth surface.
- Bacterial colonies are seen within junctional and sulcular epithelia and deep within connective tissue of gingiva.
- Junctional epithelium is now markedly thickened and it develops finger-like extensions that extend apically along root of the tooth.
- Capillaries are markedly increased, enlarged and engorged and collagen degeneration is now clearly visible in connective tissue.

◂ *What is the percentage of inflammatory cells in gingiva in gingivitis?*

◂ *Are bacteria present within gingiva in gingivitis and periodontitis?*

Periodontitis

- This is marked by further increase in inflammatory infiltrate. Plasma cells now become the predominant cell type and occupy 50–80% of the total gingival tissue volume.
- Sulcular (*pocket*) epithelium is ulcerated and many bacteria are seen in the junctional epithelium and deep within gingival connective tissue and alveolar bone.
- Junctional epithelium is ***decreased*** in length by up to ten times (*normal length of JE is 0.25–1.35 mm*) and it extends finger-like projections that are 2–3 cells thick, along the root surface. Loss of attachment at junctional epithelium's coronal end is seen.
- Degenerated collagen fibers are seen just apical to the junctional epithelium, followed by partially degenerated and then normal collagen fibers further apically.
- Bone loss can be seen at crest of the alveolar bone.

◂ *What is the percentage of inflammatory cells in gingiva in periodontitis?*

◂ *What is the length of junctional epithelium in periodontitis?*

ALERT!

How does destruction of connective tissue (*collagen loss*) occur in periodontitis?

Although remodeling (*by destruction and then new formation*) of collagen in connective tissues also occurs in health, it is increased manifold in periodontitis. Collagen is resorbed by collagenase—a collagen destroying enzyme. Collagenase is produced by:

1. Fibroblasts, PMNs and macrophages that are normally present in the gingiva.
2. Bacteria, e.g. *P. gingivalis*, etc. They:
   a. Produce collagenase
   b. Induce host defense cells to produce collagenase and enzymes that cause connective tissue destruction.

◂ *What causes destruction of collagen of periodontal tissues?*

How Periodontitis Progresses: Continuously or Intermittently

There are basically two models of progression of periodontitis:

1. Gradual Model

This model proposes that untreated periodontitis progresses ***continuously*** at an average rate.

2. Episodic Burst Model

Which of the two gradual or burst model of progression of periodontitis is more accepted? ▸

Does periodontal destruction occur continuously in periodontitis? ▸

What is the rate of progression of periodontitis? ▸

This is the ***more accepted*** model. This model proposes that untreated periodontitis progresses ***episodically***, i.e. there are phases of progress of periodontitis (*episodes of periodontal destruction*) followed by phases of relative clinical health (*inactivity or quiescence*). Alternate phases of periodontal destruction and relative clinical health continue till periodontitis is treated. For implications of episodic nature of periodontitis *see* page 155.

Average rate of progression (***attachment loss***) of grade A and B periodontitis (*chronic periodontitis, 1999 classification*) is ***0.2 to 0.3 mm per year.*** Grade C periodontitis (*aggressive periodontitis, 1999 classification*) progresses many times faster than grade A or B periodontitis.

CLINICAL UTILITY AND SHORT ANSWER

Write the factors that increase susceptibility of an individual (*host*) to gingivitis and periodontitis.

Several factors have in role in producing gingivitis and periodontitis in an individual (*Fig. 6.17*). These are:

1. Heredity (*inherited immune defects*).
2. Individual's inability to maintain good oral hygiene (*physical handicaps, mentally challenged individuals, trigeminal neuralgia, etc.*)
3. Presence of local factors that support plaque retention and maturation (*overhanging restorations, furcation defects, inadequate plaque control, etc.*). This allows plaque to establish at these sites.
4. Behavioural and environmental factors:
   a. Smoking.
   b. Severe psychological stress.
   c. Systemic illnesses, e.g. diabetes, etc. (*these produce an immune compromised state in the host*).
   d. Diseases or use of medicines that suppress the immune system (*e.g. long term corticoid use, HIV infection, etc.*).
   e. Super infection by some viruses has been suggested to cause initiation and/or worsening of periodontitis by modifying the host's response to the local subgingival bacteria.

POCKET

What is a pocket? ▸

Definition: A ***pathologically*** deepened sulcus is called a pocket.

In other words, a sulcus which has become deep due to plaque induced inflammation (disease) is called a pocket.

What is normal depth of gingival sulcus? ▸

- Depth of the normal gingival sulcus is variable. It is normally between 0.5–3.0 mm (*average depth is 1.8–2.0 mm*) (*see Chapter 2, 'Gingiva', Figs 2.4, 2.5, 2.6 and 2.7*). A periodontal probe is used for recording probing depth (*PD*) and clinical attachment loss (*CAL*) (*with 0.25 N probing pressure*).

What is walking the probe? ▸

Which of the two maximum or minimum recorded PD and CAL must be used for making a diagnosis? ▸

- As pocket depths are variable **(Fig. 10.1, diag. A)**, PD and CAL values must be taken at several sites approximately 1 mm apart. This is called ***walking the probe*** **(Fig. 10.1, diag. B)**. ***Maximum*** recorded PD and CAL values are taken into consideration for making a periodontal diagnosis (*2018 classification*).

What is the maximum acceptable depth for a normal sulcus? ▸

- According to the 2018 classification, all sulci more than 3 mm deep are considered abnormal. However, as an exception to this rule, in previously treated but now stable cases of periodontitis, 4 mm deep pockets with no BOP (*bleeding on probing*) are considered normal.
- To prevent periodontal loss, it is important to diagnose periodontitis in its early stages and especially when the disease is 'silent', i.e. is not producing many and severe clinical features (*incipient periodontitis*).

Clinical Features of Pockets

What are the clinical features of pockets? ▸

When a sulcus deepens and converts to pocket (*sulcus becomes diseased and gingiva shows signs of inflammation*), its base may lie coronal or apical to the CE junction of the tooth. As discussed previously, if the base of the pocket is coronal to the CE junction, i.e. CAL is not present, the pocket is called a gingival pocket. If, however the base of the pocket is apical to the CE junction, i.e. CAL is present, the pocket is called a periodontal pocket (Fig. 10.4) (*see section on classification of pockets presented later in this Chapter*).

- Clinical features of false pockets (*gingival pockets*) are the same as those of gingivitis (*chronic plaque induced gingivitis; see section on gingivitis presented later in this Chapter*).
- Clinical features of true pockets (*periodontal pockets*) are the same as those of periodontitis (*chronic plaque induced periodontitis; see section on periodontitis presented later in this Chapter*).

◂ *What are the clinical features of gingival pockets?*

◂ *What are the clinical features of periodontal pockets?*

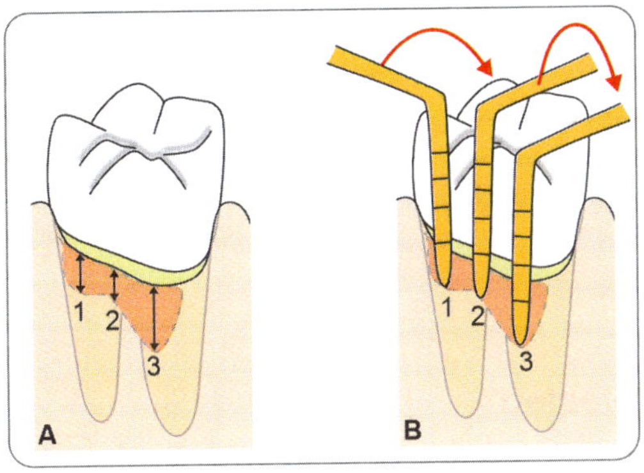

Fig. 10.1: Probing depths are variable at different sites of the same tooth surface (*diag. A, sites 1, 2 and 3*). PD and CAL values must be taken at several sites approximately 1 mm apart. This is called walking the probe (*diag. B, sites 1, 2 and 3*).

CLINICAL UTILITY AND SHORT ANSWER

How much is 0.25 N force—the recommended force for periodontal probing?

Probing pressure must not exceed 0.25 N force as it will then push the probe tip apically down to the alveolar bone crest and will ***add*** approximately ***2 mm*** to the actual sulcus depth making the reading faulty (*pocket depth + biologic width*) (*see Chapter 2, 'Gingiva', and Fig. 2.5*).

As a convenient way to know the correct probing pressure, the tip of the probe is pressed onto the bulb of one's finger, a 0.25 N force is just enough force that produces a ***slight depression*** in the bulb of the finger.

◂ *What will happen if more than 0.25 N force is applied for periodontal probing?*

How does a Sulcus Deepen?

The gingival sulcus deepens due to combined effects of infection caused by plaque microorganisms and the harmful effects of an individual's (*host's*) immunity. Deepening of sulcus occurs in three ways (Fig. 10.2):

1. Coronal movement of crest of gingiva (*false pocket formation*) due to increase in size of gingiva caused by inflammation (*exudate accumulation and fibrosis*) (Fig. 10.2, *yellow arrow*).
2. Apical movement of base of the sulcus beyond the CE junction (*true pocket formation*) (Fig. 10.2, *red arrow*).
3. Combination of the above two mechanisms (Fig. 10.2, *yellow + red arrow*).

◂ *In how many ways does a sulcus and/or pocket deepen?*

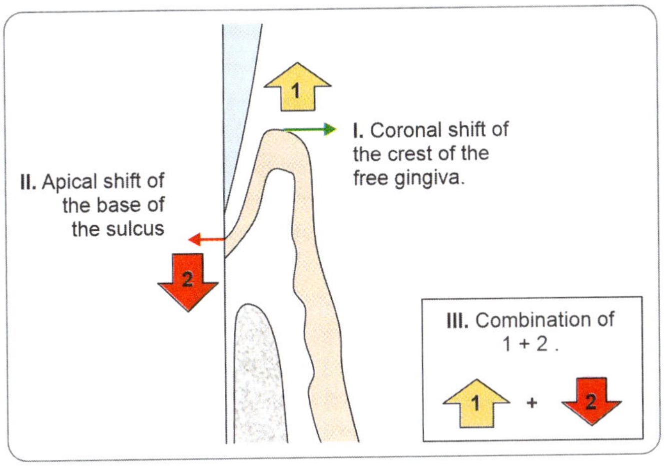

Fig. 10.2: A sulcus can deepen in three ways

CLINICAL UTILITY AND SHORT ANSWER

How deepening of sulcus leads to gingival inflammation and pocket formation

Plaque causes gingival inflammation which results in increase of size of gingiva and deepening of the sulcus to form a pocket. Increase in depth of sulcus changes the environment within the sulcus and makes it suitable for colonization by disease producing (*periodontopathogenic*) bacteria. This happens because of:

1. Change of aerobic environment of a shallow sulcus to anaerobic environment in a deeper sulcus. This favours colonization of anaerobic microorganisms which cause gingivitis and periodontitis.
2. A deep sulcus is inflamed and has more GCF (*gingival crevicular fluid—which is an exudate produced in inflammation*) and food debris. Both GCF and food debris provide nutrition to bacteria and thus support bacterial growth. As bacteria increase in numbers, they produce more gingival inflammation, this converts the sulcus to a pocket and also causes further pocket deepening **(Fig. 10.2, *yellow and red arrows*)**.
3. When a probing depth of the sulcus becomes more than 3–4 mm, the sulcus becomes difficult to clean either by natural mechanisms or cleansing methods used by the individual. This causes increase in number of plaque bacteria within the pocket which further leads to more inflammation and increase in pocket depth. Thus, a vicious cycle is established.

How can Pockets be Detected?

Pockets can be detected by:

Which is the easiest way to detect pockets?

1. Probing with periodontal probe. This is the ***simplest, easiest, most widely used*** and ***preferred method*** of detecting pockets.

Can PD and CAL be known from radiographs?

2. Manipulating digital radiographs by altering their contrast and brightness can make the image of gingiva in the ***interdental*** areas show up distinctly on the same digital radiograph **(Fig. 10.3 A and A')**. The pocket depth in the interdental radiograph can be known by subtracting 2 mm from the distance from crest of the gingiva to crest of alveolar bone (*measured using tools in the software*) (*base of the pocket is 2 mm coronal to crest of alveolar bone; this 2 mm space is biologic width*) **(diag. 10.3, C)**.
3. Injecting radiopaque dyes into sulcus or pocket and then taking radiographs will give a fair idea about the sulcus or pocket boundaries ***only*** in the ***interdental*** areas. ***No*** information can be gained on the buccal and lingual/palatal sides as images of the injected dye overlap image of teeth.
4. Perioscopy with a perioscope (*dental endoscope*) can be used to get an illuminated and magnified view of soft tissue walls of a sulcus or pocket and root of the tooth.

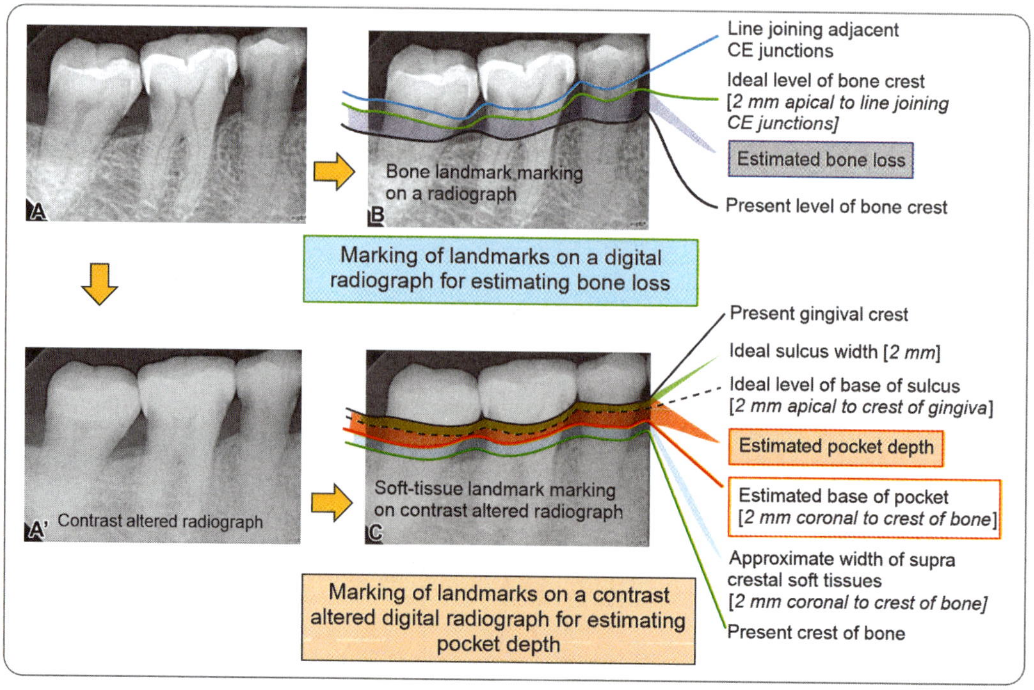

Fig. 10.3: Estimation of bone loss (*diag. B*) and pocket depth (*diag. C*) (*soft tissue and bone land marks*) on a digital radiograph.

Classification (*Types*) of Pockets

Pockets are of the following types:

1. *False Pocket or Gingival Pocket* (also called 'Pseudo' or 'Relative' Pocket)

◂ *What are the other names of a gingival pocket?*

a. Base of pocket is ***coronal*** to CE junction, i.e. there is no CAL (*clinical attachment loss*) **(Fig. 10.4, *diag.* 2)**.
b. Pocket formation occurs due to deepening of sulcus ***only*** by coronal movement of crest of marginal gingiva **(Fig. 10.4, *diag. 2, orange arrow*)**.
c. No bone resorption is seen (*due to periodontitis*).

2. *True Pocket or Periodontal Pocket*

◂ *What is the other name of a true pocket?*

a. Base of pocket is ***apical*** to CE junction, i.e. CAL is present **(Fig. 10.4, *diags 3 and 4*)**.
b. Pocket formation occurs due to deepening of sulcus by apical movement of base of the sulcus (*junctional epithelium*) apical to the CE junction **(Fig. 10.4, *diags 3 and 4, red arrow*)**.
c. Periodontal pocket formation is accompanied by resorption of alveolar bone.
d. Periodontal pockets are further classified as suprabony, infrabony, simple, complex and compound subtypes (*see below*).

◂ *What is the difference between a false and true pocket?*

***Periodontal pockets* are further classified according to:**

A. According to the number of tooth surfaces involved:
   i. **Simple pocket:** When pocket is present only on ***one*** of the four surfaces of the tooth **(Fig. 10.5, diag. 1)**.
   ii. **Compound pocket:** When pocket involves two or more surfaces of the tooth and the pocket opens into oral cavity along ***each*** of these involved surfaces **(Fig. 10.5, diag. 2)**. Base of a compound pocket can be reached in a straight line (*using a probe*) on each of the involved tooth surfaces.
   iii. **Complex** or **Spiral** or **Tortuous pocket:** When pocket originates on one surface of a tooth and continues ***spirally*** around the tooth to involve two or more surfaces of the tooth but opens into oral cavity ***only*** on the surface from which it started **(Fig. 10.5, diag. 3)**. A probe cannot reach the base of the pocket in a straight line.

◂ *What are compound pockets?*
◂ *What are the other names of a compound pocket?*
◂ *What is the difference between compound and complex pockets?*

B. Position of base of the pocket relative to crest of alveolar bone:
   i. **Suprabony** or **Supra-crestal** or **Supra-alveolar pocket:** When base of pocket is coronal to crest of the alveolar bone and there is horizontal bone loss **(Fig. 10.6, diag. A)** (*also see Chapter 18, 'Resective and Regenerative Bone Surgery for Periodontal Bone Defects' and Fig. 18.3, page 320*).
   ii. **Infrabony** or **Intrabony** or **Sub-crestal** or **Intra-alveolar pocket:** When base of pocket is apical to crest of alveolar bone, i.e. base of pocket lies in between the root surface on one side and the resorbed alveolar bone surface on the other side **(Fig. 10.6, diag. B)** and there is vertical bone loss (*also see Chapter 18, 'Resective and Regenerative Bone Surgery for Periodontal Bone Defects' and Fig. 18.3*).

◂ *What are supra bony pockets?*
◂ *What are infra bony pockets?*
◂ *What is the difference between supra and infra bony pockets?*

3. *Combined Pocket*

a. When pockets deepen due to combination of coronal movement of gingival margin and apical movement of base of the pocket **(Fig. 10.2)**.
b. ***Most true pockets are combined pockets.***

◂ *What are combined pockets?*

ALERT!

- A pocket can have varying depths along its course.
- Pockets can involve one or more tooth surfaces of the same tooth.
- Different pocket types can be present on different surfaces of a tooth.
- Pockets of different depths and types can be present on adjoining proximal surfaces of the same interdental space between two adjoining teeth.

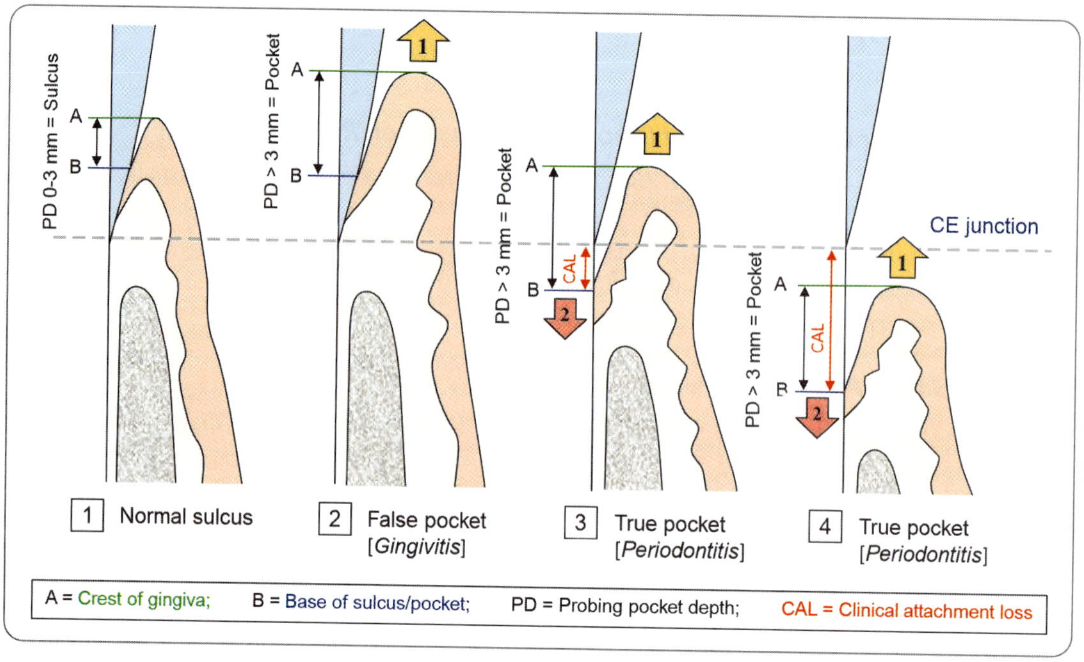

Fig. 10.4: True and false pockets. Diagram 1 represents a normal sulcus with its base on the enamel. Diagram 2 represents false (*gingival*) pocket formation due to coronal shifting of crest of the gingiva (*orange arrow*); note that base of the pocket is on the enamel, i.e. there is no CAL. Diagram 3 represents true (*periodontal*) pocket formation and clinical attachment loss (*CAL*) due to apical shifting of base of the pocket apical to the CE junction and coronal shift of crest of gingiva due to increase in its size caused by inflammation (*orange arrow*). Also note that in diagram 3, although crest of gingiva is on enamel, a true pocket is there because base of pocket is on root. Diagram 4 also represents true (*periodontal*) pocket formation where both base of the pocket and crest of the gingiva are on the root of the tooth.

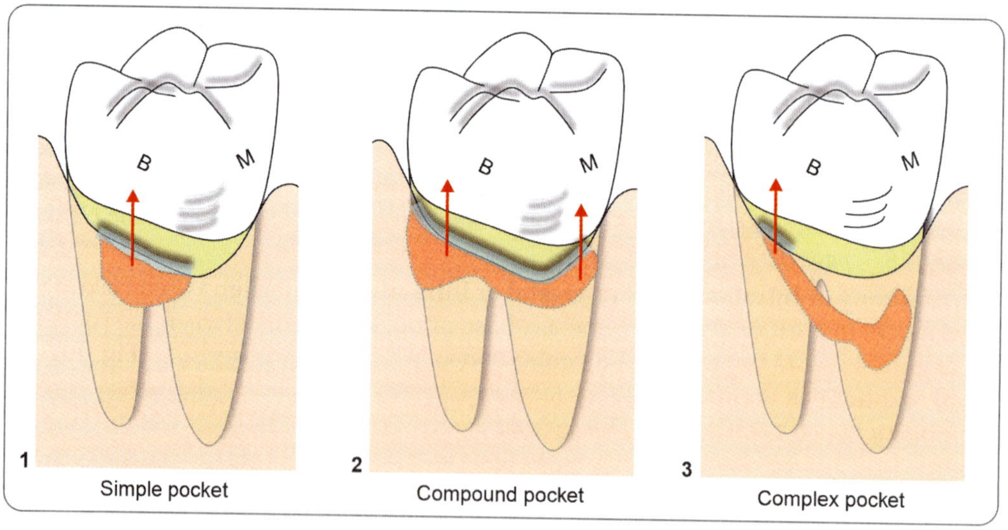

Fig. 10.5: Simple, compound and complex true pockets. In a simple pocket, only one of the four tooth surfaces (*diag.1, buccal surface (B) is involved*) and the pocket opens into the oral cavity on the same tooth surface (*diag. 1, blue line and red arrow*). In a compound pocket, two of the four tooth surfaces are involved (*diag.2, buccal and mesial surfaces (B and M) are involved*) and the pocket is in direct communication with the oral cavity along each of the involved surfaces (*diag. 2, blue line and red arrows*).

In a complex pocket, the pocket originates at one surface of a tooth (e.g. *buccal surface (B), in diag.* 3) and continues spirally around the tooth to involve other tooth surface/s (e.g. *mesial surface (M), in diag.* 3) but the pocket opens into the oral cavity only through the surface from which it started (*buccal surface (B), in diag.* 3); i.e. although the pocket involves surface M also, it does not open into the oral cavity on surface M.

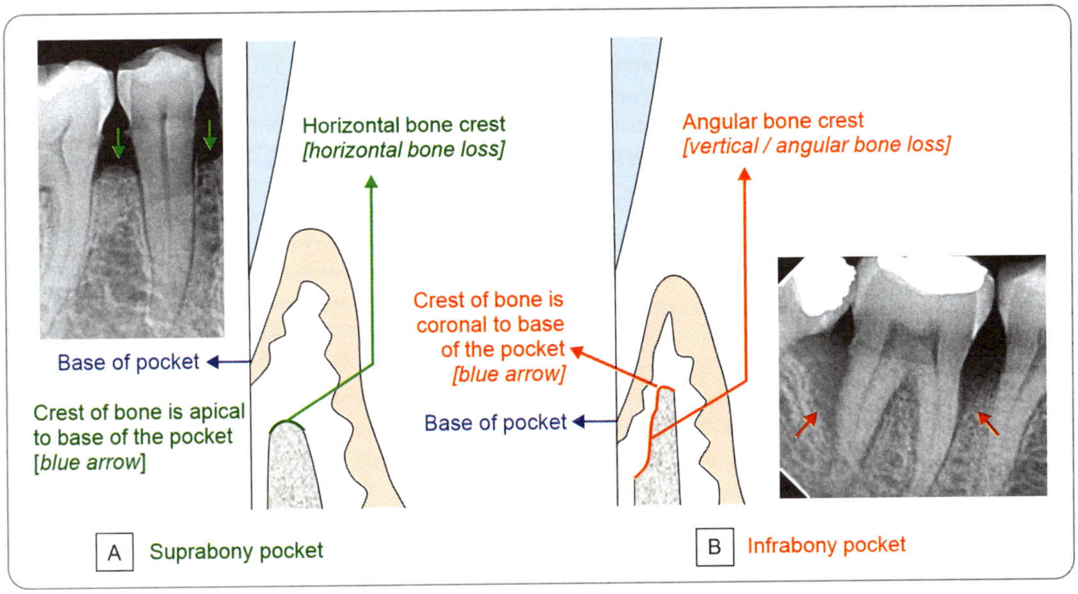

Fig. 10.6: Suprabony pocket (*horizontal bone loss, green arrows*) and infrabony pocket (*vertical bone loss, red arrow*).

CLINICAL UTILITY AND SHORT ANSWER

Differences between suprabony and infrabony pockets

Suprabony	*Infrabony*
1. Base of pocket is located coronal to crest of alveolar bone.	1. Base of pocket is located apical to crest of alveolar bone.
2. Lateral wall of pocket is made entirely of soft tissue (*gingiva*).	2. Coronal part of lateral wall of the pocket is made of soft tissue (*gingiva*) while its apical part is made of partially resorbed alveolar bone crest that is covered by pocket epithelium.
3. Crest of alveolar bone is horizontal, i.e. there is horizontal bone loss.	3. Crest of the alveolar bone is angular i.e. there is angular or vertical bone loss.
4. Transseptal fibers run horizontally over crest of resorbed interdental alveolar bone septum.	4. Transseptal fibers run obliquely over crest of partially resorbed interdental alveolar bone septum.
5. On facial and lingual/palatal surfaces PDL fibers follow their normal course apical to the base of the pocket.	5. On facial and lingual/palatal surfaces the PDL fibers follow an angular course over the angular bone crest apical to the base of the pocket.

Tooth Surface Wall of the Pocket

A pocket has *three* boundaries:

1. Tooth surface wall
2. Gingival wall
3. Floor made by junctional epithelium.

◂ *What are the boundaries of a pocket?*

The tooth side wall (*tooth surface*) of a periodontal pocket shows distinct zones from coronal to the apical end:

1. Tooth structure (*enamel/cementum/dentine or their combinations*)
2. Calculus
3. Attached plaque (*plaque deposited over calculus or tooth surface*)
4. Unattached plaque (*plaque suspended in the sulcus or pocket*)
5. Junctional epithelium
6. Zone showing partial destruction of connective tissue fibers and diseased connective tissue.
7. Zone of healthy connective tissue.

Area of the tooth covered by zones 4, 5, 6, and 7 is also called '***Plaque Free Zone***'.

◂ *What is plaque free zone?*

ALERT!

- The tooth surface wall of the pocket is nonliving, it therefore does not show any inflammatory changes.
- Bacterial endotoxins get ***absorbed*** and ***adsorbed*** into and on the root surface. These ***endotoxins leak out*** of the root surface and promote inflammation (*periodontitis*) in the adjoining gingiva.
- Acid produced by plaque bacteria causes formation of areas of demineralization on the root. Such areas are brownish in colour and have a leathery consistency.

Periodontal Pockets are Healing Lesions

Is healing activity seen in active periodontitis?

- In untreated (*ongoing*) periodontitis, both periodontal damage and healing go on side by side. Although, ***healing is happening all the time, it does not reach completion*** till periodontitis is successfully treated.

Is damage due to periodontitis ongoing during periods of remission of periodontitis?

- Untreated (*ongoing*) periodontitis may show periods of remission, in which severity of periodontitis decreases.
- In such periods of remission, healing activity becomes predominant and shows up as decrease in severity of clinical features of gingivitis and periodontitis while mild disease activity (*periodontitis*) continues in the background.

Is healing activity going on in periods of active progression of periodontitis?

- In periods of disease progression, the reverse happens. This cycle continues till it is stopped by treatment.

ALERT!

Endotoxins and bacteria from periodontal pockets not only cause periodontitis but also affect our systemic health.

How do endotoxins affect our health?

- Endotoxins can enter a patient's blood stream via gingival vessels and can cause several serious systemic problems like atherosclerosis, low birth weight babies, pre-term births, difficult sugar control in diabetics, etc.
- Antibiotics cannot remove endotoxin present on and within the root. It has to be ***removed physically*** by scaling and root planing; this can cause exposure of root dentin and lead to tooth root hypersensitivity after scaling and root planing.
- Incomplete scaling and root planing are the main reasons for continuation and our inability to treat periodontitis even after 'treatment'.

GINGIVITIS AND PERIODONTITIS PRESENT ALL THE FIVE SIGNS OF INFLAMMATION

What are the five cardinal signs of inflammation?

The five cardinal signs of inflammation are: change in color, increase in size, increase in temperature, pain and loss of function.

- Inflammation in gingivitis and periodontitis alters the normal features of periodontal tissues.

Which features of inflammation are easily noticeable in gingiva in gingivitis and periodontitis?

- Such alterations are easily visualized in the gingiva as changes in color, contour, consistency, surface texture, size and position of gingiva. Change in colour and increase in size are the ***most noticeable*** and ***easily recognized*** in ***gingiva***.

Change in Color

How does the colour of gingiva change in gingivitis and periodontitis?

Normal base colour of gingiva is light pink. In acute (*initial*) inflammatory phase, gingiva becomes red due to increase in blood supply. Later, when chronic inflammation sets in, gingiva attains a bluish-red color (*due to stagnation of blood flow which leads to increased de-oxygenation of blood*).

(*Change in color is not recordable in PDL, alveolar bone and cementum*).

Increase in Size

Why does size of gingiva increase in gingivitis and periodontitis?

Swelling of gingiva causes increase in its size. This occurs due to accumulation of exudate (*inflammatory fluid*) in gingiva.

(*Increase in size is not recordable in other periodontal tissues,* i.e. *PDL, alveolar bone and cementum*).

Increase in Temperature

This is caused by increased blood supply (*vascularity*) of the inflamed gingiva. Temperature is only recorded in the gingival sulcus using specialized equipment.
(*Increase in temperature is not recordable in other periodontal tissues, i.e. PDL, alveolar bone and cementum*).

◂ *Why does temperature of gingiva increase in gingivitis and periodontitis?*

Pain

There is usually ***no*** pain associated with gingivitis or periodontitis. Pain is not there because exudate and pus typically do not get localized to form acute abscesses (*in gingiva*) and large ulcers do not form (*in sulcular epithelium*).
(*Pain may be recordable in PDL as tenderness but is not recordable in other periodontal tissues*, i.e. *alveolar bone and cementum*).

◂ *Do individuals with gingivitis or periodontitis usually complain of pain in the affected areas?*

Loss of Function

Loss of function of the periodontal tissue is indirect. In gingiva, it is caused primarily due to increase in its size and loss of its tone and consistency. Loss of function is more noticeable in periodontal ligament and alveolar bone as mobility of teeth, etc.

CLINICAL FEATURES OF GINGIVITIS (*CHRONIC PLAQUE INDUCED INFLAMMATORY GINGIVAL ENLARGEMENT*)

Gingivitis is plaque induced gingival inflammation of the gingiva. It is characterized by false pocket formation, i.e. base of pocket is coronal to CE junction.

As inflammation induces both destructive (*disease*) and constructive (*healing*) changes, the clinical picture of gingiva in gingivitis depends on the interplay of these two processes. The clinical features of gingivitis are:

◂ *What is the main distinguishing feature of gingivitis from periodontitis?*

1. Presence of ***false pockets***, i.e. base of the pocket is ***coronal*** to CE junction and there is ***no*** CAL (*clinical attachment loss*). ***This differentiates gingivitis from periodontitis*** **(Fig. 10.4, diag. B)**.
2. ***Increase*** in rate of flow of GCF (*gingival crevicular fluid—an inflammatory exudate; it increases with increasing severity of inflammation*). However, it is measurable only with special instruments that are usually not available in most dental clinics around the world.
3. ***Increase*** in temperature of gingiva (*measured in the sulcus*). However, it is measurable only with special instruments that are usually not available in most dental clinics around the world.
4. Color of the gingiva changes from ***pink to bluish-red***. Appearance of red patches on surface of the gingiva may also be seen. This change in color is ***not*** very obvious in intensely ***pigmented gingiva*** or if there is high degree of keratinization.
5. ***Bleeding on light probing*** (*slight provocation*). Inflammation causes blood vessels to become engorged, friable and liable to rupturing. Such vessels get injured easily due to thinning of sulcular/pocket epithelium (*due to inflammation*).
   According to the 2018 classification, it is ***normal*** for an otherwise periodontally healthy patient to have mild gingival inflammation (gingivitis) at one or two sites and mild bleeding on probing (*BOP*) at less than 10% sites in the entire mouth.
6. ***Increase in size*** of gingiva. It occurs due to accumulation of gingival exudate and fibrosis. As size of gingiva increases, crest of gingiva moves coronally. This causes increase in sulcus depth (*probing depth—PD*).
7. ***Loss*** of knife edge deflecting contour of marginal gingiva and interdental papilla (*due to accumulation of exudate*). ***Gingival margin becomes round and bulbous.*** A life saver like bulge called ***'McCall's festoon'*** may form around involved teeth **(Fig. 10.8)**.
8. Consistency of gingiva changes from ***firm and resilient to soft and pitting on pressure*** (*due to inflammation*). As disease progresses, gingiva becomes soggy, puffy, markedly soft, flaccid and friable.
9. Loss of surface stippling (*if stippling was present on the gingiva earlier; see Chapter 2, Gingiva and Fig. 2.18*). Stippling is lost due to inflammation of gingiva. This makes surface of gingiva smooth and shiny.

◂ *Do rate of flow of GCF and temperature increase in gingivitis?*

◂ *In which cases changes in colour of gingiva are difficult to identify?*

◂ *Why does bleeding on probing occur in gingivitis?*

◂ *Does presence of bleeding on probing always lead to a diagnosis of gingivitis?*

◂ *What is a McCall's festoon?*

◂ *What is the consistency of gingiva in gingivitis?*

What are Stillman's clefts? ▶

10. ***Stillman's clefts*** may also form in marginal gingiva. (*Stillman's clefts are apostrophe like breaks or clefts in the gingival margin*) (Fig. 10.9).

What is milking of a pocket? ▶

11. Pus may be expressed by applying digital pressure on the gingiva in some cases with deep pockets; this is called 'milking the pocket' (Fig. 10.12).
12. As the marginal gingiva swells up, it moves ***coronally***. This causes further deepening of the ***false pocket*** and increase in probing depth (*PD*).

Is alveolar bone loss present in gingivitis? ▶

13. ***No alveolar bone loss*** attributable to plaque induced inflammation is present. Bone loss due to other causes like TFO, prominent position of tooth in the arch, cervical caries, etc. may be present.

When is pain present in gingivitis? ▶

14. ***No pain or tenderness*** are usually reported by the patient. Pain and tenderness occur only if abscess formation occurs.
15. Gingivitis is slowly progressing.

Is gingivitis reversible? ▶

16. The clinical features of gingivitis are ***reversible*** with treatment (*scaling, root planing followed by adequate plaque control*).

ALERT!

- Plaque induced inflammation of gingiva (*gingivitis*) can also occur in a successfully treated and now stable case of periodontitis in which base of pocket is located apical to CE junction (*CAL is present*).
- The presence of gingivitis (*gingival inflammation*) in case of periodontitis (*CAL is present and base of pocket is apical to CE junction = periodontitis*) can be confusing.
- Therefore to avoid confusion, the 2018 classification, terms such cases as gingival inflammation in a stable case of periodontitis (*instead of gingivitis in a case of periodontitis*) (*see Chapter 10A 'Making Clinical Diagnosis of Gingivitis and Periodontitis Using The 2018 Classification'* and Figs 10A.4 and 10A.7).

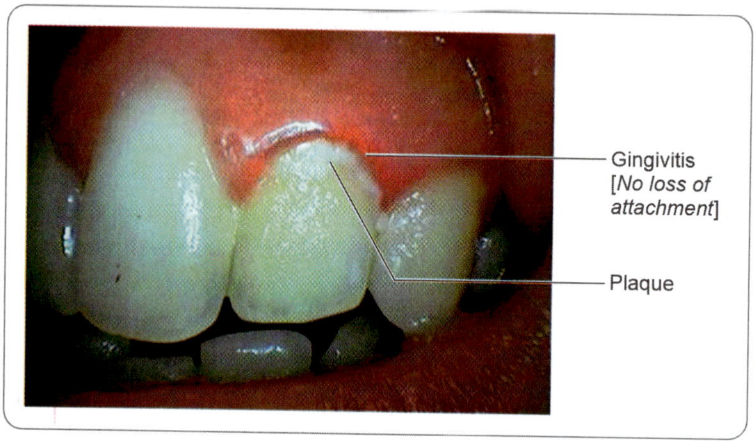

Fig. 10.7: Gingivitis

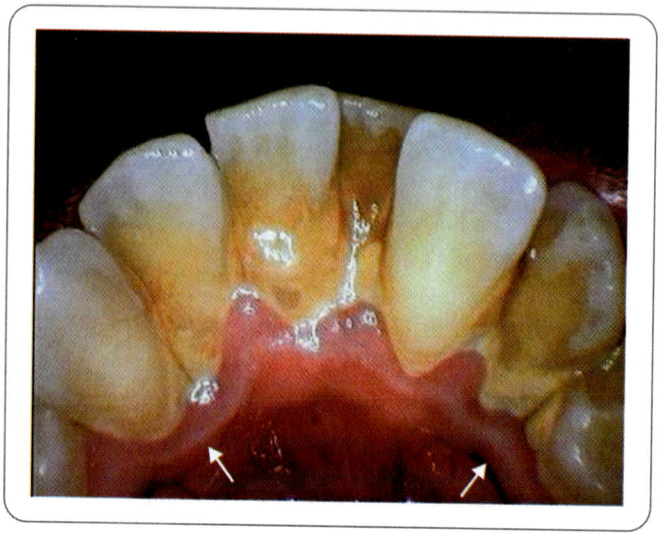

Fig. 10.8: McCall's Festoon (*white arrows*)

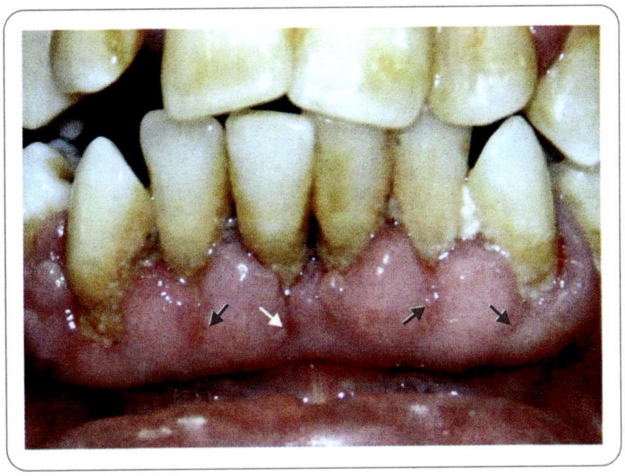

Fig. 10.9: Stillman's clefts in periodontitis. They are more often seen on the buccal surface. These maybe simple (*black arrows*) when the cleft does not branch or they can be compound (*white arrow*) when the cleft shows branching.

CLINICAL UTILITY AND SHORT ANSWER

As gingivitis or periodontitis set in, which clinical features of gingiva change first?

Initial changes associated with gingivitis or periodontitis can be noticed first in two clinical features of the gingiva with a naked eye: These are:

1. Change in color of gingiva which changes from light pink to dark pink or red.
2. Loss of knife edge deflecting contour of the marginal gingiva which changes to a rounded, bulbous and non-deflecting contour.

CLINICAL UTILITY AND SHORT ANSWER

How much force should be applied on a probe while checking bleeding on probing (*BOP*)?

A probing force of 0.25 N is recommended. This is just enough force to produce a slight depression in the bulb of a finger when a probe tip is pressed on it. A probing pressure of 0.15 N is recommended around implants.

CLINICAL FEATURES OF PERIODONTITIS

Because periodontitis is an ***extension*** of gingivitis into deeper periodontal tissues, it therefore presents clinical features of gingivitis in ***addition*** to clinical features that are specific to periodontitis. The clinical features of periodontitis are:

◂ *Are clinical features of gingivitis also seen in periodontitis?*

1. ***All*** clinical features from point number 2–13 in list of clinical features of gingivitis (*see page 145*).
2. Presence of ***true pockets*** (*base of the pocket is* ***apical*** *to CE junction*) and CAL (*clinical attachment loss*). ***This differentiates periodontitis from gingivitis.***
3. Marginal gingiva and attached gingiva may be reddish-blue in color due to chronic inflammation. At times, especially in severe or stage III or IV periodontitis, a patch of reddish-blue colour running from crest of marginal gingiva to the attached gingiva or even up to the alveolar mucosa is seen (Fig. 10.11). In ***milder*** stage I or II periodontitis, colour change may ***not*** be easily identifiable.
4. Varying degrees of alveolar ***bone loss*** is present. This bone loss may be horizontal or vertical (Fig. 10.14).
5. Gingiva is swollen to varying degrees and crest of the gingiva may be rolled out.
6. As periodontitis worsens, gingival recession can be seen (Fig. 10.10).
7. Bleeding on probing (*BOP*) from gingiva is ***present***. However, gingival bleeding may be absent if pockets are fibrotic. Bleeding is more in stage III or IV (*severe*) periodontitis.
8. Free gingiva and interdental papilla may be semi-firm or ***flaccid***. Loss of facio–lingual continuity of the buccal and lingual interdental papillae may be seen (Fig. 10.13, diag. D).

◂ *What is the main distinguishing feature of periodontitis from gingivitis?*

◂ *Does gingiva show a change in colour in periodontitis?*

◂ *Is alveolar bone loss always present in periodontitis?*

◂ *Is BOP always present in periodontitis?*

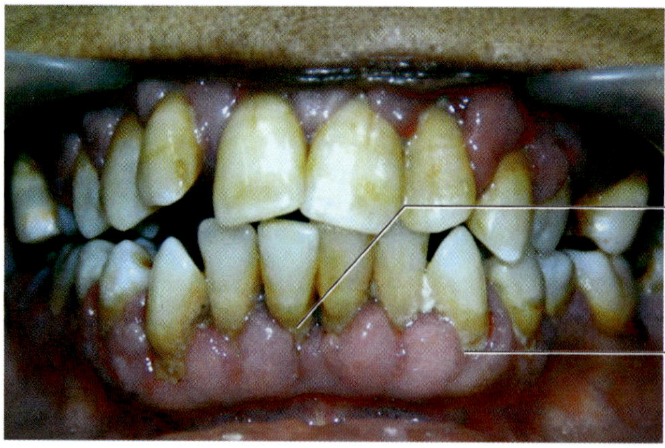

Fig. 10.10: Periodontitis

9. Pus may be expressed from the pocket by applying finger pressure on the pocket wall. This is called 'milking the pocket' (Fig. 10.12).
10. Tooth or teeth in question may be ***mobile*** to varying degrees.

In which teeth is pathologic migration most commonly seen in periodontitis? ▸

11. Pathologic migration of affected teeth may be seen. ***Disto-labial*** migration and ***extrusion*** of anterior teeth is common (Fig. 10.13, diag. A).
12. Food impaction in interdental areas and pockets is a common finding. Patients complain of an ***urge to dig out*** stuck food with a pointed object (*tooth pick*, etc.) or suck out such impacted food. After removing impacted food, patient feels relief from pressure and pain.

Is pain a common finding in periodontitis? ▸

13. Some patients may complain of ***dull ache*** or ***gnawing*** pain in the teeth and gingivae especially after eating food. Acute and severe pain is ***not*** a feature of periodontitis; if pain is present, it is usually because of food impaction or periodontal abscess formation.
14. Patients complain that mastication of food has become difficult; patients prefer to use the lesser involved side for eating food.
15. Foul breath (*halitosis*) and foul taste. These worsen with worsening of periodontitis. Most patients get to know of foul breath only when a close associate or relative points it out to them. In order to get rid of their foul breath, patients may have started to brush their teeth (*if they did not do so earlier*) or may have increased frequency and time of tooth brushing. Some patients start to use mouth fresheners and plaque control mouth washes frequently.
16. Involved teeth may have become hypersensitive due to gingival recession (Fig. 10.10). If plaque microorganisms gain entry into pulp of the tooth (*via lateral accessory canals*), such teeth may show associated pulpal disease (*see Chapter 21, Interdisciplinary Interrelationships and Supportive Periodontal Therapy and Figs 21.2 and 10*). Such teeth may lose their vitality due to degeneration of the pulp and then present with periapical abscesses (*retrograde pulpitis*).

When gingivitis extends deeper into periodontal tissues and causes attachment loss and true pocket formation, the disease is called periodontitis. A few facts pertaining to periodontitis must always be kept in mind when managing a case of periodontitis:

Does gingivitis always occur before periodontitis? ▸

- Gingivitis always occurs ***first*** and leads to (*precedes*) periodontitis.
- Plaque induced gingival inflammation also occurs during initial phase of recurrent periodontitis. To avoid confusion, the 2018 classification, terms such cases as gingival inflammation in a stable case of periodontitis (*instead of gingivitis in a case of periodontitis*) (*see Chapter 10A 'Making Clinical Diagnosis of Gingivitis and Periodontitis Using The 2018 Classification' and Figs 10A.4 and 10A.7*).

Does presence of bleeding on probing always lead to a diagnosis of periodontitis? ▸

- It is normal to have up to 10% sites with gingival inflammation and bleeding on probing (*BOP*) in a previously treated but now stable case of periodontitis. If more than 10% sites have BOP, the case is then diagnosed as recurrent periodontitis (*2018 classification*).

- *All* cases of periodontitis have CAL (*clinical attachment loss*) due to plaque mediated inflammatory disease (*see Chapter 2, Fig. 2.7*).
- CAL can however also occur due to other reasons, e.g. prominent root surfaces of teeth (Fig. 10A.1), cervical caries, crown lengthening, etc. In such cases:
  - If such teeth do not exhibit gingival inflammation, they are diagnosed as clinically healthy cases with reduced periodontium not due to periodontitis.
  - If, however such cases present inflammation in the gingiva, then, diagnosis of 'gingival inflammation on reduced periodontium not due to periodontitis' is made.
  - If in such cases CAL increases due to plaque induced inflammation, a diagnosis of periodontitis will be made (*2018 classification*) (Fig. 10A.3).

◄ *Is CAL always present in periodontitis?*

◄ *What are the other causes for CAL?*

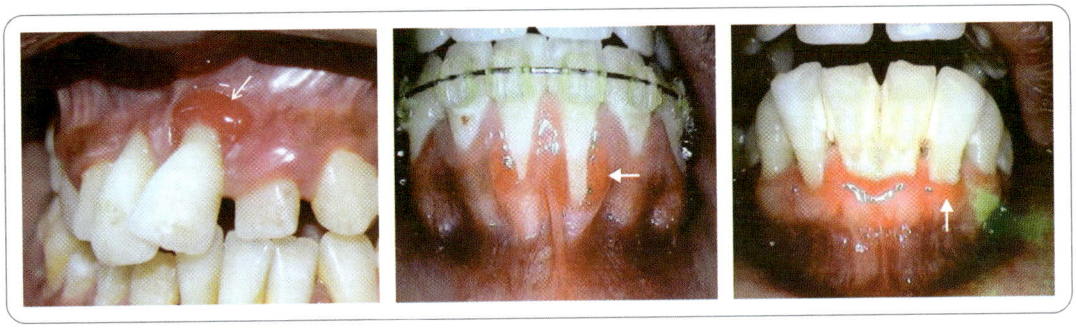

Fig. 10.11: In stage II, III or IV periodontitis, a zone of reddish-blue colour (*white arrows*) running from crest of marginal gingiva to the attached gingiva or even up to the alveolar mucosa may be seen.

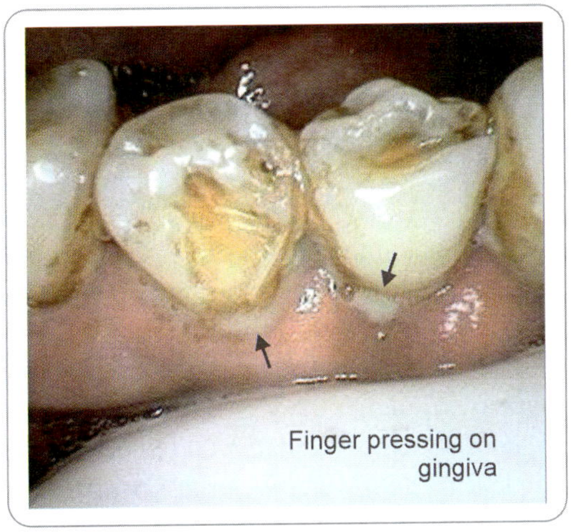

Fig. 10.12: 'Milking' the pocket. Sometimes, in severe stage II, III and IV periodontitis, pressing over the gingiva with deep pockets will express pus out of the pockets (*black arrows*). Although, amount of pus expressed is not related to severity of periodontitis, however, this when shown to the patient, serves as a very good educational and motivational tool.

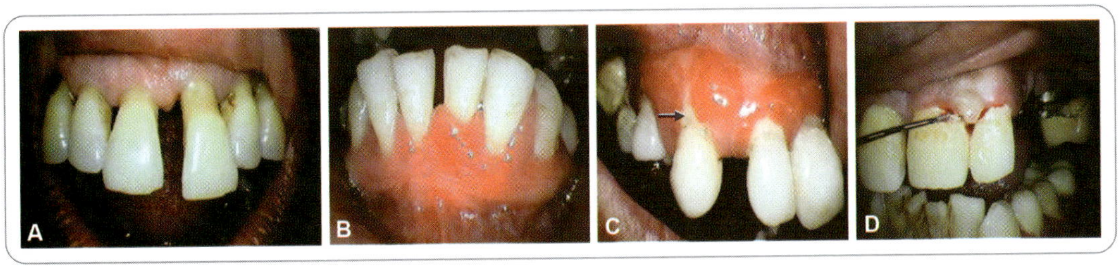

Fig. 10.13: Extrusion of teeth, distolabial migration, diastema (*gap*) formation or its worsening, recession (*diags A, B and C*), suppuration (*pus formation and expression; black arrow, diag. C*), gingival enlargement (*diags B, C and D*), flaccid gingiva with loss of facio-lingual continuity of interdental papillae (*diag. D*), etc. are common features of stage II, III and IV periodontitis (*severe periodontitis*).

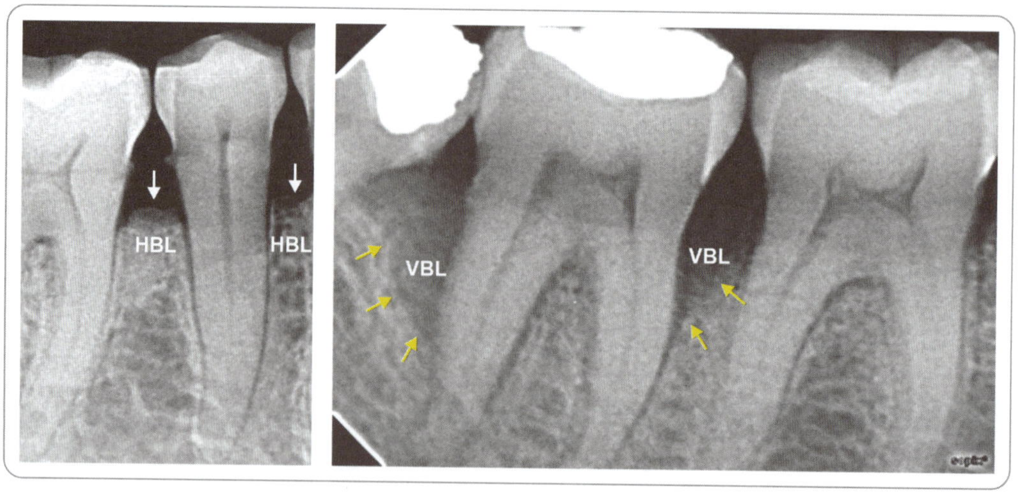

Fig. 10.14: Different sites in the same patient and around the same tooth will present different amounts of bone loss in periodontitis. This bone loss may either be horizontal (*HBL, white arrows diag. A*) or vertical (*VBL, yellow arrows diag. B*).

Can pus be expressed from all pockets in a case of periodontitis? ▸

ALERT!

Suppuration is demonstrable (*milking of a pocket*) only at approximately 5% of sites with periodontitis (Fig. 10.12).

Does periodontitis occur at all sites in the mouth? ▸

ALERT!

Periodontitis is site specific.

Periodontitis is a ***site-specific disease***. It may be active at a particular site or sites whereas other sites in the mouth may be normal. It occurs at a site, in direct response to plaque accumulation and calculus deposition at that particular site only.

Classification of Periodontitis

According to the multi-dimensional staging and grading system of the 2018 classification, periodontitis can be classified as:

Staging of periodontitis classifies periodontitis based on which parameters? ▸

Periodontitis is classified into how many stages in the 2018 classification? ▸

1. Based on ***severity and complexity of management*** **(Fig.10.15)**
   i. **Stage I** (*initial or mild periodontitis*).
   ii. **Stage II** (*moderate periodontitis*).
   iii. **Stage III** (*severe periodontitis with potential for additional tooth loss*).
   iv. **Stage IV** (*severe periodontitis with potential for loss of dentition*).

Grading of periodontitis classifies periodontitis based on which parameters? ▸

Periodontitis is classified into how many grades in the 2018 classification? ▸

2. Based on ***risk of rapid progression and anticipated treatment response*** **(Fig. 10.16)**
   i. **Grade A** (*slowly progressing periodontitis; periodontal destruction is little and is relatable to amount of plaque deposits*).
   ii. **Grade B** (*periodontitis with moderate rate of progression; periodontal destruction is moderate and relatable to amount of plaque deposits*).
   iii. **Grade C** (*periodontitis with fast rate of progression*).

Periodontitis is classified into which two types based on extent of periodontitis? ▸

3. Based on ***extent***
   i. **Localized** (*30% or lesser number of teeth involved*).
   ii. **Generalized** (*more than 30% teeth involved*).

If periodontitis is present only in relation to molars and incisors what is it called? ▸

4. Based on distribution (*area of involvement in the mouth*).
   i. **Molar-incisor distribution** (*periodontitis restricted to molar and incisor region only; other teeth are uninvolved*).

Grade C Periodontitis

What is grade C periodontitis? ▸

Grade C periodontitis (*2018 classification*) is unique and totally different from grade A and B periodontitis in many aspects. However, it has ***not*** been found to be different enough for it to be classified as a separate disease entity in the 2018 classification. Due to its unique

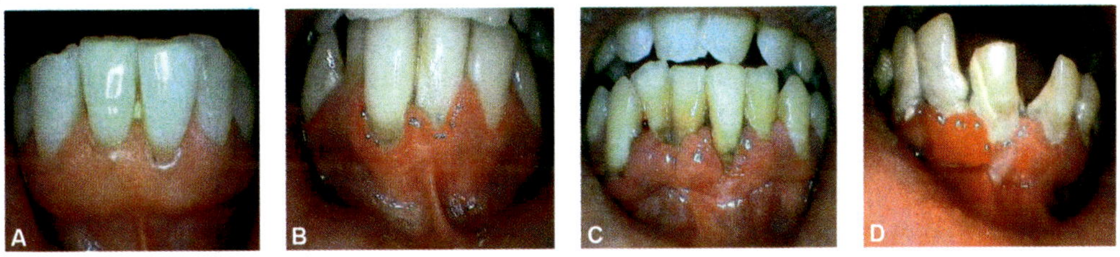

Stage I periodontitis
CAL =1-2 mm
RBL= Coronal third [<15%]
PD = ≤4 mm maximum
Mostly horizontal bone loss

Stage II periodontitis
CAL = 3-4 mm
RBL = Coronal third [15-33 %]
PD = ≤5 mm maximum
Mostly horizontal bone loss

Stage III periodontitis
CAL = ≥5 mm
RBL = Middle 1/3rd of root or more
PD = ≥6 mm maximum
Vertical bone loss ≥3 mm
≤4 teeth lost due to periodontitis

Stage IV periodontitis
≥5 teeth lost to periodontitis
In addition to stage III complexity masticatory dysfunction, secondary occlusal trauma, bite collapse, less than 20 remaining teeth

Fig. 10.15: Stage I to IV periodontitis

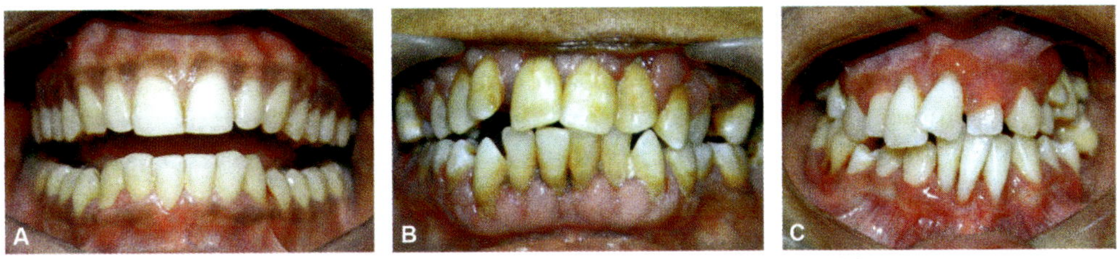

Grade A periodontitis
Note that plaque and calculus caused periodontitis [*lower arch*] is mild and its severity is relatable to amount of local factors present

Grade B periodontitis
Note that a lot of plaque and calculus have produced a lot of periodontitis *i.e.*, severity of periodontitis is relatable to amount of local factors present

Grade C periodontitis
Note that there is ***no*** visible plaque or calculus but a lot of periodontitis *i.e.*, severity of periodontitis is not relatable to amount of local factors present

Fig. 10.16: Grade A, B and C periodontitis. In grade A and B periodontitis (*diags A and B*), periodontal destruction and severity of periodontitis is usually co-relatable to the number and amount of local factors (*plaque calculus, etc.*). In grade C periodontitis (*diag. C*), this co-relation is generally missing and there are too little local factors to explain the great amount of disease. In grade C periodontitis with molar-incisor pattern (*periodontitis restricting to all 1st molars and all incisors—localized aggressive periodontitis; 1999 classification*), this correlation maybe totally absent.

clinical features, it deserves special mention in this text. Grade C periodontitis fits the description of aggressive periodontitis (*1999 classification, AAP*) in some aspects. Earlier to 1999 classification, aggressive periodontitis has also been called rapidly progressing periodontitis, juvenile periodontitis, paradontosis, etc.

When compared to grade A and B periodontitis, grade C periodontitis:

- Progresses at a very fast rate.
- Does not respond to standard periodontal treatment.
- Is usually present in patients with certain systemic diseases and conditions, e.g. diabetes, immune defects, etc.
- Grade C periodontitis especially with molar-incisor pattern, is considered to be an ***extreme variant*** type of periodontitis that is caused by a combination of immune defects and specific microorganisms.

Peculiar and Differentiating Clinical Features of Grade C periodontitis (and comparison of features of grade A and grade B periodontitis with those of grade C periodontitis)

Clinical features in fast progressing grade C periodontitis are ***more evident*** in later stages of the disease, i.e. stage II, III and IV.

◂ *How fast do grade A, B and C periodontitis progress?*

1. Grade C periodontitis has a very fast rate of progression. It is usually 3–4 times faster than grade A and B periodontitis. Grade A and B periodontitis show ***no*** or up to ***2 mm bone loss*** in ***5 years***. In untreated cases of Grade C periodontitis ***more than 2 mm*** bone loss can be seen in a period of ***5 years*** (*stages III and IV (stages of disease showing severe periodontal loss) are reached very fast*).

If clinical exam reveals that periodontal destruction is far in excess of identifiable local factors, what does it suggest?

2. Periodontal destruction is ***far in excess*** of identifiable local etiological factors like plaque and calculus, i.e. periodontal destruction is ***not*** relatable to amount of plaque and calculus deposits. (*Periodontal destruction is relatable to number and amount of local factors like plaque and calculus deposits in cases of grade A and B periodontitis*).
3. Huge amount of periodontal destruction (*deep pockets and accompanying severe bone loss*) occurs very fast and affected teeth reach poor prognosis stage early during the course of disease. (*Grade A or B periodontitis are relatively slowly progressing and patients get a lot of time during the course of disease to get treated. Therefore, teeth reach poor prognosis stage relatively late*).

What is the usual age of onset of grade C periodontitis with molar incisor presentation?

4. Grade C periodontitis, especially if it has a molar-incisor presentation or if associated with severe systemic diseases and conditions, usually has an early or circumpubertal age of onset (*around the age of puberty*, i.e. *between 12–14 years of age*).
(*Grade A and B periodontitis usually affects older individuals but can also occur in individuals in the younger age group*).

If severe periodontal loss is present without accompanying features of gingival inflammation, what does it point to?

5. Grade C periodontitis usually presents with ***vertical bone loss*** and ***infrabony pockets*** (*especially in cases with molar-incisor presentation of periodontitis*). However, despite the severe periodontal loss, features of gingival inflammation may not be present at all or these if present, may be very mild.
[*Features of inflammation (gingivitis) and degree of tissue destruction are more co-relatable in cases of grade A and grade B periodontitis*].

Which radiographic features are characteristic of periodontitis with molar-incisor presentation?

6. Grade C periodontitis with molar-incisor pattern presents with:
   a. Bone loss around permanent incisors.
   b. A unique ***semi-lunar*** or ***cup*** or ***arc shaped bone*** loss in relation permanent 1st molars (*when disease reaches stage II, III and IV*) of both sides (*bilateral symmetry*). This is a sure-shot sign of (***pathognomonic of***) grade C periodontitis with molar-incisor pattern (*earlier called as localized aggressive periodontitis—1999 classification*) (**Fig. 10.17**).

(*Other cases of localized or generalized grade A, B or C periodontitis do not show such typical bone loss patterns seen in grade C periodontitis with molar incisor pattern*).

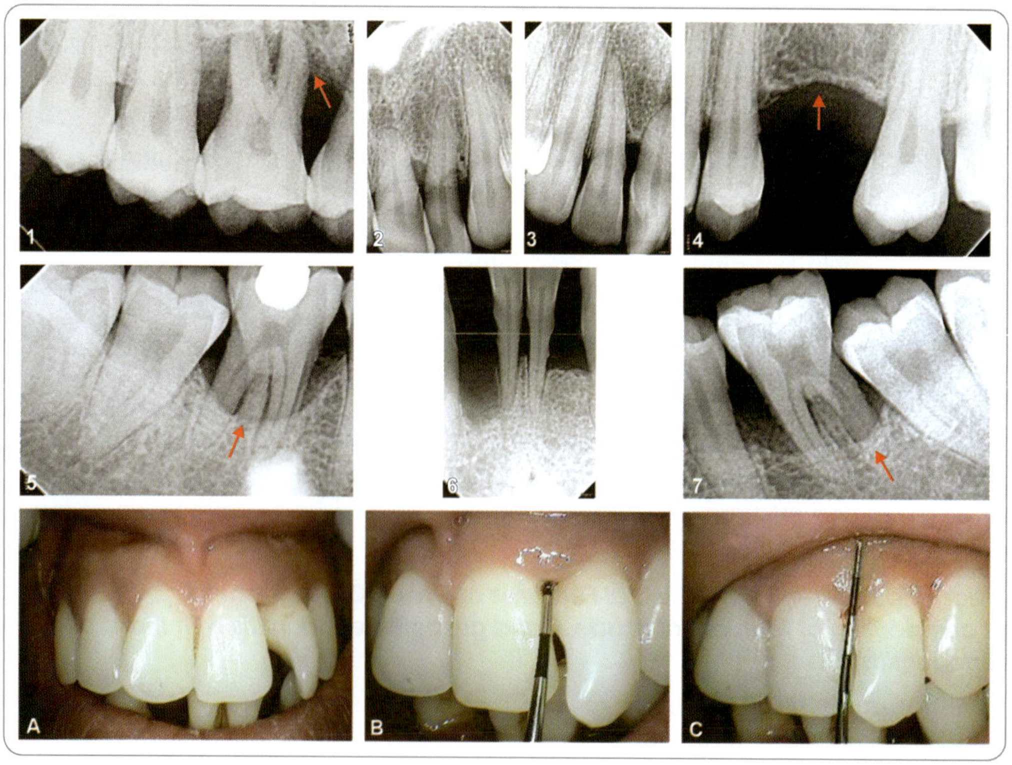

Fig. 10.17: Typical features of a case of grade C periodontitis with molar-incisor pattern (*was called localized aggressive periodontitis earlier in the 1999 AAP's classification*). This disease starts around puberty (*12–14 years*). Severe bone loss is seen around permanent maxillary and mandibular incisors on both sides of the mouth. A typical semi-lunar/arc shaped/cup like bone loss pattern (*red arrows*) is seen around permanent 1st molars on both right and left sides (*mirror image*) of the mouth.

7. Grade C periodontitis with molar-incisor pattern may not progress to involve other teeth (i.e. *may not progress to become generalized*). This self-limiting of disease is called ***'burn-out phenomenon'***. Grade C periodontitis with molar-incisor pattern may however progress to become generalized only in around **25–30%** of cases.

   (*All cases of grade A and B periodontitis, may involve all teeth and increase in severity over time*).

◂ What is burn out phenomenon?

8. Pathologic migration of anterior teeth (*disto-labial migration*) is seen at an ***early age*** and very soon after disease starts (*as disease occurs at an early age and is fast progressing, stage III and stage IV (severe disease) are reached very fast*).

   (*All cases of grade A and B periodontitis, especially stage III and stage IV cases may present pathologic migration of teeth*).

◂ Does pathologic migration occur in early or late stages of grade C periodontitis?

9. Grade C periodontitis may occur simultaneously in children (*blood relations*) of the same family. This suggests role of hereditary factors in etiopathogenesis (*especially in cases with molar-incisor pattern*). It can also be due to cross infection (*of periodontopathogens*) from a case of grade C periodontitis to an un-infected person (*siblings are most likely to be affected*). (*Grade A and B periodontitis can also be seen in closely related family members; this too can be explained on the basis of cross infection and hereditary predisposition*).

◂ Do grade A, B and C periodontitis occur in siblings?

CLINICAL UTILITY AND SHORT ANSWER

In grade C periodontitis with *molar-incisor pattern*, what is the reason for *'burn-out phenomenon'* (*periodontal loss to remain restricted to permanent 1st molars and incisors only*)**?**

◂ Why does periodontal loss remain restricted to permanent 1st molars and incisors only in grade C periodontitis with molar-incisor pattern?

Grade C periodontitis with molar-incisor pattern at times does not progress to involve other teeth; this self-limiting of disease is called 'burn-out phenomenon'. Although reasons for this are ***not*** clearly known, the following explanations have been given for this:

1. Permanent 1st molars and incisors erupt at 6–7 years age and are the first permanent teeth to erupt in the oral cavity. These teeth are therefore the 1st permanent teeth to get colonized (*infected*) by microorganisms causing periodontitis. Once the infection has occurred, immune system mounts a defensive immune reaction against it. This immune reaction, stops further spread of infection (*periodontitis*) to other oral sites, but is ***not*** capable of completely eliminating the infecting microorganisms from the already colonized sites, i.e. 1st permanent molars and incisors. Therefore, other permanent teeth (*other than permanent 1st molars and incisors*) do not get infected (*periodontitis*) even though active infectious sites are present in their neighborhood (*Zambon, et al 1983*).
2. After microorganisms infect 1st permanent molars and incisors and cause periodontitis, antagonistic microorganisms (*that oppose and compete against disease causing microorganisms*) establish themselves in the oral cavity. These antagonistic microorganisms then stop further spread of infection (*periodontitis*) by blocking colonization of new sites on permanent teeth erupting after the permanent 1st molars and the incisors (*Hillman JD, et al 1982*).
3. The permanent 1st molars and incisors have some (*unidentified*) physical or developmental defects in cementum (*of their roots*) that allow their colonization by microorganisms causing periodontitis witn molar-incisor pattern (*Lindskog, et al 1983*). They are thus prone to periodontitis.
4. After periodontitis has occurred in 1st molars and incisors, the causative microorganisms, for some unknown reasons, lose their disease-causing ability (*e.g. leukotoxin production*). This prevents colonization of new sites (*Slots, et al:1982*).

Role of Immunological Factors in Grade C Periodontitis

Some immune defects have been suggested to contribute to grade C periodontitis:

◂ What is the role of immunological factors in causing grade C periodontitis?

1. **Functional defects in PMNs and monocytes:** Such defects impair migration of these cells to site of infection and also affect their ability to kill microorganisms. This allows infection to establish and continue.
2. **Production of higher quantities of PGE2 (*prostaglandin E2*) by monocytes in patients with grade C periodontitis:** PGE2 causes increased destruction of periodontal tissues; it is produced in response to lipopolysaccharides of bacteria that cause periodontitis, etc. (*lipopolysaccharide is a component of bacterial cell wall that is released after death of bacteria*).

Role of Environmental and Genetic Factors in Grade C Periodontitis

How does smoking affect periodontitis?

Several environmental factors act like as risk factors for grade C periodontitis:

- **Smoking:** Periodontitis is more severe in smokers than non-smokers. Also, healing is slower in smokers; therefore, periodontitis is relatively more difficult to treat in such patients.
- **Genetic defects:** Grade C periodontitis runs in families; this means that certain genetic defects that run in a family predispose members of that family to grade C periodontitis. It has been found that coloured races are more prone to grade C periodontitis. The exact nature of the genetic defects is presently unknown.
- **Diabetes:** It is a known risk factor for periodontitis. Diabetic individuals develop immune defects that contribute to severity and rate of progression of grade C periodontitis.

DIAGNOSIS AND CLASSIFICATION OF GINGIVITIS AND PERIODONTITIS

The reader is referred to Chapter 10-A for detailed description of steps in making a diagnosis and staging and grading of periodontitis using 2018 classification.

FIBROTIC POCKETS

How do fibrotic pockets form?

What are fibrotic pockets?

In some cases of gingivitis and periodontitis, healing activity (*proliferative and fibrotic activity*) exceeds the amount of damage produced by inflammation. In such cases, gingival wall of the pocket becomes ***fibrotic*** and does ***not*** show inflammatory features on the ***oral*** surface. However, the inner surface of this gingival wall (*tooth side facing surface*) presents the same exudative-degenerative features as the gingival walls of an ordinary pocket (*inflammatory pocket described earlier*).

Clinical Features of Fibrotic Pockets

What do fibrotic pockets look like?

When compared to an ordinary pocket, gingiva of the fibrotic pocket wall presents the following ***altered features*** (*also see section on pocket presented earlier in this Chapter*) **(Fig. 10.18)**:

1. Colour is light pink. A faint red discolouration may however be seen at the crest of the gingiva.
2. Contour is relatively more bulbous.
3. Consistency is firm and leathery.
4. Surface stippling is coarser.
5. Bleeding on probing is less likely or if it occurs, it is mild.
6. Fibrotic pockets usually cannot be treated with plaque control or scaling and root planing. Such pockets may need to be surgically excised to reduce pocket depth to less than 3 mm.

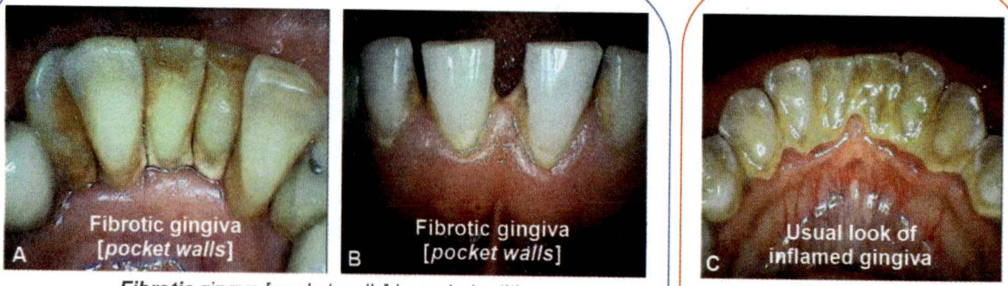

Fibrotic gingva [*pocket walls*] in periodontitis
Note gingiva is pink in colour, enlarged and shows stippling

Inflamed gingiva [*pocket walls*] in periodontitis.
Note gingiva is red, enlarged and has a smooth surface [*shows no stippling*]

Fig. 10.18: Fibrotic pockets. Gingiva with fibrotic pockets is pink in colour, has coarse stippling and is firm looking despite presence of stage II grade B periodontitis (*Figs A and B*). Compare this with the usual look of inflamed gingiva in Fig. C.

PROGRESSION (*INCREASE IN SEVERITY AND SPREAD TO OTHER TEETH*) OF PERIODONTITIS IS NOT CONTINUOUS

Episodic–Burst Model of Progression of Periodontitis (*Burst Hypothesis—Socransky et al 1984*)

This is the most ***accepted*** model that explains how periodontitis worsens at a particular site and progresses to other sites. According to it, periodontitis is:

◄ *What is the burst hypothesis?*

- **Site specific:** This means that periodontitis at a particular gingival site is independent of periodontitis or health at another site, i.e. it is not affected by and has no effect on periodontitis or health at another site.
- **Episodic:** This means that progression of periodontitis at any given site happens in short bursts of activity over a few days/weeks and these periods of activity are interspersed with periods in which no or very low disease activity is seen. In other words, worsening and spread of periodontitis is ***not continuous***.

◄ *Is progress of periodontitis continuous?*

Thus, severity of periodontitis increases due to:
1. Appearance of periodontitis at new sites.
2. Increase in periodontal loss at sites with pre-existing periodontitis.
3. Both the above.

Clinical Implications of Episodic Nature of Periodontitis

◄ *What is the clinical importance of burst hypothesis?*

- A clinician must always remember that if a ***significant reduction*** in clinical features of periodontitis occurs without treatment, this is often due to a ***period of remission*** of periodontitis rather than healing and cure of periodontitis.
- In such periods of remission, most patients and some clinicians may believe and misdiagnose the periodontal condition of a patient as normal.
- Therefore, one must not rely on the 'look' of the gingiva alone, but make an accurate diagnosis by careful clinical examination.
- Repeated periodic clinical checkups are also important for this reason.

Periods of Active Periodontitis are Clinically Recognized by:

1. Appearance or increase in severity of features of gingival inflammation, i.e. change in colour, contour, consistency, size and position of crest of gingiva (*features of gingivitis discussed earlier in this chapter*).
2. Bleeding on slight provocation (*probing*).
3. Alveolar bone loss (*assessed over a period of time*).

◄ *How can it be known whether periodontitis at a particular site is progressing or not?*

Periods of Remission of Periodontitis are Clinically Recognized by:

◄ *What are the clinical features of gingiva if periodontitis is in remission phase?*

1. Decrease in GCF (*gingival crevicular fluid*) flow rate and return of gingival sulcus temperature to normal.
2. Reduced or no gingival bleeding on probing (*BOP*).
3. Shrinking and reduction in size of enlarged gingiva. This causes gingival recession and reduction in depth of pocket (*because of decrease in inflammation within gingiva*).
4. Color of gingiva changes from reddish-blue to pink.
5. Consistency of the gingiva becomes firmer.
6. Surface stippling may reappear.
7. Bulbous gingival contour reduces and deflecting contour of the gingiva may be regained. Gingiva may partially re-attain its scalloped contour.
8. Alveolar bone loss stops and new bone formation may be seen in some areas of bone loss.

ALERT!

Can rate of progression of periodontitis and possibility of future damage at a particular site be accurately predicted?

If periodontitis remains untreated, continued periodontal loss leading to loss of the tooth will occur. However, to what extent and in how much time will periodontitis worsen at a particular site ***cannot*** be accurately predicted. Rate and degree of progression of periodontitis is dependent on patient's immunity, contributing factors of periodontitis, quality of plaque, etc.

CLINICAL UTILITY AND SHORT ANSWER

Which defense mechanisms of the sulcus area protect against initiation and worsening (*progression*) of periodontitis?

The following defense mechanisms give protection against periodontitis:

1. Up to 3 mm probing depth (*PD*). As probing depth increases, G –ve anaerobic bacteria start to colonize the sulcus and cause periodontitis.
2. Outward flow of gingival crevicular fluid (*GCF*) from sulcus into the oral cavity physically flushes out bacteria and their toxins from the sulcus or pocket. GCF also has chemical constituents that kill bacteria.
3. Intact sulcular and junctional epithelia (*epithelial barrier*) restricts invasion of microbes into gingiva.
4. Continuous shedding of superficial epithelial cells (*junctional, sulcular and outer gingival epithelia*) helps shed off invading microbes along with the superficial epithelial layers (*the shed off epithelial cells are continuously replaced by new cells from basal layer of the epithelium*).
5. Immune and inflammatory response of the gingiva (*pocket and periodontal tissues*), e.g. presence of live PMNs within the lumen of the sulcus/pocket, etc.

REVIEW QUESTIONS

1. What is the difference between gingivitis and periodontitis?
2. Write terms used to describe periodontal disease?
3. What are the five signs of inflammation? Do they appear in gingiva in gingivitis and periodontitis?
4. What are the clinical features of plaque induced gingivitis and periodontitis?
5. Write a note on histopathology of periodontium in health and subsequent stages leading to periodontitis.
6. What are McCall's festoons and Stillman's clefts?
7. What is a pocket? How can pockets be identified? Classify pockets.
8. What are the clinical features of gingival pockets (*false pockets*)?
9. What are the clinical features of periodontal pockets (*true pockets*)?
10. How is a gingival pocket (*false*) different from a periodontal (*true*) pocket?
11. How does gingival sulcus deepen to form a pocket?
12. What are the differences between supra-bony and intra-bony pockets?
13. What are the differences between simple, compound and complex pockets?
14. Classify periodontitis based on its extent and severity.
15. What are the stages that gingiva passes through during conversion of healthy gingiva to periodontitis? Or How does a sulcus deepen to form a periodontal pocket?
16. Write a note on pathogenesis of periodontal pockets and periodontitis.
17. At what stage does junctional epithelium shift apically during progression of periodontitis?
18. Write the defense mechanisms of gingiva that restrict progression of periodontitis.
19. What are the clinical implications of burst hypothesis (*episodic nature of periodontal disease*)?
20. Is progression of periodontitis continuous after its initiation?
21. How are periods of activity and remission of periodontitis clinically recognized?
22. Does periodontitis progression show site and subject variability?
23. What are the changes seen in root surface wall of the pocket in an established periodontal pocket (*periodontitis*)?
24. What is 'plaque free zone'?
25. Despite host defenses, why does the healing not reach completion and periodontitis continue to progress? Or Comment on the statement 'periodontal pockets are healing lesions'.
26. What is the etiology of grade C periodontitis?
27. Write the clinical features of grade C periodontitis.
28. Compare and contrast the clinical features of generalized grade C periodontitis and grade B periodontitis. OR What are the differences and similarities between grade C periodontitis and grade A and B periodontitis?
29. In grade C periodontitis with molar-incisor pattern, what are the reasons for periodontal lesions to remain restricted to permanent 1st molars and incisor area only?
30. What are fibrotic pockets?

Making Clinical Diagnosis of Gingivitis and Periodontitis using the 2018 Classification

The 2018 classification provides criteria for diagnosis of periodontal health, gingivitis and periodontitis. Main advantage of the 2018 classification is that it takes severity of periodontitis, complexity of treatment and patient's periodontal and overall oral rehabilitation needs into consideration for classifying periodontal disease. This helps in treating periodontal disease better. To do this, the 2018 classification has made big changes and introduced new terminology:

1. Chronic and aggressive periodontitis are ***no longer*** considered as separate diseases; they have been combined into a ***single*** disease entity called ***periodontitis***.
2. Criteria and definitions have been given for gingival health, gingivitis and periodontitis at a particular site (*site level diagnosis*) and for the entire mouth (*case level diagnosis*).
3. Periodontium providing less than normal support to a tooth (*presence of CAL*) has been termed ***reduced periodontium***. It can occur due to:
   a. Periodontitis.
   b. Other causes like tooth position (*causing apical placement of crest of bone and gingiva*) crown lengthening procedures done on that tooth, caries, etc.

◂ *Are chronic and aggressive periodontitis considered separate or same disease entities in the 2018 classification?*

◂ *What is reduced periodontium?*

DIAGNOSIS IS MADE AT TWO LEVELS (*SITE LEVEL AND CASE LEVEL*)

When using the 2018 classification, diagnosis is ***first*** made at individual sites around teeth. This is called ***site level diagnosis***. Information from site level diagnosis is then used to make case diagnosis. This is called ***case level diagnosis***. Steps in making diagnosis using 2018 classification are presented below:

◂ *What is site level diagnosis?*

◂ *What is case level diagnosis?*

STEP I: MAKING SITE LEVEL DIAGNOSIS

(To know whether there is gingival health, gingivitis or periodontitis at a particular site in the mouth)

2018 classification acknowledges the fact that, condition of gingiva at a particular site may be different from the overall diagnosis, e.g. gingiva may be healthy at some sites while the case may be that of gingivitis or periodontitis. Therefore, to make a case diagnosis, clinical gingival health or disease is ***first*** assessed at site level (*at individual sites in the entire mouth*) and then, information from all the sites is used to make a case level diagnosis. Steps in making a site level diagnosis are:

◂ *Is site level diagnosis made before or after case level diagnosis?*

Step Ia: Know if CAL is present at a particular site; this helps us know whether sites have intact or reduced periodontium

1. *Intact Periodontium*

Periodontium which has ***never had periodontitis*** and exhibits ***no CAL*** (*clinical attachment loss*) ***or RBL*** (*radiographic bone loss*) and ***base of the sulcus is located on the enamel***, is called intact periodontium.

◂ *What is intact periodontium?*

2. Reduced Periodontium

What is reduced periodontium? ▸

When periodontium exhibits ***CAL and RBL and base of sulcus is located on the anatomical root*** (*cementum*) of the tooth, it is called reduced periodontium. Reduced periodontium can be there due to:

What are the causes for reduced periodontium? ▸

What is the difference between reduced periodontium due to periodontitis and that due to other causes? ▸

i. **Periodontitis:** Here, CAL and RBL are present and base of sulcus is located on the anatomical root (*CAL*) as result of ***periodontitis*** (Fig. 10A.1, diag. A).

ii. **Other causes not related to periodontitis** (*non-periodontitis patient*)**:** Here, CAL and RBL are present and base of sulcus is located on the anatomical root of the tooth not as a result of periodontitis but because of prominence of tooth's root, crown lengthening procedure done on the tooth to increase length of crown to place a restoration, caries, etc. (Fig. 10A.1, diag. B).

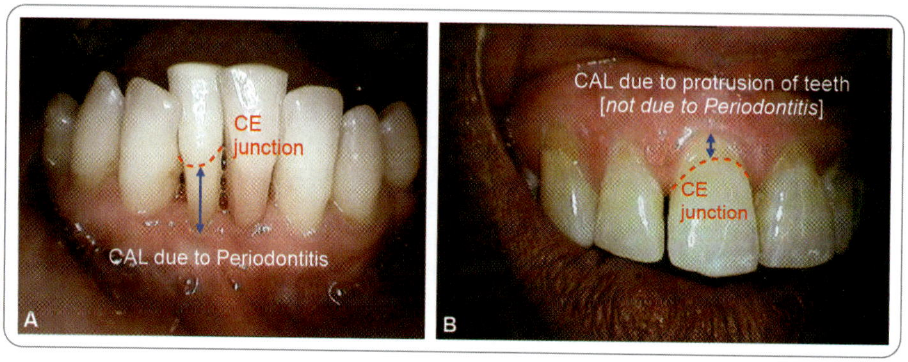

Fig. 10A.1: Reduced periodontium. Knowing the reason of CAL helps identify the reason for reduced periodontium, i.e. whether reduced periodontium is there due to periodontitis or it is due to other causes. This helps make site level and then case level diagnosis.

Step Ib: Determination of <u>*Site Level*</u> Gingival Health, Gingivitis or Periodontitis

Before starting this exercise, remember:

At which sites must site level diagnosis be done to reach case level diagnosis? ▸

- *Site level diagnosis must be made for **all** sites in the entire oral cavity.*
- *It is important to know the reason for reduced periodontium at a particular site because CAL (clinical attachment loss) may be present due to reasons other than periodontitis, e.g. tooth position, etc.*
- *Different sites in the mouth could have different characteristics. For example, there could be:*
  a. *Sites with intact periodontium that are healthy or have gingivitis.*
  b. *Sites with reduced periodontium due to periodontitis.*
  c. *Sites with reduced periodontium due to other causes.*
  d. *Sites that have had periodontitis but have been treated successfully, etc.*

A. Features of Gingival Health at a <u>Site</u> with Intact, Reduced Periodontium in a Non-periodontitis Patient and Reduced Periodontium due to Periodontitis

What are the features of site level clinical gingival health over intact periodontium? ▸

1. **Clinical gingival health at a <u>site</u> with <u>intact periodontium</u>** (*no history of previous periodontitis; no CAL*) **(Fig. 10A.2, diag. A)**:
   i. Base of sulcus is located ***coronal*** to CE junction.
   ii. No CAL or RBL (*bone crest is located at its normal position,* i.e. *1–3 mm apical to CE junction*) (*0–3 mm is biologic width*).
   iii. PD (*probing depth*) is less than 3 mm.
   iv. BOP, gingival redness, gingival swelling, etc. are ***not*** present at that site.

What are the features of site level clinical gingival health over reduced periodontium in a non-periodontitis patient? ▸

2. **Clinical gingival health at a <u>site</u> with <u>reduced periodontium in a non-periodontitis patient</u>** (*no previous history of periodontitis; CAL is present but it is not due to periodontitis, rather it is due to other causes like prominent root, crown lengthening, etc.*) **(Fig. 10A.3, diag. A, black arrow)**:
   i. Base of sulcus is located ***apical*** to CE junction.
   ii. CAL and RBL are ***present*** and bone crest is located apical to its normal position, i.e. ***more*** than 3 mm apical to CE junction.

iii. PD is ***less*** than 3 mm.
iv. BOP, gingival redness, gingival swelling, etc. are ***not*** present at that site.

3. **Clinical gingival health at a _site_ with _reduced periodontium in a stable (previously treated) periodontitis patient_** (*CAL due to periodontitis is present*) (Fig. 10A.4, white circles):
   i. Base of sulcus is located ***apical*** to CE junction.
   ii. CAL and RBL are ***present*** and bone crest is located apical to its normal position, i.e. ***more*** than 3 mm apical to CE junction.
   iii. ***No*** BOP, gingival redness, gingival swelling, etc. are present at that site.
   iv. PD is ***less*** than **_4 mm_** (*in stable (previously treated) case of periodontitis, up to 4 mm PD instead of 3 mm PD is considered normal*).

◂ *What are the features of site level clinical gingival health over reduced periodontium in a stable periodontitis patient?*

B. *Features of Gingivitis or Periodontitis at a Particular Site*

1. **Gingivitis at a _site_ with _intact periodontium_** (*no history of previous periodontitis ever; no CAL*) (Fig. 10A.2, diag. B, black arrow):
   i. Base of false pocket is located ***coronal*** to CE junction.
   ii. ***No*** CAL or RBL (*bone crest is located at its normal position,* i.e. *1–3 mm apical to CE junction*) (*0–3 mm is biologic width*).
   iii. PD (*of false pocket*) can be variable.
   iv. BOP, gingival redness, gingival swelling, etc. are ***present*** at that site.

◂ *What are the features of site level gingivitis over intact periodontium?*

2. **Gingivitis at a _site_ with _reduced periodontium in a non-periodontitis patient_** (*no history of previous periodontitis ever; CAL is present but it is not due to periodontitis rather, it is due to other causes like prominent root, crown lengthening, etc.*) (Fig. 10A.3, diag. B, black arrow):
   i. Base of sulcus is located ***apical*** to CE junction.
   ii. CAL and RBL are ***present*** with bone crest located more than 3 mm apical to CE junction.
   iii. BOP, gingival redness, gingival swelling, etc. are ***present*** at that site.
   iv. PD is ***less*** than 3 mm (*if PD is more than 3 mm then it becomes a site with periodontitis as BOP, etc. are present*).

◂ *What are the features of site level gingivitis over reduced periodontium in a non-periodontitis patient?*

3. **Gingival inflammation (*recurrent gingivitis in treated periodontitis patient*) at a _site_ with _reduced periodontium in a stable (previously treated) periodontitis patient_** (*CAL due to periodontitis is present*) (Fig. 10A.4, black circle):
   i. Base of sulcus is located ***apical*** to CE junction.
   ii. CAL and RBL from previous but treated periodontitis are ***present*** but there is no ongoing increase in CAL and RBL (*bone crest is located **more** than 3 mm apical to CE junction*).
   iii. PD is ***less*** than 3 mm.
   iv. BOP, gingival redness, gingival swelling, etc. are ***present*** at that site (*if BOP is present and PD is more than 3 mm then it becomes a case of recurrent periodontitis; if BOP is **not** present, sites with PD up to 4 mm are counted as healthy sites*).

◂ *What are the features of site level gingivitis over reduced periodontium in a stable periodontitis patient?*

4. **Periodontitis at a _site_** (*CAL due to periodontitis is present*) (Fig. 10A.2, diag. C)
   i. Base of sulcus is located ***apical*** to CE junction.
   ii. CAL, RBL (*bone crest located **more** than 3 mm apical to CE junction*) and ***active*** plaque induced gingival inflammation at that site are present.
   iii. PD is usually more than than 3 mm.
   iv. BOP, gingival redness, gingival swelling, etc. are ***present*** at that site (*except in some cases of grade C periodontitis where severe periodontal loss is present without gingival inflammation*).

◂ *What are the features of site level periodontitis?*

5. **Recurrent periodontitis at a _site_ with _reduced periodontium in a previously treated periodontitis patient_** (*CAL due to periodontitis is present*) (Fig. 10A.7, diag. C):
   i. Base of sulcus is located ***apical*** to CE junction.
   ii. CAL and RBL are present (*bone crest located **more** than 3 mm apical to CE junction*) with ***active*** plaque induced inflammation at that site (*CAL and RBL due to previous periodontitis + increase in CAL and RBL due to fresh plaque induced periodontitis*).
   iii. PD is ***more*** than 3 mm.
   iv. BOP, gingival redness, gingival swelling, etc. are ***present*** (*except in some cases of grade C periodontitis where severe periodontal loss is present without gingival inflammation*).

◂ *What are the features of recurrent periodontitis at a particular site in a previously treated periodontitis patient?*

Site level health, gingivitis and periodontitis

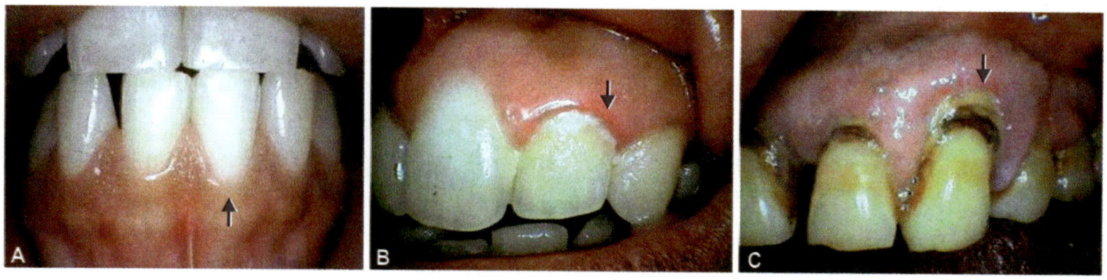

Gingival health

i. Base of sulcus is coronal to CE junction.
ii. PD less than 3 mm with no BOP.
iii. No gingival redness, gingival swelling, etc.
iv. No CAL due to periodontitis.
v. No bone loss [*bone crest located 1-3 mm apical to CE junction*].

Gingivitis

i. Base of sulcus is coronal to CE junction.
ii. PD variable but usually less than 3 mm with BOP
iii. Gingival redness, gingival swelling, etc.
iv. No CAL due to periodontitis
v. No bone loss [*bone crest located from 1-3 mm apical to CE junction*].

Periodontitis

i. Base of sulcus is apical to CE junction.
ii. PD variable
iii. CAL due to periodontitis present with bone crest located more than 3 mm apical to CE junction
iv BOP may be present
v. Gingival redness, gingival swelling, etc. may be present.

Fig. 10A.2: Features of ***sites*** (*black arrows*) with periodontal health (*diag. A*), gingivitis (*diag. B*) over intact periodontium and periodontitis (*with CAL only due to periodontitis*) (*diag. C*).

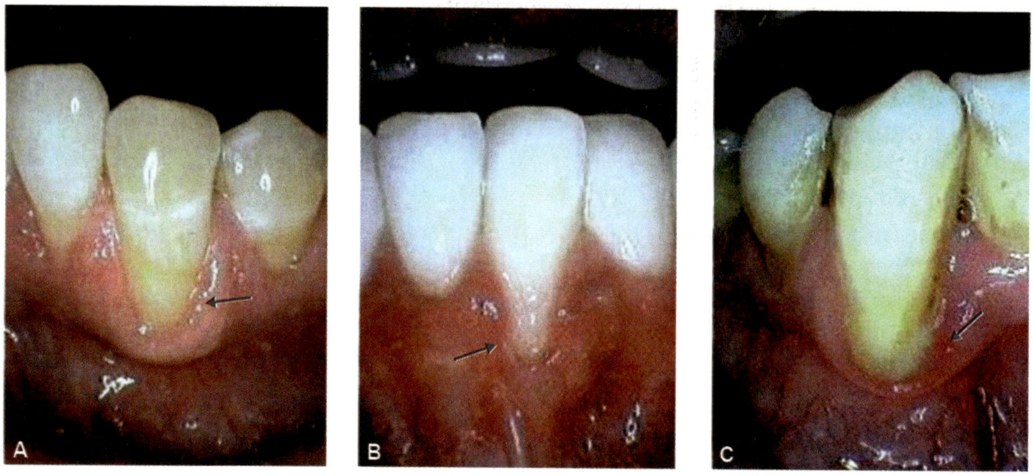

Gingival health

i. Base of sulcus is apical to CE junction.
ii. PD less than 3 mm with no BOP
iii. No gingival redness, gingival swelling, etc.
iv. CAL due to tooth position
v. Possible bone loss

Gingivitis

i. Base of sulcus is apical to CE junction.
ii. PD less than 3 mm with BOP
iii. Gingival redness, gingival swelling, etc.
iv. CAL due to tooth position
v. Possible bone loss

Periodontitis

i. Base of sulcus is apical to CE junction.
ii. CAL due to tooth position and periodontitis
iii. PD variable and BOP may be present
iv. Gingival redness, gingival swelling, etc. may be present
v. Possible bone loss

Fig. 10A.3: Features of ***sites*** with periodontal health, gingivitis and periodontitis over reduced periodontium. Diag. A and B show teeth with reduced periodontium (*CAL*) because of prominent tooth position and ***not*** due to periodontitis. Diag. C shows tooth with reduced periodontium (*CAL*) both due to prominent position of tooth and periodontitis.

ALERT!

Stage I (*initial*) periodontitis is clinically very similar to gingivitis. In such cases, diagnosis of periodontitis is made only on the basis of presence of base of sulcus apical to CE junction, i.e. CAL and true pocket formation (*known by periodontal probing*).

ALERT!

If CAL is present, it means periodontal loss has occurred. CAL (*shifting of base of sulcus apical to CE junction*) can occur due to:

1. Periodontitis
2. Other causes such as: prominent position of tooth, root caries, crown lengthening by bone removal, etc.

Despite presence of periodontal loss (*presence of base of sulcus apical to CE junction*), the 2018 classification allows cases with CAL to be classified ***clinically*** as either:

1. Health
2. Gingivitis
3. Periodontitis

However, ***only*** for **epidemiological** purposes, according to the 2018 classification, a site with CAL, either due to tooth position or periodontitis, will always be ***diagnosed*** as periodontitis (Fig. 10A.3, diags A, B and C).

STEP II: DETERMINATION OF *CASE LEVEL* GINGIVAL HEALTH, GINGIVITIS OR PERIODONTITIS

(To know whether the patient is a case of gingival health, gingivitis or periodontitis)

*Case level diagnosis is made **after** site level diagnosis. Diagnostic information (site level diagnosis) obtained from several/all individual sites in the patient's mouth is used to make a case level diagnosis.*

A. Diagnosis of Case Level Gingival Health is made based on the following findings:

1. ***Case level*** **gingival health *over intact periodontium*** (*no history of previous periodontitis ever*) (10A.6, diag. A):
   i. Base of sulcus is located ***coronal*** to CE junction at ***all*** sites in the entire mouth.
   ii. ***No*** CAL or RBL are present at all sites in the mouth.
   iii. PD is variable but is ***less*** than 3 mm.
   iv. BOP, gingival redness, swelling, etc. may be present at ***less than 10% sites*** in the entire mouth. (*2018 classification accepts that it is normal for a periodontally healthy patient to have mild inflammation of gingiva and mild BOP at few sites*).

◂ What are the features of case level gingival health?

◂ If one or two sites in the mouth have slight redness of gingival crest and BOP can this case be diagnosed as normal?

2. ***Case level*** **gingival health over *reduced periodontium in a non-periodontitis patient*** (*no history of previous periodontitis ever; CAL is present but it is not due to periodontitis rather, it is due to other causes like prominent root, crown lengthening*, etc.):
   i. Base of sulcus is located ***apical*** to CE junction only at sites where reduced periodontium due to reasons other than periodontitis is present. At other sites, base of sulcus is located ***coronal*** to CE junction.
   ii. CAL and RBL are ***present*** only at sites where there is reduced periodontium; at all other sites there is ***no*** CAL and RBL.
   iii. PD is ***less*** than 3 mm.
   iv. Mild BOP, gingival redness, swelling, etc. maybe present at ***less*** than 10% sites. (*2018 classification accepts that it is normal for a periodontally healthy patient to have mild gingival inflammation and mild BOP at few sites in the mouth*).

◂ What are the features of case level gingival health over reduced periodontium in a non-periodontitis patient?

3. ***Case level*** **gingival health *over reduced periodontium in a stable (previously treated) periodontitis patient*** (*in successfully treated patient of periodontitis; CAL due periodontitis is present*) (Fig. 10A.7, diag. A):
   i. Base of sulcus is located ***apical*** to CE junction at sites where reduced periodontium either due to previous periodontitis or other causes is present. CAL and RBL are present at sites with reduced periodontium but are not increasing with time.
   ii. Base of sulcus is located ***coronal*** to CE junction at sites where there is intact periodontium (*i.e. sites do not have reduced periodontium*) or show periodontal healing and recovery after periodontal therapy.

◂ What are the features of case level gingival health over reduced periodontium in a stable periodontitis patient?

iii. BOP, gingival redness, swelling, etc. may be present, at less than 10% sites in the entire mouth and these sites have up to 3 mm PD (*2018 classification accepts that it is normal for a periodontally healthy patient to have mild gingival inflammation and BOP at few sites in the entire mouth*).

iv. PD up to 4 mm (*but preferable to be less than 3 mm*) is acceptable, but none of these sites (*with 4 mm PD*) have BOP or gingival inflammation.

B. Diagnosis of Case Level Gingivitis is made based on the following findings:

What are the features of case level gingivitis over intact periodontium? ▶

1. ***Case level*** **gingivitis** ***over intact periodontium*** (*no history of previous periodontitis ever; no CAL*) (Fig. 10A.2, diag. B)
   - i. Base of sulcus is located ***coronal*** to CE junction at all sites in the mouth.
   - ii. No CAL and RBL are present at any site in the mouth (*bone crest is located up to 3 mm apical to CE junction; 0–3 mm is biologic width*).
   - iii. PD is variable but is less than 3 mm at all sites in the mouth.
   - iv. BOP is present at more than 10% sites in the mouth.
   - v. Gingival redness, gingival swelling, etc. maybe seen at sites with BOP.

What are the features of case level gingivitis over reduced periodontium in a non-periodontitis patient? ▶

2. ***Case level*** **gingivitis** ***over reduced periodontium in a non-periodontitis patient*** (*no history of periodontitis ever; CAL is present but it is not due to periodontitis; rather, it is due to other causes like prominent root, crown lengthening, etc.*) (Fig. 10A.6, diag. B):
   - i. Base of sulcus is located ***apical*** to CE junction at sites where reduced periodontium is present, i.e. CAL and RBL are present at such sites but CAL and RBL are not due to periodontitis. At such sites, bone crest is located more than 3 mm apical to CE junction.
   - ii. Base of sulcus is located ***coronal*** to CE junction at other sites that do not have reduced periodontium.
   - iii. PD at ***all*** sites whether with intact or reduced periodontium is ***less*** than 3 mm (*if more than 3 mm PD is found at two or more sites, such a case becomes a case of periodontitis*).
   - iv. BOP is present at more than 10% sites in the entire mouth.
   - v. Gingival redness, gingival swelling, etc. maybe seen at sites with BOP.

What are the features of case level gingivitis over reduced periodontium in a stable periodontitis patient? ▶

3. ***Case level*** **gingival inflammation (*recurrent gingivitis in a treated periodontitis patient*)** (*possible recurrent periodontitis; see II D*) ***over reduced periodontium in a stable (previously treated) periodontitis patient*** (*successfully treated patient of periodontitis; CAL due periodontitis*) (Fig. 10A.7, diag. B):
   - i. Base of sulcus is located ***apical*** to CE junction, i.e. CAL and RBL from previous periodontitis are present and bone crest is located more than 3 mm apical to CE junction at sites with reduced periodontium.
   - ii. Base of sulcus is located ***coronal*** to CE junction at sites that do not have reduced periodontium or show periodontal healing and recovery after periodontal treatment.
   - iii. BOP is present at ***more*** than 10% sites.
   - iv. PD is less than 3 mm at all sites with BOP (*at sites with BOP, if PD is more than 3 mm then it becomes a case of recurrent periodontitis*).
   - v. Gingival redness, gingival swelling, etc. are seen at sites with CAL and BOP.

C. Diagnosis of *Case Level* Periodontitis *in a Patient who has never been Treated for Periodontitis before*

(Patient has CAL due periodontitis but has not had any treatment for periodontitis earlier) (Fig. 10A.6, diag. C):

What are the features of case level periodontitis in a patient who has never been treated for periodontitis? ▶

- i. Presence of interdental CAL and interdental RBL and/or more than 3 mm buccal or lingual CAL due to periodontitis (*with PD more than 3 mm*) at ***more than two non-adjacent*** sites.
- ii. PD is usually ***more*** than 3 mm at these sites.
- iii. Bone crest is located more than 3 mm apical to CE junction at these sites.

iv. Features of plaque induced gingival inflammation (*features of gingivitis, i.e. BOP, gingival redness, gingival swelling, etc.*) are present at these and other sites of the mouth.
v. Base of sulcus is located ***apical*** to CE junction at sites with CAL.
vi. Base of sulcus is located ***coronal*** to CE junction at sites with no CAL, i.e. sites that do not have periodontitis.

D. Diagnosis of Recurrent Periodontitis in a Previously Treated Periodontitis Patient

(Patient has CAL due to earlier periodontitis that was successfully treated earlier but it has now become active again) (Fig. 10A.7, diag. C):

i. Increase in CAL and RBL due to periodontitis (*CAL due to previous periodontitis + increase in CAL due to fresh periodontitis*). Bone crest is located ***more*** than 3 mm apical to CE junction.
ii. PD is likely to be more than 3 mm at sites with ongoing CAL and RBL.
iii. Base of sulcus is located ***apical*** to CE junction at sites with CAL.
iv. Base of sulcus is located ***coronal*** to CE junction at sites with no CAL, i.e. sites that never had periodontitis or show periodontal regeneration after earlier periodontal therapy.
v. Features of plaque induced gingival inflammation (*BOP, gingival redness, gingival swelling, etc.*) are likely to be present at sites with worsening CAL and RBL.

◄ *What are the features of case level recurrent periodontitis?*

CLINICAL UTILITY AND SHORT ANSWER

How is plaque induced gingival inflammation in a previously treated stable case of periodontitis different from gingivitis?

◄ *What is gingival inflammation in a previously treated case of periodontitis?*

At the basic disease level, there is ***no*** difference between the two. In both situations, there is plaque induced inflammation of gingiva, i.e. gingivitis. To understand this, consider the following:

- The 2018 classification describes a ***confusing*** but common clinical situation: When periodontitis is treated successfully, gingival health is attained (*PD up to 4 mm and no BOP*); however, base of pocket remains on root, i.e. attachment loss remains. Later if this patient does not practice good plaque control, plaque and calculus will again start to collect near gingival margins. This will cause plaque induced inflammation of marginal gingiva (*gingivitis*). If this gingivitis (*inflammation of the marginal gingiva*) does not cause any ***further*** attachment loss, i.e. no increase in CAL, PD is less than 3 mm (*not 4 mm as in case of gingival health*) and BOP is at less than 10% sites, a case level diagnosis of ***gingival inflammation over reduced periodontium*** (*reduced periodontium due to previous periodontitis*) is made.
- This plaque induced gingival inflammation on reduced periodontium in a previously treated case of periodontitis is characterized by presence of CAL due to previous periodontitis (Fig. 10A.4, black circle and 10A.7B).
- This plaque induced gingival inflammation on reduced periodontium in a previously treated case of periodontitis is practically ***similar*** to plaque induced gingival inflammation (*gingivitis*) over intact periodontium in all aspects (*all clinical features*) but for the fact, that in this case, there is CAL from previous periodontitis.
- Therefore, ***to avoid confusion***, gingivitis seen in reduced periodontium in a previously treated case of periodontitis (*characterized by true pockets and CAL due to earlier periodontitis*) is called gingival inflammation according to the 2018 classification (Fig. 10A.7B).
- If, however CAL increases and features of gingivitis like BOP are seen, this means previous periodontitis that was treated has now recurred and is now worsening. Here a diagnosis of recurrent periodontitis is made (Fig. 10A.7C).

Clinicians must not confuse a case of gingivitis over intact periodontium (*no CAL, i.e. no loss of attachment and base of sulcus on enamel of crown*) (Figs 10A.2B and 10A.6B) or that of gingivitis over reduced periodontium with CAL due to other causes such as prominent tooth roots, etc. (Fig. 10A.3B) with gingival inflammation (*gingivitis*) in a case of previously treated case of periodontitis (*reduced periodontium characterized by CAL, i.e. attachment loss and presence of base of sulcus on root and true pockets*) (Figs 10A.4 black circle and 10A.7B).

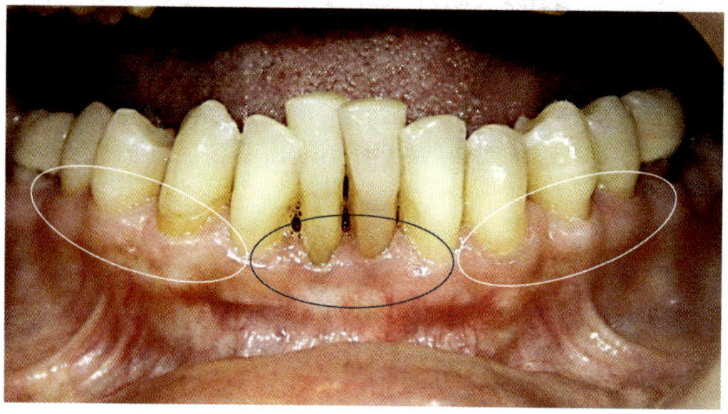

Fig. 10A.4: Gingival inflammation (*gingivitis*) in a previously treated case of periodontitis (*reduced periodontium due to periodontitis*) (*black oval outline*). Note that marginal gingiva in the area marked with black oval outline shows signs of inflammation (*slight redness, loss of knife edge contour and marginal gingival enlargement and PD is less than 3 mm*). Also note that gingiva in the surrounding areas (*area marked with white outlines*) is heathy.

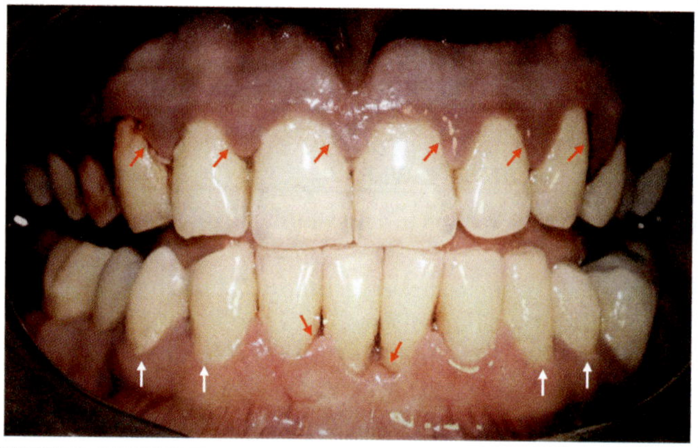

Fig. 10A.5: ***Case*** level diagnosis of periodontitis can be made the moment periodontitis is diagnosed at two or more than two non-adjacent sites (*red arrows; marked at some places only*). This rule holds even if there are some sites with gingivitis or healthy sites present in the mouth (*white arrows*).

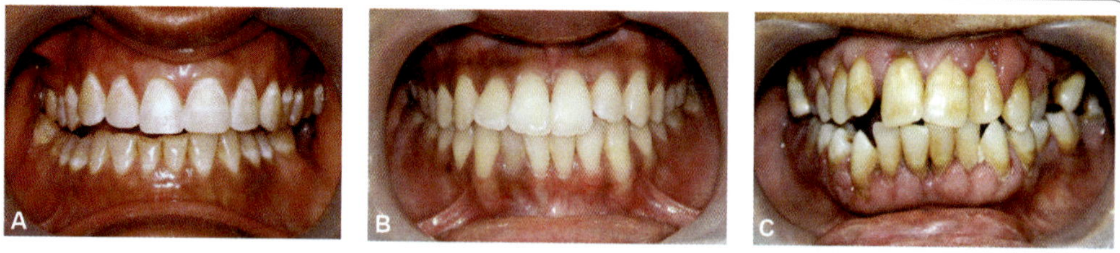

Case level health
- 1-2 areas of mild gingival inflammation
- PD less than 3 mm with BOP at less than 10% sites
- No CAL due to periodontitis [*CAL possible due to position of tooth etc.*]

Case level gingivitis
- PD variable but usually less than 3 mm and BOP at more than 10% sites. If BOP is at less than 30% sites then localized, if it is at more than 30% sites then generalized gingivitis.
- Gingival inflammation at many sites
- No CAL due to periodontitis [*CAL possible due to position of tooth etc.*]

Case level periodontitis
- CAL due to periodontitis at two or more than two non-adjacent sites.
- PD more than 3 mm at these sites
- BOP at many sites [*BOP may be absent or minimal in cases of grade C periodontitis*].
- Gingival inflammation and enlargement at many sites [*may be absent or minimal in cases of grade C periodontitis*].
- If periodontitis is at less than 30% sites then localized, if more than 30% then generalized gingivitis.

Fig. 10A.6: Features of ***case*** level health, gingivitis and periodontitis

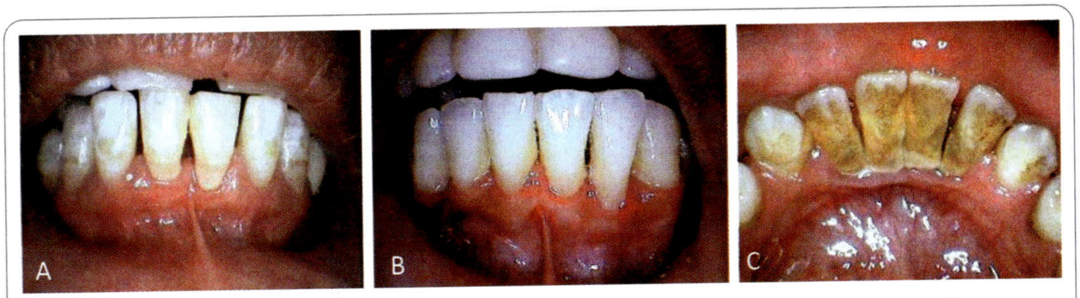

Health
- 1-2 areas of mild gingival inflammation
- PD less than 3 mm and BOP present at less than 10% sites.If there is no BOP, sites with up to 4 mm PD are normal.
- CAL due to previous periodontitis, tooth position etc.

Gingival inflammation [gingivitis]
- PD less than 3 mm
- No worsening of CAL; CAL due to previous periodontitis present.
- BOP at more than 10% sites
- Gingival inflammation at many sites

Recurrent periodontitis
- Worsening of CAL due to periodontitis.
- PD more than 3mm at sites with worsening of CAL
- BOP at many sites [*BOP may be absent or minimal in cases of grade C periodontitis*].
- Gingival inflammation and enlargement at many sites [*may be absent or minimal in cases of grade C periodontitis*].

Fig. 10A.7: Features of ***case*** level health, gingival inflammation (*gingivitis*) and recurrent periodontitis in a ***previously treated*** case of periodontitis (*over reduced periodontium due to periodontitis*).

STEP III: STAGING OF PERIODONTITIS

(If periodontitis has been diagnosed, stage, grade and add extent/distribution descriptors to it)

◂ *How is staging of periodontitis done?*

1. Staging is done to know severity, extent, rate of worsening, expected response to treatment and likely effect of periodontitis on patient's systemic health.
2. Periodontitis can have four stages: Stage I (*mild periodontitis*), stage II (*moderate periodontitis*), stage III (*severe periodontitis*) and stage IV (*very severe periodontitis*).
3. Teeth with the ***most severe destruction*** (*severest periodontitis*) determine the final stage of periodontitis assigned to the patient.
4. We can ***only assign one stage*** based on the severest periodontitis found anywhere in the mouth to a patient with periodontitis. This is true even if periodontitis of different severities is present in different teeth/quadrants of the mouth.
5. When using the 'Tooth loss' criteria for staging (Table 10A.1), all teeth previously lost and now due to be extracted due to periodontitis (*as a treatment of periodontitis*) are included in the number of teeth lost due to periodontitis.

◂ *Why is staging of periodontitis done?*
◂ *Periodontitis can be staged into how many stages?*
◂ *Which teeth, those with severest or the least severity of periodontitis are used to decide stage of periodontitis?*
◂ *Can different stages be assigned to different areas in a patient's mouth?*

Staging is done to know:

1. Severity of periodontitis (*whether periodontitis is mild, moderate or severe*).
2. Extent of periodontitis (*how many teeth in the mouth have periodontitis*).
3. Assess factors (*contributing or predisposing factors*) that will complicate maintenance of periodontal health in the long-term.

◂ *Why is staging of periodontitis done?*

Staging of Periodontitis is done in three Phases

Phase 1: Initial Staging of Periodontitis by Determining Severity of Periodontitis

In this phase we gather clinical information required to know ***severity*** of periodontitis in the mouth (*interdental CAL, RBL and tooth loss*). ***Initial*** staging of periodontitis is done as under:

◂ *How is staging of periodontitis done?*

1. Determine how many teeth in the patient's mouth have been lost (*and are due to be extracted soon*) due to periodontitis.
   i. If up to **4** teeth have been lost due to periodontitis this will ***automatically*** shift stage to stage III (*this initial staging can be modified to stage IV if complexity factors are present; see* Table 10A.1. *Staging of Periodontitis*).

ii. If more than 5 teeth have been lost due to periodontitis, the stage ***automatically*** shifts to stage IV.

iii. The first two rules apply ***irrespective*** of values of interdental CAL or RBL.

iv. If no or less than 4 teeth are lost due to periodontitis, use CAL or RBL to determine stage of periodontitis.

How is staging of periodontitis using CAL done? ▶

2. If no or less than 4 teeth are lost due to periodontitis then, initial staging of periodontitis is ***preferably*** done using CAL (*clinical attachment loss*). For this:
   i. Determine ***maximum*** interdental CAL due to periodontitis at site of ***greatest loss*** in the mouth (Figs 10A.9 and 10A.10).
   ii. Confirm CAL patterns and determine whether CAL is restricted to molars and incisors or is prevalent in other teeth also?
   iii. Stage periodontitis using maximum CAL value according to the criteria in the Table 10A.1-'Staging of Periodontitis' (*initial staging; can be modified by complexity factors*).

How is staging of periodontitis using RBL done? ▶

3. Initial staging of periodontitis can also be done using *RBL* (*radiographic bone loss*) if CAL records are ***not*** available (*patient is not in the clinic and only radiographs are available*):
   i. RBL values in the ***interdental*** areas are determined from IOPA radiographs (*full mouth series*) to know radiographic bone loss (*RBL*) in the interdental areas (Figs 3.12, 3.13 and 10A.12).

      RBL tells us the amount of bone loss that has occurred due to periodontitis in the past. It thus helps in staging periodontitis. RBL is also useful for estimating rate of bone loss which helps in grading periodontitis (described later).
   ii. Confirm RBL patterns and determine whether RBL is restricted to molars and incisors or is prevalent in other teeth also?
   iii. Stage periodontitis using RBL data according to the criteria in the Table 10A.1-'Staging of Periodontitis' (*initial staging; can be modified by complexity factors*).

Phase 2: Final Staging of Periodontitis by Determining Presence and Severity of Complicating Factors (Complexity Factors)

What is final staging of periodontitis? ▶

Initial stage of periodontitis reached from phase I exercise above can be ***raised*** to a higher level by the mere presence of certain complexity factors (*see* Table10A.1 *on staging of periodontitis*). Final stage of periodontitis is determined by factoring in these complexity factors in the information used to determine the initial stage of periodontitis. ***Final staging of periodontitis*** is done as under:

Which complexity factors can raise the stage of periodontitis? ▶

1. Identify presence of the following complexity factors that complicate treatment of periodontitis and worsen its prognosis:
   i. More than 6 mm PD
   ii. Furcation involvement
   iii. Vertical bone defects
   iv. Grade II or more mobility
   v. Trauma from occlusion
   vi. Pathologic migration, etc. (*see staging* Table 10A.1 *below*)

How many factors are required to raise the stage of periodontitis? ▶

2. Presence of even a ***single*** complexity factor (*case complicating factor*) shifts stage of periodontitis to higher stage ***irrespective of CAL*** or ***RBL*** e.g. presence of grade II or III furcation shifts stage to stage III or IV and presence of grade II mobility shifts stage to stage IV directly irrespective of CAL or RBL or other findings.
3. If ***no*** complexity factors are identified, stage of periodontitis determined earlier, i.e. initial stage is decided to be the final stage of periodontitis.

Phase 3: Describe the Extent and Distribution of Periodontitis in the Mouth for the Established Stage of Periodontitis in that Patient

After determination of final stage of periodontitis, we apply the extent/distribution describing terms 'localized' or 'generalized' to describe extent and distribution (*pattern*) of periodontitis in the mouth. The following rules are used to do this:

◂ *What is localized periodontitis?*

1. After the final stage of periodontitis has been determined, we find out how many teeth are affected by periodontitis (*percentage of teeth affected by periodontitis*).
2. The term localized is prefixed to periodontitis if ***less than 30% teeth*** are affected with periodontitis, e.g. 'Localized stage II, Grade B Periodontitis', etc.
3. The term generalized is prefixed to periodontitis if ***more than 30%*** teeth are affected with periodontitis, e.g. 'Generalized stage III, Grade C Periodontitis', etc.
4. The use of terms localized or generalized ***does not*** give information about the percentage of teeth with slight, moderate, or severe periodontitis.
5. Staging system is designed to highlight the ***severest*** periodontitis in a patient's mouth. This concept is used not only to determine the final stage of periodontitis but is also carried over to decide the use of the terms localized and generalized periodontitis.
   For example, if mild periodontitis (stage I) is present in most of the teeth in the mouth and severe periodontitis (stage III) is present only in 3–4 teeth, we will give a diagnosis of generalized stage III periodontitis to the patient. Here the term generalized describes the extent of periodontitis in the mouth irrespective of the fact that it is mild, moderate or severe. Diagnosis of stage III periodontitis instead of stage I periodontitis is made because diagnosis of periodontitis is based on presence of the severest periodontitis in the mouth.
6. The term 'molar-incisor pattern' of periodontitis is used if periodontitis is present ***only*** around molars and incisors (*other teeth are either not involved or have only mild periodontitis compared to severe periodontitis and damage in the molars and incisors*).

◂ *What is molar-incisor pattern periodontitis?*

Table 10A.1: Staging of periodontitis

	Periodontitis	***Stage 1***	***Stage 2***	***Stage 3***	***Stage 4***
Severity	Interdental CAL (*at the site of greatest loss*)	1–2 mm	3–4 mm	≥5 mm	≥5 mm
	RBL	Coronal third (<15%)	Coronal third (15%–33%)	Extending to middle third of root and beyond	Extending to middle third of root and beyond
	Tooth loss (*due to periodontitis*)	No tooth loss	No tooth loss	≤4 teeth	≥5 teeth
Complexity	Local	• Max. probing depth ≤4 mm • Mostly horizontal bone loss	• Max. probing depth ≤5 mm • Mostly horizontal bone loss	In addition to Stage II complexity: • Probing depths ≥6 mm • Vertical bone loss ≥3 mm • Furcation involvement class II or class III • Moderate ridge defects	In addition to stage III complexity: • Need for complex rehabilitation due to: • Masticatory dysfunction • Secondary occlusal trauma (*tooth mobility degree ≥2*) • Severe ridge defects • Bite collapse, drifting, flaring • < 20 remaining teeth (*10 opposing pairs*)
Extent and distribution	Add to stage as descriptor	For each stage, describe extent as: Localized (*<30% of teeth involved*); Generalized; or Molar/incisor pattern			

CLINICAL UTILITY AND SHORT ANSWER

Can stage of periodontitis regress with treatment? ▸

If a patient of periodontitis is treated and there is improvement in parameters that decided this patient's stage of periodontitis, can such a patient be shifted to a lower stage?

No; stage can increase but cannot retrogress. Even if there is improvement in parameters, staging of the patient will remain the same. However, stage will be raised to a higher level if parameters of periodontitis worsen in that patient.

Periodontitis can be graded into how many grades? ▸

STEP IV: GRADING OF PERIODONTITIS

Periodontitis can be graded into three grades: grade A (*slow progressing*), grade B (*moderately progressing*) and grade C (*fast progressing*).

Grading is done to know

Why is grading of periodontitis done? ▸

1. Rate at which periodontitis is progressing (*worsening*).
2. Its likelihood of improving with treatment (*responsiveness to treatment*).
3. Effect of periodontitis on patient's systemic health.

The Following Points Must be kept in Mind for Grading Periodontitis

What are the rules for grading periodontitis? ▸

1. Grading of periodontitis is started by ***assuming*** that it is progressing at a moderate rate, i.e. periodontitis is grade B.
2. Thereafter, specific evidence is sought (Table 10A.2, *Grading of Periodontitis*) to shift to grade to A or C if needed.

What is the importance of grading factors? ▸

3. Risk factors mentioned in the grading table (*see below*) are ***overriding*** grade modifiers (*presence of these risk factors automatically shifts grade upwards*). If these risk factors are known, final grade of periodontitis is decided easily and ***quickly***.
4. Assessing data from areas with ***maximum*** periodontal loss can help determine grade of periodontitis quickly.

Grading of Periodontitis is Done in Two Phases

Phase 1: Assessment of Primary Criteria

How is grading of periodontitis done? ▸

1. If possible (*if records are available*), determine how much CAL or RBL has occurred in the last ***5 years***. These are then used to reach a grade (*see* Table 10A.2).
2. If above is not possible, i.e. if 5-year-old records of CAL or RBL are not available, rate of progression of periodontitis can be known by dividing % of bone loss by the patient's age (*see* Table 10A.2) **(Fig. 10A.13)**.
3. Corelate amount of plaque and other local factors to amount of periodontal loss (*see* Table 10A.2) **(Fig. 10A.14)**.

Phase 2: Identification of Grade Modifying Risk Factors

How many grade modifying factors are there? ▸

What is importance of grade modifying factors in making a periodontal diagnosis? ▸

There are ***two*** grade modifying factors (*see* Table 10A.2). Presence of ***any or both*** of these will automatically shift the grade to higher grade irrespective of the grade determined using the primary criteria (*described above*). The two grade modifying factors are:

1. Smoking (*number of cigarettes smoked per day*).
2. Diabetes (*HbA1c levels* (*three-month blood glucose levels*)).

Both smoking and diabetes not only worsen severity and increase rate of progression of periodontitis but also make periodontitis less responsive to treatment and thus worsen prognosis of periodontitis. To measure the degree of a patient's sugar control (diabetic control), HbA1c is preferred over random or daily fasting blood glucose levels because HbA1c gives us average level of blood sugar over the past 2 to 3 months.

CLINICAL UTILITY AND SHORT ANSWER

Can grade increase to a higher level or decrease to a lower level after initial assessment? ▸

Can the grade of periodontitis change with time?

Yes. Grade of periodontitis can improve if grade modifying factors in a patient improve, i.e. patient reduces smoking and/or improves diabetic control (*lower blood glucose levels*). Grade of periodontitis can worsen if a patient starts or increases smoking or has poorer diabetic control (*higher blood glucose levels*).

Table 10A.2: Grading of periodontitis

	Progression:		Grade A: Slow rate	Grade B: Moderate rate	Grade C: Rapid rate
Primary criteria	Direct evidence of progression	Radiographic bone loss or CAL	No loss over 5 years	<2 mm over 5 years	≥2 mm over 5 years
	Indirect evidence of progression	% Bone loss/ age	<0.25	0.25 to 1.0	≥1
Whenever available, direct evidence should be used.		Case phenotype	Heavy biofilm deposits with low levels of destruction	Destruction commensurate with biofilm deposits	Destruction exceeds expectations given biofilm deposits; specific clinical patterns suggestive of periods of rapid progression and/or early onset disease
Grade modifiers	Risk factors	Smoking	Non-smoker	<10 cigarettes/day	≥10 cigarettes/day
		Diabetes	Normoglycemic/ no diagnosis of diabetes	HbA1c <7.0% in patients with diabetes	HbA1c ≥7.0% in patients with diabetes

DIAGNOSTIC POSSIBILITIES (*WITH RESPECT TO GINGIVITIS AND PERIODONTITIS*) ACCORDING TO THE 2018 CLASSIFICATION

◂ *What are the diagnostic possibilities in relation to health and plaque induced periodontal disease according to the 2018 classification?*

In short, therefore, according to the 2018 classification, a patient could be a case of:

1. Periodontal Health

◂ *What is periodontal health?*

This is characterized by 1–2 areas of plaque induced gingival inflammation, PD less than 3 mm and BOP at less than 10% sites.

2. Case Level Gingivitis

◂ *What is case level gingivitis?*

This is characterized by variable PD usually less than 3 mm (*false pockets*), BOP at more than 10% sites; no CAL due to periodontitis; CAL due to other reasons such as prominent root, etc. possible.

3. Case Level Periodontitis

◂ *What is case level periodontitis?*

This is characterized by interdental or buccal CAL due to periodontitis at more than two non-adjacent sites, PD variable but usually more than 3 mm (*false pocket + true pocket*, i.e. *combined pockets*); BOP may be present.

4. After Successful Treatment

A patient of gingivitis or periodontitis, could thereafter present as a case of:

i. *Periodontal Health*

◂ *What are the features of periodontal health after periodontal treatment?*

This is characterized by BOP at ***less*** than 10% sites. If case was previously of gingivitis, PD less than 3 mm is acceptable. If case was previously of periodontitis, PD less than 4 mm but with no BOP at 4 mm sites is acceptable; there is no ongoing increase in CAL.

ii. *Recurrent Gingivitis*

◂ *What are the features of recurrent gingivitis after periodontal treatment?*

This is characterized by variable PD that is usually less than 3 mm, BOP at ***more*** than 10% sites; no CAL due to periodontitis; CAL due to other reasons such as prominent root, etc. possible.

What are the features of gingival inflammation after periodontal treatment? ▸

iii. Gingival Inflammation

This is characterized by plaque induced gingival inflammation (*gingivitis*) over reduced periodontium that has CAL and RBL due to periodontitis which had been successfully treated earlier, PD less than 3 mm and BOP at ***more*** than 10% sites, there is no further increase in CAL and RBL.

What are the features of recurrent periodontitis after periodontal treatment? ▸

iv. Recurrent Periodontitis

Plaque induced gingival inflammation (*gingivitis*) over reduced periodontium that has CAL and RBL due to periodontitis which had been successfully treated earlier but now presents with BOP at ***more*** than 10% sites and further increase in CAL, RBL and PD.

Extent/Distribution Describing Terms are added to the Above Diagnostic Terms

What is localized, generalized and molar-incisor pattern periodontitis? ▸

1. When periodontitis or gingivitis is at less than 30% sites, it is called localized.
2. When periodontitis or gingivitis is at more than 30% sites, it is called generalized.
3. If periodontitis is localized to molars and incisors only, it is called periodontitis with molar-incisor pattern.

A PATIENT OF GINGIVITIS OR PERIODONTITIS COULD RECEIVE THE FOLLOWING POSSIBLE DIAGNOSIS ACCORDING TO THE 2018 CLASSIFICATION COULD BE

1. Localized or Generalized Gingivitis

The terms localized or generalized describe the extent of gingivitis in the mouth.

2. Localized or Generalized Stage I/II/III/IV, Grade A/B or C Periodontitis

The terms localized or generalized describe the extent of periodontitis in the mouth; the areas with the maximum periodontal destruction, i.e. severest periodontitis determines the assigned stage to that patient.

Can different stages be assigned to the same patient? ▸

Caution: Only one stage of periodontitis can be assigned to a patient. Therefore, even if a patient has different severities of periodontitis in the mouth, only the area with severest periodontitis will determine the diagnosis. Thus, diagnosis like 'localized stage II periodontitis with generalized stage IV periodontitis' ***cannot*** be made (*in such cases the correct diagnosis will be generalized stage IV periodontitis*), etc.

3. Molar-incisor Pattern Stage I/II//III/IV, Grade A/B or C Periodontitis

When is the term molar-incisor pattern used? ▸

The term 'Molar-incisor pattern' is used to describe the distribution and extent of periodontitis ***only*** if periodontitis is present ***only in relation to the molars and incisors*** in the mouth. If periodontitis is present both in the molars-incisor region and also in relation to other teeth of the mouth, the term 'Molar-incisor pattern' is ***not*** used and a diagnosis is made as explained in point # 2 above (Table 10A.3).

TIPS FOR STAGING AND GRADING PERIODONTITIS

To simplify making a diagnosis using the 2018 classification the following tips may be used:

1. Making a detailed diagnosis using the 2018 classification can be a difficult task and may not be possible in all clinical situations and for all patients. A clinician can however short list different diagnostic possibilities and make a quick clinical diagnosis of health, gingivitis or periodontitis using the flow chart in Fig. 10A.8A. If periodontitis is diagnosed, it can then be staged and graded as described in the later text.

What is the likely stage of mild-to-moderate periodontitis? ▸

2. Mild-to-moderate periodontitis will usually be Stage I or Stage II periodontitis.

What is the likely stage of severe-to-very severe periodontitis? ▸

3. Severe-to-very severe periodontitis will usually be Stage III or Stage IV.
4. Try to identify case complicating factors (see Table 10A.1) ***early*** during the diagnosis making exercise. These complicating factors if present will immediately shift the stage to higher level, e.g. presence of furcation defects or vertical bone defects shifts stage to III, less than 20 remaining teeth (*10 opposing pairs*) shifts stage to IV, etc.

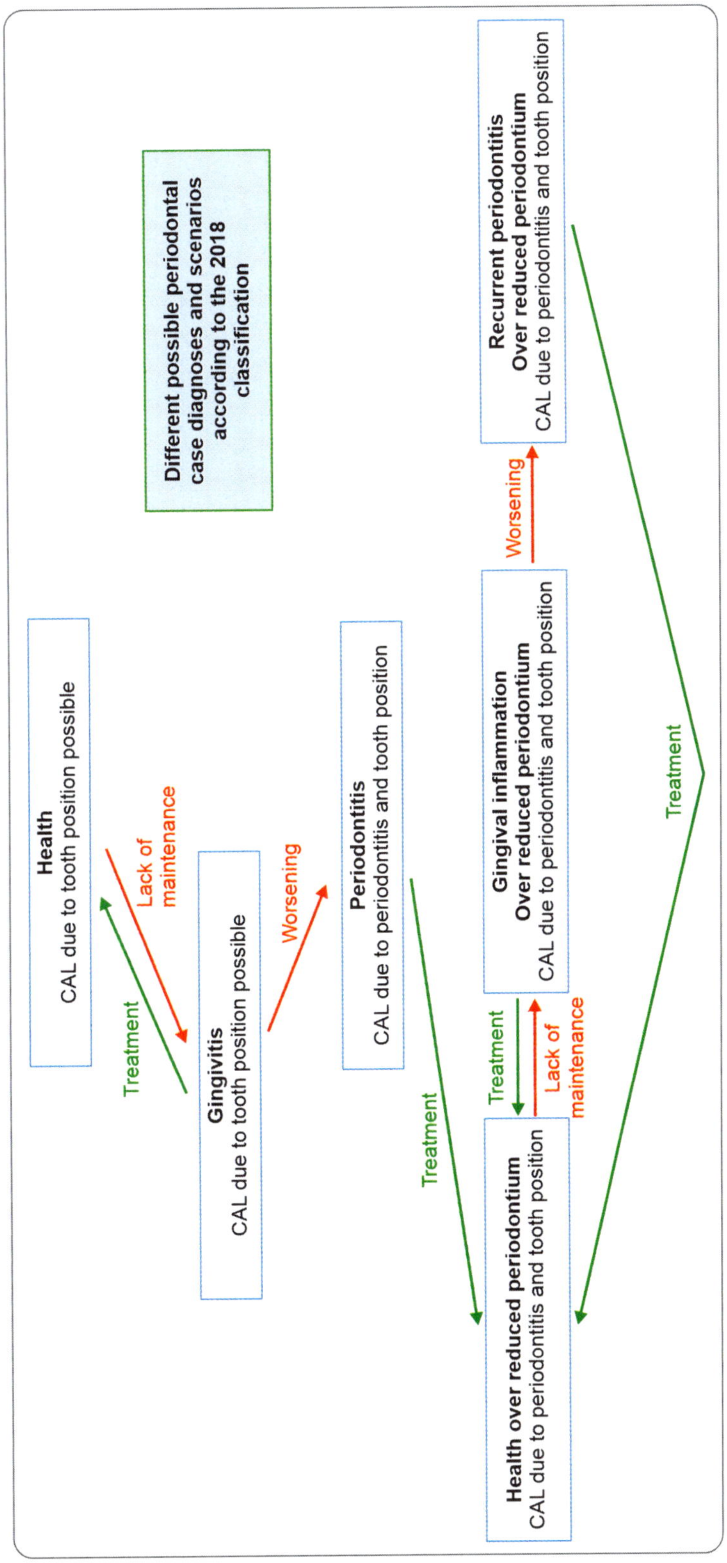

Fig. 10A.8: A periodontal case could visit a clinician at several possible stages

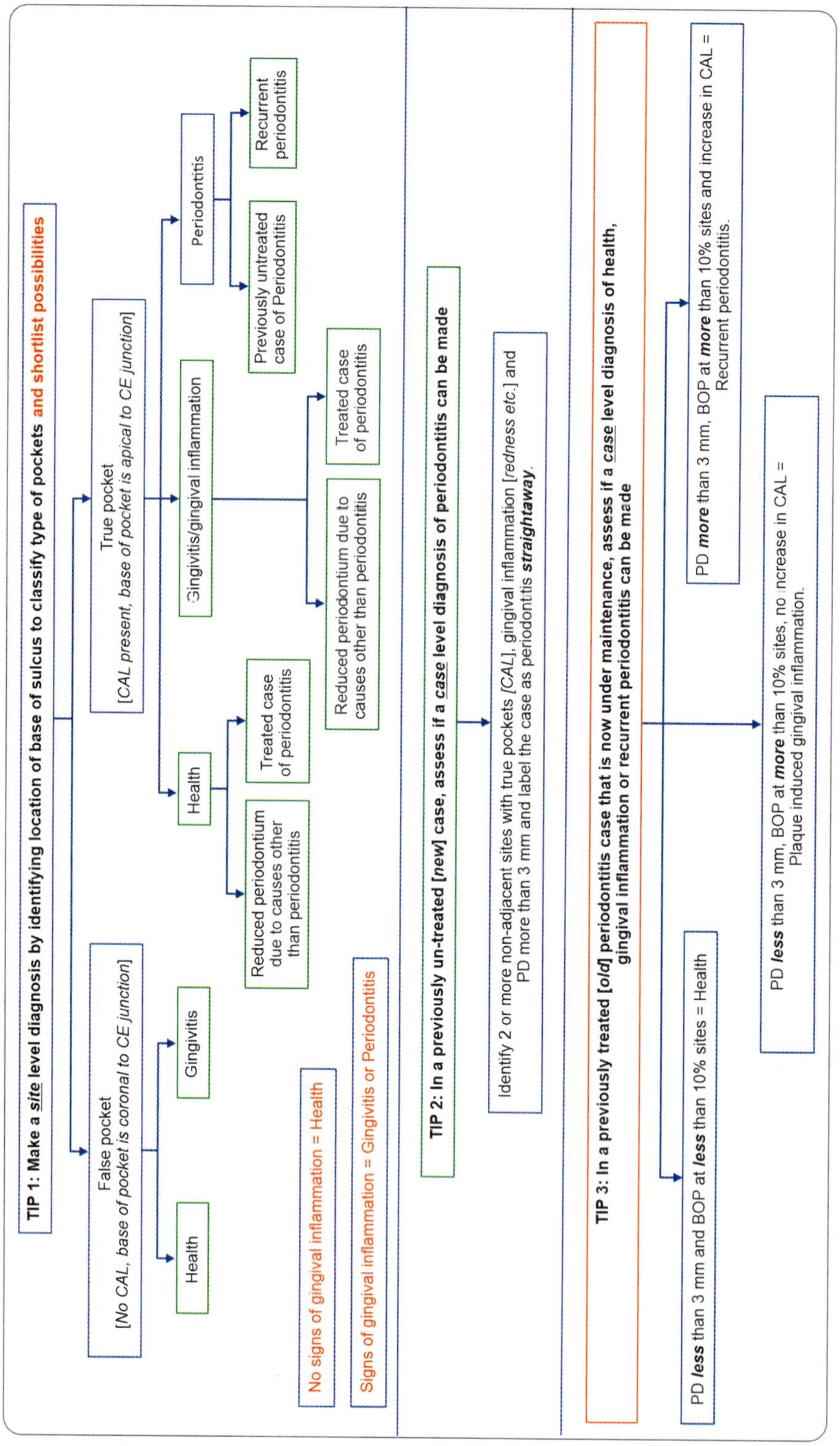

Fig. 10A.8A: Tips to make a 'working' diagnosis using the 2018 classification

5. Try to identify grade modifying factors (*see* Table 10A.2) ***early*** during the diagnosis making exercise. Identification of these grade modifying factors will immediately shift grade to higher level, e.g. if a patient gives a history of smoking more than 10 cigarettes a day or has HbA1c (*blood glucose score of more than 7*), periodontitis can then straightway be graded as grade C, etc.
6. ***Stage*** of periodontitis once established ***cannot be lowered*** even after successful treatment (*stage IV periodontitis will never lower down to stage II or II or I even after successful treatment*).
7. ***Grade*** of periodontitis once established ***will get lowered*** if grade modifying factors are managed successfully, e.g. diabetes has been successfully treated and/or patient stops smoking (*in such cases grade C can drop to grade A or B*).

◂ *What is the importance of identifying complicating factors early during making a diagnosis?*

◂ *If periodontitis has been treated, is lowering of its stage allowed?*

◂ *If periodontitis has been treated, is lowering of its grade allowed?*

Table 10A.3: Some examples of *incorrect* diagnoses that can be made using the 2018 classification in different clinical situations

S. no.	*Clinical findings*	*Incorrect diagnosis*	*Correct diagnosis*	*Comment*
1.	Generalized gingivitis with one area presenting with stage II, grade B periodontitis.	Generalized gingivitis with stage II, grade B periodontitis.	Localized stage II, grade B periodontitis.	Staging system is designed to highlight the severest disease in a patient's mouth. In this case it is periodontitis.
2.	Localized gingivitis in a small area along with generalized stage III, grade C periodontitis.	Localized gingivitis with generalized stage III, grade C periodontitis.	Generalized stage III, grade C periodontitis.	Staging system is designed to highlight the severest disease in a patient's mouth. In this case it is periodontitis.
3.	Localized gingivitis with generalized stage III, grade C periodontitis and localized stage II, grade B periodontitis at some sites.	Localized gingivitis with generalized stage III, grade C periodontitis and localized stage II, grade B periodontitis.	Generalized stage III, grade C periodontitis.	Staging system is designed to highlight the severest disease in a patient's mouth. In this case it is stage III grade C periodontitis. Different stages and cannot be assigned to different quadrants.
4.	Localized stage III, grade C periodontitis and localized stage II, grade B periodontitis at some sites.	Localized stage III, grade C periodontitis and localized stage II, grade B periodontitis.	Localized stage III, grade C periodontitis.	Different stages grades cannot be assigned to different quadrants. The severest disease determines diagnosis.
5.	Generalized stage II, grade C periodontitis and localized stage III, grade B periodontitis at some sites.	Generalized stage II, grade C periodontitis and localized stage III, grade B periodontitis.	Generalized stage III, grade C periodontitis.	Different stages cannot be assigned to different quadrants. The severest disease determines diagnosis.

CLINICAL UTILITIES FOR STAGING AND GRADING PERIODONTITIS

To simplify making a diagnosis using the 2018 classification the following clinical utilities may be used:

I. How to Measure CAL to Stage and Grade Periodontitis

Although CAL is measured clinically, however interdental CAL can also be known from a digital radiograph.

A. Measuring CAL Clinically

- CAL (*clinical attachment loss*) is the distance from the CE junction to tip of the probe that is inserted with ***0.25 N force*** into the sulcus/pocket for recording pocket depth (*ideally, the probe tip must lie at base of the sulcus/pocket but at times if gingiva is tightly adapted to the tooth probe tip may not reach the base of the sulcus*).

◂ *How is CAL measured for diagnosis of periodontitis?*

- For diagnosing periodontitis, CAL is measured at ***six sites*** around each tooth, i.e. meisobuccal, buccal, distobuccal, distolingual, lingual and mesiolingual (Fig. 10A.9, diag. 4). ***Maximum*** CAL value is taken into account for diagnosis.

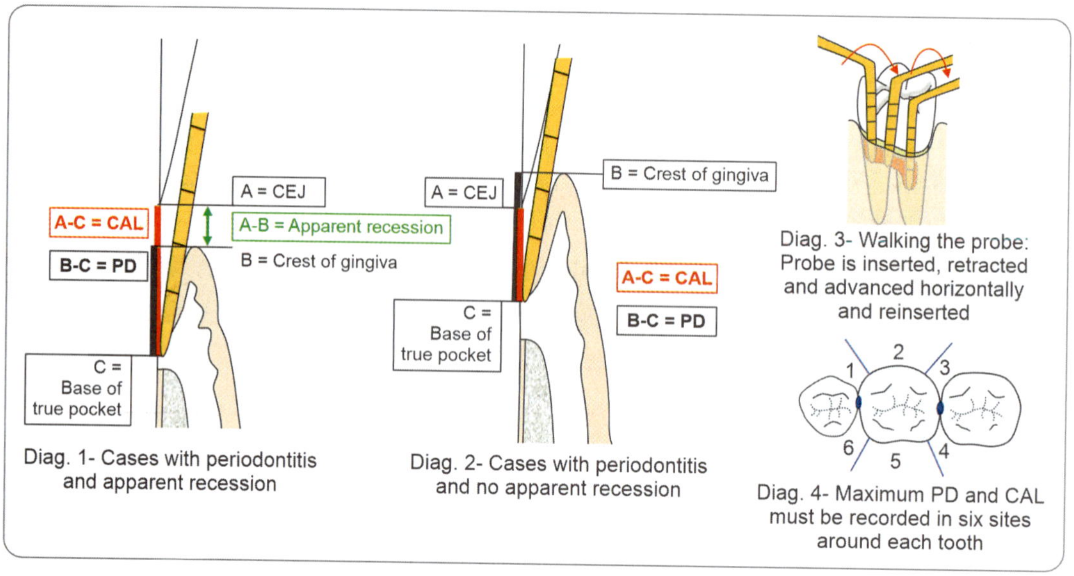

Fig. 10A.9: How to measure CAL (*clinical attachment loss*). The distance from crest of gingiva to base of pocket is probing pocket depth (*PD*). The distance from cemento-enamel junction (*CEJ*) to the tip of the probe (*base of the true pocket*) is called Clinical attachment level (*CAL*). As CAL also denotes the amount of periodontal loss, it is also called clinical attachment loss. Maximum PD and CAL are noted at six sites (*diag. 4*) by walking the probe (*diag. 3*) around each tooth.

B. *Measuring CAL Radiographically*

Can CAL be measured on a radiograph for diagnosis of periodontitis? ▸

CAL is a clinical measurement, however if clinical measurements are not possible, ***interdental*** CAL can also be easily estimated from a digital IOPA radiograph (*taken with correct X-ray geometry*). The following facts are used to measure interdental CAL (*clinical attachment loss*) on a digital radiograph:

1. Distance between alveolar bone crest and base of the sulcus/pocket is biologic width (Fig. *7.12; this space is occupied by supra-crestal connective tissue and the junctional epithelium*). Average biologic width is about 2 mm.
2. Therefore, subtracting 2 mm from the distance between interdental CE junction and the interdental bone crest is the estimated CAL (Fig. 10A.10) (*the same value is also the estimated RBL (radiographic bone loss) at that site as explained in* Fig. 10A.12).

Steps for measuring (*estimated*) CAL on a digital radiograph are:

How is CAL measured on a radiograph for diagnosis of periodontitis? ▸

1. Identify and mark the interdental CE junction on the interdental surface of the tooth where measurement has to be taken (Fig. 10A.10, CEJ).
2. Mark the present crest of the alveolar bone on the tooth root being evaluated (Fig. 10A.10, *PCB*).
3. Mark a point 2 mm coronal to the present crest of the alveolar bone (*PCB*) to denote estimated position of base of pocket (Fig. 10A.10, BP).
4. Distance between CEJ and BP is the estimated CAL.

II. How to Measure RBL to Stage (Fig. 10A.12) and Grade (Fig. 10A.13) Periodontitis

How is RBL measured for diagnosis of periodontitis? ▸

The following fact is used to measure interdental RBL (*radiographic bone loss*) on a digital radiograph:

1. Alveolar bone crest is normally located approximately ***2 mm apical*** to the CE junction.

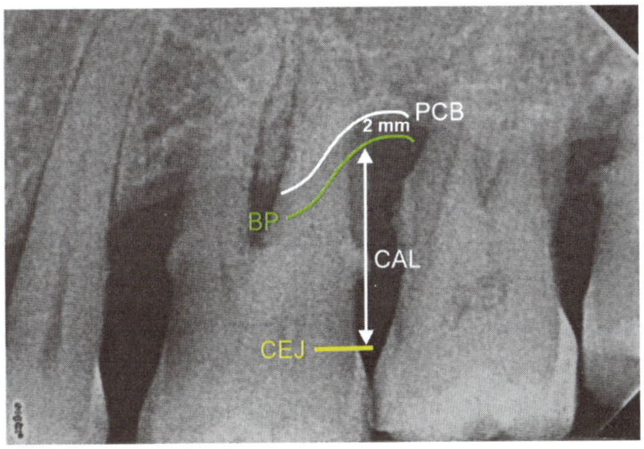

Formula

Stage I periodontitis:	CAL 1 - 2 mm
Stage II periodontitis:	CAL 3 - 4 mm
Stage III periodontitis:	CAL more than 5 mm
Stage IV periodontitis:	CAL more than 5 mm

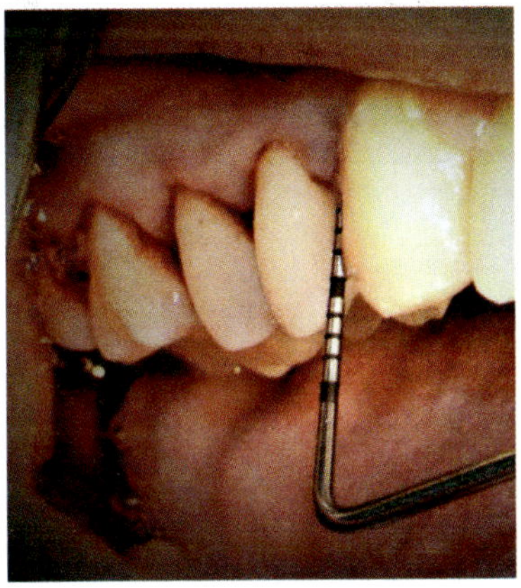

PCB = Present crest of resorbed bone
BP = Estimated level of base of pocket [*2 mm coronal to PCB*]
PCB – BP = Biologic width [*2 mm coronal to crest of bone*]
CEJ = Cementoenamel junction
CEJ – BP = CAL [*CEJ to estimated base of pocket*]

Staging periodontitis using estimated CAL in a IOPA radiograph

Staging periodontitis using CAL measurements clinically with a probe

Fig. 10A.10: Measuring CAL clinically and radiographically to stage periodontitis.

No CAL

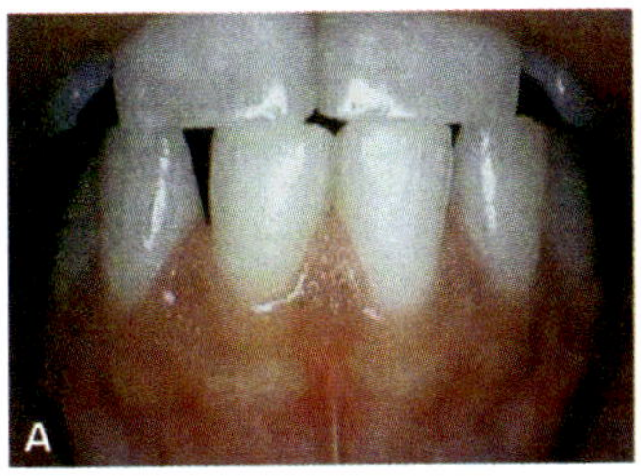

Clinical gingival health over intact periodontium
[*no history of periodontitis ever; no CAL*]:

i. PD is less than 3 mm with BOP present at less than 10% sites.
ii. No gingival redness, gingival swelling etc.
iii. No CAL is present; bone crest located not more than 2–3 mm apical to CE junction.

CAL due to protrusion of teeth
[*not due to Periodontitis*]

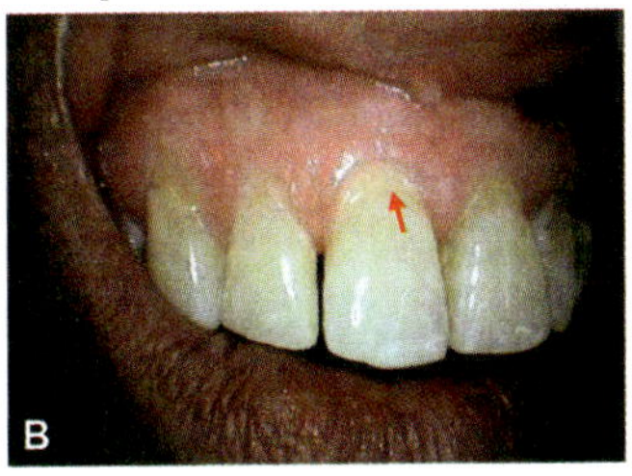

Clinical gingival health over reduced periodontium in a non-periodontitis patient
[*no history of periodontitis ever; CAL present but not due to periodontitis but due to tooth's prominent root*]

i. PD is less than 3 mm with BOP present at less than 10% sites.
ii. No gingival redness, gingival swelling, etc.
iii. CAL is present; bone crest located more than 3 mm apical to CE junction.

CAL due to Periodontitis

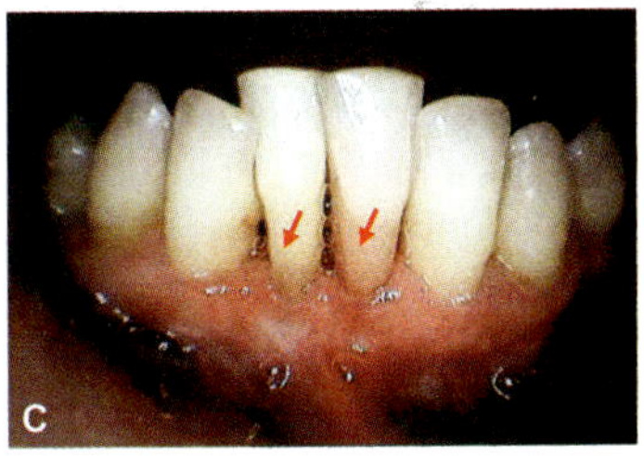

Clinical gingival health over reduced periodontium in a stable [*previously treated*] periodontitis patient
[*history of successful treatment of periodontitis; CAL due to earlier periodontitis; now gingiva is clinically healthy*]

i. PD less than 3 mm and BOP present at less than 10% sites. If there is no BOP, sites with up to 4 mm PD are normal.
ii. No or mild BOP maybe present at less than 10% sites
iii. No gingival redness, gingival swelling, etc.
iv. CAL is present; bone crest located more than 3 mm apical to CE junction.

Fig. 10A.11: Diagnostic significance of CAL. Presence of CAL does not necessarily and automatically mean periodontitis. CAL is absent in intact periodontium (*diag. A*). CAL may be present in healthy periodontium if periodontium is reduced (*gingival crest and bone crest are placed apical to CE junction*) due to causes other than periodontitis, e.g. prominent position of tooth root, crown lengthening done earlier, etc. (*diag. B, red arrow*). CAL will remain present even in a previously successfully treated and presently healthy case of periodontitis (*diag. C, red arrow*).

Steps for measuring RBL on a digital radiograph are:

1. Identify CE junction on interdental surface of the tooth where measurement has to be taken (Fig. 10A.12, *CEJ*).
2. Mark a point 2 mm apical to CEJ. This point is the ideal location of the unresorbed alveolar bone crest (Fig. 10A.12, *NBC*).
3. Mark present crest of resorbed bone (Fig. 10A.12, *PCB*).
4. Distance between NBC and PCB is the estimated RBL.

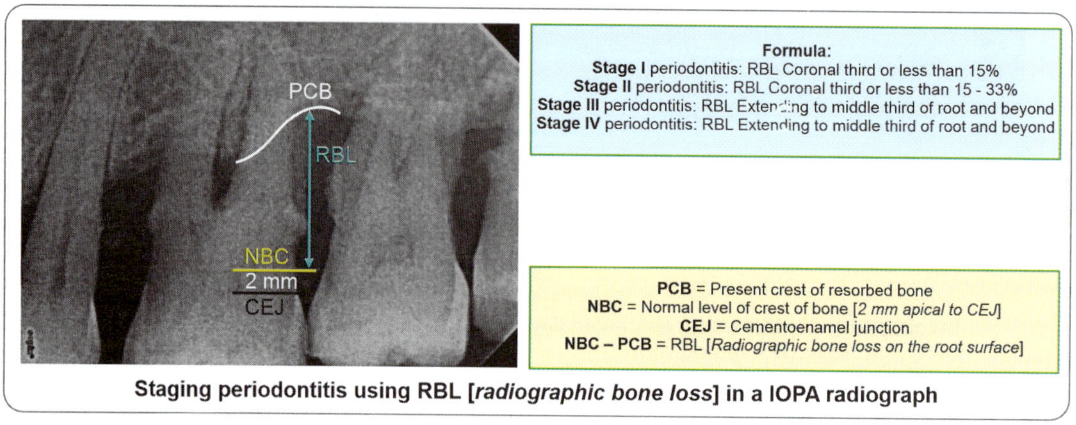

Fig. 10A.12: How to measure RBL (*radiographic bone loss*) and stage periodontitis using RBL in an IOPA radiograph.

CLINICAL UTILITY AND SHORT ANSWER

Which of the two, CAL or PD is a better way of assessing periodontal loss?

- CAL is a measure of total (*past + present ongoing*) periodontal destruction that has occurred due to periodontitis whereas PD tells us the present-day status of periodontitis.
- CAL (*clinical attachment loss*) gives ***better*** assessment of damage to the periodontium than PD (*probing pocket depth*) (*Fig. 2.7*).
- Periodontal probing for PD or CAL is often ***not*** accurate and reproduceable as pressure on the probe during probing is not accurately controllable and limited to 0.25N. Increasing the probing pressure to 0.5 N or more makes the probe cross (*JE*) junctional epithelium and stop at the bone crest. If the gingiva is inflamed, even 0.25 N force pushes the probe down to the crest of alveolar bone.
- PD is however very useful in estimating threat of worsening of periodontitis at that site. Greater PD means deeper pockets; these deeper pockets will predispose to worsening of periodontitis at that site/s.

III. How Staging of Periodontitis is Done

Can different stages be allocated to different quadrants in the same patient? ▸

Staging of periodontitis is done ***after*** diagnosis of periodontitis has been made. Staging gives us information about extent, severity and complexity of periodontitis in the ***whole*** mouth of a particular patient. Even if periodontitis of different severity (*different amount of periodontal loss*) is present in different areas of the mouth, only ***one*** stage is allocated to periodontitis in that patient (*see* Table 10A.1). Based on diagnostic information obtained from sites (*in the entire mouth*) that exhibit ***maximum*** severity of periodontitis, a patient of periodontitis can be allocated one of the four possible stages; these are:

Stage I Periodontitis (Mild Periodontitis); it is Characterized by:

What are the criteria of stage I periodontitis? ▸

1. PD less than 4 mm
2. CAL less 1–2 mm
3. Horizontal bone loss
4. Non-surgical treatment (*scaling and root planing*) is required to treat such cases.
5. Loss of teeth due to periodontitis is not expected.
6. Overall case prognosis is very good.

Stage II Periodontitis (Moderate Periodontitis); it is Characterized by:

◂ *What are the criteria of stage II periodontitis?*

1. PD less than 5 mm.
2. CAL less than 3–4 mm.
3. Horizontal bone loss.
4. Both non-surgical (*scaling and root planing*) and surgical treatment (gingivectomy, flap surgery, etc.) are needed to treat such cases.
5. Loss of teeth due to periodontitis is not expected.
6. Overall case prognosis is good.

Stage III Periodontitis (Severe Periodontitis); it is Characterized by:

◂ *What are the criteria of stage III periodontitis?*

1. PD more than 6 mm.
2. CAL more than 5 mm.
3. Horizontal bone loss is present; vertical bone loss more than 3 mm and/or furcation involvement of class II or III may be present.
4. Non-surgical (*scaling and root planing*) and surgical treatment (*gingivectomy, flap surgery, etc.*) are needed to treat such cases; regenerative therapy (*bone grafting, etc.*) may also be required.
5. 0–4 teeth have already been or are likely to be lost due to periodontitis.
6. Implant and/or restorative treatment requiring services pertaining to other dental specialities is needed.
7. Overall case prognosis is fair.

Stage IV Periodontitis (Very Severe Periodontitis); it is Characterized by:

◂ *What are the criteria of stage IV periodontitis?*

1. PD more than 6 mm
2. CAL more than 5 mm
3. Horizontal bone loss is present; vertical bone loss more than 3 mm and/or furcation involvement of class II or III may be present.
4. 5 or more teeth have been lost due to periodontitis and less than 20 teeth (*10 opposing pairs*) are present in the mouth.
5. Remaining teeth may exhibit trauma from occlusion, flaring and pathologic migration, etc.
6. Non-surgical (*scaling and root planing*) and surgical treatment (*gingivectomy, flap surgery, etc.*) are needed to treat such cases; regenerative therapy (*bone grafting, etc.*) may also be required.
7. Complex implant and/or restorative treatment requiring services pertaining to other dental specialities is needed.
8. Overall case prognosis is questionable or poor.

IV. How Grading of Periodontitis is Done

For grading periodontitis, it is essential to estimate the rate at which periodontitis is progressing (*speed at which periodontal tissues are being lost*). This can be done by using criteria that provide either direct or indirect evidence of rate of progression of periodontitis:

1. *Direct Evidence of Rate of Progression*

◂ *Which criteria are used as direct and indirect evidence for grading periodontitis?*

This is got by comparing CAL or RBL records over past 5 years (*see grading of periodontitis* Table 10A.2). Although this is the simplest method, but it is not often used as detailed 5-year-old CAL and RBL records for a particular patient are usually not available in most clinical setups.

◂ *Why are direct evidence criteria generally not used for grading periodontitis?*

2. *Indirect Evidence of Rate of Progression*

This can be obtained in two ways:

a. Using RBL to estimate rate of bone loss (*% bone loss age*) (*see* Table 10A.2 and Fig. 10A.13).
b. Comparing amount of plaque deposits with amount of periodontal destruction (*see* Table 10A.2 and Fig. 10A.14).

Why is comparing amount of plaque deposits with amount of periodontal destruction not a dependable way of grading periodontitis? ▶

In cases where direct evaluation of rate of progression of periodontitis is not possible, indirect evaluation of rate of progression of periodontitis is done. Comparing amount of plaque deposits with amount of periodontal destruction though simpler, is less accurate and less reliable. This is so because patients have a tendency to thoroughly clean their teeth and remove most of plaque prior to a dental visit. This can lead to faulty evaluation. The other more reliable method involves using interdental RBL evaluated on an accurate IOPA. This is described in detail below **(Fig. 10A.13)**. The following fact is used to measure interdental RBL on an accurate digital radiograph:

1. Bone crest is normally located approximately 2 mm apical to CE junction of the tooth (*this 2 mm space is the average biologic width, i.e. space occupied by supra-crestal gingival connective tissue*).

Steps for measuring rate of progression of periodontitis using RBL are as under:

How can rate of progression of periodontitis be measured using RBL? ▶

1. On the radiograph identify CE junction on the interdental surface of the tooth where measurement has to be taken (**Fig. 10A.13**, *CEJ*).
2. Mark a point 2 mm apical to the CE junction. This point marks level of the normal unresorbed crest of interdental bone (**Fig. 10A.13**, *NBC*).
3. Mark the present crest of the bone on the root being evaluated (**Fig. 10A.13**, *PCB*).
4. Mark the tip of the root (**Fig. 10A.13**, *TR*).
5. Measure distance from NBC to PCB in millimeters. This is the bone loss on the root (**Fig. 10A.13**, *NBC-PCB = A = RBL*).
6. Measure the distance from NBC to TR. This is the length of the root that should have been covered by bone normally *NBC-TR = B*).
7. Divide A by B and multiply by 100 to know % bone loss (**Fig. 10A.13**, *C*).
8. Divide C by the patient's age to have a numeric value (**Fig. 10A.13**, *examples 1 and 2*). If this numeric value is:
   a. Less than 0.25, it suggests slow rate of progression of periodontitis.
   b. Between 0.25 to 1.0, it suggests moderate rate of progression.
   c. More than 1, it suggests fast rate of progression.

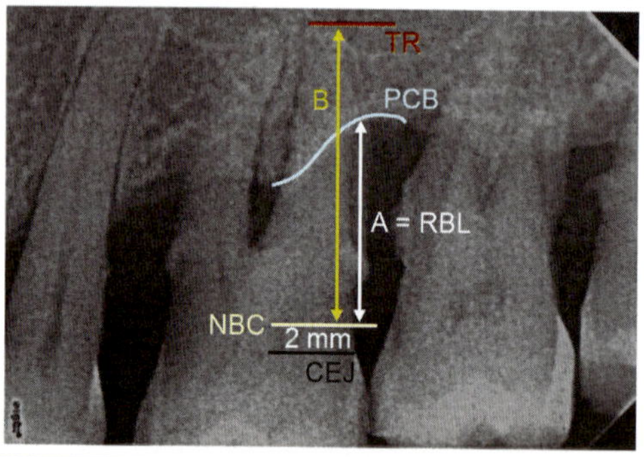

Formula:
A ÷ B x 100 = C [*% bone loss*]
C ÷ Age = rate of progression of periodontitis
Grade A periodontitis: % bone loss ÷ age < 0.25
Grade B periodontitis: % bone loss ÷ age < 0.25 – 1.0
Grade C periodontitis: % bone loss ÷ age > 1.0

Example 1
Assuming X-ray is of a patient aged 50 years and A = 7 mm, B = 11 mm
A 7 mm ÷ B 11 mm x 100 = C 63.6%
C 63.6% ÷ age 50 years = 1.27 [*means fast rate of progression*]
Diagnosis = Grade C Periodontitis

NBC = Normal level bone crest [*2 mm apical to CEJ;*]
CEJ = Cementoenamel junction
TR = Tip of root
PCB = Present crest of resorbed bone
NBC – PCB = A = RBL [*Radiographic bone loss on the root surface*]
NBC – TR = B = Total length of root minus 2 mm [biologic width]

Example 2
Assuming X-ray is of a patient aged 70 years and A = 7 mm, B = 11 mm:
A 7 mm ÷ B 11 mm x 100 = C 63.6%
C 63.6% ÷ age 70 years = 0.90
[*means moderate rate of progression*]
Diagnosis = Grade B Periodontitis

Grading periodontitis using RBL in a IOPA radiograph [*estimating rate of progression of periodontitis*]

Fig. 10A.13: Grading periodontitis using RBL in a IOPA radiograph

ALERT!

The 2018 classification allows ***early*** diagnosis and aggressive treatment of periodontitis as it is based on the ***worst*** clinical findings in particular case. For example, even if majority of the sites have no periodontitis (*no CAL*) but only gingivitis and CAL (*periodontitis*) is at present only at 2 non-adjacent sites, a diagnosis of periodontitis is made (**Fig. 10A.15**). This scales up the disease level and forces clinicians to treat periodontitis rather than 'wish-away' disease (*if a diagnosis of gingivitis is made*) by advising better toothbrushing, chemical plaque control (*mouth washes*), etc.

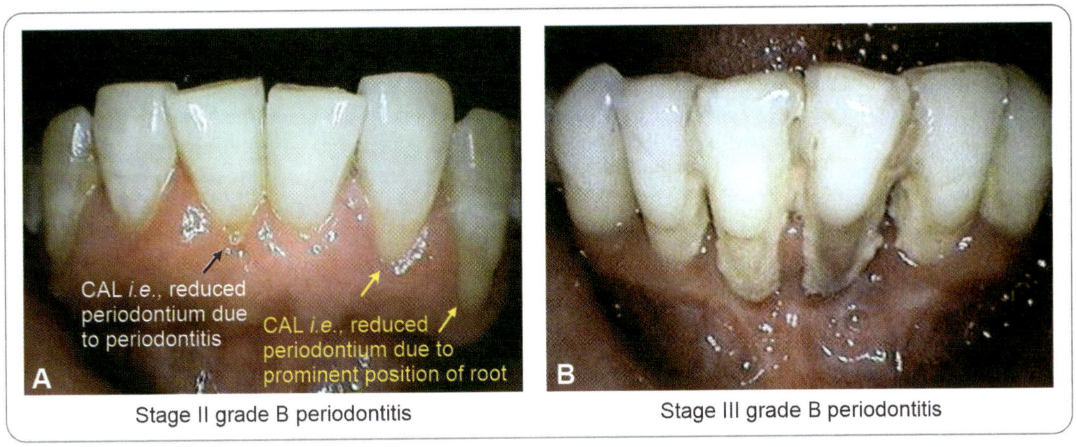

Fig. 10A.14: Grading periodontitis by comparing amount of plaque deposits (*etiologic factors*) with amount of periodontal destruction. In both these diagrams, amount of periodontal destruction is proportionate to amount of plaque and other etiologic factors (*diag. A, black arrow and diag. B*). Therefore, a diagnosis of grade B periodontitis is made in both these cases. As periodontitis in diag. A is mild, it is classified as stage II periodontitis whereas periodontitis in diag. B is of moderate severity it is therefore classified as stage III periodontitis.

Note that in diag. A, reduced periodontium is also present because of prominent position of the tooth root (*diag. A, yellow arrows*). As CAL in these areas is not due to periodontitis (*diag. A, yellow arrows*), these areas are not considered for grading.

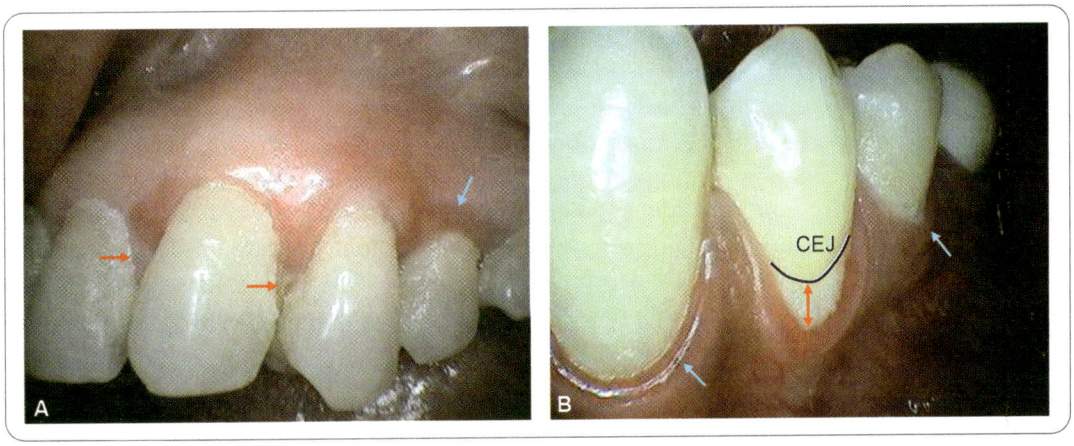

Fig. 10A.15: In both diagrams A and B, there is site level gingivitis at many sites (*blue arrows*) but since CAL due to periodontitis is present at other sites (*red arrows*) it takes priority and a diagnosis of periodontitis is made.

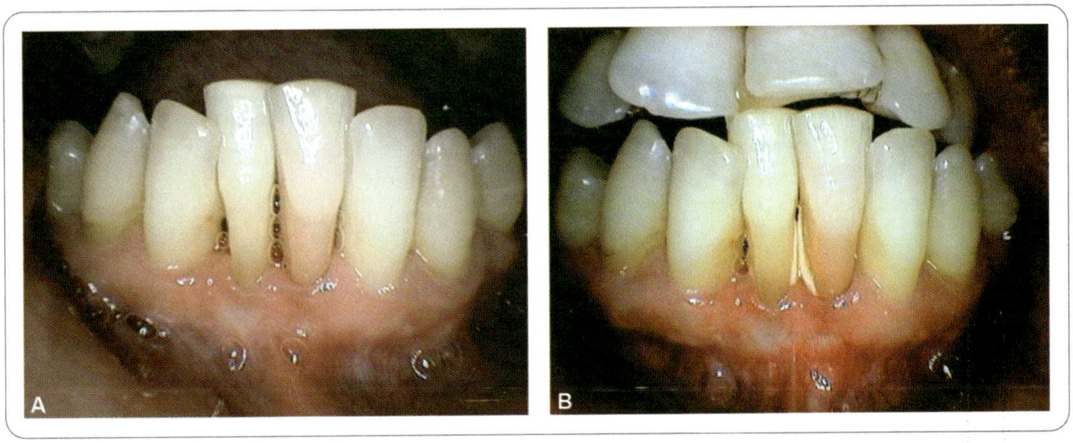

Fig. 10A.16: Clinical health (*diag. A*) and gingival inflammation (*recurrent periodontitis if CAL is increasing over time*) (*diag. B*) in a previously treated case of periodontitis.

CLINICAL UTILITY AND SHORT ANSWER

According to the 2018 classification, if after periodontal treatment, in a case of periodontitis, there is normal gingiva and a stable 2 mm deep gingival sulcus with both its base and marginal gingiva on the root of the tooth and a few sites with BOP. What will the diagnosis be, considering the fact that the gingiva and the underlying sulcus are healthy but periodontal support has been lost?

In such cases, difficulty and confusion in diagnosis arises from the fact that this case cannot be called abnormal as gingiva has now become healthy after treatment. This case also cannot be diagnosed as normal because periodontal loss (*CAL*) has already occurred and BOP—a sign of gingival inflammation is also present at few sites.

The 2018 classification (*as improvement over the 1999 classification*) provides an easy solution to such problems as it uses ***site level*** diagnosis to reach a ***case level*** diagnosis.

It recognizes that despite best plaque control efforts in such treated periodontitis cases, some sites will always have BOP (*bleeding on probing*) due to plaque induced gingival inflammation (*gingivitis*) at those sites. In such cases diagnosis is made in the following way:

1. If there is no BOP, sites with up to 4 mm PD are considered normal; if BOP is present, sites are counted as ***sites*** with gingival inflammation (*gingivitis*).
2. If ***less than 10% sites*** have plaque induced gingival inflammation but ***no*** increase in CAL, ***case level*** diagnosis of clinical health over reduced periodontium is made **(Fig. 10A.16, A)**.
3. If ***more than 10% sites*** have plaque induced gingival inflammation (*gingivitis*) but ***no*** increase in CAL, ***case level*** diagnosis of gingival inflammation over a previously treated case of periodontitis is made **(Fig. 10A.16, B)**.
4. If PD increases more than 4 mm and/or ***increase*** in CAL occurs, a diagnosis of recurrent periodontitis is made **(Fig. 10A.16, B)**.

REVIEW QUESTIONS

1. What is the difference between site level and case level diagnosis?
2. What is the difference between intact and reduced periodontium?
3. What are the features of gingival health at a site with intact periodontium, reduced periodontium in a non-periodontitis patient and reduced periodontium due to periodontitis?
4. What are the features of gingivitis at a site with intact periodontium and reduced periodontium in a non-periodontitis patient?
5. What does the term 'gingival inflammation' at a site with reduced periodontium in a stable previously treated periodontitis patient refer to?
6. What are the features of case level gingival health over intact periodontium and over reduced periodontium in a non-periodontitis and over reduced periodontium in a stable previously treated periodontitis patient?
7. What are the features of case level gingivitis over intact periodontium and over reduced periodontium in a non-periodontitis patient?
8. On which features is diagnosis of case level periodontitis made in a patient who has never been treated for periodontitis before?
9. What is case level gingival inflammation (*recurrent gingivitis in a treated periodontitis patient*)?
10. On which features is diagnosis of case level periodontitis made in a patient who has never been treated for periodontitis before? How are these different form features of recurrent periodontitis in a previously treated periodontitis patient?
11. What is staging and grading of periodontitis? Why are they done?
12. Discuss grade modifying risk factors.
13. What is radiographic bone loss? How is it measured to stage and grade periodontitis?

Chapter

11

Plaque Associated Periodontal Disease and Gingival Enlargements

Plaque is a causative and disease modifying factor in gingival and periodontal diseases. Gingival enlargement (*gingival overgrowth*) is a common feature of gingival and periodontal disease. Gingival enlargement can occur due to local reasons or it can be a local manifestation of systemic disease.

HOW ENLARGED GINGIVA AFFECTS HEALTH OF PERIODONTIUM

Enlarged gingiva affects gingival (*periodontal*) health in the following ways:

◂ *What is the clinical and etiological importance of enlarged gingiva?*

1. As gingiva enlarges, knife edge deflecting contour of the gingiva is lost and it changes to bulbous non-deflecting contour. This leads to increased plaque accumulation near crest of the gingiva and also increases food debris impaction in the sulcus. This results in inflammation of gingiva (*gingivitis and periodontitis*).

◂ *Does PD increase when gingiva gets inflamed?*

2. Inflammation of gingiva causes increase in bulk of gingiva. This leads to increase in probing depth (*PD*) of the sulcus. As probing depth increases, sulcus converts to a pocket.
3. Gingivitis and periodontitis proceed faster when PD becomes more than 3 mm.
4. Physical plaque control measures (*tooth brushing, flossing,* etc.) are less efficient in removing plaque when gingiva is enlarged. This makes plaque control more difficult thereby leading to gingivitis and periodontitis.
5. Inadequate plaque control causes worsening of gingivitis and periodontitis; thus, a vicious cycle develops.

ALERT!

The terms used to describe the location and distribution of gingival enlargement are the same as the ones used for describing gingivitis or periodontitis, e.g. localized, generalized, discrete, marginal, papillary, diffuse, acute, sub-acute, chronic, recurrent and refractory. These have been described in the Chapter 10, 'Plaque Induced Gingivitis and Periodontitis'.

GRADING OF GINGIVAL ENLARGEMENTS

The simplest and preferred grading scheme for gingival enlargements is:

◂ *How is enlargement of gingiva graded?*

Grade 0: No gingival enlargement

Grade 1: Enlargement limited only to interdental papilla

Grade 2: Enlargement involving interdental papilla and marginal gingiva

Grade 3: Enlargement covering 3/4ths or more of crown.

CLASSIFICATION OF GINGIVAL ENLARGEMENTS

◂ *How are gingival enlargements classified?*

Gingival enlargements may be classified on the basis of their ***chief*** etiology and pathogenesis as:

1. **Inflammatory enlargements**
   a. Chronic inflammatory enlargement (*gingivitis and periodontitis*)

b. Acute and sub-acute abscesses
   i. Gingival
   ii. Periodontal
   iii. Pericoronal (*pericoronitis*)

2. **Conditioned enlargements (*gingival enlargements <u>associated</u> with systemic diseases and conditions*):**
   a. Puberty enlargement
   b. Pregnancy enlargement
      i. Marginal
      ii. Angiogranuloma
   c. Vitamin C deficiency
   d. Nonspecific conditioned enlargement (*pyogenic granuloma*)
   e. Plasma cell gingivitis
3. **Enlargements <u>*caused*</u> by systemic diseases**
   a. Leukemia
   b. Granulomatous diseases (*sarcoidosis, wegener's granulomatosis*, etc.)
4. **Drug induced gingival enlargements**
5. **Idiopathic gingival enlargements (*hereditary gingival fibromatosis*)**
6. **Cysts and tumors of the periodontium (*neoplastic enlargements*)**
   a. Benign
   b. Malignant
7. **Enlargement due to mouth breathing**
8. **False enlargements** (*'false enlargement' is actually a mis-diagnosis and therefore does not qualify to be accepted as an enlargement as such*)
9. **Combined enlargements** (combinations of above).

1. Inflammatory Enlargements

1a. *Chronic Inflammatory Gingival Enlargement* (Gingivitis and Periodontitis)

What is the other name for chronic inflammatory enlargement? ▶

Chronic inflammatory gingival enlargement is also called chronic plaque induced gingival enlargement (Fig. 11.1). Chronic inflammatory gingival enlargement (*gingivitis and periodontitis*) have already been discussed in detail in Chapter 10 'Plaque Induced Gingivitis and Periodontitis'.

What are chronic periodontitis and aggressive periodontitis now called in the 2018 classification? ▶

The 2018 classification of periodontal diseases and conditions does not differentiate between chronic periodontitis and aggressive periodontitis; both these diseases have now been clubbed and are now called periodontitis (*see Chapter 10A, 'Making Clinical Diagnosis of Gingivitis and Periodontitis Using The 2018 Classification'*).

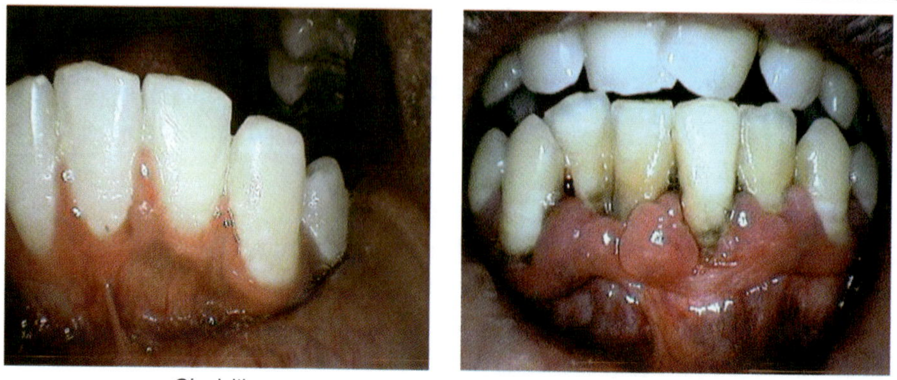

Gingivitis
[*Chronic inflammatory enlargement*]

Periodontitis
[*Chronic inflammatory enlargement*]

Fig. 11.1: Chronic inflammatory gingival enlargement

1b. Acute and Subacute Inflammatory Gingival Enlargement (Gingival, Periodontal and Peri-coronal Abscesses)

Acute inflammation in gingiva and deeper periodontal tissues can cause gingival enlargement and abscess formation (*an abscess is a **localized** collection of pus*).

◂ *What is an abscess?*

1bi. Acute gingival abscess

Localization of pus in the gingiva produces a painful acute gingival abscess (Fig. 11.2). Clinical features of an acute gingival abscess are:

◂ *What are the clinical features of a gingival abscess?*

1. The swelling has a ***sudden start*** and is restricted to marginal gingiva or interdental papillary regions.
2. Gingiva in relation to the abscess is inflamed, red in color, has a shiny surface and is tender (*painful to touch*).
3. Adjoining teeth can be painful and tender. Pain, tenderness and size of the abscess increase ***rapidly*** for one or two days. After this, the abscess becomes fluctuant and pointed and drains (*pus comes out of the abscess on its own*).
4. After pus drains from the abscess, pain, tenderness and size of abscess decrease and gingival abscesses heal leaving back no permanent damage.
5. ***No*** radiographic changes are seen.

◂ *How long does it usually take for a gingal abscess to drain?*

◂ *What are the radiographic features of a gingival abscess?*

Etiology of gingival abscess

1. Impaction of food or dental materials in gingiva. This causes:
   a. Entry of bacteria in very large numbers deep into gingiva through gingival wounds (*caused by biting into foods or mastication, impaction of dental material during dental treatment, etc.*).
   b. Food acts like a source of nutrition for bacteria leading to their growth.
   c. Foreign body reaction in the gingiva against impacted food or dental materials results in acute inflammation and abscess formation in gingiva.

◂ *What causes gingival abscess?*

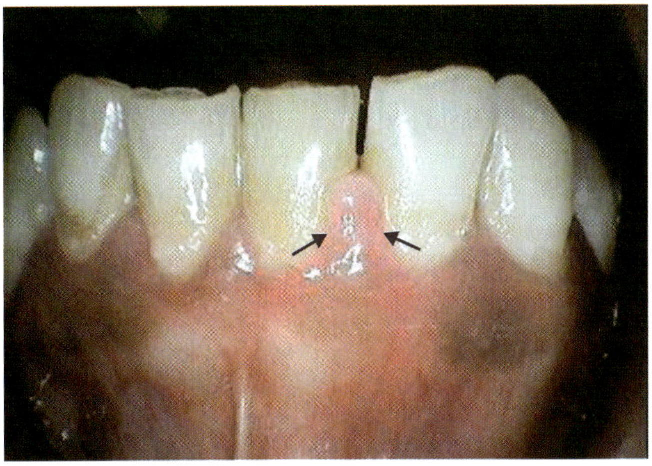

Fig. 11.2: Gingival abscess

ALERT!

***Gingival sulcus* and *interdental col* are *prone* to injury, bacterial infection and abscess formation.**

This is so because:

1. These areas are lined by ***non-keratinizing*** epithelium which is a weak barrier against entrance of bacteria (*than when compared to keratinizing epithelium*).
2. They cannot be cleaned properly either by natural or instituted measures (*tooth brushing, etc.*) due to difficult access.
3. Anaerobic conditions are more likely to be present in these areas; this facilitates growth of anaerobic bacteria that cause infection, inflammation and abscess formation.

◂ *Why gingival sulcus and interdental col are prone to injury, bacterial infection?*

1bii. Periodontal abscess

What is periodontal abscess?

What are the other names of a periodontal abscess?

A periodontal abscess is a localized pus producing (*purulent*) inflammation in deeper periodontal tissues. Although the actual inflammatory lesion may or may not involve the gingiva, it ***always*** causes enlargement of gingiva. A periodontal abscess is also called lateral abscess or parietal abscess.

ALERT!

A periodontal abscess differs from a gingival abscess ***only*** in the extent of involvement of periodontal tissues.

How does an acute abscess become chronic?

How does a chronic abscess become acute?

Clinical features of a periodontal abscess:

A periodontal abscess may be acute, sub-acute or chronic **(Fig. 11.3, diags C, D and E)**. An acute abscess may become chronic after pus drainage whereas a chronic abscess converts to an acute abscess when drainage of pus is blocked.

Periodontal abscess may also occur in association with periapical abscesses of endodontic origin. In such cases, clinical features of periapical abscesses and pulpitis (*chronic/acute*) may be present along with clinical features of periodontal abscess.

What are clinical features of an acute or subacute periodontal abscess?

a. Acute and sub-acute periodontal abscess:

1. Gingiva over the periodontal abscess presents a circular swelling and surrounding gingiva is enlarged and edematous.
2. Surface of gingiva is smooth and shiny and if abscess is ready to burst, the surface may be pointed.
3. Pus may come out spontaneously or on applying finger pressure from the abscess's sinus or from the underlying periodontal pocket.
4. Surrounding area and adjoining teeth are tender and painful (*dull throbbing and radiating pain*). Teeth may show increased mobility.
5. In severe cases, systemic signs and symptoms like fever, malaise, lymphadenopathy and external swelling of face may be there but such instances are ***not*** very common.

What are clinical features of chronic periodontal abscess?

b. Chronic periodontal abscess:

i. Clinical features are similar to but milder than those described above.
ii. A chronic periodontal abscess may become acute if drainage of pus is blocked. This results in an increase in the severity of clinical features.

CLINICAL UTILITY AND SHORT ANSWER

What is a periapical abscess?

- Periapical abscess is of pulpal origin; it occurs in relation to a tooth whose pulp has become infected (*such teeth may be vital or non-vital*) or in teeth with faulty root canal treatment (*RCT*).
- A pure periapical abscess can involve periodontal tissues when it drains out into the oral cavity. In such cases, marginal gingiva is usually not involved (*in a periodontal abscess marginal gingiva is usually involved*) **(Fig. 11.3, diags A and B)**.
- Periapical abscesses are treated with RCT.
- A periapical and periodontal abscess can also occur simultaneously—this is called endo-perio complication **(Fig. 21.9)**. In all such cases, endodontic treatment (*RCT*) must be carried out ***before*** extensive periodontal treatment is done.

How does a periodontal abscess appear on a radiograph?

Radiographic signs of acute and chronic periodontal abscesses:

1. In an ***acute*** periodontal abscess of very ***recent*** origin, ***no*** radiographic changes are seen even when clinical features (*pain, swelling, tenderness, etc.*) are severe.
2. In a ***chronic*** periodontal abscess or in an ***acute*** periodontal abscess which has ***arisen from a chronic abscess,*** radiolucent (*blackish–grey*) areas (*due to bone destruction*) are seen on the lateral side of the involved tooth root or furcation area of involved tooth.

3. In ***chronic*** periodontal abscesses occurring ***simultaneously*** and ***communicating with periapical abscesses of endodontic origin***, radiolucent areas are seen in relation to root apices, lateral sides of involved tooth root/s or furcation area of the involved tooth. No clear-cut distinction can be made radiographically between the two **(Fig. 21.9)**.

ALERT!

A periodontal abscess may present different radiological images depending on:

a. Angle at which the radiograph is taken.
b. Location of abscess in relation to other anatomical structures.
c. Stage of development of the abscess.

If an abscess is located on the buccal or lingual aspects of teeth, image of the root and lingual and buccal bony plates get superimposed on radiographic image of the abscess. In such cases, a periodontal abscess is ***not*** visible radiographically.

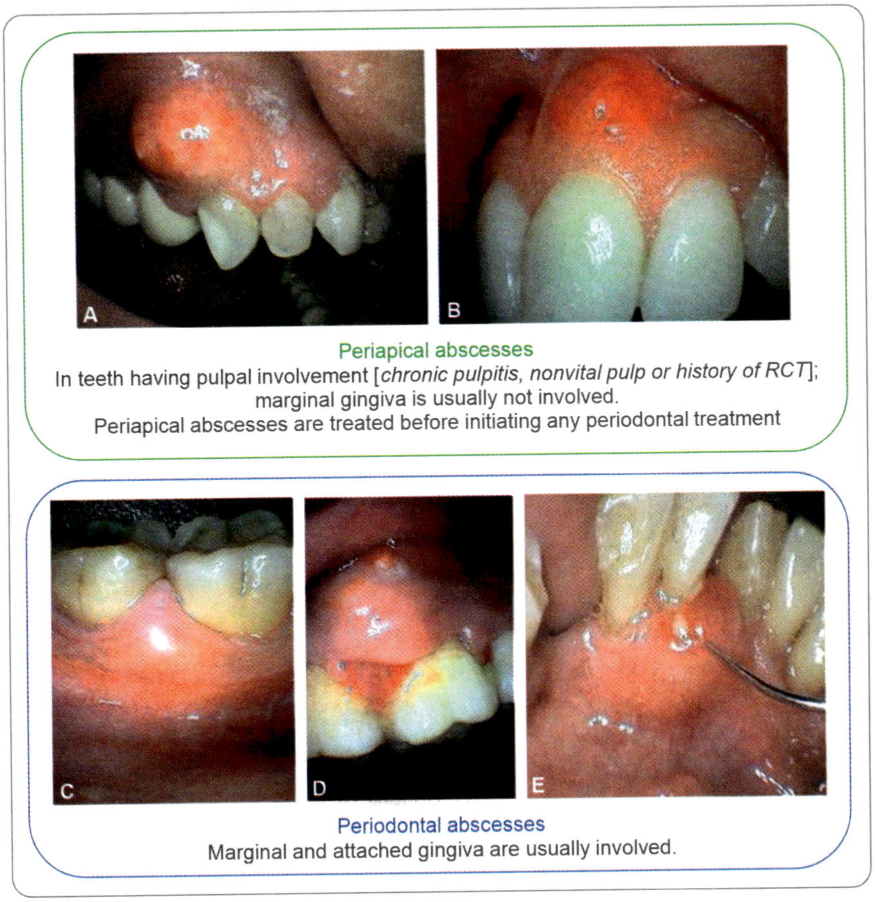

Fig. 11.3: Periapical and periodontal abscesses

Etiology and pathogenesis of a periodontal abscess

Pus produced in gingival sulcus or pockets (*as a response to plaque bacteria*) keeps coming out and drains into the mouth. If this drainage is blocked due to any reason, collection and localization of pus occurs and this results in formation of periodontal abscess. Pus localization resulting in periodontal abscess formation could occur due to:

◂ *What are the causes periodontal abscess?*

1. **Deep and lateral extension of inflammation** (*from the pocket*) into the surrounding periodontal connective tissue.
2. **Blocking of abscess's sinus or pocket opening (*drainage*)** by food debris, calculus or other foreign objects leading to restriction or complete stopping of drainage of pus.

◂ *How does a compound pocket lead to periodontal abscess formation?*

3. **Incomplete drainage of pus from a complex or compound pocket.** Complex and compound pockets **(Fig. 10.5, diags 2 and 3)** have a pouch-like cavity with a large fundus and a very small 'mouth' that opens into the oral cavity. In such pockets, if pus forms in

larger volume and greater rate than it can drain out, or if the opening of this pouch gets blocked, pus will accumulate and an abscess will form.

How does incomplete scaling cause periodontal abscess? ▶

4. **'Superficial' or incomplete scaling and root planing.** If a clinician is unable to scale or root plane the entire diseased root surface efficiently, only the gingiva opposing the superficial root surface that has been treated shrinks due to resolution of inflammation in this part of gingiva. On the other hand, pus continues to form in deeper part of the pocket opposite surface of the tooth that has not been scaled and root planed. This pus forming in deeper part of the pocket cannot now drain out as the gingiva of the coronal part of the pocket has shrunk and has closed or restricted the pocket opening through which pus was draining earlier. This causes localization and collection of pus and a periodontal abscess results.
5. **Extension of infection from an infected pulp or periapical abscess of pulpal origin deep into periodontal tissues.** Infection from infected pulps can be translocated into periodontium during bio-mechanical preparation of root canals (*BMP for RCT*) or root canal perforation. This infection causes pus formation and can result in peri-apical and/or periodontal abscesses.
6. **A periodontal abscess may form due to inflammation resulting from physical trauma to a tooth.**

ALERT!

In which clinical situations is a periodontal abscess more likely to develop? ▶

A periodontal abscess is more likely to develop in:

1. Class II and III furcations.
2. Complex pockets.
3. Deep periodontal pockets (*more than 5 mm*).
4. Endo-perio complications.
5. Patients having coexisting systemic ailments like:
   a. Severe diabetes, debilitating diseases, etc.
   b. Immune deficiencies from:
      i. Disease, e.g. AIDS, etc.
      ii. Immune suppression caused by drugs, e.g. steroids (*used for treatment of severe asthma, etc.*), cyclosporine (*used for preventing rejections of transplanted kidneys, etc.*), etc.

ALERT!

Role of diabetes in periodontal abscesses and periodontitis

Poorly controlled diabetes complicates periodontitis. Such patients have:

1. Relatively higher rate of loss of periodontal tissues (*PDL and alveolar bone*) in periodontitis.
2. Slower healing.
3. Greater tendency to formation of periodontal abscesses.

This happens because of:

a. PMN defects like defective chemotaxis, phagocytosis, etc.
b. Reduced speed of healing.
c. Increased collagen loss in periodontal tissues.
d. Increased glucose in the patient's blood and gingival fluid (*this encourages growth of microorganisms that cause periodontitis*).

CLINICAL UTILITY AND SHORT ANSWER

How is a periodontal abscess treated? ▶

What is the prognosis and treatment of a periodontal abscess?

A periodontal abscess that is not complicated by systemic disease responds well to treatment; its prognosis is therefore ***very good***. Periodontal abscesses can however reoccur in incompletely treated cases or in patients with systemic ailments. General line of treatment of periodontal abscess is as under:

1. Establish drainage. This relieves pain and is particularly important in acute abscesses. In a chronic abscess, it is important to ensure that drainage of abscess is not blocked (*this will prevent chronic abscess from converting to a very painful acute abscess*).
2. Ensure correct diagnosis. If the abscess is of endodontic origin and is draining through the periodontal tissues, ***endodontic treatment*** will be needed first. Periodontal treatment must be carried out ***after*** or along with endodontic treatment.

(*Contd.*)

(*Contd.*)

3. Antimicrobial (*'antibiotic'*) therapy will be needed if systemic signs and symptoms like cervical lymphadenopathy, fever, etc. are there.
4. If teeth are 'very' tender, occlusion may have to be relieved by selective grinding of the crown (*coronoplasty*) of affected or opposing tooth.
5. Temporary or semi-permanent splinting may be done if teeth show more than grade II mobility.
6. The 'actual' treatment of a periodontal abscess begins only ***after*** it has been converted to a chronic abscess. It includes:
   a. Root planing.
   b. Reduction of pocket depth by flap surgery or gingivectomy.
7. Prevention of recurrence of periodontal abscesses can be done by:
   a. Good plaque control and regular six monthly (*or earlier*) scaling and root planing visits.
   b. Control of diabetes and other contributing illnesses (*if present*).
   c. Completion of all planned periodontal treatments.
   d. Extraction of hopelessly involved teeth.

CLINICAL UTILITY AND SHORT ANSWER

Which of the two: Periodontal pocket reduction by flap surgery or periodontal pocket elimination by gingivectomy is more suited for treatment of a periodontal abscess?

Of the two, pocket elimination by gingivectomy is ***better*** suited and preferred because chances of recurrence of a periodontal abscess are ***lesser*** after pocket elimination.

1biii. Pericoronal abscess and pericoronitis

(*see Chapter 12 and page 209–212, Desquamative Gingivitis and Acute Gingival Infections page 209–212 also*).

◂ *What is pericoronitis?*

Definition: Pericoronitis is inflammation of gingiva in relation to crown of an ***incompletely*** erupted tooth (Figs 11.4 and 12.4).

If pus formation increases under such inflamed gingiva (*pericoronal flap*) and discharge of pus is restricted causing localization of pus, a pericoronal abscess results. Pericoronitis is of three types: Acute, sub-acute and chronic (Fig. 11. 4).

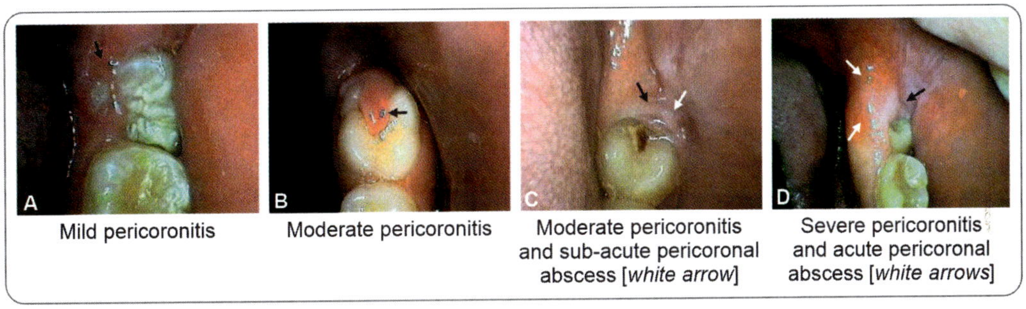

Fig. 11.4: Pericoronitis and pericoronal abscess in relation to an erupting mandibular third molar. Note inflamed operculum (*black arrows*) and food impaction under it and pericoronal abscess formation (*diags C and D, white arrows*).

Etiology and pathogenesis of pericoronitis and pericoronal abscess

◂ *Can pericoronitis be seen in relation to any erupting tooth or is it seen only in relation to mandibular third molars?*

◂ *What is an operculum in relation to a tooth with pericoronitis?*

1. Pericoronitis may occur in relation to ***any*** erupting tooth. However, it is ***more commonly*** seen in relation to erupting ***mandibular third molars***.
2. A partially erupted or impacted tooth is usually completely or partially covered with a 'loose' lid (*operculum*) of gingival tissue. The space between occlusal surface of this tooth and overlying gingival operculum allows accumulation of plaque and food debris. As a result, sometimes, moderate or severe inflammation occurs in the gingival operculum. If this inflammation is mild, it is not bothersome.
3. This inflammation is also accompanied by pus formation. If localization of pus occurs in the gingival operculum, pericoronitis and pericoronal abscess result.
4. The inflamed gingival operculum enlarges and is then physically hit and traumatized by cusps of opposing teeth. This worsens inflammation and pain in the gingival operculum.

What are the clinical features of pericoronitis and pericoronal abscess? ▸

Clinical features of pericoronitis and pericoronal abscess in relation to *mandibular third molars* (*similar clinical features with some variations are found in pericoronitis in relation to maxillary third molars and other teeth*)

1. The crown of the partially erupted tooth is completely or partially covered by a flap of gingival tissue (*operculum*) which is inflamed and maybe traumatized **(Fig. 11.4)**.
2. If operculum is chronically inflamed, patient presents with mild clinical features. In case acute inflammation occurs, severity of inflammation increases and patients usually complain of tenderness and severe pain that radiates to throat, floor of mouth, ear, forehead, etc.
3. Patient often complains of foul taste and foul odour (*from decomposing food debris and pus under the operculum*).

Why do patients with pericoronitis complain of painful mouth closure? ▸

4. If infection in the area worsens, pus formation increases manifold. This causes the operculum to become markedly red and swollen. Pain now becomes more severe.
5. The swollen operculum causes interference with jaw closure and can also get physically traumatized by teeth of opposing arch during jaw closure. This causes worsening of inflammation and existing clinical features.
6. Muscle trismus may be seen in some cases. This causes painful and restricted mouth opening.
7. Swelling and numbness of same side of the face may be there.
8. Draining lymph nodes may become palpable and tender.
9. In severe cases fever, malaise may also be there.

2. Conditioned Enlargements (*Gingival Enlargements Associated with Systemic Diseases and Conditions*)

What are conditioning factors? ▸

How do conditioning factors affect gingiva? ▸

Systemic factors like pregnancy, puberty, etc. act like response modifying factors (*conditioning factors*) in the gingiva. Under the effect of these factors, gingiva gets conditioned and responds to dental plaque in an ***exaggerated*** and ***altered*** way. The resulting gingival enlargements are called conditioned enlargements.

CLINICAL UTILITY AND SHORT ANSWER

What are conditioning factors?

- Conditioning factors are systemic factors that act as response ***modifying*** factors at the local gingival level.
- Conditioning factors are ***not*** etiological factors (i.e. *causative factors*), but they when present, affect the gingiva (*target tissue*) in such a way that they modify and exaggerate gingiva's response to the already present (*same quality and quantity*) plaque and other contributing etiological factors.

2a. *Pregnancy Gingivitis and Periodontitis*

Does pregnancy cause pregnancy gingivitis? ▸

Pregnancy itself ***does not*** cause gingival enlargement but only conditions and modifies (*exaggerates*) response of gingiva to pre-existing (*already present*) local etiological factors.

General clinical features of pregnancy gingivitis (Fig. 11.5) and pregnancy periodontitis (Fig. 11.6):

How are clinical features of pregnancy gingivitis different from those of plaque induced gingivitis? ▸

- Clinical features of pregnancy gingivitis and pregnancy periodontitis are ***similar to*** and are ***exaggerated*** versions of clinical features of plaque induced gingivitis (*see chapter 10, Plaque Induced Gingivitis and Periodontitis*) **(Fig. 11.5)**.
- All clinical features of gingivitis and periodontitis that were not easily identifiable till the patient became pregnant now become pronounced and easily identifiable, e.g. bleeding gums, etc. (*that was not present before pregnancy*). If gingivitis or periodontitis were present earlier, their ***severity worsens.***
- Severity of clinical features of gingivitis and periodontitis is much more than what is expected in that particular case, i.e. severity of local factors is ***not*** relatable to identifiable local factors present in the mouth (*this proves the disease is a conditioned response*).

Till which month during pregnancy are features of pregnancy gingivitis seen? ▸

- Severity of clinical features of gingivitis and periodontitis worsen till 8th month of pregnancy. Thereafter the clinical features improve automatically to some extent.

- When treated, clinical features (*gingivitis and periodontitis*) show improvement only to a limited extent. Pregnancy gingivitis and pregnancy periodontitis are usually ***not*** completely treatable till a few weeks after childbirth.

◂ *Can pregnancy gingivitis and periodontitis be treated?*

Clinical presentation of pregnancy gingivitis

There are ***two*** distinct clinical types of gingival enlargements related to pregnancy:

i. Marginal enlargement
ii. Angiogranuloma (*tumor-like enlargement*).

◂ *How many types of gingival enlargements are associated with pregnancy?*

2ai. Marginal enlargement

1. It is seen in ***10–70%*** of all pregnant females (Fig. 11.5).
2. Enlargement is confined to marginal and interdental gingiva.
3. Gingiva bleeds ***profusely*** after slight injury (*slight provocation like probing, etc.*).
4. There is also an increased tendency to spontaneous gingival bleeding (*without provocation*).
5. As severity of gingivitis increases, gingiva becomes friable and tendency to bleed worsens.
6. Colour of the involved gingiva is dark bluish-red. Small blood capillaries on surface of gingiva are prominent.
7. Gingiva is soft, pitting on pressure and smooth.

◂ *Do all pregnant females have pregnancy gingivitis?*

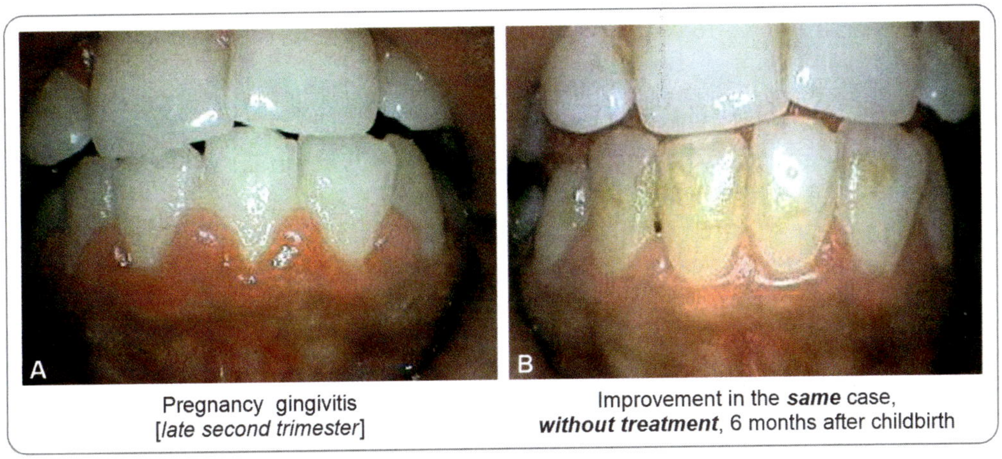

Fig. 11.5: Pregnancy gingivitis. Note that gingivitis is severe despite small amount of local factors (*indicating that this a conditioned enlargement*) (*diag. A*). This patient refused dental treatment during her pregnancy and reported back for dental treatment 6 months after childbirth. At this time gingivitis is seen to be markedly better and degree of gingivitis is now co-relatable to the local factors (*effect of conditioning effect of pregnancy is no longer there*) (*diag. B*).

◂ *What are the clinical features of marginal enlargement seen in pregnancy gingivitis?*

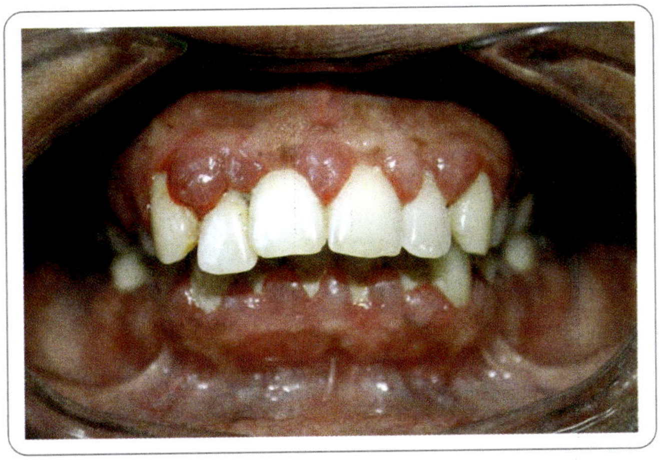

Fig. 11.6: Pregnancy periodontitis. Note that degree of gingival inflammation is much more that what can be attributed to present local etiological factors (*plaque, calculus deposits, etc.*). This suggests conditioning effect of pregnancy.

Is angiogranuloma a tumor/neoplasm? ▸

2aii. Angiogranuloma (*Tumor-like pregnancy enlargement*)

The term angiogranuloma is ***misleading*** as it suggests that this is a neoplasm (*tumor*) ***whereas it is not***.

In what percentage of pregnant females is angiogranuloma seen? ▸

1. It is seen only in 2–5% of all the pregnant females.

Where does angiogranuloma usually occur? ▸

2. It usually occurs on the interdental papilla and rarely on marginal gingiva.
3. It is a bead like, protruding out and localized (*discrete*) enlargement. It may be flattened and its base is either sessile or pedunculated (*mushroom-like*). Flattening of the enlargement occurs due to pressure of the cheek, lips or tongue.
4. Its surface is smooth and dotted by small pinpoint, irregular red patches.

What are the clinical features of angiogranuloma? ▸

5. It is semi firm in consistency. As severity of inflammation increases, it may become soft and friable.
6. Pain is usually not there; however, if ulceration occurs under the fold of the enlargement, patient may complain of vague discomfort.

Does angiogranuloma cause resorption of underlying bone? ▸

7. Angiogranuloma does not depress underlying alveolar bone. It therefore does not cause bone resorption due to its pressure.

2b. *Puberty Enlargement*

What is puberty? ▸ *What is puberty enlargement?* ▸

Puberty is the time in life when an individual becomes sexually mature; it occurs between 10–14 years in girls and 12–16 years in boys. Puberty gingivitis is caused by change in levels of an individual's hormones during puberty (Fig. 11.7).

Clinical features of puberty enlargement:

In which sex and age group is puberty enlargement seen? ▸

1. Puberty enlargement may be seen in both girls and boys in the age group of 10–17 years.
2. Its clinical features are practically the ***same*** and slightly exaggerated versions of clinical features of plaque induced gingivitis (*inflammatory enlargement*) (*see Chapter 10, Plaque Induced Gingivitis and Periodontitis*).
3. Severity of gingivitis and periodontitis is much more than what is expected in that particular case, i.e. size of gingival enlargement is larger than expected (*exaggerated response*) and is not relatable to the amount of local factors present in the mouth (*this proves the disease is a conditioned response*).
4. Gingiva is bulbous and enlargement is usually confined to the marginal and interdental gingiva.

Can puberty enlargement be treated? ▸

5. Enlargement cannot be completely treated and is recurrent till puberty phase is over (*it does not respond completely to periodontal treatment*).
6. After puberty phase is over (*end of conditioning factor*) the enlargement may reduce automatically.

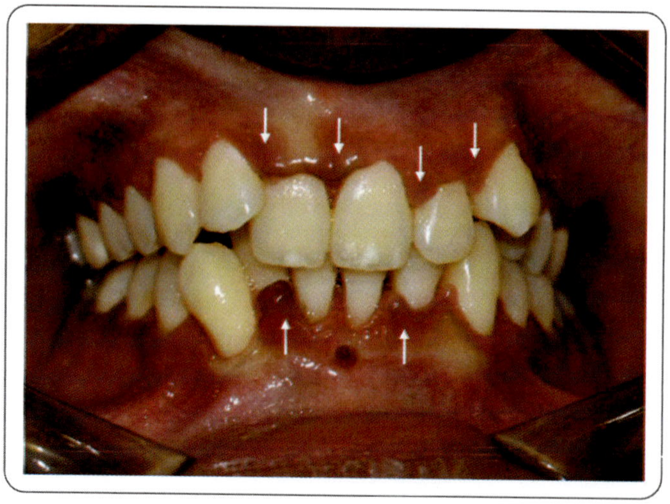

Fig. 11.7: Puberty gingivitis in 14-year-old male patient. Note that degree of gingivitis is far in excess and not relatable to plaque and other local factors (*suggesting conditioning effect of puberty*).

CLINICAL UTILITY AND SHORT ANSWER

Can biopsy help in diagnosis of pregnancy and puberty enlargement?

No. The histopathological picture of ***pregnancy and puberty enlargement*** (*conditioned enlargements*) is very similar to that of plaque induced gingivitis. Therefore, it cannot form the basis of diagnosis.

◂ *Why can't biopsy help in confirmative diagnosis of pregnancy and puberty gingivitis and periodontitis?*

2c. *Vitamin C Deficiency Induced Gingival Enlargement*

The general (*systemic*) clinical condition caused by ***severe*** vitamin C deficiency is called ***Scurvy***.

◂ *What is scurvy?*

Clinical features of vit. C induced gingival enlargement:

1. Vitamin C deficiency induces a conditioned enlargement in the gingiva which is clinically almost ***similar*** to one seen in puberty and pregnancy.
2. Typical features of vit. C induced gingival enlargement are ***only*** seen in patients with ***severe*** and ***prolonged*** vitamin C deficiency; as such cases are ***rare***, vitamin C deficiency induced gingivitis is ***not*** commonly seen.
3. It may occur at any age.
4. Enlargement is usually seen in marginal gingiva.
5. Gingiva is smooth, shiny, friable and red. In some cases, desquamation of epithelium occurs. This leads to formation of pseudomembrane.
6. Spontaneous hemorrhage from gingiva after slight provocation is present. Such hemorrhage is also noticeable at other sites of body (*purpura, ecchymosis, bleeding into joints, etc.*).

◂ *Is scurvy and vit. C induced gingival enlargement common?*

CLINICAL UTILITY AND SHORT ANSWER

Can biopsy be used to diagnose vitamin C deficiency induced gingival enlargement?

No. Histopathological features of vit. C induced gingival enlargement are not specific enough to reach a diagnosis.

◂ *Why can't biopsy help in confirmative diagnosis of vit. C deficiency induced gingival enlargement?*

2d. *Nonspecific Conditioned Enlargement (Pyogenic Granuloma or Granuloma Pyogenicum)*

(*The name* ***Granuloma pyogenicum or Pyogenic granuloma*** *should* ***not*** *be used for this lesion as it is* ***not*** *a true granuloma nor is it truly pyogenic (pus producing). The use of these terms is therefore discouraged*).

◂ *Why must the terms Granuloma pyogenicum or Pyogenic granuloma not be used for referring to nonspecific conditioned enlargement?*

These enlargements usually occur in healthy patients and are believed to arise after minor oral trauma; however, the exact cause (*conditioning factor*) is not known.

Clinical features of nonspecific conditioned enlargement:

1. The lesion may be sessile or pedunculated and lobulated.
2. Enlargement may be marginal or diffused. It usually originates from interdental gingiva and occurs more commonly in the maxilla.
3. It has bluish red colour.
4. Older lesions may show surface ulcerations which may be covered by a pseudomembrane. Hemorrhage and exudation may be seen on surface of the ulcerated lesion.
5. Size of enlargement may increase rapidly.
6. Recurrence of lesions after excision is ***common***.

◂ *Does nonspecific conditioned enlargement recur after treatment?*

CLINICAL UTILITY AND SHORT ANSWER

Can biopsy be used to diagnose nonspecific conditioned enlargement?

No. Histopathological features of nonspecific conditioned enlargement are not specific enough to reach a diagnosis.

2e. *Plasma Cell Gingivitis*

Plasma cell gingivitis is believed to be allergic in origin (*allergy to food articles, or cosmetics, etc.*). It usually appears as a mild marginal enlargement of the gingiva **(Fig. 11.8)**.

Clinical features of plasma cell gingivitis:

Which other ailments often occur along with plasma cell gingivitis?

1. Marginal enlargement of gingiva is seen. Enlargement often ***extends*** into attached gingiva.
2. Enlarged gingiva is red and friable and has a granular surface.
3. Cheilitis (*inflammation of lips*) and glossitis (*inflammation of tongue*) are often also seen simultaneously.
4. Lesion maybe localized or may spread out to involve large areas of gingiva.

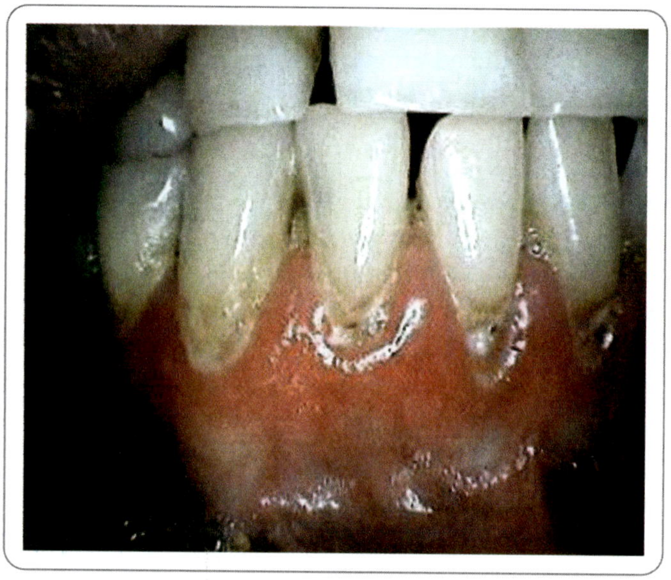

Fig. 11.8: Plasma cell gingivitis

CLINICAL UTILITY AND SHORT ANSWER

Can biopsy help in confirmative diagnosis of plasma cell gingivitis?

Can biopsy be used to diagnose plasma cell gingivitis?

Yes, biopsy can be useful in diagnosing a case of plasma cell gingivitis.

Specific features of plasma cell gingivitis (*seen in addition to HP features of chronic gingivitis; page 137*) are:

1. Spongiosis (*intercellular edema within epithelium*)
2. Infiltration by plasma cells (*antibody producing B-lymphocytes*) in connective tissue (*this suggests the lesion is allergic in nature*).

3. Enlargements Caused by Systemic Diseases

3a. *Leukemic Enlargement*

Leukemic enlargement is a conditioned and exaggerated response of gingival tissues to local irritation from the leukemic infiltrate (*abnormal WBCs*) present in gingiva.

- All patients with leukemia ***do not*** have gingival enlargement.
- Enlargement of gingiva is ***more common*** in patients with acute or sub-acute leukemia (*not common in chronic leukemia*).
- Patients with leukemia are prone to severe periodontitis; this can be managed by regular scaling and root planing.

Clinical features of leukemic enlargement

1. Leukemic enlargement presents with similar and slightly exaggerated clinical features of plaque induced gingivitis (*inflammatory enlargement*) (*see Chapter 10, Plaque Induced Gingivitis and Periodontitis*).

2. Gingival enlargement may be localized or generalized and may be marginal or diffused. If it is tumor like (*discrete*) then it is often present on the interdental papilla.
3. Gingival surface is bluish red and shining.
4. Gingiva may be friable.
5. Bleeding on slight provocation or spontaneous bleeding (*without provocation*) may be there.
6. Necrotizing ulcerative gingivitis (*NUG*) may be seen in relation to involved tissue.

CLINICAL UTILITY AND SHORT ANSWER

Can biopsy be used to diagnose leukemic enlargement of gingiva?

Yes, specific **histopathological features of leukemic enlargement are:**

1. Immense infiltration of gingival connective tissue by leukemic infiltrate. Some leukemic cells are even seen in the gingival epithelium.
2. Leukemic infiltrate's type varies with type of leukemia.
3. Edema is seen both in connective tissue and epithelium.
4. Isolated areas showing NUG like features may be seen.
5. Capillaries are engorged. Connective tissue shows degeneration to varying degrees.

◄ *Can biopsy help in confirmative diagnosis of leukemic enlargement of gingiva?*

3b. *Enlargements Caused by Granulomatous Diseases*

3bi. Wegener's granulomatosis

◄ *What is strawberry gingivitis?*

- Oral lesions of Wegner's granulomatosis make the gingiva red, friable and sometimes nodular. As this lesion looks like a ripe strawberry, it is also called ***strawberry gingivitis***.
- It is an ***uncommon*** disease (*form of vasculitis,* i.e. *inflammation of small and medium blood vessels*) that can occur in many organs (*especially respiratory system and kidneys; head neck region is also involved in more than 90% of cases*).
- Its exact cause is unknown but is thought to be an autoimmune disorder.
- This vasculitis restricts blood flow which results in damage to tissues.

3bii. Sarcoidosis

- Oral lesions usually occur in the tongue; if gingiva is involved, it may appear to be reddish-pink in color, enlarged and painless. Sarcoidosis is characterized by formation of abnormal non-caseating granulomas of unknown origin.
- Lesions of sarcoidosis commonly involve the lungs and lymph nodes.

CLINICAL UTILITY AND SHORT ANSWER

All conditioned enlargements cannot be treated completely by scaling and root planing, why then is it important to perform these procedures for such patients?

Although conditioned enlargements cannot be treated completely with scaling and root planing still, scaling and root planing must be done frequently and at regular intervals as this will reduce the severity of the inflammatory component of the disease (*gingivitis and periodontitis*) and will also delay its worsening to severe stages again in the future (*till conditioning factor is present*).

4. Drug Induced Gingival Enlargements

Many medicines (*drugs*) used for treating systemic diseases can cause gingival enlargements. Some commonly used drugs known to cause gingival enlargements are:

1. Anticonvulsants (*used to treat epilepsy*), e.g. phenytoin, mephenytoin, etc.
2. Immuno-suppressants (*used in patients with autoimmune diseases, organ transplants,* etc.), e.g. cyclosporine, tacrolimus, etc.
3. Anti-hypertensives (*calcium channel blockers, used to treat high blood pressure*), e.g. amlodipine, nifedipine, etc.

Clinical features of drug induced gingival enlargement

Phenytoin induced gingival enlargement was the first drug induced enlargement to be identified (*phenytoin is used for treatment of epilepsy*), its features are described in detail below. It must be remembered that ***all drug induced gingival enlargements*** present ***similar clinical features*** therefore, diagnosis is based solely on history of drug intake. Clinical features of phenytoin enlargement (*and other drug induced enlargements*) are (Figs 11.9 and 11.10):

Are clinical features of different drug induced gingival enlargements immensely different? ▸

1. Enlargement is painless to start.
2. Initially, enlargement is bead like and first appears on interdental gingiva or marginal gingiva. Attached gingiva is ***rarely*** involved by drug induced gingival enlargements (Fig. 11.9).

How commonly is attached gingiva involved by drug induced gingival enlargements? ▸

3. The bead like enlargements increase in size and unite to become larger. Enlargements may then cover clinical crown of the tooth to varying degrees. If the enlargement covers a significant portion of the clinical crown, it may then interfere with occlusion and mastication (Fig. 11.11, *blue arrows*).

In which areas of the mouth are drug induced enlargements the severest? ▸

4. Drug induced enlargements are often ***generalized*** but are of ***maximum severity*** in ***anterior*** region. Usually both upper and lower teeth are equally involved.
5. Gingival enlargements ***almost always*** occur in ***dentulous areas*** of the mouth. Sometimes gingival enlargements may reduce in size automatically after extraction of teeth.
6. They slowly increase in size and ***recur*** after surgical removal.
7. Drug induced gingival enlargements seem to ***'erupt' from under the gingival margin*** (*free gingiva*). Usually, a linear groove can be seen to separate the gingival enlargement and marginal gingiva (Fig. 11.9).

What are the clinical features of drug induced enlargement that does not have clinically identifiable inflammation in it? ▸

8. If the enlargement is ***not*** clinically complicated by inflammation, it is firm, pink, resilient, minutely lobulated and shows no increased tendency to bleed (Fig. 11.11, *white arrow*). Enlargement however makes adequate plaque control difficult leading to inflammation in the gingiva.
9. If plaque induced inflammation increases in severity and becomes clinically evident, the enlargement becomes a combined enlargement, i.e. it also has component of plaque induced inflammation in addition to the drug induced enlargement. Therefore, all clinical features of plaque induced gingivitis and periodontitis (*see Chapter 10, Plaque Induced Gingivitis and Periodontitis*) can be also be seen (Fig. 11.11, diag. C, *black arrow*). These include:

What are the clinical features of drug induced enlargement that has clinically identifiable inflammation in it? ▸

   a. Change in color of the gingiva from pink to dark pink or bluish red.
   b. Loss of firmness and resiliency of gingiva. This makes gingiva soft and friable.
   c. Increased tendency to bleed on probing or spontaneous bleeding.
   d. Dull pain.
   e. Smoothening of the minutely lobulated gingival surface to produce a smooth and shiny surface (*due to ballooning out of the gingiva*), etc.

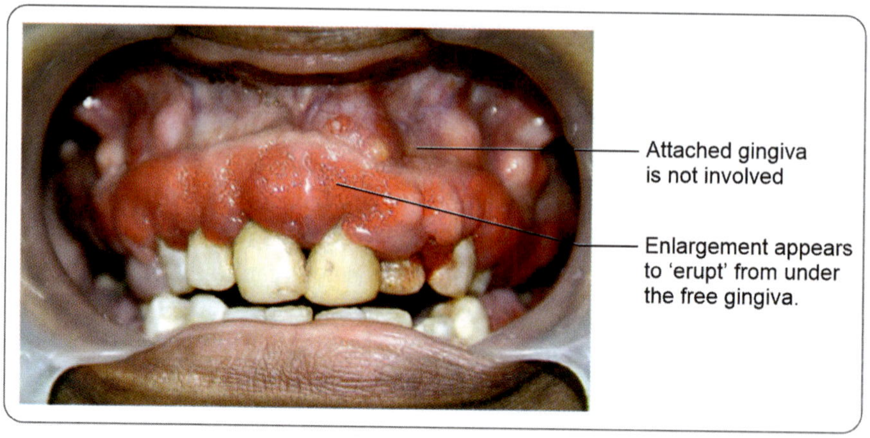

Fig. 11.9: Drug induced (*phenytoin*) gingival enlargement. All drug induced gingival enlargements have almost similar clinical features.

ALERT!

- Marginal and interdental gingiva are involved in ***drug induced*** gingival enlargements, while attached gingiva is ***rarely*** involved (Fig. 11.9).
- In ***idiopathic*** gingival enlargements (*described in subsequent text below*), enlargement is diffuse, i.e. marginal, interdental and attached gingiva are ***always collectively involved*** (Fig. 11.11, diags A and B; compare with diag. C).
- Involvement of attached gingiva is the ***chief*** distinguishing clinical feature between drug induced and idiopathic gingival enlargements.

◄ *How can drug induced gingival enlargements be clinically differentiated from idiopathic gingival enlargements?*

CLINICAL UTILITY AND SHORT ANSWER

Can biopsy be used to diagnose different drug induced gingival enlargements?

No. Histopathological features of all drug induced gingival enlargements are almost similar. Therefore, definitive diagnosis of which drug has caused the enlargement cannot be made from a biopsy specimen of the enlargement. Histopathological features ***common*** to all drug induced gingival enlargements are:

1. Acanthosis (*thickening of stratum basale and stratum spinosum*)
2. Large rete pegs extending deep into connective tissue.
3. Hyperplastic connective tissue with dense collagen bundles, increased amorphous ground substance and fibroblasts in connective tissue.
4. Increased number of normal blood vessels in connective tissue.
5. Chronic inflammatory cells (*especially plasma cells*) seen in larger numbers.
6. Granulation tissue is seen in grossly inflamed enlargements.

ALERT!

- Diagnosis of which drug has caused gingival enlargement is based only on history of drug intake by the patient.
- Good plaque control can reduce the rate of increase of size of drug induced enlargements.

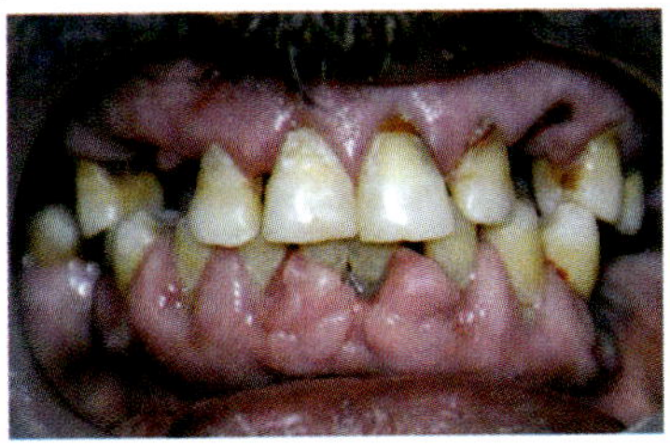

Antihypertensive induced gingival enlargement

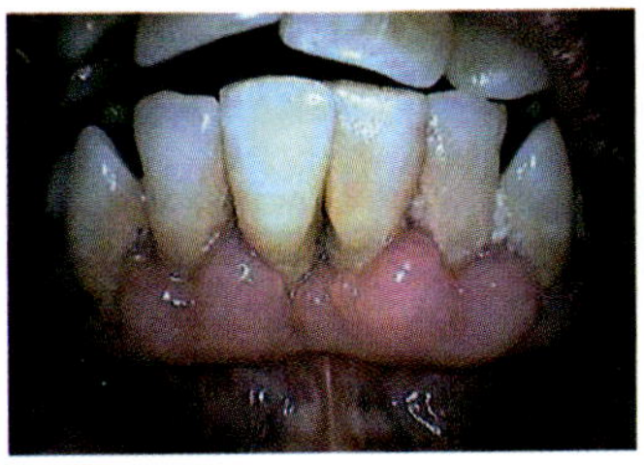

Immunosuppressant induced gingival enlargement

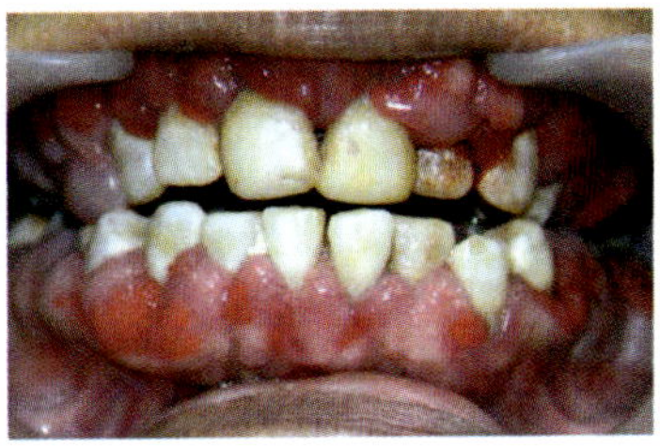

Anticonvulsant [*phenytoin*] induced gingival enlargement

Fig. 11.10: Gingival enlargements caused by different drugs are similar and cannot be differentiated clinically or histologically. As the gingiva enlarges, probing pocket depth (*PD*) increases (*pockets deepen*). This is leads to plaque induced inflammation over and above the enlargement caused by the drug.

5. Hereditary Gingival Fibromatosis (*Idiopathic Gingival Enlargement*)

These enlargements are relatively ***uncommon***. Although exact cause of hereditary gingival fibromatosis (*idiopathic enlargement*) is unknown, it is thought to occur because of:

◄ *Are idiopathic enlargements common?*

1. Genetic tendency. Hereditary gingival fibromatosis (*idiopathic gingival enlargements*) are commonly seen in more than one blood relation, i.e. closely related family members like real brothers and sisters, parents and their children.
2. Plaque is believed to be an aggravating factor and acts along with the genetic predisposition of the patient to predispose to this enlargement.

◄ *Does plaque cause idiopathic enlargements?*

Clinical features of Hereditary gingival fibromatosis (*idiopathic gingival enlargement*)

1. The enlargement involves marginal gingiva, interdental papilla and attached gingiva, i.e. it is ***diffuse***. This is one of the ***chief*** diagnostic features of idiopathic enlargements and is helpful in its differential diagnosis from drug induced enlargements (Fig. 11.11, diags A and B, *yellow arrows; compare with diag. C*).

◄ *Which of the two, drug induced or idiopathic enlargements are diffuse in presentation?*

2. Both or either of the jaws may be affected.

In which areas of the mouth do idiopathic enlargements occur commonly?

3. Enlargement is more common on buccal side of anterior teeth of both jaws but can extend to posterior regions also. Hereditary gingival fibromatosis (*idiopathic gingival enlargement*) may be localized to a particular region of the mouth; unaffected regions of the same mouth may have normal gingiva.
4. Consistency and surface of the enlargement is variable:
   a. In some cases, the enlargement may have a soft consistency, smooth surface and may be friable **(Fig. 11.11, diag. A)**.
   b. In some other cases, it may be firm and lobulated with prominent stippling and have a leathery consistency **(Fig. 11.11, diag. B)**.
5. Color of the enlargement is also variable **(Fig. 11.11, diags A and B)**:
   a. When enlargements do not have clinically identifiable plaque induced inflammation, enlargement is usually pink and minutely pebbled **(Fig. 11.11, diags A and B**, *white arrows*).
   b. When inflammation is clinically evident, enlargement is soft, friable and reddish blue (**Fig. 11.11, diags A and B**, *black arrows*).
6. As enlargement progresses, it covers clinical crown of the tooth (**Fig. 11.11, diag. B**, *blue arrows*). In severe cases, entire crown may be covered and it may then interfere with mouth closure and mastication. Very large enlargements distort the facial appearance of the patient. Enlargements on the lingual side interfere with speech and swallowing.
7. Inflammatory changes are usually seen on margin of the enlargement. Here, gingiva is enlarged due to combination of idiopathic and inflammatory enlargement.

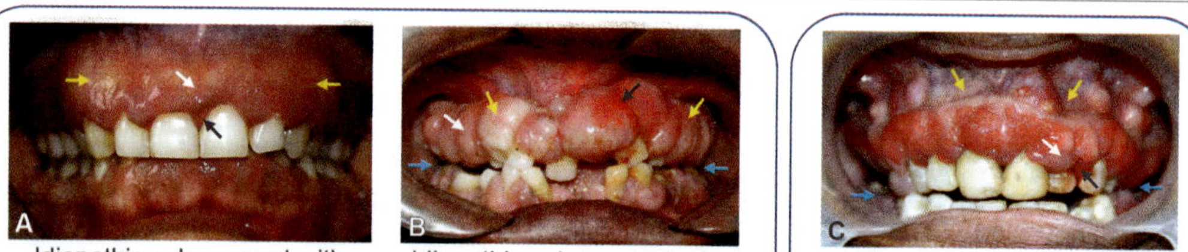

Fig. 11.11: Hereditary gingival fibromatosis (*idiopathic gingival enlargement*) and comparison of its clinical features which those of drug induced gingival enlargements. Note that only the free gingiva and interdental papillae are involved in drug induced enlargements, i.e. attached gingiva is not involved (*diag. C, yellow arrows*). Idiopathic enlargements are diffuse i.e. marginal gingiva, interdental papilla and attached gingiva are all involved (*diag. A and B, yellow arrows*) and generally more severe than drug induced enlargements.

CLINICAL UTILITY AND SHORT ANSWER

Can biopsy be used to diagnose idiopathic enlargement of gingiva?

No. Histopathological features of idiopathic enlargement are not specific enough to lead to a definite diagnosis. The histopathological features include:

1. Epithelium is thickened and acanthotic.
2. Rete pegs are longer than normal.
3. Connective tissue is relatively avascular and enlarged.

6. Cysts and Tumors Occurring in the Periodontium (*Neoplastic Enlargements*)

Are gingival tumors common?

Majority of enlargements seen in gingiva are inflammatory in nature. Tumors of the gingiva are not very common. Only a small percentage of tumors of the gingiva are truly neoplastic in nature (*benign or malignant*). Gingiva can also get involved secondarily with benign or malignant growths arising in the neighboring tissues, e.g. floor of mouth, alveolar bone, tongue, etc.

For detailed descriptions of such enlargements, the reader is referred to texts of oral pathology. Some relatively common pathologies arising from or affecting the periodontium and gingiva are discussed here.

6a. *Benign Tumors of Gingiva (Epulis)*

Of all oral neoplasms, only about 8% occur in relation to gingiva. Some common benign gingival enlargements are:

6ai. Fibroma

They are painless slow growing, firm and rounded tumors but may sometimes be soft. They are usually pedunculated and are composed of numerous collagen bundles (Fig. 11.12, diag. A).

6aii. Papilloma

They are usually solitary painless epithelial overgrowths that are viral in origin (*caused by human papilloma virus HPV-6 and HPV-11*). Gingival papillomas are small and have a flattened irregular wart or cauliflower-like surfaces.

◂ *What is a papilloma?*

◂ *Which viruses cause papillomas?*

6aiii. Peripheral Giant Cell Granuloma

They may be sessile or pedunculated, painless and usually ***do not*** cause involvement and destruction of underlying bone. They commonly arise from either interdental papilla or marginal gingiva. These may have a smooth or irregular surface and may have a regularly outlined or a multi-lobulated indented surface. They are pink to bluish-red in colour and may be firm or spongy in consistency. Peripheral giant cell granulomas are believed to be healing responses of gingiva to local injury (*this has not been proved*). Complete removal leads to uneventful recovery.

◂ *Where does peripheral giant cell granuloma occur?*

◂ *What is the etiology of peripheral giant cell granuloma?*

6aiv. Central Giant Cell Granuloma

Central giant cell granuloma is similar to peripheral giant cell granuloma but these arise in the jaw bone rather than in gingiva. As these arise in the jaw bone, they produce a deformity of the jaw bone's surface and thus of the gingiva also.

◂ *What is the difference between central and peripheral giant cell granuloma?*

6av. Leukoplakia

Leukoplakia is a white lesion of oral tissues that is caused by smoking or use of chewing tobacco. It must be remembered that:

◂ *What is leukoplakia?*

- Leukoplakia is a ***benign*** lesion (*but may be pre-malignant; about 20% of leukoplakias may convert to malignant lesions*). Biopsy of all leukoplakias that do not regress after treatment within two-three weeks must ***always*** be done. Chronic leukoplakia must always be periodically examined for malignant changes.
- When it occurs on the gingiva, it is a flat, white and scaly lesion with irregular margins and surface (Fig. 11.12, diag. B).
- Lesions ***similar*** to leukoplakia can occur due to other etiological factors also, e.g. chronic irritation (*frictional keratosis*), candidiasis, etc.

◂ *What percentage of leukoplakia lesions convert to malignant lesions?*

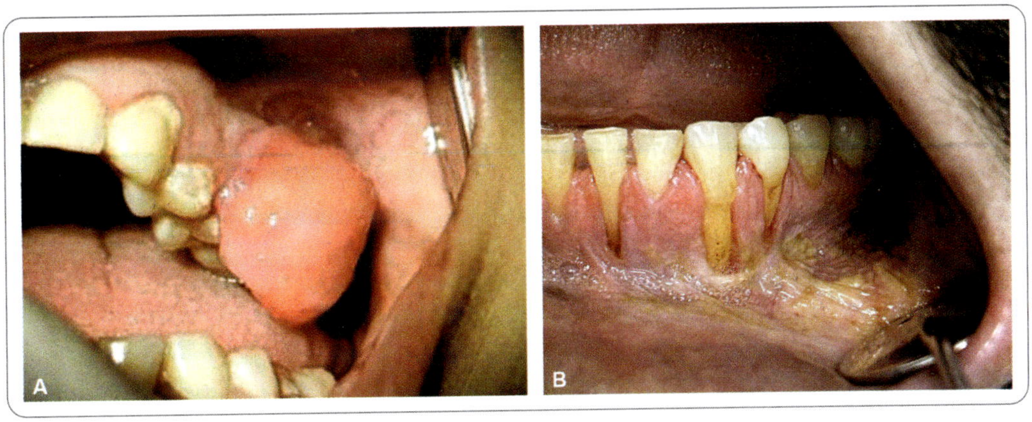

Fig. 11.12: Gingival fibroma (*diag. A*) and leukoplakia (*diag. B*)

6avi. Gingival cysts

How does a gingival cyst arise? ▸

Gingival cysts are different from periodontal cysts (*that originate in the periodontal ligament and the alveolar bone*). Gingival cysts arise from impaction of odontogenic, sulcular or surface epithelium into the connective tissue. Usually, they are very small and therefore remain undiagnosed. These do not recur after complete removal.

6avii. Eruption cyst

What is the difference between a gingival and eruption cyst? ▸

An eruption cyst can occur over an un-erupted tooth. It appears like a bluish (*or red, if filled with blood*) fluid filled enlargement over an erupting tooth. Eruption cysts occur commonly over deciduous anterior teeth, but may occur over permanent teeth also.

6b. *Malignant Tumors of the Gingiva*

Is gingiva a common site for malignant tumors? ▸

Gingiva is ***not*** a very common site of development of malignant tumors (*oral cancer*). Metastasis of tumors that are growing at other sites also does ***not*** occur commonly to the gingiva. Some malignant tumors of the gingiva are:

6bi. Carcinoma

Which is the commonest malignant tumor seen in the gingiva? ▸

Squamous cell carcinoma is the ***commonest*** malignant tumor of gingiva. Being symptom free in early stages, it goes unnoticed and undiagnosed or mis-diagnosed in many patients. It is locally invasive and may show metastasis in the immediate surrounding areas; metastasis to far sites, e.g. lung and liver is not commonly seen.

6bii. Malignant melanoma

Malignant melanoma is a rare rapidly growing tumour that originates from melanoblasts of gingiva. It usually occurs on the hard palate. It is dark in color and is often preceded by hyperpigmentation of the tissue at the site of its occurrence. This tumor shows early metastasis to other sites.

6biii. Sarcoma

In which disease is Kaposi's sarcoma commonly seen in the gingiva? ▸

Sarcomas are of various types and are rarely seen in the gingiva. Kaposi's sarcoma afflicting the gingiva is usually seen in AIDS (*Acquired immunodeficiency syndrome*) patients.

7. Enlargement due to Mouth Breathing

In individuals who breath through their mouths, gingiva of maxillary anterior labial and palatal regions gets dried due to passage of air. Due to chronic air drying, gingiva gets inflamed and appears red, enlarged, edematous and shiny (Fig. 11.13).

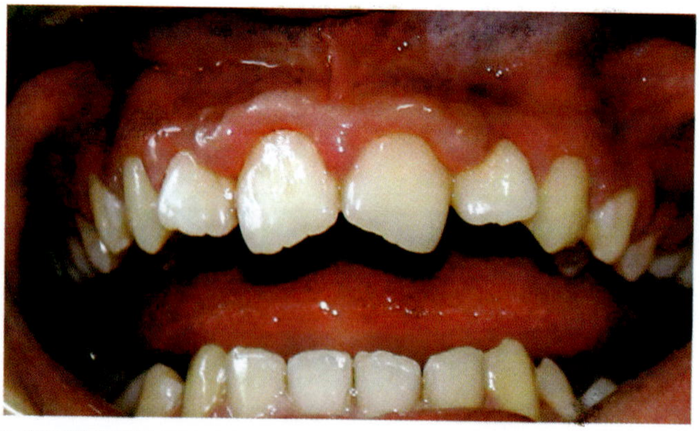

Fig. 11.13: Gingival enlargement due to mouth breathing

8. False Enlargements

What are false enlargements? ▸

Although false enlargements make the gingiva appear enlarged, they are ***not*** actually true enlargements of the gingiva. Gingiva that appears enlarged due to increase in bulk of the underlying bone or tooth is called 'false enlargement'.

In false enlargements, gingiva is normal but presents with increased size and a consequent change in contour of the gingiva is seen. Plaque induced inflammation in gingiva can add associated features of plaque induced inflammation (*gingivitis/periodontitis*) over such false enlargements. False gingival enlargements may be of *two* types:

◂ *What causes false enlargements?*

a. **Due to enlarged underlying alveolar bone:** Alveolar bone can be enlarged due to increased occlusal loads, tori and bone exostosis (Fig. 11.14, A and C). Bone may also be enlarged due to bone pathologies, e.g. central giant cell granuloma, ameloblastoma, etc.
b. **Due to underlying teeth:** As a tooth erupts out of the gingiva, its labial bulge is often identifiable and can be felt on the outer surface of the gingiva. This sometimes causes a big bulge on gingiva that appears like an enlargement (Fig. 11.14, B). Such bulges (*false enlargements*) are commonly seen over erupting maxillary incisors and canines (*both deciduous and permanent*). Blanching of gingiva may be noticed in the bulge on stretching lips This bulge (*false enlargement*) reduces as tooth erupts and gingiva over it recedes. False enlargements over an erupting tooth are also called developmental enlargements.

◂ *What are developmental enlargements?*

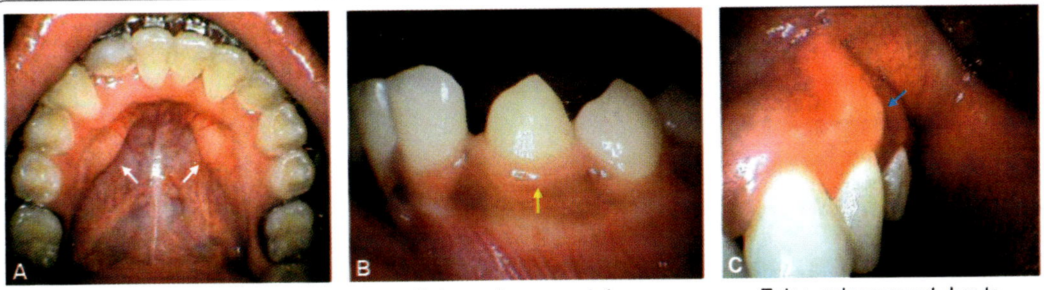

A: Lingual tori; B: False enlargement due to erupting tooth; C: False enlargement due to buttressing bone formation

Fig. 11.14: False enlargements

CLINICAL UTILITY AND SHORT ANSWER

How are false enlargements treated?

- False enlargements (*uncomplicated by any other pathology or inflammation*) often require ***no*** treatment as in reality the gingiva is not enlarged.
- False enlargements due to bulge of an erupting tooth will self-correct after eruption of the tooth.
- False enlargements occurring due to increased bulk of alveolar bone can be corrected surgically by correction of contours of alveolar bone during flap surgery.

9. Combined Enlargements—Combinations of the Above

A clinician must remember that classification of gingival enlargements is done for convenience. Classifying a gingival enlargement using the above classification is based on the ***single most prominent*** clinical and histopathological feature of the lesion and it does not necessarily completely depict the complete nature and other contributing and causative etiological factors of any enlargement in question. In the above context, it is important to remember that:

- ***All gingival enlargements are combined in nature, i.e. all enlargements are caused by a combination of enlargement due to fibrosis and inflammation*** (Fig. 11.15). This means:
  - Plaque induced gingivitis and periodontitis (*inflammatory enlargement*) have a component of enlargement caused by fibrosis (*non-inflammatory*).
  - All drug induced, idiopathic (*non-inflammatory*) and neoplastic gingival enlargements usually have a component of plaque induced inflammation (*inflammatory enlargement*).
- Gingival enlargements may also be caused due to inflammation, fibrosis and a specific disease occurring simultaneously.
- The above facts necessitate a multipronged diagnostic and treatment approach for managing a case of gingival enlargement.

◂ *What are combined enlargements?*

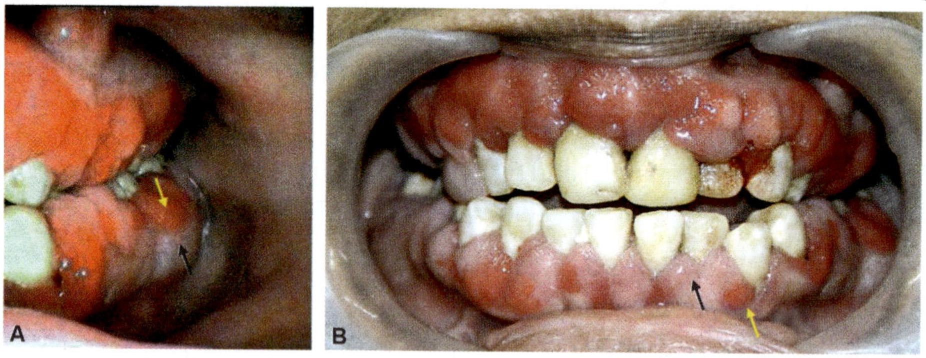

Combined enlargement [*drug induced + inflammatory enlargement*]

Fig. 11.15: Combined gingival enlargements. Non-inflammatory enlargements, e.g. drug induced enlargements (*diags A and B, black arrows*) usually also have a component of inflammation in them due to ongoing plaque induced gingival inflammation, i.e. inflammatory enlargement (*diags A and B, yellow arrows*). Such enlargements are therefore combined enlargements.

Review Questions

1. Classify gingival enlargements. How does an enlarged gingiva affect overall health of the periodontium?
2. What are inflammatory enlargements? Write their clinical features.
3. Write etiology and clinical features of acute inflammatory gingival enlargement.
4. What is a periodontal abscess? How is it different from a gingival abscess?
5. What are the clinical features of a periodontal abscess? What are the radiographic signs of a periodontal abscess? Write the etiology and pathogenesis of a periodontal abscess.
6. Why are the gingival sulcus and the interdental col area more prone to bacterial infiltration?
7. Which of the two: Periodontal pocket reduction versus periodontal pocket elimination procedures is more suited for treatment of a periodontal abscess?
8. What is pericoronitis? Write the etiopathogenesis of pericoronitis and pericoronal abscess. What are the clinical features of pericoronitis/pericoronal abscess?
9. What are conditioning factors? What are conditioned enlargements?
10. Write the chief characteristics of pregnancy gingivitis (*and periodontitis*). What is angiogranuloma?
11. What is puberty enlargement? Write its clinical features.
12. Write a note on vitamin C deficiency induced gingival enlargement (*gingivitis*).
13. Write a note on non specific conditioned enlargement (*granuloma pyogenicum/pyogenic granuloma*).
14. What is plasma cell gingivitis?
15. What are drug induced gingival enlargements? Write the clinical features of phenytoin induced gingival enlargement.
16. Write on hereditary gingival fibromatosis (*idiopathic gingival enlargement*). How is it different from drug induced gingival enlargements?
17. What are false enlargements?

Chapter

12

Desquamative Gingivitis and Acute Gingival Infections

Desquamative gingivitis is ***not*** a disease but, a ***common clinical feature*** (*clinical presentation*) of a number of ***different diseases*** in the gingiva. Although chronic infections of the gingiva are more common, the gingiva may also have acute infections. Chronic gingival infections are usually mild. On the other hand, acute gingival infections can cause severe pain and systemic manifestations like fever, lymphadenopathy, etc.

◂ *Is desquamative gingivitis a disease?*

DESQUAMATIVE GINGIVITIS

Desquamative gingivitis is an unusual form of gingivitis that is ***not*** caused by plaque and is characterized by intense redness (*erythema*), ulceration and desquamation (*increased shedding*) of gingival epithelium. Milder forms of desquamative gingivitis may be totally asymptomatic, while patients with severe forms can present with mild-to-severe burning and pain.

◂ *What is desquamative gingivitis?*

CLINICAL UTILITY AND SHORT ANSWER

What is the difference between desquamation and exfoliation?

Exfoliation is physiologic shedding of cells of epithelium.

Desquamation refers to increased rate of shedding of epithelium cells as an effect of disease.

The following must always be kept in in mind while managing a case of desquamative gingivitis:

- Desquamative gingivitis is a common clinical feature of ***several*** diseases that are of different etiologies, e.g. oral lichen planus (*OLP*), pemphigus, etc.
- Underlying cause of desquamative gingivitis is ***not*** clearly identifiable in about ***1/3rd*** of the cases.
- 2/3rd cases of desquamative gingivitis are oral manifestations of ***skin diseases***. Gingival lesions may be present without any skin lesions in about 50% of cases.
- Of all skin diseases that can cause desquamative gingivitis, ***majority*** of cases are of ***lichen planus, pemphigus*** or ***pemphigoid***. Other skin diseases/conditions that can present as desquamative gingivitis are: linear immunoglobulin A (*IgA*) disease, lupus erythematosus, etc.

◂ *Is desquamative gingivitis related to one or several diseases?*

◂ *What percentage of cases of desquamative gingivitis can be related to skin diseases?*

◂ *A majority of cases of desquamative gingivitis are associated with which two skin diseases?*

Diseases Commonly Manifesting as Desquamative Gingivitis

1. *Oral Lichen Planus (OLP)*

- Lichen planus is primarily a skin disease. Lesions are commonly seen on scalp, nail beds, genitals and mucosal surfaces of oral cavity.
- It may occur in up to 4% of the population at any given time.
- ***Females*** in their middle age and older are ***twice*** as likely to be affected by OLP than males.
- Only 50% of OLP patients have coexisting skin lesions of lichen planus.

◂ *What is lichen planus?*

◂ *In whom is OLP more common—in males or females?*

Clinical features of OLP

1. OLP lesions usually occur ***bilaterally*** on buccal mucosa (*cheek mucosa*) and gingiva (Fig. 12.1).

How many types of OLP lesions are there? ▶

2. Oral lesions of OLP may be of the following types: Reticular, atrophic, ulcerative, patch or plaque, papular and bullous.

Which are the commonest type of OLP lesions on gingiva? ▶

3. Reticular, atrophic and ulcerative lesions are the ***commonest*** lesions on buccal mucosa. While lesions on the gingiva are usually combinations of reticular and atrophic types. Often lesions of ***more*** than one type are present in the same patient.

What are striae of Whickham? What is their diagnostic significance? ▶

4. Reticular lesions have a lace like pattern of ***crisscrossing white lines*** called ***striae of Whickham*** on them. These lesions are:
   i. ***Least*** symptomatic.
   ii. ***Always*** found at the periphery of lesions of other types of OLP.
   iii. Presence of striae of Wickham is the ***chief*** diagnostic feature of OLP.

What are the commonest clinical features of OLP? ▶

5. Usual complaints of patients with OLP are burning sensation in the affected areas of the mouth and sensitivity to hot and spicy foods.
6. Disease shows periods of complete remission and acute exacerbation repeatedly.

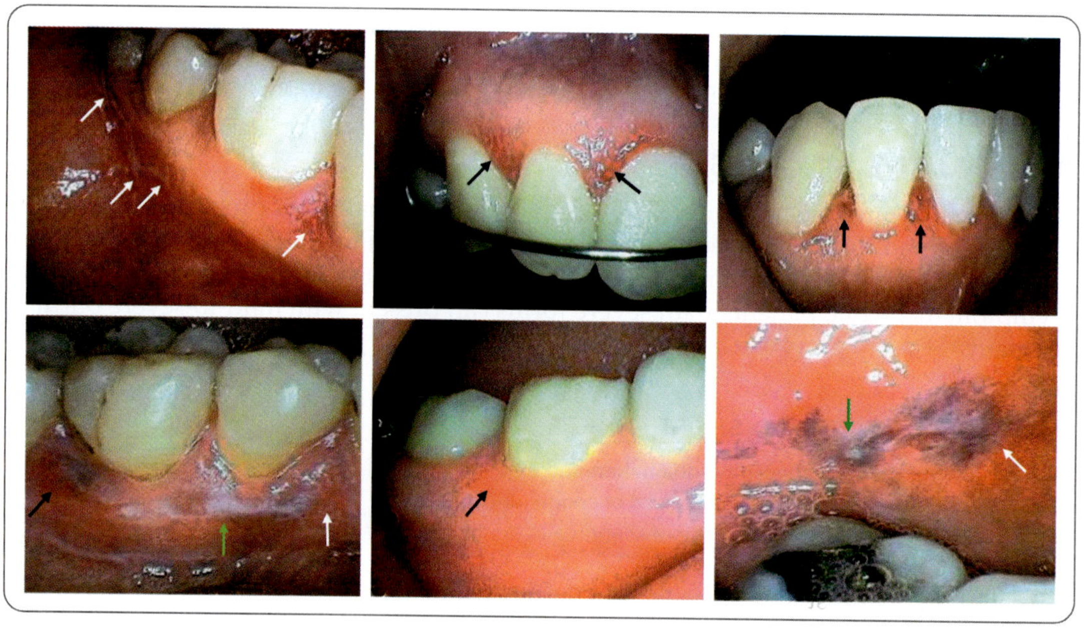

Fig. 12.1: Clinical presentations of oral lichen planus. OLP is commonly seen in the buccal vestibule and on gingiva. Of the many types of OLP lesions, reticular (*white arrows, diag. A, D and F*), atrophic (*black arrows, diag. B, C, D and E*) and patch (*green arrows, diag. D and F*) are the most common types.

How is OLP treated? ▶

Treatment of OLP

- Topically applied steroids, e.g. fluocinonide 0.05%, clobetasol 0.05%, etc. are the drugs of choice. Topically applied tacrolimus 0.1% (*immunosuppressant*) can also be used for treatment of OLP.
- Systemic steroids (*prednisolone 40 mg for 7 days followed by 10–20 mg for 14 days and then tapered off*) may be used in cases with very severe symptoms.
- As a general rule, topical antifungal medicines (e.g. *clotrimazole*) must also be used at the same time to prevent oral candidiasis that may arise as a side effect of steroids or tacrolimus use.
- As reticular lesions are asymptomatic, they usually require ***no*** treatment.

2. *Pemphigoid*

What is pemphigoid? ▶

The term pemphigoid comprises a group of ***many*** vesicle (*or bullae*) and ulcer producing, immune mediated diseases of skin and mucus membranes.

- Separation of upper layers of epithelium from underlying tissues at the basement membrane of epithelium occurs in pemphigoid.
- Oral lesions of pemphigoid often belong to either ***bullous pemphigoid*** or ***mucus membrane pemphigoid*** (*cicatricial pemphigoid*) types.

◂ *Oral lesions of pemphigoid are usually of which types?*

- When the disease does not produce a scar (*on healing*) it is called bullous pemphigoid, if it produces a scar, it is called mucous membrane pemphigoid (*cicatricial pemphigoid*).

◂ *What is the difference between bullous pemphigoid and mucous membrane pemphigoid?*

- Desquamative gingivitis and vesicles (*or bullae*) that rupture to produce ulcers are most ***prominent*** features of these diseases.
- Histology and immunofluorescence studies are helpful in making a diagnosis and can help differentiate this disease from other diseases.

Treatment of pemphigoid

- Same as that of OLP.
- Cases that do not respond to this treatment regimen and if affiliated lesions are also present in the eyes, nose, vagina, etc. must be referred to medical specialists for further treatment.

◂ *What is the treatment of oral lesions of bullous pemphigoid and mucous membrane pemphigoid?*

CLINICAL UTILITY AND SHORT ANSWER

What is the difference between vesicle and bulla?

- Both vesicles and bullae are blisters, i.e. circumscribed (*bounded*) fluid filled elevations of skin or mucus membrane.
- If diameter of the blister is ***less than 0.5 cm, it is called vesicle.***
- If the diameter of the blister is ***more than 0.5 cm*** it is called a ***bulla***.

◂ *What is a bulla?*

3. *Pemphigus*

- Pemphigus is a group of auto-immune diseases that produce vesiculo-bullous lesions on skin and mucus membranes.
- ***Pemphigus vulgaris*** is the ***commonest*** type (*it has a 10% mortality rate*).
  - It usually affects women in their 40s.
  - Skin lesions generally appear one year ***after*** oral lesions.
  - Oral vesicles or bullae rupture to form painful ulcers.

◂ *What is the commonest type of pemphigus?*

Treatment of pemphigus

- Treatment of pemphigus is usually ***not*** in the purview of a dental surgeon.
- If there are only oral lesions and no skin lesions are present, the oral lesions can be managed by topically applied steroids, e.g. fluocinonide 0.05%, clobetasol propionate 0.05%, etc. or systemic steroids.

4. *Chronic Ulcerative Stomatitis*

This disease presents with chronic oral ulcerations that rupture to form ulcers with a red (*erythematous*) halo.

◂ *What is chronic ulcerative stomatitis?*

- Gingiva, lateral borders of tongue and hard palate may be involved.
- It occurs most commonly in women in their 40s.

Treatment of chronic ulcerative stomatitis

- Same as that of OLP.
- Hydroxychloroquine sulfate 200–400 mg per day has been shown to effective in producing lasting complete remission.

◂ *How is chronic ulcerative stomatitis treated?*

ALERT!

- A patient suffering from desquamative gingivitis, occurring as result of any disease, needs to examined repeatedly during the treatment phase.
- Such patients are recalled and reevaluated every week initially and then after 2–4 weeks till clinical features begin to subside.

Desquamative gingivitis has a ***tendency*** to ***recur***, therefore medications may need to be restarted if disease shows recurrence.

ACUTE GINGIVAL INFECTIONS

Necrotizing Ulcerative Gingivitis (*NUG*)

What is NUG? ▸ *What is old name of NUG?* ▸ *What are necrotizing periodontal diseases?* ▸

NUG is an ***uncommon*** disease (*in its classical form; as described below*) and causes severe inflammation and necrosis of gingiva. It is the mildest disease in a group of diseases called ***necrotizing periodontal diseases***. NUG was earlier called ANUG (*acute necrotizing ulcerative gingivitis*). The other diseases in this group are necrotizing ulcerative periodontitis, necrotizing stomatitis and the most extreme, cancrum oris (*Noma*).

Etiology of NUG

What causes NUG? ▸ *Which bacteria are implicated in the etiology of NUG?* ▸ *Can NUG be caused only by a bacterial infection?* ▸ *Which predisposing factors are implicated in the etiology of NUG?* ▸

NUG is believed to be caused by bacterial infection in a ***severely stressed*** (*immune compromised*) patient.

- NUG lesions have primarily ***anaerobic bacteria*** and ***fuso-spirochetal bacteria***. However, as these bacteria are also normally present in a normal person's mouth, NUG ***cannot*** be only caused by a bacterial infection.
- It is believed that NUG occurs in individuals in whom certain ***pre-disposing co-factors*** are also present along with high numbers of causative bacteria. These factors include chronic malnutrition, extreme psychological stress and immunosuppression, etc.
- Most patients of NUG also present a history of preexisting gingivitis, local injury to gingiva and smoking.

CLINICAL UTILITY AND SHORT ANSWER

What are the other names of NUG?

NUG was also called ANUG (*Acute necrotizing ulcerative gingivitis*), Vincent's angina, Trench mouth, Ulceromembranous gingivitis, Fusospirochetal gingivitis in the past.

Clinical features of NUG

1. History

i. ***Sudden*** and ***rapid*** onset.

Are patients with NUG likely to suffer from stress? ▸

ii. Patients usually gives a history of going through a phase of extreme ***psychological stress*** when NUG started. This extreme psychological stress can be caused by sudden and drastic change in living habits, working without adequate rest in very stressful situations, e.g. army men in war zones, a bout of debilitating disease, e.g. acute respiratory tract infection, etc.

Which factors predispose to NUG? ▸

iii. Many patients of NUG are heavy ***smokers*** and have ***poor nutritional status***.

What is the likely outcome of NUG? ▸

iv. If NUG is not adequately treated and if predisposing causes of NUG continue (*stress and poor nutrition*, etc.), NUG may become chronic or recurrent. In extreme cases, it may progress to necrotizing ulcerative periodontitis (*NUP*) or gangrenous stomatitis and cancrum oris (*Noma*).

Is NUG associated with AIDS? ▸

v. NUG and other necrotizing periodontal diseases are fairly ***common*** in patients having ***HIV infection (AIDS)***.

2. Oral signs and symptoms

How do lesions of NUG look? ▸

i. Lesions of NUG are ***punched-out, crater like depressions*** at the crest of ***interdental papillae***. As NUG increases in severity, these lesions may lead to complete loss of interdental papilla. Necrosis of gingiva may then extend to marginal and attached gingiva also.

What is the pseudomembrane covering a lesion of NUG composed of? ▸

ii. Lesions of NUG may be covered with grey ***loosely*** adhering ***pseudomembranous slough*** and are demarcated from adjoining gingiva by marked linear erythema (*line like redness or halo*). The pseudomembranous slough is made of fibrin meshwork, necrotic epithelial cells, PMNs and microorganisms. If pseudomembranous slough is removed, underlying gingiva is red, shiny and bleeds easily.

iii. Lesions are very sensitive to touch. Constant ***radiating*** and ***gnawing pain*** is felt in the involved gingivae. Pain is worsened upon eating coarse, spicy or hot foods.

What are the chief complaints of a patient with NUG? ▸

iv. Patients complain of ***increased salivation*** and drooling (*unintended spilling of saliva over the lower lip*). Saliva is ***thick*** and ***pasty***. There is ***'metallic' taste*** in the mouth. Salivation is markedly increased.

v. Patient's breath is extremely foul and has a ***'fetid odour'*** (*from rotting necrotic gingival tissue in the mouth*).

vi. NUG does ***not*** cause deepening of sulcus and pocket formation (*because marginal gingiva that forms outer wall of pocket is necrosed and is not there*). After healing, gingival recession due to apical shifting of crest of the gingiva may be seen.

◂ *Does NUG cause pocket formation and gingival recession?*

3. Systemic (*extra oral*) clinical features (*systemic features are more severe in children*)

i. Patients are usually mobile, i.e. ambulatory.

ii. Mild-to-moderate ***fever*** with increased pulse rate. High fever may be present if NUG is severe.

iii. Leukocytosis (*increased in total leukocyte count (TLC) in blood; PMNs are especially increased*).

◂ *What are the systemic features of NUG?*

iv. Local ***lymphadenopathy*** (*enlargement of lymph nodes*).

v. Patients have loss of appetite and general tiredness (*lassitude*). Some patients may also have constipation, gastro-intestinal disorders, headache, insomnia (*inability to sleep*) and mental depression.

vi. If NUG is very severe, the above clinical features show corresponding increase in severity. Such patients may then become so sick that they may become bed ridden, i.e. non-ambulatory (*unable to easily move around*).

Histopathology of gingival lesion of NUG

◂ *What are the histopathological features of NUG?*

- Acute inflammation of necrotizing nature that involves both gingival epithelium and connective tissue is the key finding.
- Surface epithelium is destroyed and replaced by pseudomembranous slough (*fibrin, necrotic epithelial cells, PMNs and microorganisms*).
- PMN infiltration in intercellular spaces of epithelium is marked.
- Connective tissue is hyperaemic and has numerous engorged capillaries. There is dense infiltration of PMNs. Plasma cells are also seen in the periphery of the PMN infiltrate.

Diagnosis of NUG

◂ *How is NUG diagnosed?*

◂ *Can NUG be diagnosed with bacterial culture or histopathology?*

- Diagnosis is primarily based on characteristic clinical findings, history and response to antimicrobials. Other specific diagnostic tests, e.g. bacterial cultures, histopathology (*biopsy*), etc. are ***not*** useful in establishing a definitive diagnosis.
- A clinician can prescribe a course of antimicrobials (e.g. *metronidazole*, etc.) to a patient suspected of having NUG. As NUG responds extremely well to antimicrobials (*within 3–4 days*), improvement in lesions proves that the disease was NUG.

Treatment of NUG

Initial phase treatment—management of acute local and systemic features

◂ *How is NUG treated?*

The 'initial phase' treatment is required ***only if*** the patient has high fever, malaise, lassitude, severe local pain, inability to eat normal food, etc. This is done by reducing microbial load and removing necrotic tissue to facilitate healing. Initial phase treatment is performed as under:

- Remove pseudomembranous slough. For this, first isolate the NUG lesion with cotton rolls and apply topical anesthesia. Pseudomembranous slough is then gently wiped off with a small ball of cotton held in a tweezer.
- The area is then gently irrigated with **3%** hydrogen peroxide diluted with equal amount of warm water (*hydrogen peroxide releases oxygen that kills anaerobic bacteria that cause NUG and bubbling of oxygen physically loosens surface slough and debris*).
- Only easily accessible supragingival calculus is removed using a manual scaler (*NUG is common in HIV +ve patients, ultrasonic scalers may be used only after reviewing the patient's history for likelihood of underlying HIV infection*).

  At this stage, deep scaling is ***not done*** as it will injure gingiva (*surgical trauma*) and will cause extension of infection deep into uninvolved gingival tissues.

◂ *Why is hydrogen peroxide used to irrigate lesions of NUG?*

◂ *Why must ultrasonic scalers not be used in patients of NUG?*

◂ *Why must deep scaling not be done during initial acute phase of NUG?*

- Antipyretic-analgesics, e.g. paracetamol, ibuprofen etc. are prescribed for fever and pain. Antibiotics like metronidazole (*400–500 mg orally, every 8 or 12 hours*) or amoxicillin (*500 mg orally every 6 hours*), etc. are also prescribed for at least 10 days.
- Patient is also advised to:
  - Stop smoking and alcohol intake. Take a nutritious bland diet (*no spices*) and adequate rest.
  - Rinse with 3% hydrogen peroxide diluted with equal amount of water every 2–3 hours (*chlorhexidine, povidone iodine, etc. mouth rinse may also be used*).
  - Tooth brush with light strokes.
- After the above treatment systemic clinical features should subside within 2–4 days.

Which general instructions are given to a patient of NUG?

How long does the initial acute phase of NUG usually last?

Second phase treatment—management of local lesions of NUG

When can scaling for treatment of periodontitis be done in a patient of NUG?

After 2–4 days of first phase treatment, patient's systemic health improves remarkably.

- Further scaling of the area can now be done after irrigating the area (*as described above*). Gingivitis or periodontitis are treated after two weeks of acute phase.
- Patient is asked to take nutritious balanced diet and maintain stress free lifestyle.
- Any identified systemic illness must be managed by medical specialists. Patient is recalled every week till NUG lesions have healed completely.

Subsequent treatment—correction of deformities caused due to necrosis of gingiva (*NUG lesions*)

Gingival defects left behind after healing of NUG lesions usually auto-correct themselves within few weeks. If they do not, corrective surgery may be done. Any kind of surgery must not be performed till there is complete resolution of NUG.

Primary Herpetic Gingivostomatitis (*PHG*)

What causes primary herpetic gingivostomatitis?

Which of the two primary or secondary herpetic gingivostomatitis occurs in children?

Why is primary herpetic gingivostomatitis not common in adults?

How is secondary HSV-I infection different from primary HSV-I infection?

- Primary herpetic gingivostomatitis (*acute herpetic gingivostomatitis*) is a viral infection caused by the herpes simplex virus type-1 (*HSV-1*).
- PHG usually occurs in infants and children (*less than 6 years of age*) but can occur in adults as well.
- ***Secondary*** infection of HSV-1 is common in adolescents and adults and causes herpes labialis, herpes genitalis, ocular herpes, etc. (*PHG is not common in adolescents and adults as in all likelihood, they will have had a primary exposure to HSV-1 during childhood*).
- After primary infection by HSV-1 is cured, the virus survives and stays latent in the local nerve ganglia. Later, usually in response to prolonged exposure to sun, physical trauma, fever, emotional stress, etc. HSV-1 gets re-activated and comes out of the nerve ganglia. It then travels down nerves and causes recurring secondary infection at the ***same*** sites where primary lesions were present.
- Secondary lesions of herpes (*HSV-1 infection*) usually occur on the palate as irregular ulcers and on lips (*herpes labialis*) (Fig. 12.3). Secondary HSV-I infection is ***milder*** than primary. Involvement of gingiva is not seen in secondary infections.

Oral signs and symptoms

Which oral sign is pathognomonic for herpetic gingivostomatitis?

How long does vesicle stage of PHG last?

What is the look of herpetic ulcers?

- PHG can occur in both males and females.
- PHG first appears as small, discrete, spherical grey vesicles on gingiva, palate (Fig. 12.2), labial and/or buccal mucosa, pharynx, sub-lingual mucosa or tongue. Presence of palatal lesions (***vesicles and ulcers***) is pathognomonic (*a sign or symptom that is specifically indicative of a particular disease*) for HSV 1 infection (*primary or secondary herpetic gingivostomatitis*).
- The vesicle stage lasts for about 24 hours, is usually ***asymptomatic*** and therefore goes ***un-noticed*** and undiagnosed.
- After the first day, vesicles rupture and ***painful*** ulcers form. These ulcers have irregular margins, depressed pale-yellow central region and raised red margins. Ulcers are surrounded by a red elevated halo. The involved areas become sensitive to touch and

thermal changes. Because of this, patients, especially infants and children, refuse to eat or drink anything (*even bland food and plain water*).

- As ulcers mature, they show confluence (*join*) and lead to formation of clusters of large ulcerated areas that are very ***painful***. Patients complain of generalized 'soreness' of the mouth.
- Involved gingiva shows diffuse enlargement, redness (*erythematous*), is shiny and bleeds easily. Interdental papilla, marginal gingiva and attached gingiva are all involved.
- Lesions of PHG usually heal within 7 to 10 days without scarring.
- Gingival erythema and edema persists for several days.

◂ *Are lesions of PHG painful?*

◂ *How long does it take for PHG lesions to heal?*

Extraoral and Systemic Signs and Symptoms

- In some cases, PHG may be accompanied by high fever (*101°F to 105°F*), malaise and cervical lymphadenitis (*inflammation and enlargement of lymph nodes of neck; such lymph nodes are tender*).

◂ *What are the systemic features of PHG?*

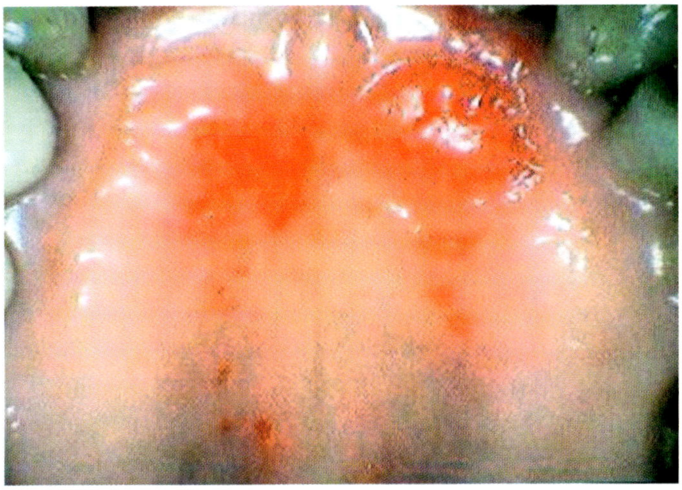

Fig. 12.2: Palatal lesions in herpetic gingivostomatitis. Palatal lesions are pathognomonic (*indicative*) of herpetic gingivostomatitis.

Histopathology

Presence of ***Tzanck*** cells (*multinucleated giant cells resulting from swelling of cells and nuclear enlargement*), acantholysis (*loss of intercellular connections* (e.g. *desmosomes*, etc.*) resulting in loss of cohesion between epithelial cells*) and intraepithelial vesicle formation are characteristic features.

◂ *What are Tzanck cells?*

Diagnosis

Diagnosis of PHG is ***usually*** made on basis of ***history*** and ***clinical features***. In most clinical situations, histopathology is usually of no help as the disease will have run its full course (*7–10 days*) by the time histopathological reports are available. A clinician has to often differentially diagnose between ulcers caused by PHG and aphthous ulcers or other diseases and conditions that cause ulcers.

◂ *How is PHG diagnosed?*

Treatment of primary and secondary herpetic gingivostomatitis

Although herpetic gingivostomatitis is a self-limiting disease that is eventually controlled by the body's immune system within 2 weeks. To manage the severe clinical features associated with it the following measures may be undertaken:

- Topical antivirals like 5% Aciclovir, etc. to control growth of virus.
- Antipyretics, e.g. paracetamol to control fever and pain.
- Soft, bland and nutritious diet.

◂ *How is herpetic gingivostomatitis treated?*

CLINICAL UTILITY AND SHORT ANSWER

How can PHG be differentiated from other similar diseases?

Differential diagnosis between primary herpetic gingivostomatitis (*PHG*) and other diseases causing similar oral lesions:

What is the difference between aphthous ulcers and ulcers seen in PHG? ▶

Primary herpetic gingivostomatitis	***Acute aphthous ulcers***
1. Ulcers seen in PHG have ***irregular*** margins (*due to rupture of vesicles*).	1. Margins of aphthous ulcers are ***smooth***.
2. PHG ulcers or lesions occur simultaneously on the ***hard palate*** and ***keratinized gingiva***.	2. Aphthous ulcers ***do not*** occur on ***hard palate*** (*and on other areas of the oral cavity covered by keratinized mucosa*).
3. Systemic features like fever, malaise, etc. are seen in PHG.	3. These systemic features are not present.

Primary herpetic gingivostomatitis	***Erythema multiforme***
1. It is caused by herpes simplex I virus.	1. It is an allergic reaction to medication or infection and is seen on the skin.
2. Lesions are vesicular and can involve any part of oral mucosa.	2. Vesicular and hemorrhagic lesions involve the oral mucosa and tongue.
3. Gingival involvement is common	3. Gingival involvement is not common
4. These lesions are usually not present in the eyes and skin.	4. Lesions could also be present in eyes and skin (*target lesions*).
5. Lesions are commonly seen on the hard palate.	5. Lesions are usually ***not*** seen on the hard palate.

Primary herpetic gingivostomatitis	***Lichen planus***
1. It is caused by herpes simplex I virus.	1. It is an autoimmune disease.
2. Has a short history (*acute disease*).	2. Has a long history (*chronic disease*).
3. Stria of Wickham are not present.	3. Bullous and ulcerative types of oral lichen planus might be confused with PHG. Stria of Wickham (*crisscrossing white lines*) are ***always*** present at the ***periphery*** of lesions of ***all*** types of OLP.
4. Systemic features like fever and malaise are seen in PHG.	4. Oral Lichen planus does not present any systemic features.

Primary herpetic gingivostomatitis	***Desquamative gingivitis***
1. It is caused by herpes simplex I virus.	1. It is a shared (*common*) ***clinical feature*** of several diseases but in most cases, it is usually related to Lichen planus or Pemphigus.
2. Palatal lesions are common and pathognomonic, i.e. confirm diagnosis of PHG.	2. Palatal involvement is generally not there or if present limited only to the marginal and adjoining attached gingiva.
3. Lesions are ulcers with irregular raised margins and are surrounded by a red halo.	3. Lesions of desquamative gingivitis are usually covered by very thin (*atrophic*) epithelium and therefore give a raw and red look. Sometimes frank ulcerations may also be seen.
4. Systemic features like fever and malaise may be seen in PHG	4. Systemic features seen are not present.
5. PHG is acute short duration disease.	5. Desquamative gingivitis is a chronic disease.

ALERT!

Is PHG communicable? ▶

Infection caused by HSV-1 viruses whether primary (*primary herpetic gingivostomatitis*), secondary (*herpes labialis*) or recurrent (*recurrent herpes labialis*) are ***highly*** communicable and contagious. Any individual can get the disease by coming in contact with an active lesion (*including dental surgeons when working on a patient*).

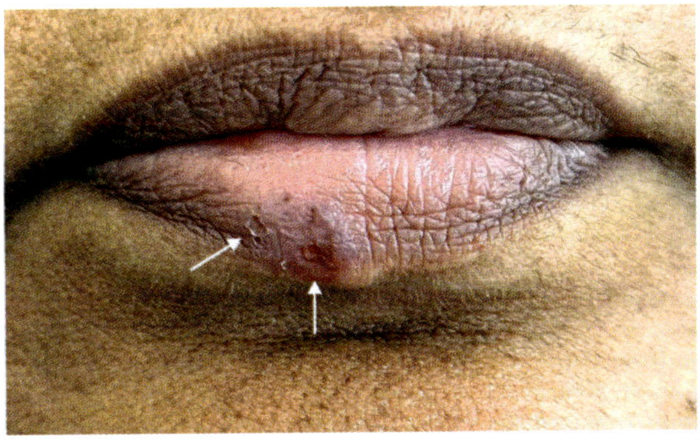

Fig. 12.3: Herpes labialis *(recurrent herpes simplex virus I infection)* on the lower lip of a 58-year-old female. This patient gave a classical history of recurrent ulcerations on her lower lip usually following a bout of fever at the start of every winter season.

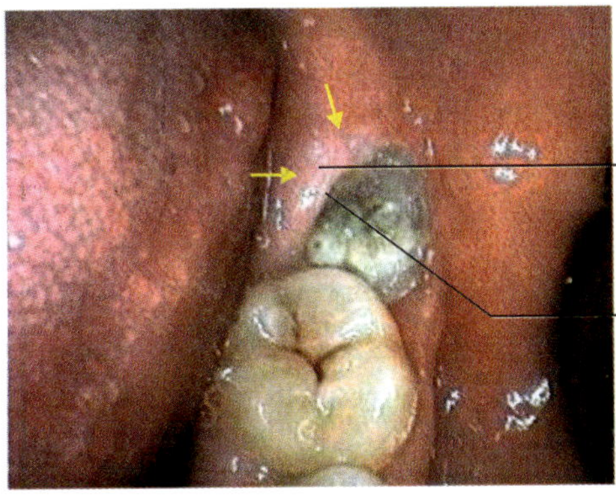

Fig. 12.4: Pericoronitis. As operculum gets swollen, its size increases. A swollen operculum is likely to getting injured by hits form cusps of opposing teeth *(yellow arrows)*. This injury further increases the inflammation in the operculum.

Pericoronitis

(see Chapter 11, Plaque Biofilm Associated Periodontal Disease and Gingival Enlargements, page 187 also).

CLINICAL UTILITY AND SHORT ANSWER

Pericoronitis can get complicated and may spread to oro-pharyngeal region and base of tongue. Complicated pericoronitis can sometimes lead to peritonsillar abscesses, cellulitis and Ludwig's angina.

Treatment of Pericoronitis

(especially when occurring in relation to erupting mandibular third molars)

Treatment of pericoronitis is dependent on its stage and decision of retaining the tooth over which the pericoronal tissue is inflamed.

Non-surgical management of pericoronitis

◂ *How is pericoronitis treated conservatively?*

- Area under the operculum is ***gently*** irrigated with equal volume of warm water and 3% hydrogen peroxide. This will flush out food debris and pus from under the pericoronal flap. Oxygen released by dissociation of hydrogen peroxide will kill bacteria present under the operculum.
- The operculum is then gently lifted with a scaler and debris under the operculum is gently removed.
- If acute pericoronal abscess has formed and gingival flap is ***fluctuant,*** a postero-anterior incision is made in it to establish drainage (*after local anesthesia*).

- If systemic complications like fever are there or if inflammation is very severe, antibiotics, e.g. amoxicillin 500 mg tid or ciprofloxacin 500 mg bd or metronidazole 400 mg tid, etc. may be prescribed for 5–7 days.
- If gingival tissue over the erupting tooth is getting traumatized by cusps of opposing tooth, the opposing tooth's offending cusp may be slightly reduced.
- Within a few days of treatment, the patient becomes comfortable. Decision to excise overlying gingival tissue and operculum and/or extract the under lying tooth is now made.

Surgical management of pericoronitis

(see also Chapter 17B, Periodontal Flap Surgery; Flap modifications for the retro-molar (behind the molar/distal molar) areas; Distal wedge procedure and Fig. 17B.14).

When is it recommended to extract the third molars to treat pericoronitis? ▸

- If the underlying tooth is not likely to erupt in its normal position, it is preferable to extract such teeth soon after acute phase of pericoronitis has subsided. In case of mandibular third molars, if possible, teeth are preferably extracted before their roots are fully formed.

What is the biggest drawback of extracting third molars? ▸

- It must also be remembered that extraction of third molars frequently leaves a 'huge' bone defect distal to the second mandibular molars **(Fig. 12.5)**. This results in formation of deep distal bone defects and pockets in relation to second mandibular molars.

How is pericoronitis treated surgically? ▸

- If the tooth is likely to erupt in its normal position or if for other reasons the tooth is decided to be retained, ***operculum and surrounding gingival tissue*** covering and surrounding the tooth must be excised to prevent repeated episodes of acute pericoronitis. This is done as under:
  - After attaining local anesthesia, the pericoronal flap, i.e. ***operculum and gingival tissue distal to the erupting third mandibular molar*** is removed using BP knives (*#15, 11 and 12*) and/or periodontal knives (*e.g. Orban's knife, etc.*) and curettes. Thus, a wedge of tissue distal to third molar is removed.
  - It must be ensured that after removal of gingival tissue no pocket remains distal to the third molar (*as it will invite recurrence of pericoronitis/continued periodontitis*) **(Fig. 12.6, diags E, F and G)**.
  - Sutures may be given, antibiotics may not be necessary in all cases, analgesics are however prescribed.

CLINICAL UTILITY AND SHORT ANSWER

What is operculectomy? ▸

Why is operculectomy not preferrred? ▸

Operculectomy is the excision of ***only*** the operculum that covers the crown of a tooth (*rather than excising adjoining gingival tissue constituting the entire pericoronal flap*). It is a simple but an ***incorrect*** way of excising pericoronal flaps over mandibular third molars (*Fig. 12.5, diags B, C and D*). This is so because, performing only an operculectomy will leave back a deep pocket distal to the third molar. This will invite frequent reoccurrence of pericoronitis and continued periodontitis in the region.

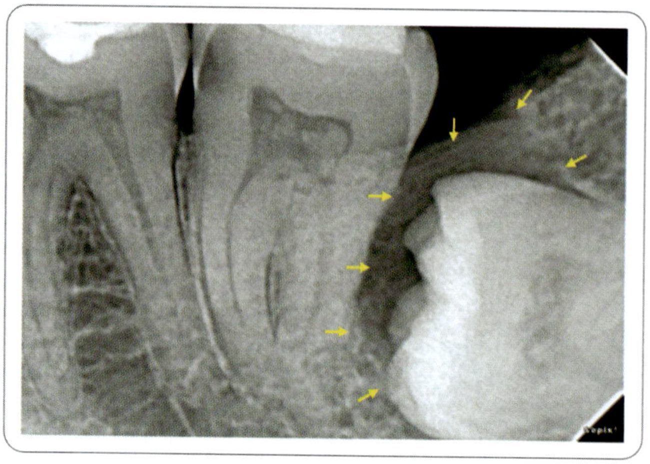

Fig. 12.5: Extraction of third molars frequently leaves a 'huge' bone defect distal to the second mandibular molars (*yellow arrows*). This defect can jeopardize the health of second molar in the long term.

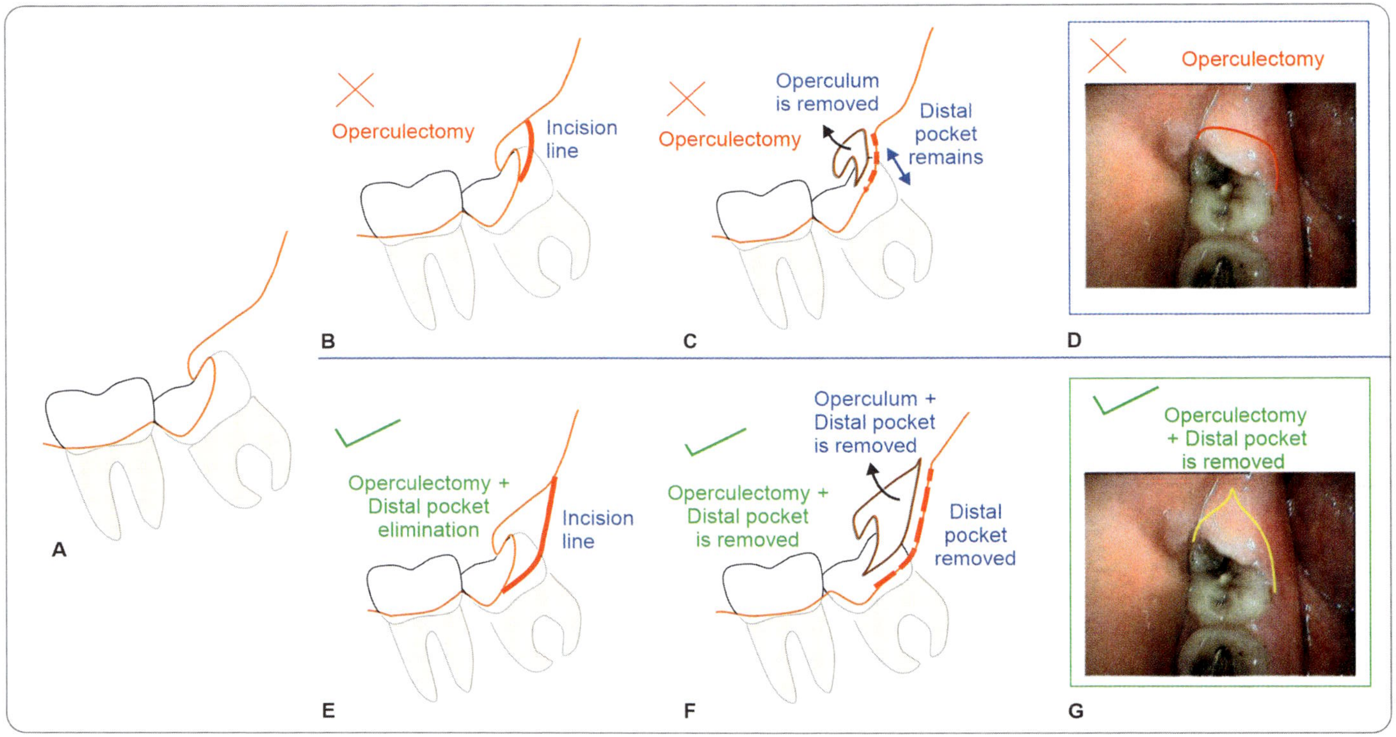

Fig. 12.6: Operculectomy, i.e. excision of only the operculum covering an erupting tooth (*diags B, C and D*) is a simple but incorrect way of removing pericoronal tissue over mandibular third molars. Correct technique of excising pericoronal tissue involves operculectomy and excision of gingival tissue forming the distal pocket (*diags E, F and G*).

Review Questions

1. What is the difference between desquamation and exfoliation? Name some diseases commonly associated with desquamative gingivitis.
2. Write the clinical features of oral lichen planus and its treatment.
3. What is pemphigus? Write the treatment of oral pemphigoid and oral pemphigus.
4. Write the management of chronic ulcerative stomatitis.
5. Name other diseases closely resembling desquamative gingivitis.
6. What are the other names by which necrotizing ulcerative gingivitis (*NUG*) is referred to? Write a note on NUG.
7. How can NUG be diagnosed and treated?
8. Write a note on primary herpetic gingivostomatitis. Write its differential diagnosis.
9. Write a note on clinical features, diagnosis and treatment of pericoronitis.

Chapter 13

Planning and Initiating Periodontal Treatment

I. Diagnosis and Diagnostic Aids
II. Prognosis
III. Rationale
IV. Treatment Plan

Management of a periodontal case must be carefully and scientifically planned. It involves making a diagnosis, establishing prognosis, justifying the planned treatment (*rationale*) and instituting the treatment plan.

I. DIAGNOSIS AND DIAGNOSTIC AIDS

Careful examination of the ***entire*** oral cavity is very important before making a periodontal diagnosis. Several tests, radiographs and diagnostic aids are used to make a diagnosis. Periodontal examination to make a correct periodontal diagnosis includes:

1. Recording a patient's detailed ***dental*** and ***medical*** history.
2. Reviewing past dental and medical history of the patient.
3. Discussing findings and diagnosis with the patient.

◂ *What does periodontal examination include?*

Patient's History (*Dental and Medical History*)

A detailed history helps make a diagnosis and know the prognosis (*prediction of the outcome of treatment and course of disease*). Patient examination starts from the moment a clinician sees (*even though at a distance*) or talks to the patient on a phone This way a clinician quickly assesses the general health of the patient; further information is acquired during the consultation visit. Oral examination must include examination up to the pharyngeal region and oral cancer screening in addition to detailed examination of the oral cavity. Photographic and other records must be made and maintained. History taking includes:

◂ *When does patient examination start?*

◂ *What does oral examination include?*

1. **Recording of:**
   i. **Reason for consultation**, e.g. pain, tooth mobility, foul breath, etc.
   ii. **History of present illness.**
   iii. **Past dental history**, i.e. past dental illnesses and treatments, last visit to a dental clinic, etc.
2. **Extra oral and Intra oral examination:**
   i. Assessment of normal features of gingiva (*colour, contour, consistency, surface texture, position and size*) and identification of changes in these.
   ii. Assessment of gingival health by assessing bleeding on probing (*BOP*).
   iii. Correlation of plaque and calculus deposits with type and severity of disease.
   iv. Assessment of clinical attachment level (*CAL*), probing depth (*PD*) and gingival recession.
   v. Evaluation of gingiva, alveolar bone and bone defects and identification of muco-gingival defects and complications (*recession, reduced/inadequate zone of attached gingiva, etc.*).

vi. Examination of teeth for crowding, caries, defective restorations, attrition, abrasion, erosion, abfraction, plunger cusps, malocclusion, tenderness, pulpal (*endodontic*) status, hypersensitivity, perio-endo lesions, furcation involvements, etc.
vii. Assessment of suitability and status of existing prostheses and appliances.
viii. Assessment of occlusion for hyper occlusal contacts and malocclusion.
ix. Detecting and grading mobility in teeth and/or dental implants.
x. Palpation of lymph nodes (*sub-mandibular, sub-lingual, jugulodigastric groups, etc.*) and jaws, face muscles and TM joints.
xi. Assessment of deviation of the mandible during mouth opening, etc.

2. **Radiographic examination** (*Bitewing, IOPA, OPG, CBCT, etc.; Bitewing radiographs are **not** ideal for periodontal diagnosis; they are used only if apical regions of the teeth are not to be viewed*).
3. **General physical examination and assessing correlation between systemic and periodontal health.**
4. **Assessment of dentition and alveolar bone for suitability to receive crowns, prostheses appliances and dental implants.**

Radiographic Examination for Periodontal Case Management

The following radiographs can be used for periodontal diagnosis:
1. Bitewing
2. Intra oral periapical (*IOPA*)
3. Orthopantomogram (*OPG*)
4. Cone beam computed tomography (*CBCT*).

Bitewing Radiographs

Why a bitewing radiograph cannot be used for periodontal diagnosis? ▶

- These radiographs provide images of only coronal halves of both upper and lower teeth in a ***single*** radiograph.
- As the 2018 classification mandates staging and grading of periodontal disease by taking into account the amount of bone loss and relating it to tooth root length (*that requires viewing of the entire length of the tooth*), these radiographs are ***not suitable*** for periodontal diagnosis.
- These can however give the clinician a good perspective of carious lesion of teeth visible in the radiograph and some idea about their periodontal health.

Intra Oral Peri Apical (IOPA) Radiographs

Why is a IOPA radiograph ideal for periodontal diagnosis? ▶

- Complete teeth and surrounding structures can be visualized in an IOPA radiograph, they are therefore ***ideal*** radiographs for making a periodontal diagnosis (*as per requirements of the 2018 classification*).

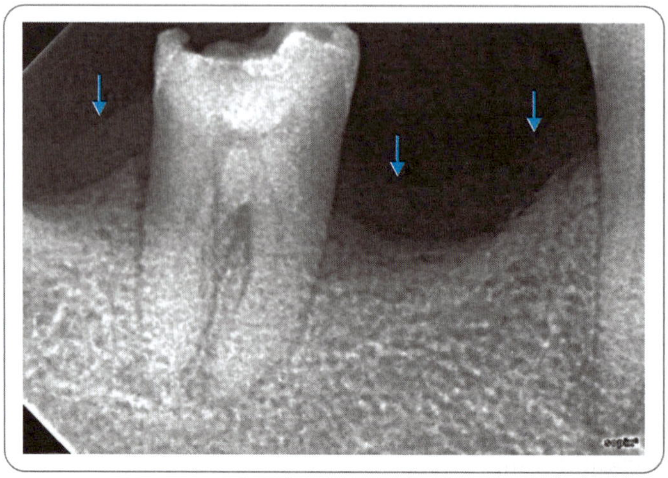

Fig. 13.1: Appearance of gingiva (*blue arrows*) in an IOPA radiograph.

ALERT!

Soft tissue is usually not visible in a radiograph; however, more so on a digital radiograph (*RVG*), soft tissue can be clearly identified especially after adjusting contrast of the RVG. PD (*pocket depth*), CAL (*clinical attachment loss*) and amount of bone loss can be easily known from such radiographs and without clinically examining the patient. This can also help stage and grade periodontitis according to the 2018 classification. Technique for this has been explained in Chapters 10 and 10A. (*see Figs 10.3, 10A.10, 10A.12, and 10A.13*).

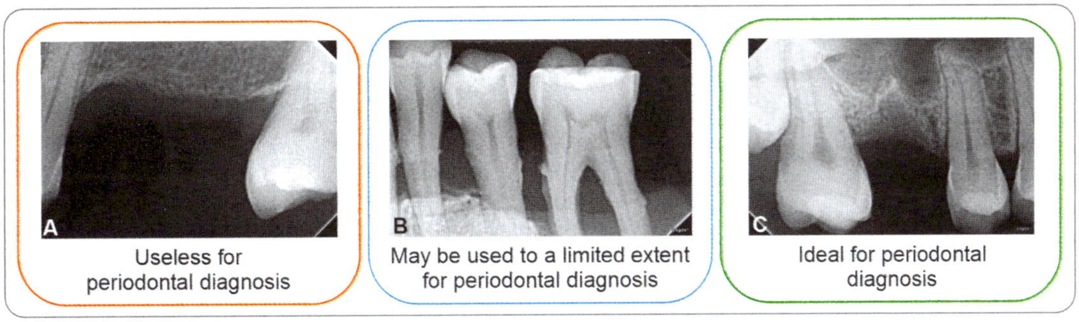

Fig. 13.2: Examples of IOPA radiographs that can and cannot be used for periodontal diagnosis. IOPA radiograph in diag. A cannot be used as it does not show teeth or surrounding anatomical structures completely. IOPA radiograph in diag. B may be used for limited and specific needs as more than 90% of the teeth structure and surrounding anatomical structures are visible. IOPA radiograph in diag. C shows entire structure of teeth and surrounding anatomical structures; it is therefore ideal for periodontal diagnosis.

Orthopantomogram (OPG)

- Although an OPG gives a complete view of jaws and teeth in a single radiograph; however, it is still ***not*** the ideal radiograph for periodontal diagnosis (**Fig. 13.3,** red marked areas) because:
  - i. It does not show detail.
  - ii. Images are about 25% magnified and geometrically distorted.
  - iii. Images of adjoining teeth and anatomical structures are often overlapped and some structures may appear distorted or deviated in an OPG.
  - iv. Anterior region of the jaws (*teeth and bone*) are not clear as image of spinal column is superimposed over their images.

◂ Why is OPG not ideal for periodontal diagnosis?

- Despite the above disadvantages, OPG is a very useful radiograph for assessing position of unerupted or impacted teeth, maxillary sinuses, mandibular canals for implant planning, caries, restorations, etc.

◂ In which situations is the OPG best used for periodontal diagnosis?

- OPG is also used for diagnosis in patients who ***cannot*** open their mouth (*IOPA radiograph cannot be taken in such patients*).

Cone Beam Computed Tomography (CBCT)

- It is similar to the traditional computed tomography (*CT*) scans. CBCT scans are viewed using special software on a computer. Images of anatomical structures in the scan can be enlarged and marked for diagnosis and treatment planning.

◂ What is CBCT?

- CBCT has multiple uses in periodontics, these include:
  - i. ***Accurate measurements*** of structures and distance between points of interest (*dimensions of available bone and proximity to anatomical structures, etc.*) for implant planning, etc. **(Fig. 13.5)**.
  - ii. 3-D imaging of tooth and bone architecture and defects.

◂ How is CBCT useful in periodontics?

- Disadvantages of CBCT:
  - i. High radiation dose. CBCT exposes a patient to a ***higher*** radiation dose as compared to OPG or IOPA radiographs.
  - ii. Distortion of some structures and appearance of artefacts around metal structures (*crowns, implants, etc.*).
  - iii. High cost.

◂ What are the disadvantages of CBCT?

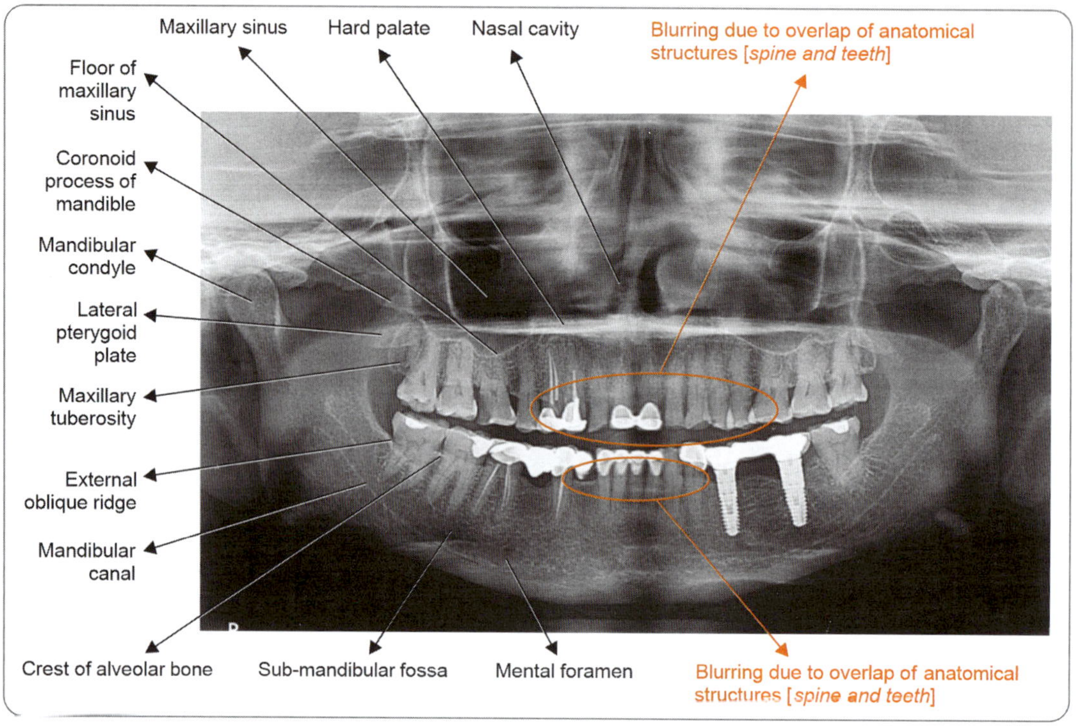

Fig. 13.3: OPG (*orthopantomogram*). An OPG shows a two-dimensional half-circle view (*ear to ear*) of the jaws, TM joints, maxillary sinuses and the neck region. In this diagram, some commonly used landmarks for periodontal diagnosis and implantology have been labelled for the right side.

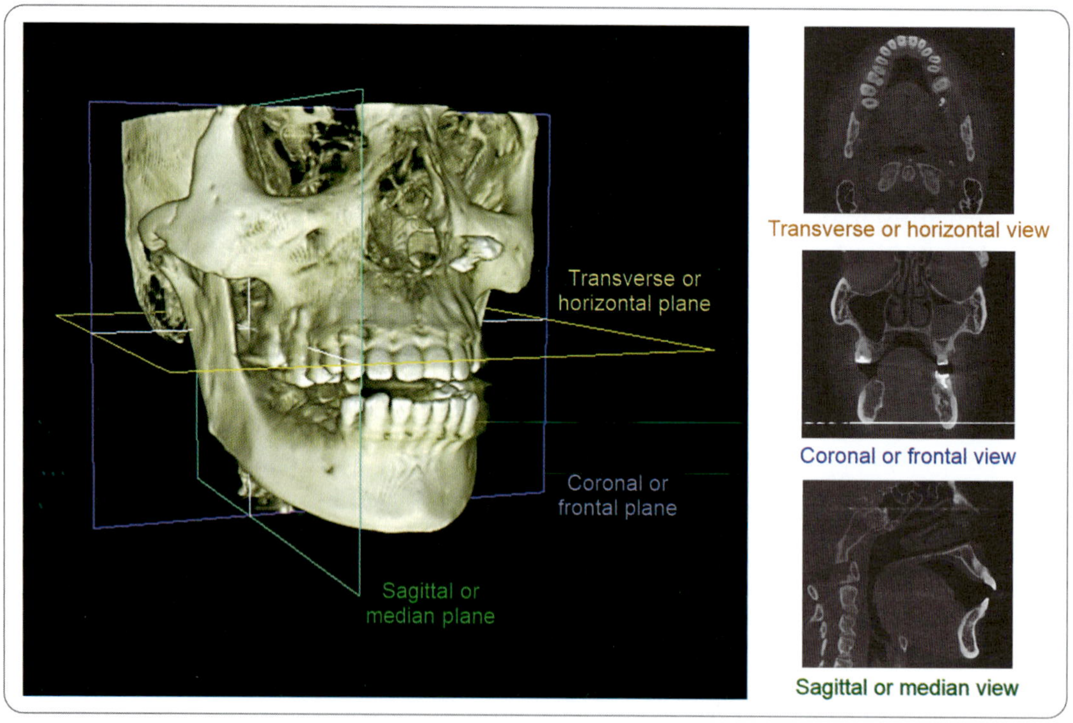

Fig. 13.4: A 3-D reconstructed CBCT image of maxilla and mandible and planes of the body—sagittal (*median*), transverse (*horizontal*) and coronal (*frontal*).

Periodontal Probing

What information can be attained by periodontal probing?

- Periodontal probing is the most ***commonly*** used and ***simplest*** diagnostic procedure used for periodontal diagnosis. It is done with a periodontal probe.
- Probing is done to know the ***clinical*** probing depth (*PD*) of sulcus or pocket (*see Chapter 2, Fig. 2.6*) and clinical attachment level or clinical attachment loss (*CAL*) (*see Chapter 2, Fig. 2.7*).

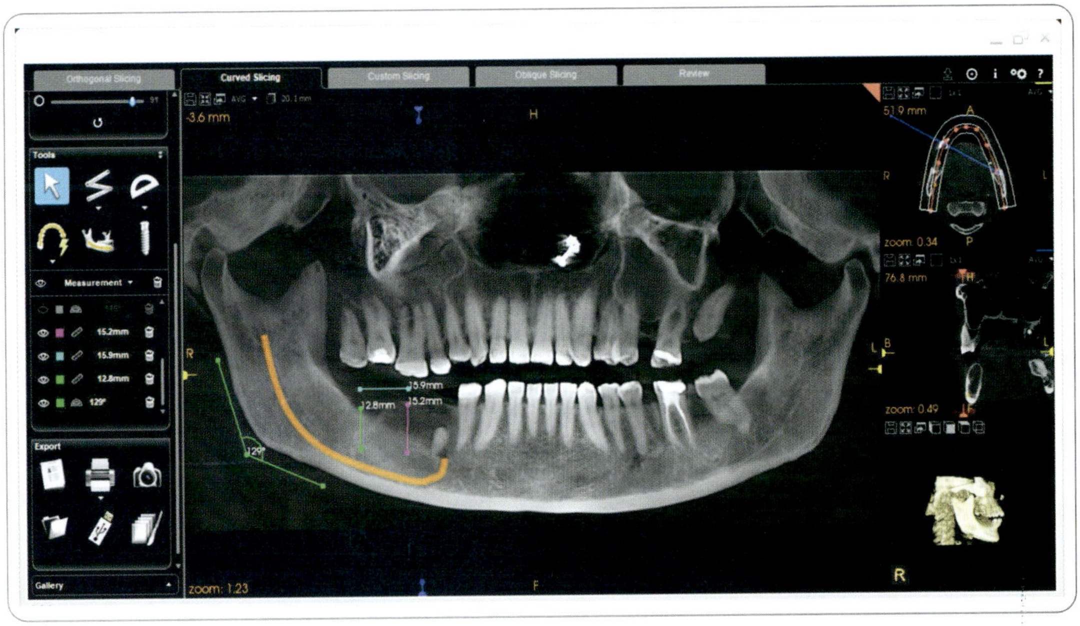

Fig. 13.5: Accurate measurements of angles and distance between points of interest can be easily and accurately done on a CBCT image. Structures like the mandibular canal, mental foramen etc. can be marked for easy reference. This makes planning and surgery for implant placement easier.

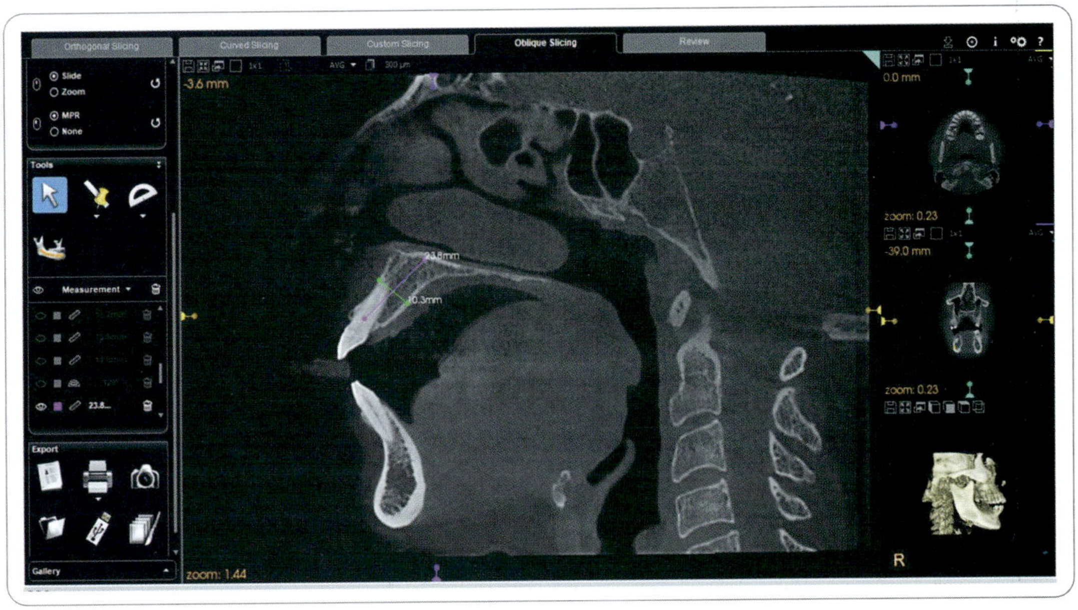

Fig. 13.6: Measurements made on sectional images of a CBCT scan are *more* accurate than measurements made on reconstructed 'OPG like' images in the same CBCT scan (*Fig. 13.5*).

- For these, a probe is inserted parallel to the long axis of the tooth into the sulcus/pocket under ***light pressure*** (*0.25 N force*) till ***light resistance*** is felt. The average depth of the normal gingival sulcus is 1.8–2.0 mm; however, PD more than 3 mm is considered abnormal and must be corrected (*2018 classification*).
- To probe the furcation area of multirooted teeth (*molars and premolars*) a Naber's probe is used. It is the ideal probe for probing furcations (Fig. 13.10, diags A and. B).
- It is important to remember that a dental explorer has a sharp pointed tip (*end*), it therefore cannot replace and be used in place of periodontal probes for periodontal probing.
- Healthy gingiva may be so firmly adapted to the tooth that it may sometimes not be possible to insert a probe into it (*see Chapter 2, Fig. 2.5, page 6*).

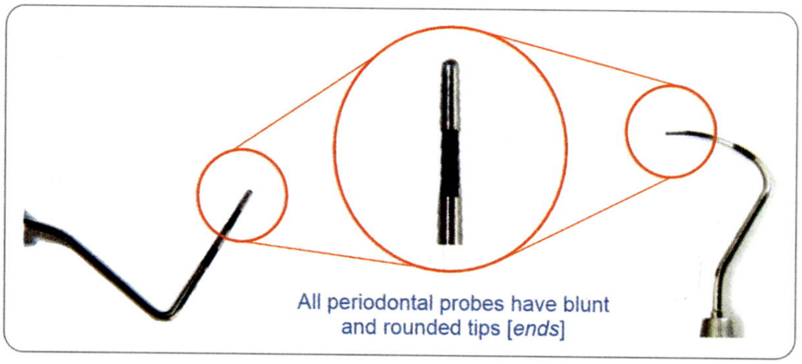

Fig. 13.7: Periodontal probes have a blunt and rounded tip

Walking the Probe

Why is it important to walk the probe?

What is walking the probe?

- Base of the sulcus or pocket is ***not*** located at the same distance from the CE junction at different sites even on the same surface of a tooth **(Figs 13.8 and 13.9, diag. A)**.
- Therefore, PD, CAL and gingival recession measurement values will be different at different locations; these must therefore be recorded at several locations approximately 1 mm apart all around the tooth in question. This is called ***'walking the probe'*** **(Fig. 13.9, diags A and B)**.

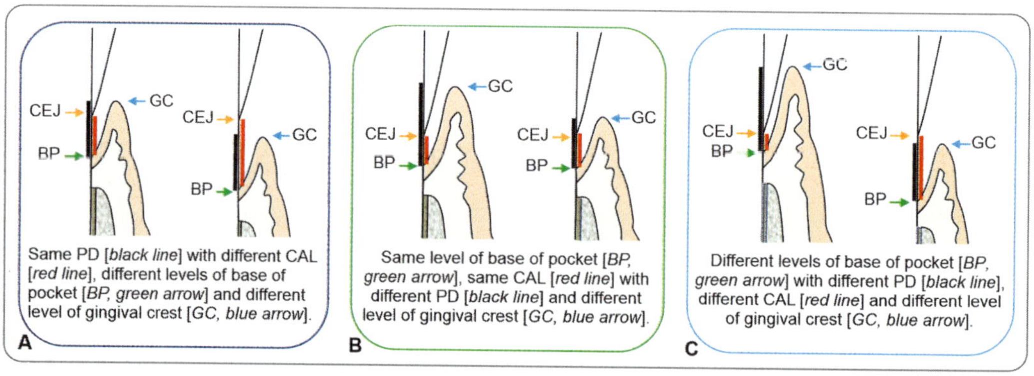

Fig. 13.8: Probing depth, CAL and level of gingival crest are not necessarily interrelated. Level of base of pocket (*BP, green arrow*), gingival crest (*GC, black arrow*), depth of pocket (*PD, black line*) and clinical attachment level (*CAL, red line*) are variable in different pockets.

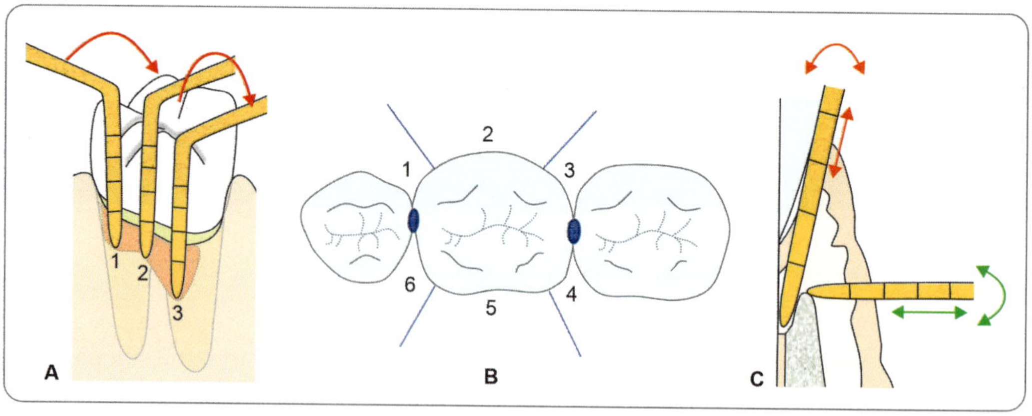

Fig. 13.9: Walking the probe (*diag. A and B*) and transgingival probing (*diag. C*). Walking the probe helps determine *maximum* PD and CAL in relation to a tooth. For this, a probe is inserted upto the base of the sulcus, retracted 1–2 mm and advanced about a millimetre horizontally and then reinserted into the pocket. The probe is advanced millimetre-by-millimetre all around the tooth surface. Maximum PD and CAL must be recorded in six zones (*diag. B*) all around the tooth circumference. Measurement in zones 1, 3, 4 and 6 (*diag. B*) must be taken by slanting the probe to reach under the contact area.

Transgingival probing and bone sounding (diag. C) help us know the morphology of crest of the alveolar bone or extent and configuration of infrabony component of the pocket (*bone loss*) without lifting a flap.

Transgingival Probing (Bone Sounding)

What is transgingival probing? How is it done?

- Transgingival probing is done to know anatomic location and morphology of crest of the alveolar bone, shape of infrabony area of the pocket (*bone loss*) and furcation defects ***without*** lifting a periodontal flap.
- To do this, after anaesthetizing the area, a periodontal probe is first inserted horizontally into the gingiva and then vertically into the sulcus till alveolar bone is felt.
- The probe tip is then moved vertically and horizontally to 'feel' and map the bone anatomy and the bone defect **(Fig. 13.9, diag. C, red and green arrows)**. Transgingival probing is done at multiple locations in the area of interest.

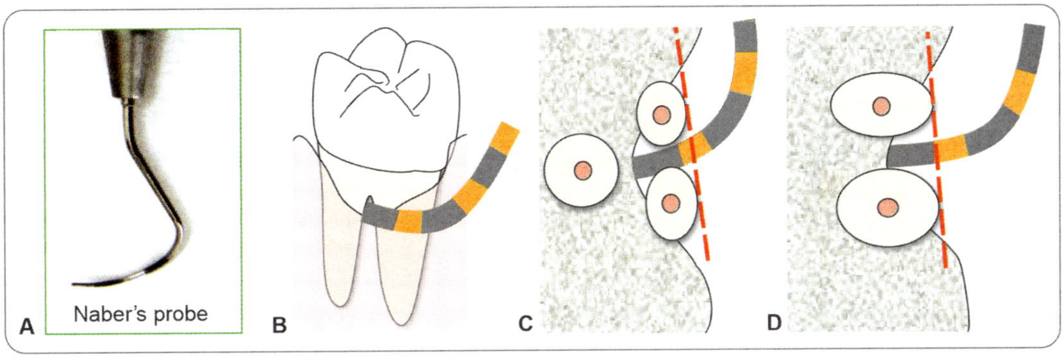

Fig. 13.10: Probing of furcation. A Naber's probe is used to probe furcations. The naber's probe is a curved, colour-coded probe that has markings at 3 mm intervals (*diag. A*). Measurements are made from an imaginary line (*red line*) connecting prominences of root surfaces of the tooth making the furcation (*diags C and D*). If furcation entrance is covered by gingiva, assessing the furcation depth is difficult.

Steps in Making a Periodontal Diagnosis

Step 1: Initial Interaction

Why is it important to give full attention to the first interaction with a patient?

Making of a diagnosis starts from the first interaction with the patient. This first interaction may happen during a telephone call or personal visit of the patient to the clinic. This includes:

i. Assessment of needs, goals, socioeconomic status and psychology of the patient. This helps us to have a clear understanding of the patient's concerns, fears, frame of mind, and seriousness to get treatment.
ii. Assessment of medical conditions that the patient might have.

Step 2: First Diagnosis Visit

The following work is done during first diagnosis visit:

i. Gathering general information about patient and the reason of consultation (*first few minutes of interaction*).
ii. Recording dental and medical history
   a. Taking clinical pictures for diagnosis and record keeping.
   b. Making diagnostic casts.
   c. Ordering radiographs and medical tests, requesting medical opinion of suspected systemic diseases and conditions.
   d. Making a provisional or if feasible, final diagnosis.

Which tasks are accomplished during the first and second diagnostic visits?

Step 3: Second Diagnosis Visit (If Required)

The following work is done during second diagnosis visit:

i. Review of information gathered during the initial interaction and first visit and corelating it to radiographic findings, medical test reports (*ordered earlier*), etc.
ii. Ordering more specific radiographs, dental and medical tests if required.
iii. Confirmation or modification of the provisional diagnosis and communicating the diagnosis and its basis to the patient and/or caretaker.

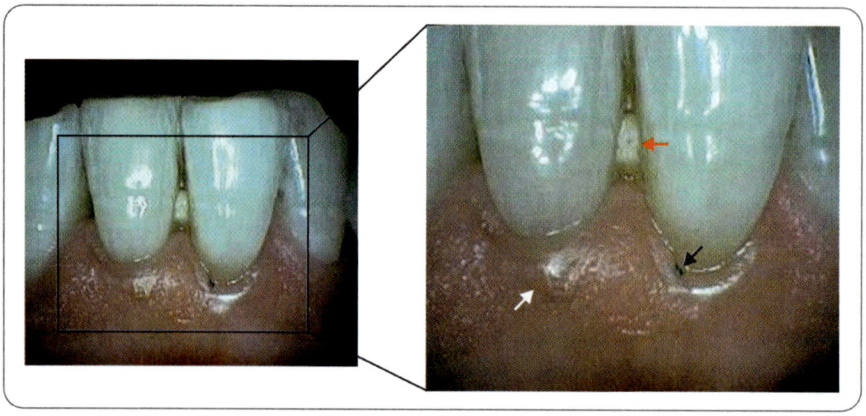

Fig. 13.11: To identify even the smallest etiological factors, thorough clinical examination is very important. In this case, note that despite presence of normal colour, arcuate contour and absence of clinical gingivitis, there is a slight protuberance in the free gingiva in relation to tooth # 41 (*white arrow*). This protuberance is due to subgingival calculus (*white arrow*). Also note impacted food in the gingival sulcus in relation to tooth # 31 (*black arrow*) and between tooth # 41 and # 31 (*red arrow*).

CLINICAL UTILITY AND SHORT ANSWER

Why taking medical history is important while planning dental treatment?

Knowledge of medical history of a patient (*systemic disease*) is important because oral cavity and the periodontium being part of the body are automatically affected by systemic disease and medication. A two-way inter-relationship exists between oral and systemic health:

1. Systemic disease or conditions can cause or complicate dental diseases or conditions, e.g. puberty gingivitis, immune deficiency due to AIDS, etc.
2. Dental diseases or conditions can cause or complicate systemic disease or conditions, e.g. periodontal disease complicating diabetes control, etc.

CLINICAL UTILITY AND SHORT ANSWER

Which common patient complaints can suggest the possibility of periodontal disease?

1. Vague dull pain in relation to a tooth.
2. Frequent food impaction at a particular site.
3. Feeling that teeth are loose (*tooth mobility*), migration, formation of gaps between teeth and tooth loss.
4. Bleeding from gingivae.
5. Bad breath and bad taste in the mouth.
6. Irritation and itching in the gingiva, especially in the interdental region and an urge to insert a pointed object (*toothpick*) in gingiva to relieve it.

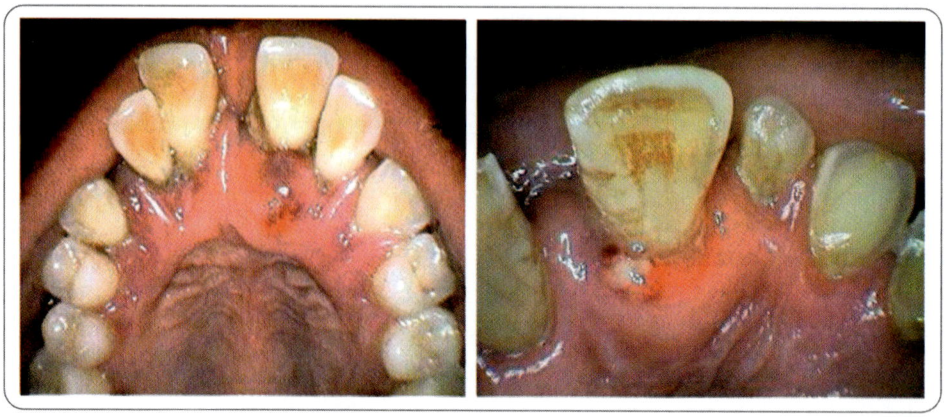

Fig. 13.12: Recurrent and multiple periodontal abscesses seen in both these cases were diagnosed to be because of untreated periodontitis complicated by uncontrolled diabetes.

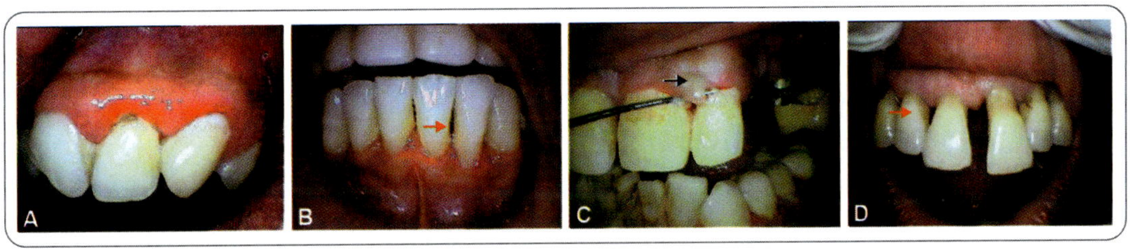

Fig. 13.13: Common signs of periodontitis include bleeding on probing, gingival enlargement (*diag. A*), redness (*diag. A*), flacid gingiva (diag. C, *black arrow*), gap formation between teeth and gingival recession (*red arrow, diags B and D*), clinical attachment loss (*diags A, B, C and D*) and flaring of teeth (*diag. D*).

Tooth Mobility

Definition: Tooth mobility is horizontal or vertical (*axial*) movement of a tooth due to an occlusal or other applied force.

◂ *Define tooth mobility.*

- When examined clinically, ***all*** healthy teeth including those with no periodontal loss, exhibit a less than ***1 mm*** mobility in the horizontal direction. This is called ***physiologic mobility***.

◂ *What is physiologic mobility?*

- If horizontal tooth mobility is more than 1 mm (*physiologic mobility*) or if tooth mobility is noticeable in the vertical direction, it is a cause for concern and its reason must be ascertained.

◂ *When is tooth mobility a cause for concern?*

- Mobility of a tooth can be assessed by trying to move the tooth in all directions after holding the tooth between the back of the handle of one instrument and the clinician's finger or backs of handles of two instruments **(Fig. 13.14)**. Magnitude of the tipping movement is assessed at the tip of the crown. Sophisticated mechanical and electronic devices called ***mobilometers*** (*periodontometers*) are also available for assessing tooth mobility.

◂ *How is tooth mobility assessed?*

◂ *What are mobilometers or periodontometers?*

◂ *What are the types of tooth mobility?*

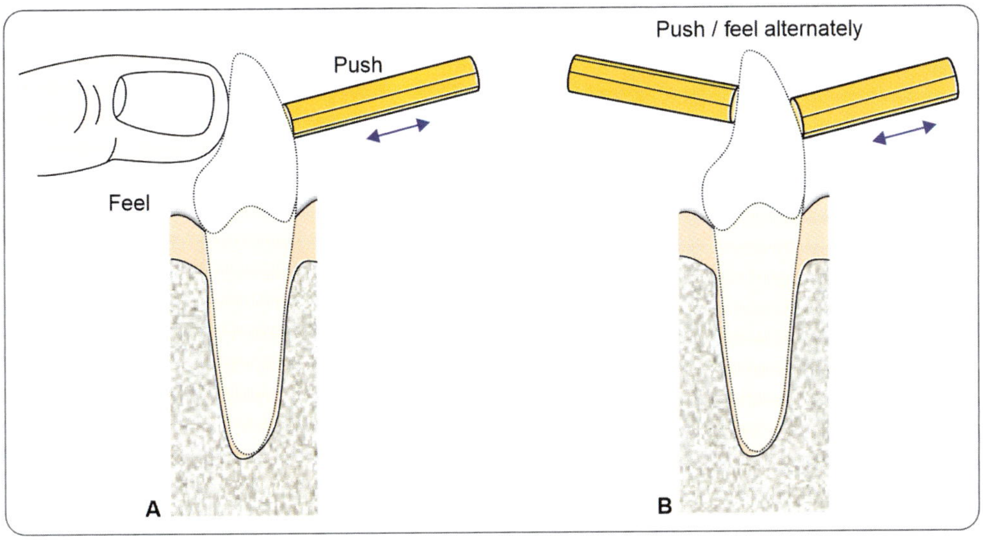

Fig. 13.14: Tooth mobility can be assessed either by holding the crown of a tooth between a back of an instrument handle and the operator's finger (*diag. A*) or between back of handles of two instruments and then trying to move it in all directions (*diag. B*).

Types of Tooth Mobility

There are two types of tooth mobility. These are:

1. **Physiologic:** It is the slight amount of tooth mobility seen in a tooth with a normal and healthy periodontium. When assessed clinically, Grade 1 can be termed as physiologic mobility.
2. **Pathologic:** Mobility more than grade I mobility, due to any cause, is termed pathologic mobility.

3. *Grading of Tooth Mobility*

How is tooth mobility graded?

The simplest and most used grading scheme is **(Fig. 13.15)**:

Grade 0: No mobility

Grade I: 0.2–1 mm mobility (*measured horizontally at the crown tip*)

Grade II: 1 mm to 2 mm mobility (*measured horizontally at the crown tip*)

Grade III: More than 2 mm mobility (*measured horizontally at the crown tip*) and/or ***any*** movement of the tooth in vertical direction or rotation.

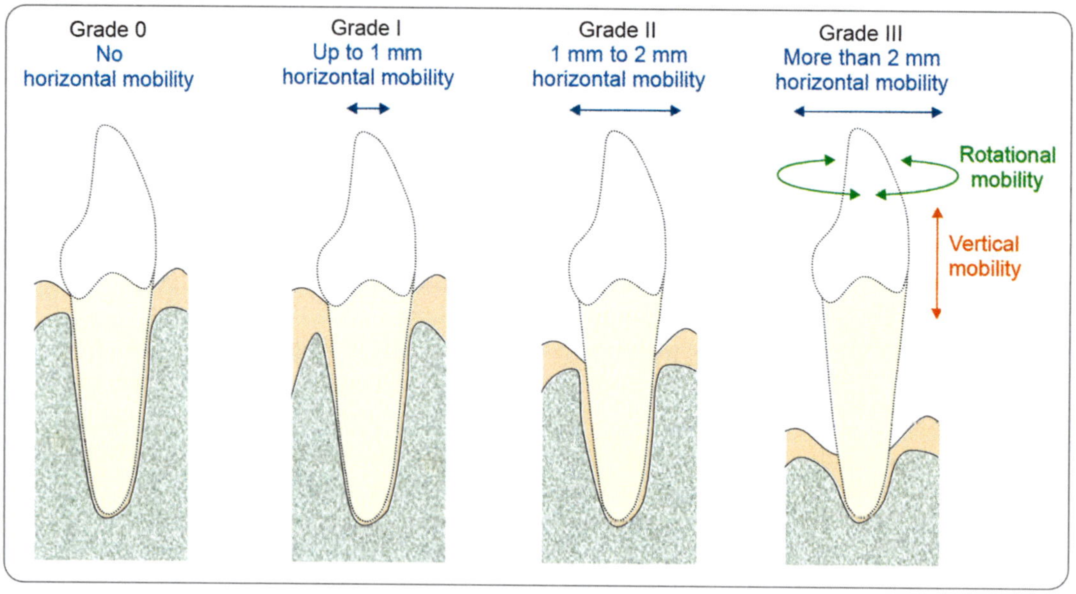

Fig. 13.15: Grading of tooth mobility

Causes of Increased Tooth Mobility

What are the causes of increased tooth mobility?

1. Loss of height of alveolar bone (*tooth support*) due to periodontitis.
2. Inflammation and abscess formation in the PDL due to periodontitis, pulpitis, etc. These result in destruction of PDL fibres and leads to increased tooth mobility.
3. Increased mobility is noticed for a few days after periodontal surgery (e.g. *flap surgery*).
4. TFO (*trauma from occlusion due to bruxism, orthodontic movement*, etc.). In initial (*destructive*) stages of TFO, mobility increases due to loss of vertical height of alveolar bone (*lamina dura or the alveolar bone proper*) and damage to the PDL. In the adaptive phase (*later stages*), increase in mobility results from widening of the PDL.
5. Fractures of teeth.
6. Pathological lesion of jaws. Diseases resulting in resorption of root or supporting alveolar bone, e.g. cysts, tumours, etc. will lead to increased mobility.
7. Increased mobility is also seen in teeth that are not in use, e.g. teeth without antagonist.
8. Pregnancy and prolonged use of oral contraceptive use (*in women*), etc.

ALERT!

On which factors does tooth mobility depend?

Factors on which mobility of a tooth depends:

1. Remaining height of supporting alveolar bone, width of periodontal ligament, shape and number of roots **(Fig. 13.16)**.
2. Mobility occurs more commonly in the bucco-lingual direction rather than in the mesio-distal direction.
3. It is greater in mornings than in evening.
4. It is greater in children than in adults.
5. It is greater in females than in males.
6. Ankylosed teeth show no mobility whereas normal teeth have physiologic horizontal mobility less than 1 mm.

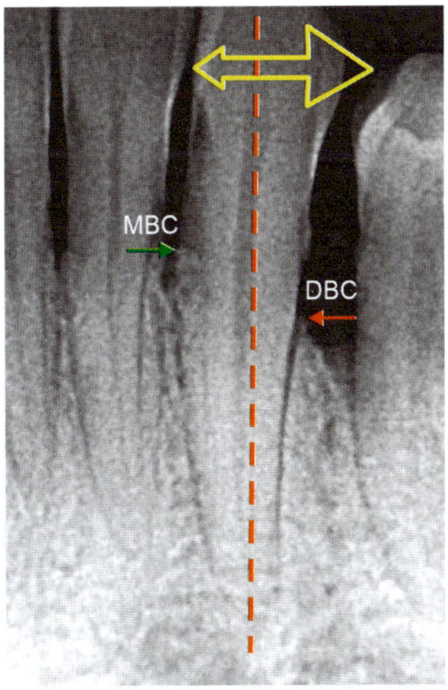

Fig. 13.16: Tooth mobility is more towards the side with greater bone loss (*on which bone crest is located more apically*). In this radiograph, distal bone crest (*DBC, red arrow*) in relation to tooth # 33 is located more apically than the mesial bone crest (*MBC, green arrow*). Therefore, this tooth will show more distal mobility as compared to mesial mobility (*yellow arrow*).

Advanced Diagnostic Test Systems

Advanced diagnostic tests may provide additional information about local mediators of inflammation, periodontal pathogens, metabolic products of host and/or microorganisms (*specially bacteria*), host response to periodontopathogens (*immunological*), genetics, etc. As our knowledge of these is limited, the available advanced diagnostic tests do not provide us with much clinically usable information. Advanced diagnostic tests are therefore ***not*** done in routine clinical practice. Some advanced test systems used for periodontal diagnosis are:

◂ *Why are advanced diagnostic test systems not routinely used for periodontal diagnosis?*

◂ *Name some advanced diagnostic test systems.*

1. Identification of microbes by direct viewing, bacterial culturing, DNA probes, etc. These help us know the relative numbers of identifiable bacteria of different species present in plaque sample. Antibiotic sensitivity can also be known.
2. Tests that help to confirm presence of particular microbes in a plaque sample, e.g. immunological assays, enzymatic tests, e.g. BANA test (*N-benzoyl-d L-arginine-2-napthylamide*), etc.
3. Biopsy can help identify some specific diseases, e.g. cancerous lesions.

II. PROGNOSIS OF TEETH WITH PERIODONTAL DISEASE

Definition: Prediction of the likely course, duration and outcome of a disease is called prognosis.

◂ *What is prognosis?*

- Prognosis tells us the ***likelihood of recovery*** from a disease and expected time to be taken for this.
- It is established ***after*** making the diagnosis but ***before*** making a treatment plan.

◂ *What does prognosis tell us?*

◂ *When is prognosis determined?*

Types of Prognoses

Prognosis assigned to the dentition (*overall prognosis*) or to the individual tooth is affected by the clinician's experience and level of training in a particular field. The following prognoses can be assigned: excellent, good, fair, poor, questionable and hopeless.

◂ *Is prognosis of periodontitis dependent on the clinician?*

1. *Excellent Prognosis can be assigned if:*

i. Periodontium is healthy or there is mild gingivitis at some sites but there is no periodontitis, i.e. no CAL or bone loss attributable to periodontitis is present. Even if CAL and bone loss are present, they are due to other reasons, e.g. prominent position of tooth in the arch, etc.
ii. Patient is a non-smoker or smokes very occasionally and is not a diabetic. There are no other complicating systemic or environmental factors that can predispose to periodontitis.

◂ *When is an excellent prognosis assigned?*

iii. Present dental disease is easily treatable.
iv. Patient is expected to get all prescribed treatment done and follow all instructions regarding plaque control and follow up visits.

2. Good Prognosis can be assigned if:

When is good prognosis assigned? ▸

i. Mild gingivitis or Stage I grade A periodontitis is present and CAL due to periodontitis is up 2 mm. There is no tooth loss due to periodontitis or caries.
ii. Radiographic bone loss (*RBL*) is less than 15%, i.e. bone crest is located in the coronal 1/3rd of the root (*visualized in interdental areas*).
iii. Grade I mobility is present in some teeth.
iv. TFO if present is mild and easily treatable.
v. No or mild grade I-II furcation involvement is present but it can be treated and thereafter maintained easily by the patient (*see Chapter 20; 'Furcation Involvement and Its Management'*).
vi. Complicating systemic or environmental factors which can predispose to or complicate periodontitis are present but are treatable, e.g. controlled diabetes.
vii. Patient is a non-smoker or smokes very occasionally.
viii. Dental disease is easily treatable and patient is expected to get all prescribed treatment done and follow all instructions regarding plaque control and follow up visits.

3. Fair Prognosis can be assigned if:

When is fair prognosis assigned? ▸

i. Stage II grade B periodontitis is present and CAL due to periodontitis is up 3–4 mm.
ii. Radiographic bone loss (*RBL*) is between 15–33%, i.e. bone crest is located in the coronal 1/3rd of the root (*visualized in interdental areas*).
iii. Grade I-II mobility is present in some teeth but these areas are easily treatable.
iv. TFO is mild-moderate.
v. No or moderate grade II–IV furcation involvement is present but it can be treated and thereafter maintained easily by the patient.
vi. Complicating systemic or environmental factors which can predispose to or complicate periodontitis are present but are treatable, e.g. controlled diabetes.
vii. Patient smokes less than 10 cigarettes (*or equivalent amount of tobacco in some other form*) per day.
viii. Present dental disease is treatable. However, patient compliance is doubtful, i.e. patient may not get all prescribed treatment done and may not also completely follow all instructions (*including plaque control and follow up visits*).

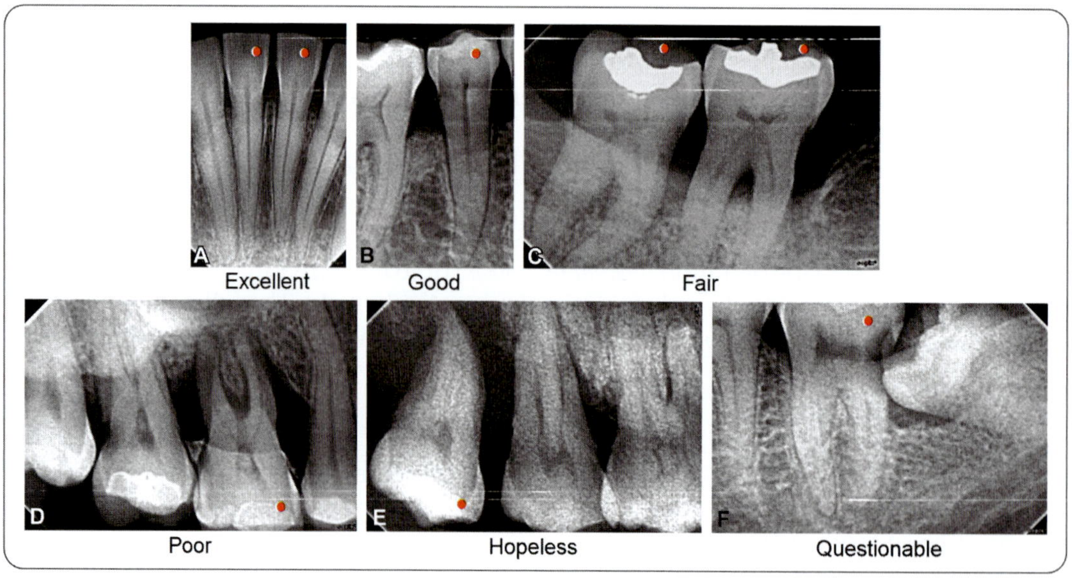

Fig. 13.17: Examples of different types of prognoses (*applicable to teeth marked with red dots*)

4. Poor Prognosis can be assigned if:

i. Stage III–IV grade C periodontitis is present and CAL due to periodontitis is more than 5 mm.

ii. Radiographic bone loss (*RBL*) extends to middle 3rd of the root and beyond (*visualized in interdental areas*).

iii. Grade II–III mobility is present in some teeth.

iv. TFO is moderate-severe.

v. Severe grade II–IV furcation involvement is present and assess to these furcation areas is limited (*this will not allow adequate treatment and hygiene maintenance after treatment*).

vi. There are complicating systemic or environmental factors that can predispose to or complicate periodontitis and these may or may not be easily manageable, e.g. un-controlled diabetes, autoimmune diseases, immune defects, etc.

vii. Patient smokes more than 10 cigarettes per day (*or smokes equivalent amount of tobacco in some other form*).

viii. Present dental disease is not easily treatable and patient compliance is doubtful, i.e. patient is not expected to completely follow all instructions (*including plaque control and follow up visits*).

◂ *When is poor prognosis assigned?*

◂ *Why is poor prognosis assigned if severe furcation involvement is present?*

5. Hopeless Prognosis can be assigned if:

i. Stage IV grade C periodontitis is present.

ii. Remaining teeth/tooth have grade III mobility.

iii. Severe grade III or IV furcation involvement is present.

iv. Severe and difficult to treat systemic factors of enormous clinical significance are present and all causative or contributing etiologic factors and dental disease ***cannot*** be corrected and/or patient is not cooperative.

◂ *When is hopeless prognosis assigned?*

6. Questionable Prognosis can be assigned if:

Questionable prognosis is assigned if the overall prognosis is good–fair but certain systemic or local contributory factors, whose control is dependent on outcome of dental treatment, patient dependent or patient's systemic health dependent, are present and long-term prognosis of teeth depends on these factors. For example:

- In a diabetic patient with moderate bone loss, long term prognosis will remain good–fair if diabetes remains controlled and patient follows all instructions. If the clinician is unsure that patient will fulfil these conditions, prognosis in such cases is questionable.
- A tooth has good prognosis but this is dependent on successful management of another tooth. In Fig. 13.17, dia., F, good prognosis of 2nd molar (*marked with red dot*) is dependent not only on extraction of impacted 3rd molar (*that is the cause of distal caries of 2nd molar*) but also on the long-term successful management of the distal bone defect (*and deep pocket*) that extraction of 3rd molar will leave behind. The second molar is assigned a questionable prognosis.

◂ *What is questionable prognosis?*

◂ *Give examples of cases with questionable prognosis.*

Prognosis is determined at two levels:

A. Overall prognosis

B. Individual tooth prognosis

◂ *How many types of prognoses are determined for any patient?*

A. Overall Prognosis

Some factors affect both overall and individual tooth prognosis. All factors affecting individual tooth prognosis affect overall prognosis in an indirect way. The overall prognosis helps determine:

- If it will be advisable and worth while to try to save the remaining teeth in the mouth.
- Can the remaining teeth be saved with treatment.
- Determination of overall prognosis is done ***before*** determining prognosis for individual teeth.

◂ *What does the overall prognosis tell us?*

◂ *Overall prognosis is dertermined before or after individual tooth prognosis?*

Factors on which overall prognosis depends are:

How does stage and grade of periodontitis affect prognosis?

1. *Stage and Grade of Periodontitis (Severity and Rate of Worsening of Periodontitis)*

i. This factor affects both overall and individual tooth prognosis.
ii. More severe periodontitis (*e.g. stage III and IV, grade C periodontitis*) has worse the prognosis because:
   - It results in faster periodontal loss which leads to loss of teath.
   - It is ***difficult*** to treat.
   - It is more likely to ***recur*** early.

iii. Location of base of pocket in relation to CE junction (*false vs. true pocket*), type of pockets (e.g. *simple, compound or complex*), pocket depth, amount and type of associated bone loss (*infra or supra bony*) affect both the rate at which periodontitis progresses and outcome of treatment they thus also affect the overall prognosis of the case.

2. *Age of the Patient*

In two patients with similar periodontal loss why is prognosis better in the older patient?

- In two patients having comparable levels of periodontal destruction arising from periodontitis, prognosis is generally ***better*** in ***older*** of the two patients.
  This is because, the given amount of periodontal loss has occurred in the younger patient in a ***shorter*** time while the same amount of periodontal loss occurred in longer time in the older patient. This means periodontitis is progressing ***faster*** and is more destructive in nature in the younger patient.

3. *Local Environmental Factors*

i. **Rate of deposition and composition of plaque:**
   - Individuals who show higher plaque formation and whose bacterial plaque is rich in periodontopathogenic microorganisms show more severe periodontal disease and vice versa.

How does calculus affect prognosis?

ii. **Type, amount and rate of deposition of calculus:**
   - Calculus promotes gingivitis and periodontitis by providing a surface for plaque formation (Fig. 13.18).
   - It also keeps plaque in close vicinity and in touch with the sulcular and junctional epithelium through which infectious microorganisms enter the gingiva easily.
   - Subgingival calculus has greater potential to cause periodontitis than supragingival calculus.
   - Higher rate of calculus formation also leads to more periodontitis.

iii. **Type of occlusion, shape of dental arch, crowding of teeth, carious lesions, etc.:**
   - If these factors increase plaque accumulation and reduce plaque control more gingivitis and periodontitis will result.

iv. **Smoking:**
   - It increases severity of periodontitis.
   - Rate of healing is slower in smokers.

How do iatrogenic factors affect prognosis?

v. **Iatrogenic factors:**
   - High restorations can cause TFO (*trauma from occlusion*). Which can worsen periodontal health and complicate treatment.
   - Rough and unpolished surfaces of restorations, over or under-contoured and overhanging restorations, etc. favour plaque and food debris deposits leading to initiation and maintenance of periodontitis, etc.

4. *Patient Compliance*

Does patient compliance have a role in prognosis?

- Patient's compliance and cooperation are necessary for completing all planned treatment and maintenance of oral health thereafter (Fig. 13.19).
- As a ***general rule***, if a patient is not frightened at the very thought of losing teeth, does not report for the timely maintenance visits, does not afford indicated and recommended treatment or cannot for some reason maintain good plaque control etc., such patients are not good candidates for receiving comprehensive periodontal treatment. In such cases, only essential and limited treatment maybe planned.

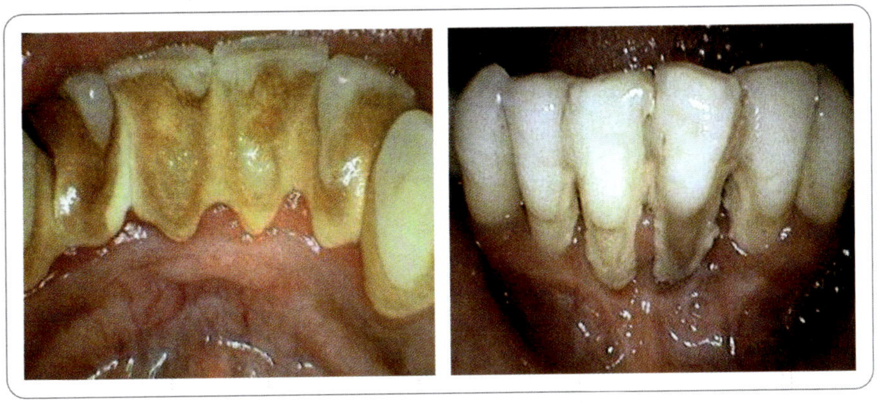

Fig. 13.18: Heavy calculus deposits seen on mandibular incisors. Calculus forms at a very fast rate in some individuals. Such individuals are more prone to severe periodontitis.

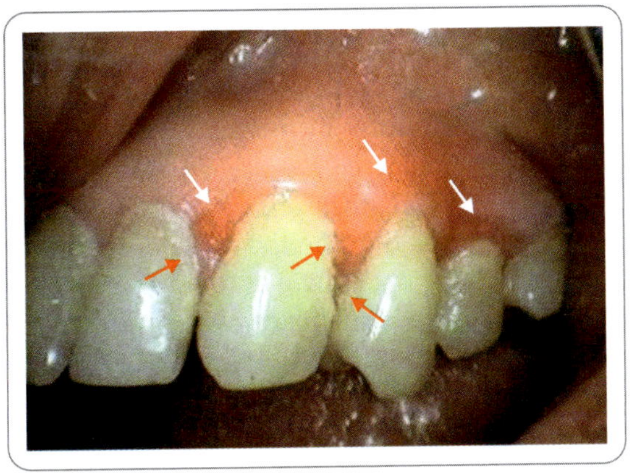

Fig. 13.19: Plaque deposits (*poor plaque control*) (*red arrows*) in a patient suffering from atrophic (*painful*) lesions of oral lichen planus (*white arrows*). If a patient cannot maintain adequate level of oral hygiene, long-term prognosis of such cases is not good.

5. *Systemic Factors*

- Untreated systemic ***ill health*** has huge effect on the overall prognosis of the dentition.
- Medicines used to treat systemic illnesses can also have adverse effects on periodontal health (*e.g. corticoids used for treatment of autoimmune diseases*).
- If systemic health of a patient does not allow comprehensive periodontal treatment (*e.g. unstable cardiac condition, etc.*), prognosis of periodontitis automatically becomes unfavourable.

6. *Genetics*

- Genetic defects in some individuals lead to more severe and destructive forms of periodontitis (*e.g. individuals with down's syndrome, severe autoimmune diseases, etc.*).
- Correction of such genetic defects is not possible, therefore periodontitis in such individuals has an unfavourable overall prognosis.

◄ *Why do patients with genetic defects that affect periodontitis have a poor prognosis?*

7. *Stress*

- It decreases body immunity.
- Patients with chronic psychological stress are also more likely suffer from TFO.
- They also may have severe periodontitis and are less likely to get it treated thereby resulting in unfavourable prognosis.

◄ *How does stress affect prognosis?*

8. *Possibility of Restoring a Fully Functional and Aesthetic Dentition with Remaining Natural Teeth and Prosthetic Replacements*

- Suitability of the remaining teeth to act as healthy and functional abutments is essential for restoring dentition with adequate function.

- If the dentition or group of teeth do not fit in the prosthetic rehabilitation plan for the patient, they must be extracted even if otherwise healthy. If this is not done, they will adversely affect the overall prognosis of the dentition.

B. Individual Tooth Prognosis

When is individual tooth prognosis determined? ▶

Individual tooth prognosis is determined ***after*** determining overall prognosis. Factors on which prognosis of an individual tooth depends are:

1. *Tooth Mobility*

- The most common causes of tooth mobility are bone loss, inflammation in PDL and TFO.
- Although grade I and II mobility can be treated and managed satisfactorily, grade III mobility usually cannot be managed satisfactorily.
- If tooth mobility cannot be corrected, prognosis of the tooth becomes poor (Figs 13.14, 13.15, 13.16 and 13.20).

2. *Type and Depth of Pockets, Bone Loss and Position Crest of Alveolar Bone on Different Surfaces of the Same Tooth*

- Severe bone loss if accompanied by presence of compound or complex pockets, particularly if these are infrabony, make periodontitis around that tooth more complicated. This makes treatment more difficult.

Why is mobility and prognosis more dependent on the more coronal bone crest? ▶

- If level of crest of alveolar bone on different surfaces of the same tooth is different, mobility of that tooth is more dependent on the more coronal bone crest, i.e. mobility of this tooth is lesser due to the support provided by the more coronally placed alveolar bone crest (*mobility is lesser than what is expected when looking at the more apical crest*). This improves prognosis of the tooth (Fig. 13.16 and 13.20).

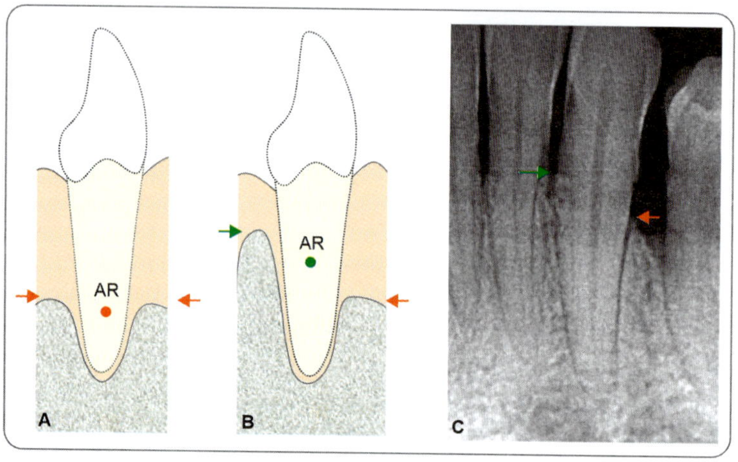

Fig. 13.20: Height of alveolar bone crest on the lesser involved surface (*green arrows, diags B and C*) is taken into consideration for determining prognosis. When level of crest of alveolar bone on different surfaces of the same tooth is not the same (*diags B and C, green arrow vs. red arrow;*) the more coronal bone crest (*green arrow, diag. B and C*) helps maintain the axis of rotation (*AR*) of that tooth (*diags A and B*) at a more occlusal level and thus reduces mobility of that tooth (*compare red dot in diag. A to green dot in diag. B*).

3. *Individual Tooth Morphology*

- A tooth's morphology affects prognosis by either predisposing the tooth to disease or reducing chances of complete cure by obstructing treatment.

Why do narrow furcations and closely placed roots have poorer prognosis? ▶

- Narrow furcations (*in multi-rooted teeth*), closely placed roots, root concavities etc. increase plaque deposition, reduce effectivity of oral hygiene measures and do not allow effective instrumentation for treatment of periodontitis in these areas (*SRP; due to difficult access to these areas*) (Fig. 13.21). Such situations affect prognosis of the tooth in a negative way.

Which teeth have lesser peri-cemental area? ▶

- If a tooth has short roots, e.g. lower incisors, it will have lesser peri-cemental area (*area of anatomical root*), such a tooth will have lower occlusal load bearing capacity and will also be more susceptible to TFO.

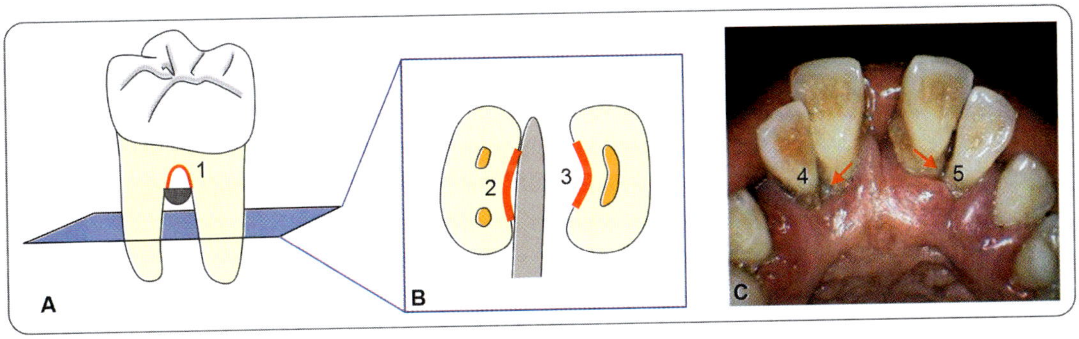

Fig. 13.21: Furcation regions that are narrower than the blade of the scaling instrument (*diag. A, grey semicircle and red lined area 1*), root concavities (*diag. B, red lined areas 2 and 3*) and surfaces of closely placed roots of teeth (*diag. C, areas 4 and 5*) may not be reachable by scalers, curettes or ultrasonic scaler tips. As a result, SRP and oral hygiene maintenance by the patient in such areas is difficult or even impossible. This predisposes such areas to continued periodontitis and worsens prognosis of such teeth.

4. Teeth with Caries, Root Resorption and Nonvital Teeth

- Teeth mutilated by extensive caries and/or pulpal involvement and those with extensive resorption of their roots (*due to any cause*, e.g. *high orthodontic forces, pathologic processes, idiopathic external resorption*, etc.) have a questionable prognosis that is dependent on severity of damage and the probability adequate treatment (**Fig. 13.22**).
- A ***nonvital tooth has similar prognosis as that of a vital tooth*** if it has been satisfactorily endodontically treated.
- Periodontal healing is similar in both vital and successfully endodontically treated teeth.

◂ *Is the periodontal prognosis of nonvital tooth similar to that of a vital tooth?*

◂ *Is the periodontal healing similar in non-vital and vital teeth?*

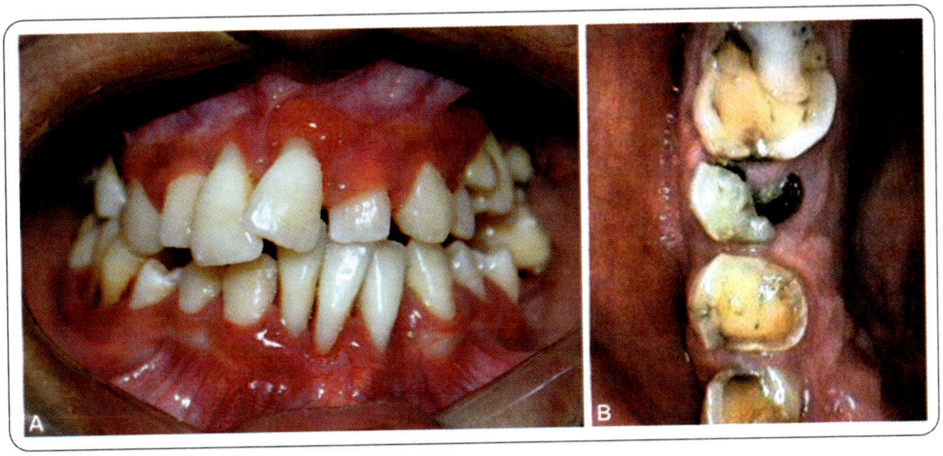

Fig. 13.22: Mucogingival problems like inadequate attached gingiva, high frenal attachments, severe periodontitis, systemic contributing factors that cannot be treated adequately (*diag. A*), teeth mutilated by caries (*diag. B*), etc. contribute to increased severity of periodontitis and worsen prognosis of affected teeth.

5. Mucogingival Problems in Relation to a Tooth

- Inadequate width of attached gingiva, location of base of pocket apical to muco-gingival junction, etc. may jeopardise periodontal health of teeth and make treatment complicated and difficult.
- Prognosis of such teeth is dependent on severity of mucogingival problems and degree to which these are corrected.

6. Location and Restorative Importance of a Tooth

- As premolars, 1st and 2nd molars and other teeth that are to serve as abutments (*teeth adjacent to edentulous areas in the arch*) have to bear additional (*greater*) occlusal forces, ***more rigid*** standards are employed for determining prognosis of such teeth.

◂ *Why are more rigid standards employed for determination of prognosis of abutment teeth?*

7. Restorability and Value of the Tooth in the Prosthetic Plan

How does the value of a tooth in prosthetic plan after prognosis? ▸

How does restorability of a tooth affect prognosis? ▸

- If a tooth does not fit into or obstructs a prosthetic plan, it should be extracted to improve overall prognosis (*even if the tooth has a good individual prognosis*).
- If a tooth requires extensive treatment which the patient does not afford or it has poor prognosis, extracting it will improve the overall prognosis.
- Attempts to treat and retain a tooth with hopeless prognosis (*for some more time*) are likely to worsen the overall prognosis.

8. Furcation Involvement

How does furcation involvement affect periodontal treatment and prognosis? ▸

- When furcation area of a multirooted tooth has periodontitis, such a tooth is said to have a 'furcation involvement' (*see Chapter 20; 'Furcation Involvement and Its Management'*).
- As plaque control is difficult in furcation areas of teeth, it leads to faster periodontal loss (*faster progress of periodontitis*).
- As furcations areas are narrow and are located in posterior teeth, they have a relatively more difficult access. This makes treatment relatively more difficult (*even impossible in some situations as instrumentation is impossible*) **(Fig. 13.21, diag. A)**.

Why is prognosis of a multirooted tooth better than that of a single rooted tooth with similar bone loss? ▸

- If, however, such problems (*difficult instrument access and plaque control*) can be successfully managed, prognosis of furcation involved multirooted teeth is usually better that that of single rooted teeth with similar bone loss. This is so because multi-rooted teeth have greater number of roots. More number (*more peri-cemental area*) and widely placed roots of multirooted teeth provide them more stability and increase their load bearing capacity.
- In general, if surgical access to the furcation is good, treatment can be done and oral hygiene can be adequately maintained, prognosis of all grades of furcation involvement (*grade I to IV*) is good.

III. GOALS AND RATIONALE (*JUSTIFICATION*) OF PERIODONTAL TREATMENT

Goals of Periodontal Treatment

(*Why is periodontal treatment undertaken?*)

Periodontal treatment not only improves an individual's dental health it also benefits and improves the individual's general (*systemic*) health. There are ***three basic goals*** of periodontal therapy:

What are the goals of periodontal treatment? ▸

Goal 1: Treating periodontal disease, e.g. gingivitis, periodontitis, TFO, etc.

Goal 2: Reducing the possibility of progression of gingivitis and periodontitis (*reducing and maintaining pockets to preferably less than 3 mm but certainly not more than 4 mm*).

Goal 3: Improving the health and aesthetics of oral tissues and gingiva and providing a patient, a comfortably functioning and aesthetic natural or implant supported dentition that can be maintained both by the patient and the dental surgeon.

Rationale (*Justification*) of Periodontal Treatment

(*Why must periodontal treatment be done? How will it benefit the patient?*)

What is the rationale of periodontal treatment? ▸

Adequate and scientifically performed periodontal treatment will result in numerous health benefits, these include:

1. **Healthy changes in periodontium (*local changes*) expected after periodontal treatment**
   a. **Histological changes:** Restoration of normal histology of periodontal tissues (*gingiva, PDL, alveolar bone and cementum*).

What clinical changes can be expected to take place after periodontal treatment? ▸

   b. **Clinical changes:**
      - Resolution of inflammation in the periodontal tissues and reestablishment of normal (*physiologic*) features of gingiva (*this will help maintain gingival and periodontal health in future*).
      - Reduction in probing pocket depth (*PD*), clinical attachment level (*CAL*) and bleeding on probing (*BOP*).
      - Improved alveolar bone health and bone height (*to some extent*). This reduces tooth mobility and reduces secondary trauma from occlusion.

- Reduction in patient complaints like food impaction, pain, irritation in gingivae, etc.
- Improvement in ease of mastication.
- Increased life of teeth.

2. **Positive changes (*improvement*) in systemic health expected after periodontal treatment**
   - Decrease in bacteraemia (*bacteria circulating in blood stream that come from infected pockets*). This will reduce chances of infection and adverse effects of bacterial products at other sites and organs of the body.
   - Improvement in blood sugar control and diabetes (*leading to reduced insulin requirement, better blood sugar level control with the same or lower medication and precautions, etc.*).
   - Reduced chances of atherosclerosis, lung infections, stroke, low birth weight and premature babies, etc.

◂ *What improvements can be expected in a patient's health after periodontal treatment?*

IV. THE TREATMENT PLAN

A ***detailed*** plan of required treatment/s and their sequence is essential ***before*** initiating periodontal treatment. Treatment plan is based on diagnosis, treatment needs, prognosis and all future possibilities.

◂ *Name the factors on which a treatment plan is based?*

Some important points to be kept in mind while formulating a treatment plan are:

- Treatment of all oral (*periodontal, prosthetic, orthodontic, etc.*) and systemic diseases (*e.g. treatment of diabetes, etc.*) and conditions must be incorporated in all treatment plans. Untreated systemic diseases can complicate periodontitis and reduce long-term survival of teeth.
- Periodontal health and usability of teeth to be retained after treatment are more important than the number of teeth retained in the mouth. 'Heroic' attempts for saving dentitions/individual teeth with poor prognosis are doomed to fail.
- The treatment plan must be clearly explained to the patient in the language he/she understands and approval of the same must be ensured. Emphasis should be laid on teeth that can be saved with treatment and their importance to the overall health of the dentition. Even when discussing teeth with poor prognosis, stress should be laid on benefits of extracting such teeth.
- At times, changes in treatment plan are necessary due to change in local and systemic conditions and treatment needs of the patient.
- Long-term oral health maintenance is dependent on patient's quality of post treatment plaque control and regularity of periodic dental maintenance visits for examination, prophylaxis, etc.

Establishing a 'Baseline' of Periodontal Disease before Starting Treatment

For measuring long-term progress or improvement of disease, we must establish ***reference points*** or ***parameters*** with which future parameters can be compared. This is called 'Establishing a Baseline'. Some commonly used parameters are BOP, PD, CAL, RBL, grades of furcation defects, tooth mobility, amount of smoking (*e.g. cigarettes or equivalent tobacco smoked every day*), severity of diabetes, plaque and calculus scores, etc. Relevant medical and dental information and history, evaluation of outcome of previous treatment is also useful in establishing baselines.

◂ *What is establishing a baseline?*

Such baseline information helps set short-term goals, plan and select therapies and home care procedures and products for a particular patient. Baseline data is also useful for making strategies for maintaining an individual's periodontal health in the future keeping in mind current oral condition, expectations, capabilities and values.

Making a Treatment Plan

A common specific treatment plan ***cannot*** be prescribed for all patients; a widely accepted plan of treatment is presented hereunder:

1. *Initial Visit(s)*

What is done during the initial patient visit?

i. For a patient with ***severe*** pain or another emergency:
   i. Make a provisional diagnosis.
   ii. Treat diseases or conditions requiring immediate treatment, e.g. acute abscesses, acute pulpitis, etc.

   After acute pain has been settled, follow undermentioned schedule.

ii. For a patient with ***no*** pain or other emergency:
   i. First make a ***provisional*** diagnosis. This may require:
      a. Ordering radiographs and diagnostic tests, etc.
      b. Getting opinion of other specialists regarding oral and systemic health.
   ii. Discuss provisional diagnosis and possible treatment plan with patient. Caution the patient that the diagnosis and treatment plan may change after test reports and specialist opinion are available.
   iii. Educate—motivate—instruct the patient regarding plaque biofilm and its ill effects, give instructions on maintaining oral hygiene and diet suggestions for maintenance of oral and systemic disease control, etc.
   iv. After test reports, radiographs and opinions from other specialists are available, if required, modify the initial diagnosis to make a ***final*** diagnosis
   v. Now make a ***final*** treatment plan and discuss diagnosis and treatment plan with patient.

2. *Phase-I Therapy or Etiotrophic Phase (Cause Related Therapy)*

What treatments are done during phase-I therapy?

This may include some or all of the following:

i. Scaling and root planing (*SRP*).
ii. Restoration of caries and correction of other defects in teeth that prevent adequate plaque control, e.g. correction of overhanging margins of restorations and crowns, etc.
iii. Extraction of teeth with poor or hopeless prognosis.
iv. Temporary or 'permanent' splinting of teeth.
v. Endodontic treatment (*if required*).
vi. Placing temporary or permanent crowns and prostheses.
vii. Orthodontic treatment for correcting crowding of teeth and tooth malposition that predisposes and contributes to periodontal and other oral disease.

2a. Assess results attained after phase-I treatment (*assessment of results of treatment must be done after allowing a reasonable time for healing to take place; this could range from few weeks to few months*).

Assess results and re-examine for:

What must a clinician look out for during reassessment of results of phase-I therapy?

- *Inadvertently left calculus and caries.*
- *Improvement in plaque control and oral disease including periodontitis (as per 2018 classification of periodontal disease); there should be:*
  - *No BOP (bleeding on probing) at most sites.*
  - *BOP if present, is there at less than 10% sites.*
  - *Reduction in PD (probing depth) to less than 3mm at all sites.*
- *Reattainment of normal clinical features of gingiva (colour, contour, consistency, surface texture and size of gingiva).*

*If the results of treatment done so far are **not** satisfactory and the above have **not** been attained proceed for phase II of treatment.*

3. *Phase-II Therapy or Surgical Phase (Corrective Periodontal Therapy)*

What is done during phase-II of the treatment plan?

This may include some or all of the following:

i. Refinement of previous treatment plan if necessary.
ii. Extraction of teeth, if their condition has not improved significantly after treatment done during phase-I (i.e. *if their prognosis has not converted to good or fair*).
iii. Periodontal surgery for correction of gingival and alveolar bone defects and periodontal conditions that have not improved significantly after phase-I treatment.
iv. Implant placement.

3a. *Assess results attained after phase II treatment* *(assessment of results of treatment must be done after allowing a reasonable time for healing to take place; this could range from few weeks to few months).* ***Assess results and re-examine for:***

- *Adequacy of plaque control and maintenance of oral hygiene.*
- *Accomplishment of goals of surgery and assessment of improvements in efficiency of dentition after surgery.*
- *Improvement in periodontal health (as per 2018 classification of periodontal disease); there should be:*
  - *No BOP (bleeding on probing) at most sites.*
  - *BOP if present, is there at less than 10% sites.*
  - *Reduction in PD (probing pocket depth) to less than 3 mm.*
  - *PD of 4 mm at some sites is acceptable but these sites should have no BOP; if this is present such sites must be re-treated to reduce PD to less than 3 mm.*
  - *Exploring teeth for any remaining calculus and caries.*

If above ***have been attained*** *proceed for phase III.*

◄ *What must a clinician look out for during reassessment of results of phase-II therapy?*

4. Phase-III Therapy or Restorative Phase (Placement of Final Restorations and Prosthetic Replacements)

i. Temporary restorations and crowns or prosthetic replacements, splints, etc. if were placed earlier (*during phase I*) are replaced with final ones.

◄ *What treatments are done during phase-III therapy?*

4a. Assess results attained after treatment done so far and re-evaluate health status of the entire oral cavity

- *Ensure that desired improvement in efficiency of dentition has occurred.*
- *Confirm that all restorations, crowns or prostheses are being tolerated well by oral tissues.*
- *Assess if any additional treatment or re-treatment required.*

5. Phase-IV Therapy or Maintenance Phase (Periodic Recall)

◄ *What is done during phase-IV therapy?*

This includes the following:

i. Recording any change in medical history and start or stop or modification in dose of medication that the patient is taking for systemic diseases.
ii. Re-assessing quality of oral hygiene and re-educating, re-motivating and re-instructing patients in oral hygiene measures.
iii. Examining ***entire*** oral cavity and reassessing results of treatment done earlier and maintenance of periodontal health by the patient (*see Chapter 10A for criteria of health and periodontal disease in a treated case of periodontitis*). Ensure that:
   a. PD is maintained less than 3–4 mm.
   b. Ensure that bleeding on probing (*BOP*) if present, it is there only at less than 10% sites.
   c. No site with 4 mm probing depth (PD) has BOP; if this is present such sites must be re-treated to reduce PD to less than 3 mm (*as per 2018 classification of periodontal disease*).
iv. Oral cancer screening.
v. Oral prophylaxis (*scaling and root planing done for prevention of gingivitis and periodontitis*).

ALERT!

- Excellent plaque control and periodic scaling (*prophylaxis*) after surgery ***improves*** healing after surgery.
- Do ***not*** measure pocket depth until at least ***three months*** after surgery (*this will injure newly formed attachment apparatus between gingival connective tissue and cementum and reduce chances of new attachment*).
- Slight ***increase*** in tooth mobility is expected during 1st three weeks after surgery (*due to the presence of inflammation in PDL*).
- New bone formation in a healing periodontal wound occurs till the third week after surgery but bone remodeling continues for nine months to two years.
- Teeth that have undergone periodontal surgery may become ***hypersensitive*** (*especially to cold*) for a few days to many weeks.
- When bone is surgically exposed during a flap surgery, ***0.25 mm*** of surface bone is always ***lost*** (*resorbed*) even if no bone surgery is performed.

Factors Affecting Decision of Type of Periodontal Surgery to be Performed in a Particular Case

Different clinicians may have different opinions regarding the best surgical method to treat a particular case. Many factors affect the choice of surgical procedure in a particular patient, these are:

Enumerate the factors on which choice of type of surgery depends. ▶

1. Patient's age, general (*systemic*) health and aesthetic concerns.
2. Patient's present status of oral hygiene, willingness and capability of complying with specific oral hygiene instructions.
3. PD, CAL, type of pockets, comparative level of base of pockets in the arch (*of several teeth plotted on a diagnosis chart*).
4. Degree of already present gingival recession.
5. Degree and type of bone loss (*one, two or three walled bone defects*) and remaining length of tooth root with bone support.
6. Overall dental treatment plan, goals and patient's expectations.
7. Eagerness to get treated as per ideal treatment plan and patient's affordability of recommended treatment, etc.

How do we Measure Severity of Periodontitis?

The commonly used clinical parameters are:

How is severity of periodontitis measured? ▶

1. At the ***individual tooth*** level severity of periodontitis is gauged by:
   - PD (*probing pocket depth*). This tells us the ***present status*** of health or disease.
   - CAL (*clinical attachment loss or level*). This tells us the damage produced by periodontitis ***in the past.***
   - Furcation involvement and its grade.
   - Degree of tooth mobility.
2. To know the severity of periodontitis at the ***case level*** (*entire mouth*), staging and grading of periodontitis using the 2018 classification is done (*see Chapter 10A*).

Remember:

Presenting clinical parameters of gingival health are markers of past or present gingival disease? ▶

Why must absence of clinical signs of gingivitis not be mistaken for gingival health. ▶

1. The above clinical parameters are markers of ***past and present*** disease activity and ***do not*** reliably predict future progression of periodontal disease.
2. Periodontitis often affects different teeth to ***different*** degrees; therefore, periodontal assessment must be done at several sites in the mouth (*Chapter 10A, Making Clinical Diagnosis of Gingivitis and Periodontitis Using The 2018 Classification'—Making site level diagnosis*).
3. As periodontitis progresses in an episodic pattern i.e. bursts of active periodontitis are followed by inactive periodontitis phases (*periods of time when disease is be inactive*), therefore, ***absence of clinical signs of inflammation (as seen in quiescent phases) must not be mistaken for health*** **(*Chapter 10, 'Plaque Induced Gingivitis and Periodontitis'—Models of progression of periodontitis—Episodic Burst Model, page 138*).**

ALERT!

After periodontal treatment how can we know if periodontium has become healthy?

General signs of periodontal health after periodontal therapy are:

1. Absence of inflammation in the gingiva and reduction in tooth mobility.
2. No increase in gingival recession, interproximal bone loss and CAL.
3. Healthy peri-implant tissues around fully functional dental implants.

Also see parameters of gingival and periodontal health in Chapter 10A, 'Making Clinical Diagnosis of Gingivitis and Periodontitis Using The 2018 Classification'.

Factors that Affect Outcome of Periodontal Therapy

Name the factors that affect the outcome of periodontal treatment. ▶

1. Higher initial CAL and PD (*probing pocket depth*) of true pockets are generally inversely proportional to outcome of periodontal therapy.
2. Complicated local topography adversely affects outcome of therapy (*e.g. complex pockets, infrabony bone loss, etc.*).

3. Post treatment plaque control especially at surgical site is directly proportional to outcome of periodontal therapy, i.e. better the plaque control better the outcome.
4. Type of periodontal surgery performed and sequence of treatment have a bearing on the outcome of treatment, e.g. attached gingiva must be made adequate before performing a mucogingival surgery to cover recession; if this is not done, failure is certain, etc.
5. Level of training and skill of clinician.

ALERT!

Easily avoidable/correctable factors that adversely affect periodontal healing are:

1. Improper and 'rough' surgical technique:
   i. Excessive tissue manipulation and trauma during surgery.
   ii. Failure to raise a flap with adequate blood supply (Fig. 17B.4).
   iii. Incomplete SRP and debridement of wound.
2. Frequent re-treatments and surgical interventions at short intervals.
3. Improper plaque control in general but especially within a fortnight of periodontal surgery, etc.

ALERT!

Systemic factors that adversely affect periodontal healing:

1. Old age.
2. Poor systemic health, e.g. uncontrolled diabetes, immune defects, etc.
3. Nutritional deficiencies.
4. Use of medications that cause delayed and impaired wound healing, e.g. steroids, etc.
5. Severe hormonal imbalances, etc.

Healing after periodontal therapy and possible outcomes of periodontal wound healing are discussed in detail in Chapter 16—Scaling, Root Planing and Other Fundamentals of Periodontal Surgery.

Review Questions

1. What are the steps in planning and initiating periodontal treatment?
2. Which radiographs are best suited for making a periodontal diagnosis and why?
3. Why is an orthopantomogram (OPG) not the ideal radiograph for periodontal diagnosis?
4. Write a note on cone beam computed tomography (CBCT).
5. What is 'walking the probe' and transgingival probing?
6. Write on tooth mobility.
7. Write on advanced diagnostic tests used for making a periodontal diagnosis.
8. What is prognosis? Why must overall prognosis of the dentition be determined along with individual tooth prognosis?
9. Discuss factors on which overall prognosis and that of an individual tooth depends.
10. Write on rationale of periodontal treatment.
11. What is treatment plan? Write plan of treatment for a periodontal patient.
12. What are the factors on which decision of performing the type of periodontal surgery depends?
13. What are the goals of periodontal treatment? What are the factors that affect outcome of periodontal therapy?
14. What is meant by 'establishing a baseline'?

Chapter 14

Periodontal Instruments and Principles of Periodontal Instrumentation

A large assortment of instruments is available for use in periodontics. In addition to instruments meant for exclusive periodontal use, the list also includes general dental instruments like dental mirrors, explorers, tweezers, etc.

INSTRUMENTS AND EQUIPMENT USED IN PERIODONTICS

Classify instruments used for periodontal use. ▸

Some commonly used periodontal instruments and equipment are:

1. Scaling and Root planing (*SRP*) instruments
   a. Scalers
      i. Manual
      ii. Ultrasonic
   b. Curettes
      i. Area specific
      ii. Universal
2. Equipment used for polishing surface of teeth after SRP
   a. Polishing paste, rubber cups, bristle cups, polishing tapes, etc.
   b. Micromotor and contra-angle hand piece
3. Surgical instruments
   a. Incisional and Excisional instruments
      i. Periodontal knives, e.g. Kirkland, etc.
      ii. Bard parker blades # 11, 12, 12d, 15 and blade handles
   b. Muco-periosteal elevators
   c. Surgical periodontal chisels and surgical periodontal files
4. Other equipment
   a. Lasers
   b. Physio-dispenser for placing implants
   c. Piezo-surgical unit for bone surgery, etc.

What are the parts of an instrument? ▸

Parts of a Hand Periodontal Instrument

1. *Handle*

The part of an instrument with which it is held with fingers is called handle. It may be made of metal or plastic. Handles may have round or polygonal shape (Fig. 14.1).

2. *Working End*

What is the other name for the working end of an instrument? ▸

Terminal end of an instrument with which work of the instrument is done is called working end or blade. It may be made of metal or plastic.

3. *Shank*

How many types of shanks are there in periodontal instruments? ▸

The part which connects handle and blade of the instrument is called shank. Shanks could be:

a. **Simple:** Shank is bent only at one place, e.g. sickle scaler.
b. **Complex:** Shank is bent at two or more places, e.g. Gracey curette.
c. **Straight:** When the shank, handle and blade of the instrument are in a straight line, e.g. chisel.

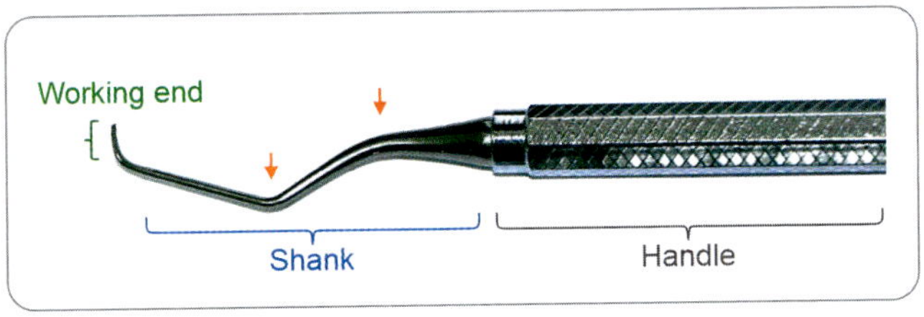

Fig. 14.1: Parts of an instrument. Shank of an instrument may be bent (*red arrows*) at one or more places and in different planes

Instruments used for Scaling and Root Planing (*SRP*)

Which instruments are used for scaling and root planing?

1. Dental mouth mirrors
2. Periodontal probes and dental explorers
3. Scalers and curettes
4. Cleansing and polishing instruments.

Dental Mirrors

Three types of dental mouth mirrors are available:

What are front surface dental mirrors?

1. **Plane surface (*back surface*):** These mirrors have their reflecting surface on the back of the mirror (*just like a looking mirror*).
2. **Front surface mirror (*metallic*):** These mirrors are made of ***metal*** whose front surface is highly polished like a mirror.
3. **Magnifying:** This is a magnifying ***concave*** mirror.

Dental mirrors can be used for:

What are the uses of a dental mirror?

1. **Indirect vision:** Used to see an area (*in the mirror*) that cannot be seen directly.
2. **Indirect illumination:** Reflecting light onto a surface that is being viewed. Trans-illumination of teeth can also be done this way.
3. **Check/Tongue retraction**.
4. **Percussion** (*tapping*) of teeth with back of the mirror handle.
5. **To evaluate mobility** of teeth (*by holding a tooth between backs of two mirror handles or between back of one mirror handle and an operator's finger, Fig. 13.14*).

Periodontal Probes

What is a periodontal probe?

A periodontal probe is a tapered, thin and rod like instrument with a rounded (*blunt*) tip (*end*) (Fig. 14.3).

- Periodontal probes have markings on them (*in millimeters*) and they may be straight or curved and round or flat (Fig. 14.2).
- Some commonly used probes are: William's probe, WHO Probe, Marquis probe, etc. (Fig. 14.2).
  - A straight periodontal probe is used for recording PD, CAL, etc. It is used by keeping it ***parallel*** to the long axis of the tooth (Fig. 13.9).
  - A curved probe (*Naber's periodontal probe*) is used for examining a furcation and for this it is inserted from the side of a multirooted tooth into its furcation (Fig. 13.10).

Name some periodontal probes.

What is a Naber's probe?

Periodontal probes are used for:

What are the uses of a periodontal probe?

1. **Measuring**
   i. Pocket or sulcus depth (*PD*) (Figs 2.5, 2.6, 2.7 and 13.9).
   ii. Clinical attachment loss and clinical attachment level (*CAL*) (Fig. 2.7).
   iii. Gingival recession, distances between any two anatomical land marks, e.g. width of the attached gingiva.
2. **Marking pockets** (*bleeding points*) **during periodontal surgery** (*gingivectomy, etc.*) (Fig. 17A.2).
3. **Determining consistency** of the gingiva.
4. **Evaluating bleeding on probing** from a pocket (Fig. 2.5).
5. **Assessing furcations** of multirooted teeth (*Naber's probe*), etc. (Fig. 13.10).

Dental Explorers

What is a dental explorer? ▸ An explorer is a tapered, thin and rod like instrument with a ***sharp*** tip (*end*). Explorers are used to detect irregularities on hard oral surfaces (*caries, calculus, restorations, prostheses, etc.*) **(Fig. 14.3)**.

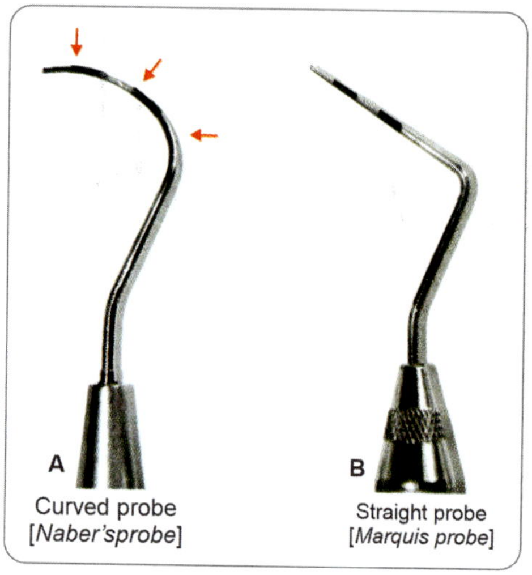

Fig. 14.2: Naber's probe. It is a curved (*red arrows*) double ended periodontal probe used for assessment of periodontal furcations (*diag. A*).

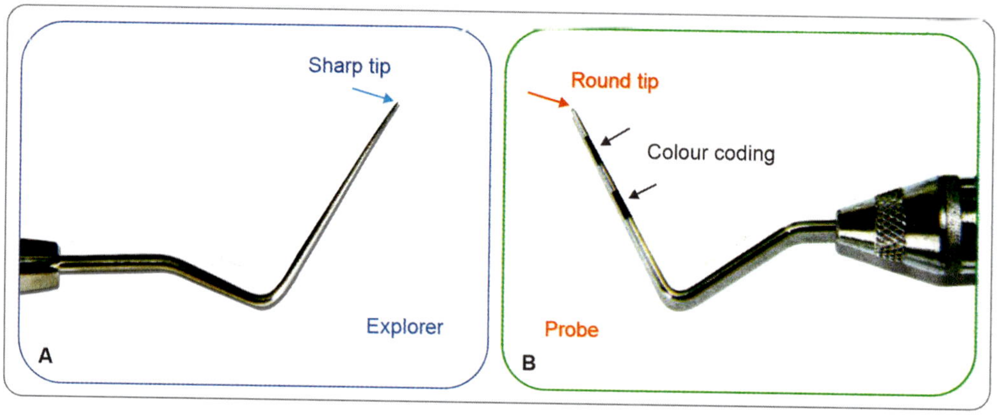

Fig. 14.3: Periodontal probe and dental explorer. A probe always has a rounded tip/end (*diag. B, red arrow*) whereas an explorer has sharp tip (*diag. A, blue arrow*). Colour coding on probes (*diag. B, black arrows*) increases visual identification of calibrations on the probe blade and makes taking measurements easy. Markings (*calibrations*) if present on the blade of an explorer will not make it a probe.

CLINICAL UTILITY AND SHORT ANSWER

What are colour coded probes?

- If a periodontal probe's calibrations are alternately coloured, it makes recording measurements easier **(Fig. 14.3, diag. B)**.
- Such probes with alternating-coloured bands are called colour coded probes.
- A colour coded probe otherwise is same as a non-colour coded probe.

CLINICAL UTILITY AND SHORT ANSWER

What is the difference between a periodontal probe and an explorer?

- The difference between a periodontal probe and explorer basically lies in their tip designs.
- Periodontal probes are used to probe soft tissues, therefore, they have ***blunt*** (*rounded*) tips **(Fig. 14.3, diag. B)**.
- Explorers are used to 'catch' hard surface irregularities they therefore have ***sharp*** tips **(Fig. 14.3, diag. A)**.

ALERT!

- Probes with greater number of markings (*calibrations*), i.e. markings at smaller distances (1 mm), are more ***difficult*** to use in the oral cavity than those with lesser number of markings, i.e. markings at larger distances (3 mm).
- Greater numbers of markings at shorter distances can probably produce more accurate measurements, but, skilled clinicians can measure distances with probes with markings after longer distances more quickly and with comparable accuracy.

Instruments for Scaling, Root Planing and Curettage

Two basic types of instruments are available for scaling and root planing:

1. **Scalers:** Sickle scaler, morse scaler, surface scaler, hoe, periodontal file, chisel, etc.
2. **Curettes:** Universal and area specific curettes.

Of the above, ***sickle scalers*** and ***curettes*** are the most ***commonly*** used hand instruments for scaling and root planing.

◂ *Which instruments are commonly used for scaling and root planing?*

Sickle Scaler

- Sickle scalers are available in different sizes. Large bladed sickle scalers are used for larger and firmer calculus whereas small bladed instruments are suitable for smaller and softer calculus deposits.
- Anterior sickle scalers have a straight shank while the posterior sickle scalers have an angled shank **(Fig. 14.4, diag. A)**.
- Sickle scalers can be used for all surfaces of all teeth.
- Specific design features of a sickle scaler are:
  - Blade is ***triangular*** in cross section **(Fig. 14.4, diag. B)**.
  - It has three surfaces:
    - Two lateral surfaces and a face **(Fig. 14.4, diag. C)**.
    - Lateral surfaces meet the face to make ***two cutting*** edges.
    - The three surfaces converge into a ***pointed tip (toe)***.
  - The shank of a sickle scaler is short and rigid.
  - The face of the sickle scaler is at 90° to the shank **(Fig. 14.4, diag. B)**.
  - The lateral surfaces make an internal angle of 70°–80° with the face of the blade.

◂ *How many cutting edges does a sickle scaler have?*

◂ *What is angle between the shank and the blade of a sickle scaler?*

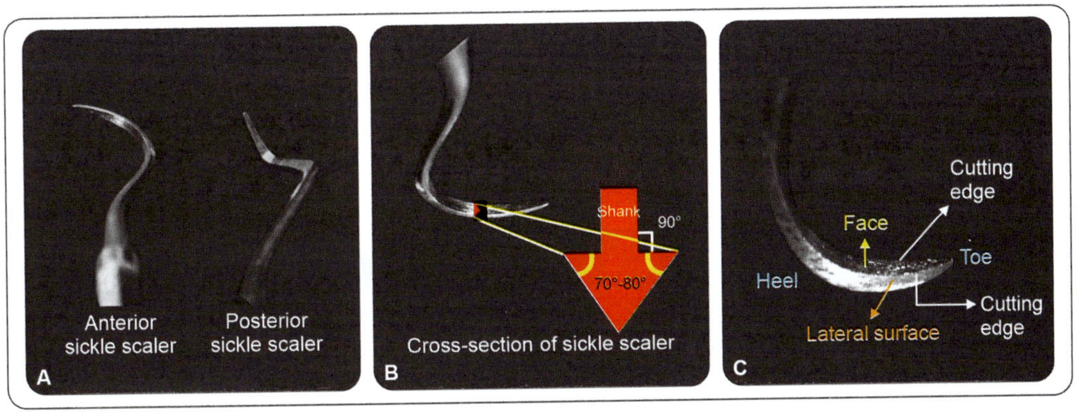

Fig. 14.4: Sickle scalers. Blade of a sickle scaler is triangular in cross section (*diag. B, red area*), pointed at the tip (*toe*) and has two usable cutting edges (*diag. C*)

Curette

It is commonly used for subgingival scaling and root planing, removal of granulation tissue and soft tissue lining of periodontal pockets. Two kinds of curettes are available:

1. Universal curettes
2. Area specific curettes.

◂ *How many types of periodontal curettes are available?*

Universal curettes

- They are designed to be used on all surfaces of teeth, i.e. anterior curettes can be used on all surfaces of anterior teeth and posterior curette can be used on all surfaces of posterior teeth (*e.g. columbia curette*). This is done by making small alterations in position of hand, finger rest and adaptation of instrument blade.
- Specific design features of a ***universal curette*** are:
  - It has ***two cutting edges*** that meet to make a ***rounded toe*** (Fig. 14.5, diag. C).
  - Its ***face is at an angle of 90° to the lower shank*** (*this allows either of the two cutting edges to be used*) and lateral surfaces make an internal angle of 70°–80° with face of the blade (Fig. 14.10).
  - Its blade is semi-circular in cross section and has a convex base.

How many cutting edges does a universal curette have? ▸

Area specific curettes

- Area specific curettes, e.g. Gracey curettes are designed to work ***only on*** particular surfaces of teeth.
- Gracey curettes provide excellent reachability and adaptability to specific surfaces of teeth for SRP. Gracey curettes are preferred over universal curettes due to this reason.
- **Only the lower cutting edge of the Gracey curette is usable** on the tooth surface for SRP (Fig. 14.6).
- The unique design features of Gracey curettes are:
  - Blades of Gracey curettes are ***offset***, i.e. the blade is at an angle of **60°–70°** to the ***lower shank*** of the instrument (Fig. 14.5, diag. B). Different shank designs make different Gracey curettes suitable for specific tooth surfaces (Fig. 14.9).
  - The cutting edges meet to make a ***rounded*** toe (Fig. 14.5, diag. C).
  - The blade of ***posterior*** Gracey curettes is curved in ***two*** planes: upward and sideward (Fig. 14.6). This blade curvature and shank angulation facilitates and limits use of a particular Gracey curette to specific tooth surfaces.

How many usable cutting edges does a Gracey curette have? ▸

Which design features of a Gracey curette make it area specific? ▸

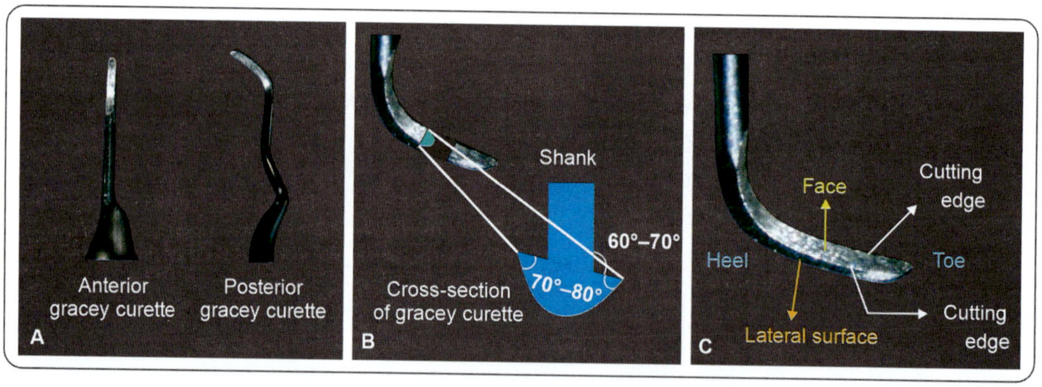

Fig. 14.5: Blades of both universal and Gracey curettes are spoon shaped and are rounded at the tip. The lateral surfaces make an angle of 70°–80° with the face of the blade.

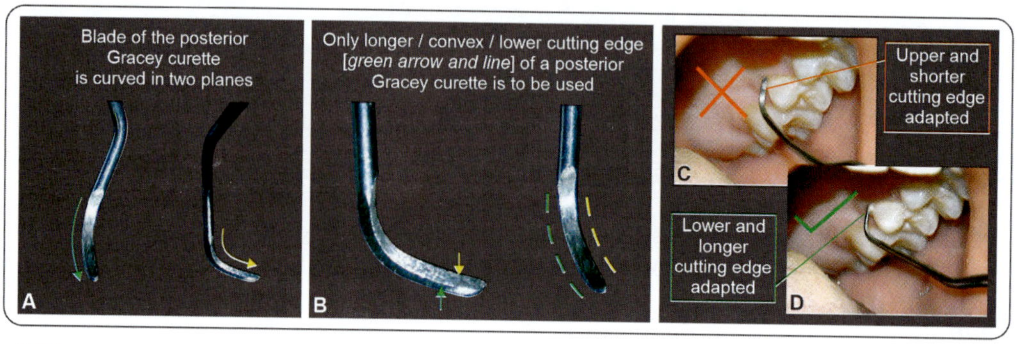

Fig. 14.6: The blade of a posterior Gracey curette is curved in *two* planes, i.e. to the side and upwards towards the shank (*diag. A, green and yellow arrows*). Only the lower cutting edge (*diag. B, green arrow and green line and diag. D*) is to be used for scaling and root planing. The correct (*lower*) cutting edge of a Gracey curette is convex and forms the larger outer curve (*diag. B, green dotted line*).

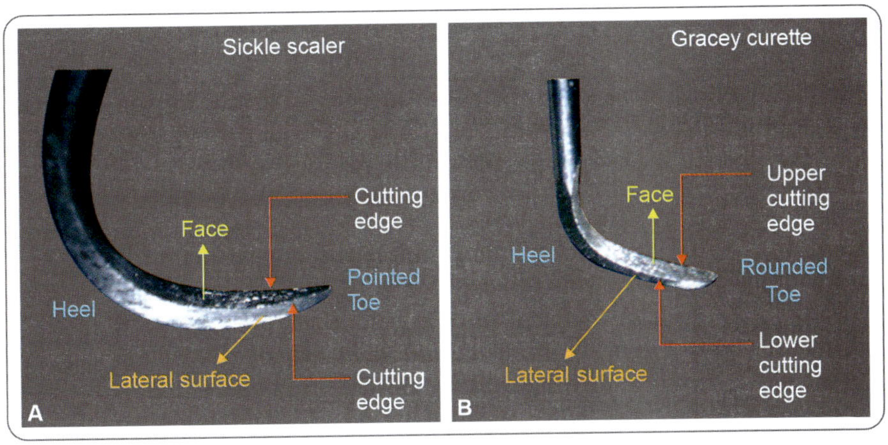

Fig. 14.7: Comparison between blades of a sickle scaler and curette

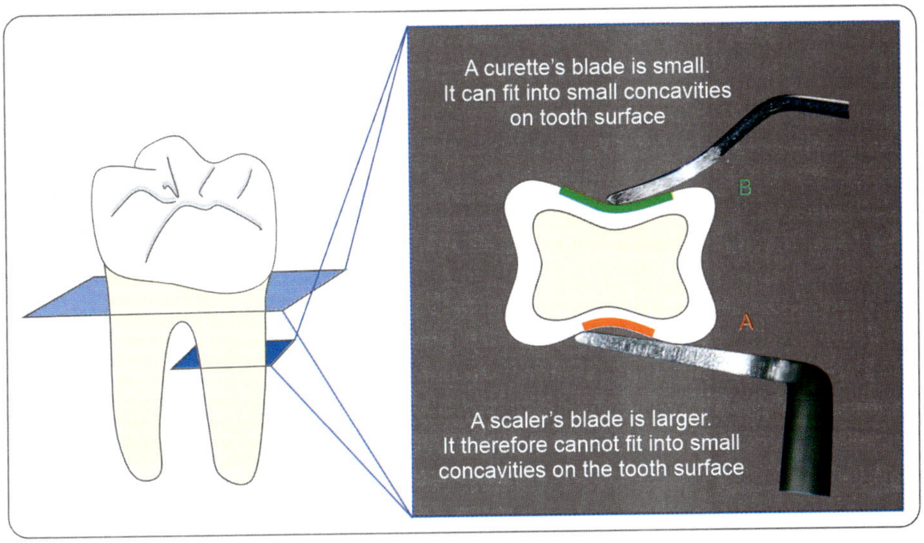

Fig. 14.8: Surfaces of teeth may not be straight, rather they may be either convex or concave. Depressions (*concavities, red and green marked areas*) in root surfaces may be so small that it is difficult and sometimes even impossible to adapt blades of larger scaling instruments like scalers into these areas (*diag. A, red marked area*). As blades of area specific curettes are relatively smaller and curved, they can easily fit into such small depressions on the tooth surfaces (*diag. B, green marked area*).

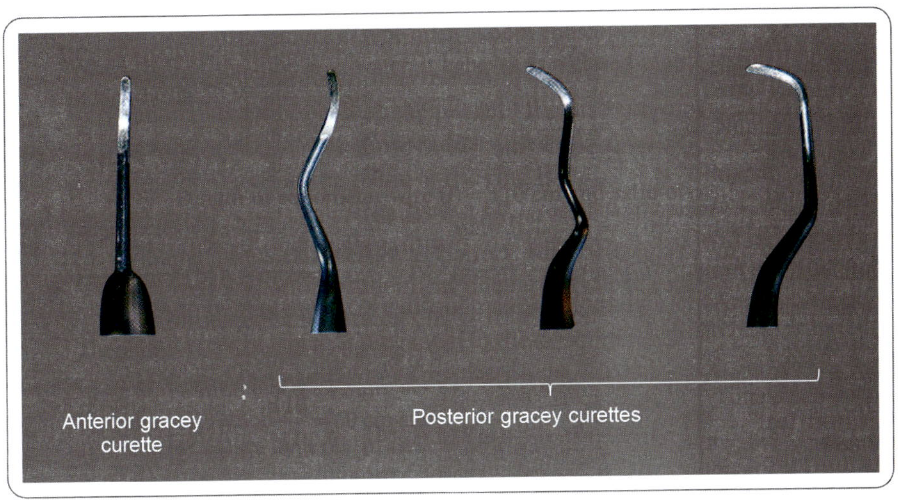

Fig. 14.9: Shanks and blades of area specific curettes are designed to reach and adapt only to particular surfaces of specific teeth.

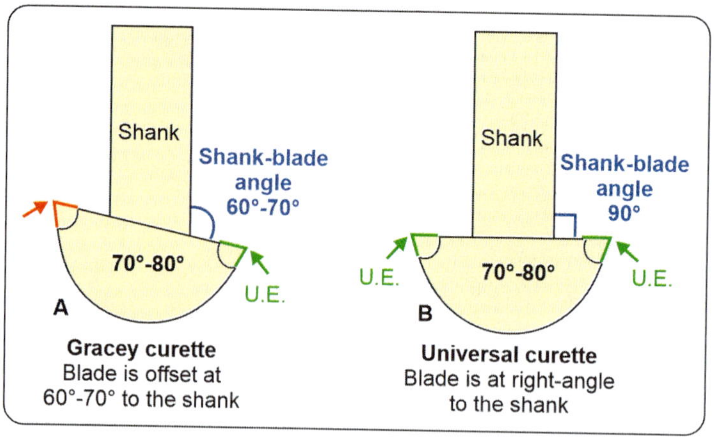

Fig. 14.10: Cross section of blades of area specific and universal curettes. Blade of Gracey curette is offset and is at 60°–70° to the shank while blade of a universal curette is 90° to the shank. In case of Gracey curette, only the lower cutting edge is usable whereas both cutting edges are usable in universal curette (*usable edge–UE, green arrows*).

Suitability of use of Gracey curettes on specific surfaces:

Can a Gracey curette be used on other surfaces of teeth that are different from the one it is designed for? ▶

Shanks and blades of area specific curettes are designed to reach and adapt only to particular surfaces of specific teeth; their shanks and blades are bent and shaped differently for this reason. An experienced clinician can however use each of the Gracey curettes on some other area different from the one they were originally designed for by changing position of the patient's head and working hand. Specific Gracey curettes that are recommended for use on particular surfaces of teeth are:

Gracey curette number	*Surfaces of teeth where usable*
1. # 1/2 and # 3/4	1. ***All*** surfaces of ***anterior*** teeth.
2. # 5/6	2. ***All*** surfaces of ***premolars***; also usable on ***all*** anterior teeth.
3. # 7/8 and # 9/10	3. ***Facial*** and ***lingual*** surfaces of ***all posterior*** teeth.
4. # 11/12	4. ***Mesial*** surfaces of ***posterior*** teeth.
5. # 13/14	5. ***Distal*** surfaces of ***posterior*** teeth.

Differences between a universal and a Gracey curette

Gracey curette	*Universal curette*
1. Several blade designs are there; each is usable on specific tooth surfaces (Fig. 14.9).	1. There is one blade design for all teeth.
2. Blade of ***posterior*** Gracey curettes is curved in two directions, i.e. upward and sideward (Fig. 14.6).	2. Blade is curved only in one direction, i.e. upward.
3. Blade is ***offset*** at an angle 60°–70° to the lower shank (Fig. 14.10).	3. Blade is at an angle of 90° to the lower shank.
4. Only ***lower*** cutting-edge is usable (Fig. 14.10, diag. A, UE, green arrow).	4. ***Both*** cutting-edges are usable (Fig. 14.10, diag. B, UE green arrows).

Periodontal Hoes

What is the main disadvantage of using a periodontal hoe? ▶

- Hoes are very efficient scaling instruments but they ***tend to scratch the tooth*** surface, they are therefore ***not*** preferred for SRP.
- The periodontal hoe (*e.g. Orban's hoe # 6/7 and 8/9 and Kirkland's hoe # 14*) is used to remove large chunks of calculus that are easily accessible.
- The shank of the hoe may be slightly curved. It is used with a pull stroke while maintaining a ***two-point*** contact with the tooth surface.

Periodontal File

- Files are also used in pull strokes. Files also tend to scratch tooth surfaces they are therefore ***not*** preferred for SRP.
- A file's blade has a series of fine short hoes and can be used to remove supragingival calculus, overhanging dental restoration's margins, etc.

◂ *What is the main disadvantage of using a periodontal file?*

Polishing after SRP

- Polishing is done to remove light stains and ***smoothen*** tooth surfaces after SRP (*freshly scaled tooth surfaces get scratched during SRP; such rough surfaces encourage plaque retention*).
- Polishing can be done with a rubber cup, bristle brushes and polishing paste (*this creates progressively finer and finer scratches till a smooth surface is created*). Alternately, air polishing can be done by spraying abrasive particles (*sodium bicarbonate slurry*) using air pressure onto the tooth surface.
- If surfaces of teeth are visibly smooth and shiny, polishing may be ***avoided*** on such surfaces.

◂ *Is it essential to polish teeth every time after SRP?*

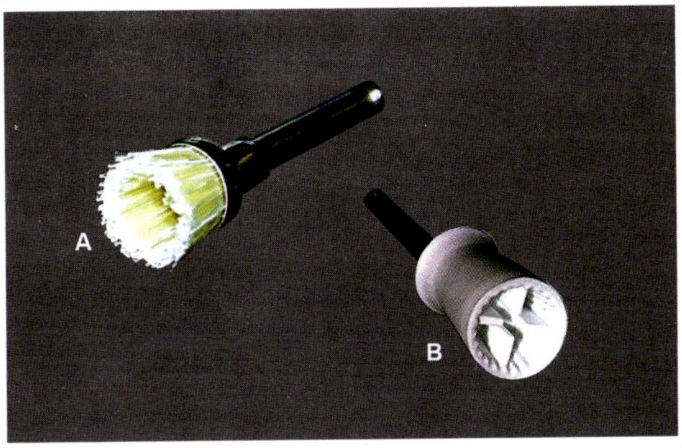

Fig. 14.11: Bristle brush (*A*) and rubber cup (*B*) can be used for polishing after SRP. When compared to rubber cups, bristle brushes are more abrasive and produce more heat during use.

Periodontal Surgical Instruments

Periodontal Knives

Kirkland and orban knives and BP blades are commonly used for periodontal surgery.

- Kirkland knife **(Fig. 14.12, diag. D)** has a ***kidney*** shaped blade which has a cutting edge across its entire periphery. It is primarily used in gingivectomy and gingivoplasty.
- Orban's **(Fig. 14.12, diag. C)** and Merrifield knives are ***spear*** shaped knives that have cutting edges on both sides of their blades. They are commonly used for interdental incisions during periodontal surgery. All these are multi-use knives and must be sharpened when they become blunt.
- BP blades #11, 12, 12d, 15, 15 c, etc. mounted over BP blade handle (*straight or angled*) are used for making incisions during periodontal surgery.

◂ *What is the shape of blade of Kirkland knife?*

◂ *What is the shape of blade of Orban's knife?*

Scissors and Tissue Nippers

Scissors are used in periodontal surgery to trim flaps, cut tissue, trim GTR membranes, remove sutures, etc. Goldman Fox, Iris, Castroviejo, etc. scissors are commonly used for periodontal surgery. Tissue nippers **(Fig. 14.12, diag. G)** are used to trim and reshape gingiva during gingivectomy and gingivoplasty.

Mucoperiosteal Elevators

These are used to elevate flaps, retract tissue, etc. (e.g. *mucoperiosteal elevators Goldman Fox, Molts*, etc.).

Surgical Chisels and Rongeur Forceps

Commonly used periodontal chisels like Ochsenbien chisels # 1–2 **(Fig. 14.13, diag. A)**, Todd-Gilmore chisels, etc. are used to remove and re-shape alveolar bone. Rongeur forceps are used to bite into and cut out small pieces of bone.

Surgical Files

Sugarman **(Fig. 14.13, diag. C)** and Schluger **(Fig. 14.13, diag. D)** periodontal files are used to smoothen rough bony ledges and remove bone for recontouring purposes.

Needle Holders and Tissue Holder

Needle holders are used to hold suture needles during suturing. Tissue holders are used to hold soft tissue during trimming and suturing.

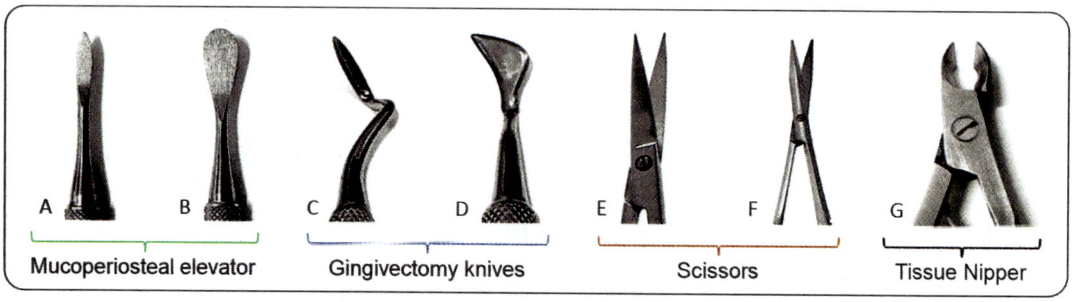

Fig. 14.12: Commonly used instruments for periodontal soft tissue surgery

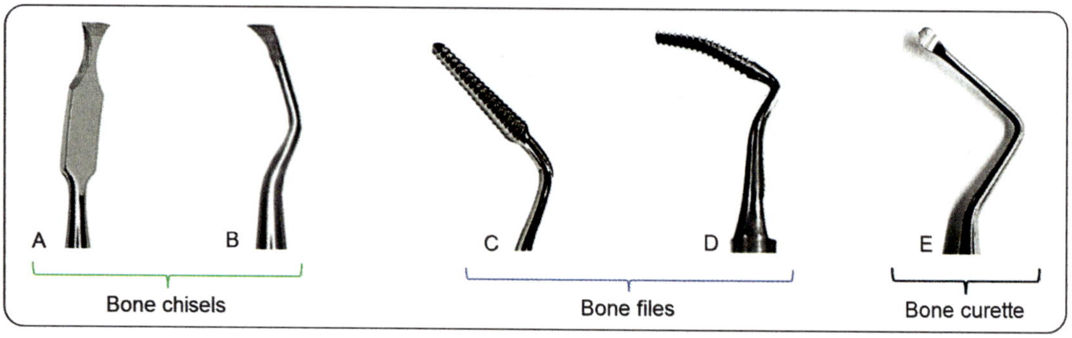

Fig. 14.13: Commonly used alveolar bone scrapping and reshaping instruments

Ultrasonic Scalers

What are ultrasonic scalers? ▶

Ultrasonic scalers are power driven scalers. In these, a scaling tip is attached to a handpiece and when switched on, the tip vibrates at an ultrasonic frequency. Tips of ultrasonic scalers vibrate at more than 20,000 cycles per second (*>20 kHz, more than human range of hearing, therefore ultrasonic*). ***Two*** types of ultrasonic scalers are commercially available: piezoelectric and magnetostrictive. Piezoelectric ultrasonic scalers are the ***more*** commonly available and preferred type.

Which type of ultrasonic scaler is preferred? ▶

Magnetostrictive Ultrasonic Scalers

- Handpiece of a magnetostrictive scaler has a shack of ferromagnetic materials with a scaling tip attached to it. When a magnetic field (*produced by **alternating** current in the handpiece of a magnetostrictive ultrasonic scaler*) is applied to this shack, it causes it to alternately change its size and then come back to normal repeatedly. This causes the scaling tip to move up and down with every change in dimension of the shack, (*more than 20,000 times per second*). Such an ultrasonically moving scaling tip is used for scaling.

- Magnetostrictive scalers usually operate at up to 45 kHz (*45,000 cycles per second*) and their scaling tips move in a ***semi-circular*** manner. Therefore ***side, back and front of the scaling tip can all be used for scaling***.
- Heat is produced due to friction between the scaling tip and tooth surface. A lot of ***heat*** is also produced ***within*** a working (*activated*) magnetostrictive handpiece. Constant and abundant spray of water (*coolant/irrigant*) is therefore required to cool the working tip area and handpiece during use. Water flowing on a working ultrasonic scaling tip also produces ***cavitation effect*** that ***adds*** to the scaling action of the scaling tip.

◂ *Which side of a magnetostrictive scaler's tip can be used for SRP?*

◂ *Why is constant spray of irrigant required during ultrasonic scaling?*

CLINICAL UTILITY AND SHORT ANSWER

What is cavitation effect?

Cavitation is formation of vapour cavities (*bubbles*) due to the movement of the ultrasonic tip in the water that is flowing over the working ultrasonic tip. These vapour cavities have lesser pressure within them as compared to the surrounding water. As a result, these vapour cavities collapse violently inwards (*implode*). This produces intense shock waves that physically dislodges soft deposits like food debris and plaque and also causes fractures in calculus making it easier to remove.

◂ *What is cavitation effect? How does it help during SRP?*

Piezoelectric Ultrasonic Scalers

- When an electrical field produced by an alternating current is applied to piezoelectric materials, it produces a change in their size repeatedly. If a scaling tip is mounted on a piezoelectric material insert in an ultrasonic scaler, it will move up and down when physical size of the piezoelectric material insert changes due to applied alternating current.
- Piezoelectric scaling units can operate up to 50 kHz (*50,000 cycles per second*) and their scaling tips move in a ***line*** like manner, i.e. in a ***linear fashion*** only. Therefore, only the ***two lateral*** sides of the scaling tip can be used for scaling and root planing. Positioning of the piezoelectric scaling tip relative to the tooth surface is consequently very important for this reason.
- Constant flow of water is required during their use to dissipate frictional heat and produce cavitation effect. Significant heat is ***not*** produced within piezoelectric scaling hand pieces.

◂ *Which side of a piezoelectric scaler's tip can be used for SRP?*

◂ *Is constant spray of irrigant required during ultrasonic scaling using piezoelectric scaling units?*

ALERT!

Two controls are available on *both magnetostrictive and piezoelectric* ultrasonic scaling units. These are:

1. **Power control:** This controls the amplitude of the scaling tip, i.e. the maximum distance the tip travels away from its rest position and therefore it controls the ***force*** at which the vibrating tip hits the tooth or calculus.
2. **Water flow control:** This controls ***amount*** of water (*coolant/irrigant*) that flows on the scaling tip. Water flow on the scaling tip acts like a lubricant, dissipates heat, is used for water lavage and produces cavitation effect.

CLINICAL UTILITY AND SHORT ANSWER

Why is it important to have a constant flow of water* (coolant) *during ultrasonic scaling?

It is ***not*** possible to perform ultrasonic scaling without a steady stream of water flowing on the scaler tip (*through the scaler's hand piece*). This water flow:

1. Dissipates heat (*frictional heat produced by scaling tip working on the tooth surface and heat generated in the magnetostrictive handpiece; no heat is produced in a piezoelectric handpiece*).
2. Acts like a lubricant making scaling smoother.
3. Flushes out microorganisms, plaque and soft debris from the site (***water lavage***).
4. Ultrasonically vibrating tip produces cavitation effect in water. Cavitation effect works in addition to and ***increases*** the mechanical scaling force of the scaling tip insert. It also has the capacity to ***break*** bacterial cell walls leading to their death.

◂ *What is the effect of cavitation on plaque bacteria?*

Advantages of ultrasonic scalers

What are the advantages of ultrasonic scalers?

1. Scaling and root planing can be done with relative ***ease*** (*especially in hard-to-reach areas*) and with more ***speed***. This reduces chair time, ***physical stress*** and ***strain*** on the patient and clinician.
2. Ultrasonic scaler tips (*inserts*) ***do not*** need sharpening. In fact, ultrasonic tips must be ***blunt*** and discarded if they become sharp. Sharp tips tend to localize ultrasonic energy and damage tooth surface.
3. Ultrasonic scalers disrupt plaque deposits both supra and sub-gingivally. Cavitation effect produced during ultrasonic scaling kills microorganisms and water lavage flushes out dead microorganisms from pockets.
4. Antiseptics can be added to the water that is being used as a coolant (*irrigant*). This allows chemical killing and control of plaque microorganisms.

Disadvantages of ultrasonic scalers

What is splatter and aerosol?

Why are splatter and aerosol health hazards?

1. **Production of contaminated splatter and aerosol:** During use, ultrasonic scalers produce a mist of droplets of water called ***splatter*** (*larger than 10 μ*) and ***aerosol*** (*smaller than 10 μ*) (Fig. 14.14). As these droplets bounce off oral surfaces, these water droplets pick up microorganisms present on these oral surfaces. These contaminated water droplets (*splatter and aerosol containing microorganisms*) spread in the vicinity of the work area and are a potential health hazard for the patient, clinician or any other person nearby. Aerosol being smaller and lighter, remains airborne for a long time, can travel longer distances and settle at farther places in a dental clinic. Communicable infectious diseases, e.g. COVID-19, HIV infection, common colds, etc. can be spread this way.

Why must SRP be checked thoroughly after ultrasonic scaling?

2. **Imperfect results:** Often ultrasonic scaling done alone does ***not*** produce a totally clean tooth surface, i.e. specks of calculus or necrotic cementum might be unintentionally left back after ultrasonic scaling. SRP must therefore be thoroughly checked and finished with hand instruments after ultrasonic scaling.
3. **Interference with working of some cardiac pacemakers:** Although newer models of pacemakers are safe, working of ***some*** older models of cardiac pacemakers may be affected due to the electromagnetic fields produced during working of an ultrasonic scaler. Piezoelectric scalers are believed to be generally ***safer*** than magnetostrictive units in this regard.
4. **Scratching of surfaces:** Ultrasonic scaling tips tend to produce scratches on tooth or implant surfaces during use. This happens more commonly if a higher power setting is used for scaling.
5. **High coolant flow:** As high-water flow is required for ultrasonic scaling; it may lead to water pooling in the oral cavity. Some patients can gag and may find it difficult to breathe due to this water pooling in the mouth.
6. **Discomfort during scaling:** Mild-to-moderate dentinal ***hypersensitivity*** (*discomfort*) may be felt by some patients during ultrasonic scaling. Some patients also feel uncomfortable due to vibration of the working scaler tip and screeching noise produced during ultrasonic scaling.

Contraindications of use of ultrasonic scalers

Why must ultrasonic scalers not be used for scaling in patients suffering with communicable diseases?

1. Due to high risk of spread of disease-causing microorganisms, ultrasonic scalers ***must not be used*** in the following situations and patients:
   a. Patients suffering from communicable diseases, e.g. COVID-19, common cold, tuberculosis, AIDS, etc.
   b. Patients with pre-existing poor systemic health can get lung infections by their own oral bacteria after inhalation of contaminated aerosol produced during ultrasonic scaling. ***Immune compromised*** patients, e.g. those suffering from uncontrolled diabetes, leukaemia, AIDS, etc. and those on ***long-term*** immunity suppressing medications like steroids, cyclophosphamide, etc. are particularly susceptible.
2. As mouth breathers can get very uncomfortable during ultrasonic scaling due to pooling of water in their mouth and throat, ultrasonic scaling may be contraindicated in some such cases.

3. Ultrasonic scaling can cause scratches on implant abutments and surfaces of restorations, e.g. composites, porcelain crowns, laminates, etc. Their use is contraindicated on these surfaces.
4. Ultrasonic scaling can cause 'debonding' of orthodontic brackets and permanent retainers, it must therefore be used with extreme care in patients undergoing active orthodontic treatment.

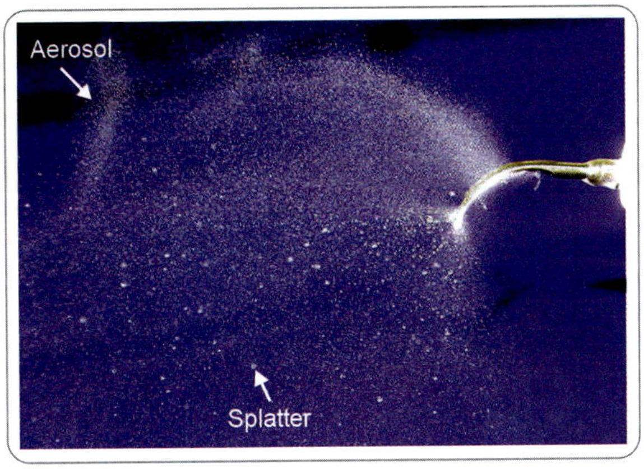

Fig. 14.14: Splatter and aerosol produced by a working ultrasonic tip

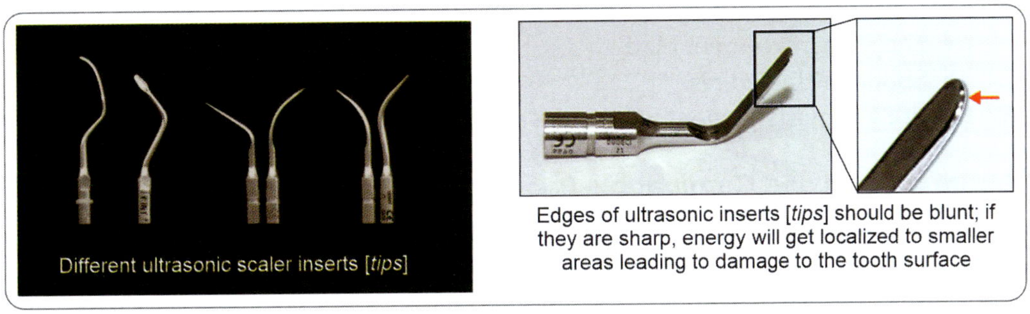

Fig. 14.15: Scaling tips (*inserts*) for ultrasonic (*piezoelectric*) scaler

Recommendations for obtaining best results with ultrasonic scalers

◂ *How can optimum results be used with ultrasonic scalers?*

1. Ultrasonic scalers must be used at the ***lowest*** possible power setting required to perform SRP.
2. Abundant water flow must be maintained on the working scaling tip.
3. Many scaling tip designs are available, the manufacturer recommended one must be selected for use on specific areas.
4. Ultrasonic scaling tips must be used in ***short*** and ***light*** back and forth strokes and must be ***constantly moved*** during use.
5. The tip of the ultrasonic scaling insert must ***not*** be used at 90° angle to the tooth surface (*this will damage the tooth surface*). Ideally, the working scaling tip surface (*in contact with the tooth*) must be almost ***parallel*** to the tooth surface (Fig. 16.2).

   ◂ *How must the ultrasonic insert be positioned on the tooth surface for SRP?*
6. Tips used for ultrasonic scaling must be in good shape and ***blunt*** (Fig. 14.15).
7. Use of barriers like masks, doctor's coats (*overalls*) for protection and covering/ maintaining disinfection of operatory surfaces are essential.
8. Scaling must be rechecked and if required, completed with hand instruments after ultrasonic scaling.
9. Water must be allowed to flow through the ultrasonic scaler for about two minutes before use. This reduces microbial contamination from biofilms that form on the walls of water tubing of the dental unit. Dental unit water lines must be disinfected repeatedly at recommended intervals.

   ◂ *Why must dental unit's water lines be flushed with water before every use?*
10. Ultrasonic scalers must not be used in patients with unshielded cardiac pacemakers (*most modern pacemakers are shielded against electrical interference*). Most research suggests

How can the clinician know that the cardiac pacemaker functioning is getting affected by ultrasonic scaler?

that piezoelectric ultrasonic scalers are safer for cardiac pacemakers. Symptoms of a cardiac pacemaker malfunction include: sudden difficulty in breathing, light-headedness, change in pulse rate, chest pain, prolonged hiccoughing, muscular twitching, etc.

PRINCIPLES OF PERIODONTAL INSTRUMENTATION

Appropriate position of clinician and patient, good visibility and well-maintained instruments are essential for adequate periodontal instrumentation. A clinician must also have good knowledge of instrument design, grasp/hold, adaptation, angle of application, hand stabilization and instrument activation to perform satisfactory instrumentation at all oral sites. There are ***four basic*** principles of periodontal instrumentation:

I. **Ensure a good and comfortable reach to the operating area:**
   - Position of patient
   - Position of clinician
   - Accessibility (*reach*)

II. **Ensure a good view of the operating field:**
   - Visibility
   - Illumination
   - Retraction
   - Maintaining a clean operating field

III. **Ensure instruments are in good condition:**
   - Shape of instrument blade
   - Sharp cutting edges

IV. **Ensure a firm instrument grip and a supported, steady working hand**

I. Ensure a Good and Comfortable Reach to the Operating Area

Position of clinician and patient and accessibility (*reach*) (Fig. 14.16).

Explain the ideal position of the clinician while working.

- Good accessibility to the operating site (*reach*) allows thorough instrumentation with ease and prevents clinician from getting tired early. It is attained by adequate patient and operator position.
- To be comfortable, the clinician must be seated with his/her feet resting ***flat*** on the floor and thighs are ***parallel*** to it. The clinician must be able to visualize the operating field while keeping his/her back straight and head erect.
- Clinician's arms should be held slightly away from the waist. The back of the dental unit should be reclined so that patient's back makes an angle of 30° to the floor.

What is the ideal height of a dental unit for periodontal treatment?

- Height of the dental unit should be adjusted so that the patient's mouth is at the same level as that of the clinician's ***elbow*** (*resting*). Head rest should be adjusted to make back of the patient's head and neck in the ***same*** plane (*preferably*). The head of the patient may then be tilted, chin raised or lowered as needed (*chin up position or chin down position*).
- Instrument tray can be positioned slightly above the patient (*seated on the dental chair*) to allow easy viewing and handling of the instruments placed on it.
- For easy maneuverability of clinician's and dental assistant's stools, ample space should be available around the dental unit on all sides (*at least 7 × 7 feet unrestricted rectangular floor area*).

II. Ensure a Good View of the Operating Field

Visibility, illumination, retraction and maintaining a clean operating field.

What is the difference between direct and indirect visibility and illumination?

- Work area may be viewed directly or indirectly (*looking at the site through a dental mirror*). Similarly, the working area may be illuminated directly or indirectly (*when light falls on working area after being reflected from a mouth mirror*). It is however **best** to work with direct vision and direct illumination.
- Retraction of cheeks and tongue is done by mouth mirrors, fingers of either or both working and non-working hand. Special retractors can also be used (*especially during*

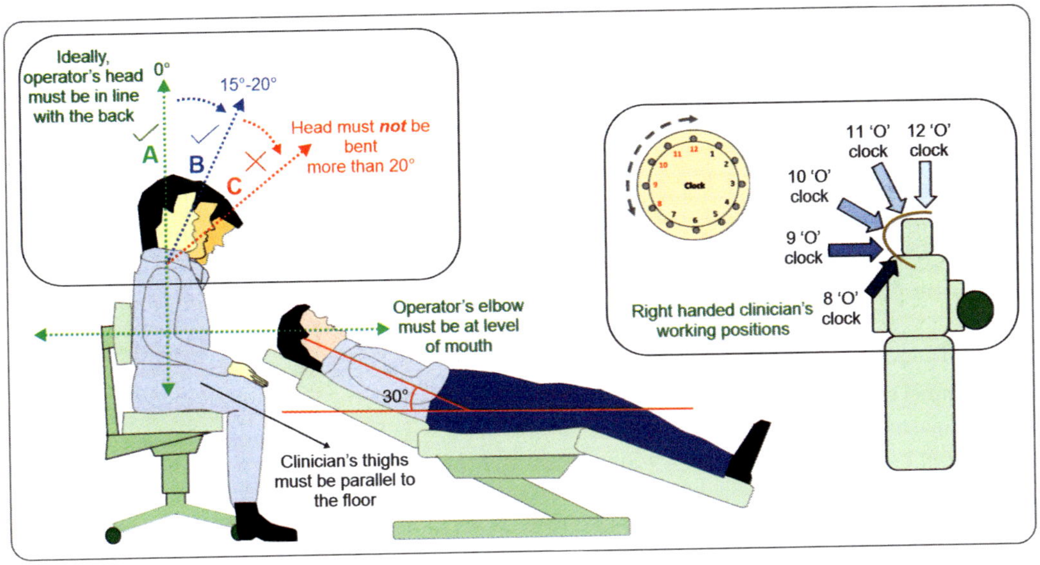

Fig. 14.16: Patient and clinician positions for comfortable periodontal instrumentation

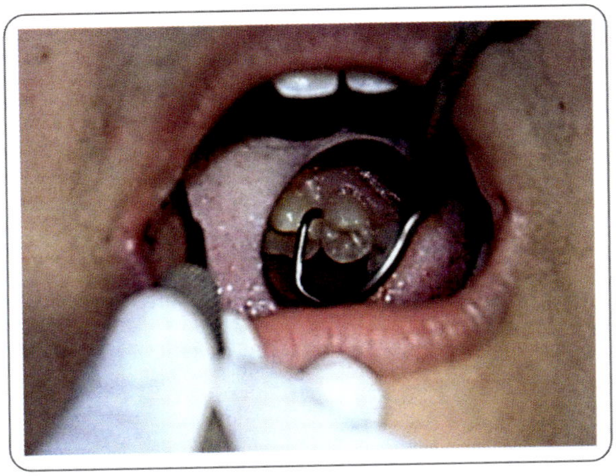

Fig. 14.17: Indirect illumination and visibility using a dental mirror

surgery). Retraction of cheeks and tongue helps attain accessibility, visibility, illumination and prevents injury to tissues surrounding the area of work.

- Adequate instrumentation of work area is impossible if operative field is covered with saliva, blood or debris (*these hinder visibility and make surfaces of teeth and instruments slippery thus reducing stability of finger rests and instrument grasp*). Therefore, adequate isolation of work area with cotton rolls, etc. and use of suction for clearing blood and pooled saliva is essential. Though not routinely advised, a stream of compressed air blown out of a three-way syringe can also be used with extreme ***caution*** to blow away blood and saliva from the work area (*doing so will also produce splashes and aerosol*).

◂ *Why is adequate retraction and maintenance of a clean operating field important?*

III. Ensure Instruments are in Good Condition

Shape of the instrument blade and its sharpness

- All-instruments will lose their shape and sharpness after repeated use or due to falls. Sharpening of dull/blunt instruments is essential but this has to be done carefully as sharpening done in an improper way can also de-shape the instrument blade.
- Instruments with de-shaped or dull/blunt blades (Fig. 14.19, diag. A) must not be used because:
  - More force is required to work with such instruments.
  - Increased working force decreases tactile sensitivity of the clinician and makes control of such instruments more difficult.

◂ *Why must dull/blunt instruments not be used?*

- This leads to improper instrumentation and poor results as dull and de-shaped scalers do not remove calculus completely.
- Calculus portions left back on the tooth surface after scaling with a dull instrument have a smooth surface (*caused by use of dull instruments*) which makes their identification and removal more difficult.
- Excessive force required for working with dull and de-shaped instruments may also result in ***sprains*** and ***injury*** in the ***clinician's fingers and wrist*** and ***carpal tunnel*** syndrome.
- Sterile sharpening stone must therefore always be available on the instrument tray during periodontal treatment.

ALERT!

Carpal tunnel syndrome (*CTS*)

What is carpal tunnel syndrome?

- The carpal tunnel is a tunnel like passage in the wrist through which nine ***flexor tendons*** and the ***median nerve*** run to the hand. The flexor tendons bend our wrist, while the median nerve provides sensation to thumb, index finger, middle finger and thumb side of the ring finger and palm.
- Any action or swelling that compresses the median nerve repeatedly and for a ***prolonged*** time can result in pain, numbness, tingling or weakness in the areas of the hand supplied by the median nerve. This is called the carpal tunnel syndrome (Fig. 14.18).
- Dentists are at ***high-risk*** of CTS.
- Clinical features of CTS include feeling of numbness in the thumb, first and middle fingers, burning and tingling sensation in the thumb side of the palm, upward radiating pain in the hand and tightening of the joints of the hand and the fingers leading to poor grip.
- To prevent CTS, the following are recommended:
  - Use ***minimum*** force while working.
  - Use instruments with good grip (*serrated and large diameter handles*).
  - Take frequent breaks and stretch hands regularly when working.

Periodontal Instrument Sharpening

What is periodontal instrument sharpening?

Definition: Grinding of surface that forms the edge of the blade till a fine and sharp cutting edge is created is called sharpening.

If the instrument blade has a sharp edge, it appears like a ***dull line*** that does ***not*** reflect light (Fig. 14.19, diag. B). If the instrument has become blunt, the cutting edge appears like a surface and starts to reflect light (Fig. 14.19, diag. A).

Evaluation of Sharpness of an Instrument Blade

How can we know whether cutting edge of an instrument is sharp?

There two ways of doing this:

1. **Visual:** The cutting edge of the instrument is examined in ***good*** light and preferably under a magnifying glass. Blunt cutting edges reflect light and appear ***shiny*** and ***rounded***. Sharp cutting edges appear dull and non-reflecting (Fig. 14.19).
2. **Test stick:** Test stick or a plastic saliva ejector is used for this. Instrument is held parallel to test stick or a plastic saliva ejector and its cutting edge is pressed against the stick and released. A sharp cutting edge will bite into the test stick or plastic saliva ejector and produce a metallic sound when it is disengaged. A blunt instrument edge glides over surface of the test stick or plastic saliva ejector and does not bite into it.

Sharpening of Periodontal Instruments

How many types of sharpening stones are used for sharpening periodontal instruments?

Sharpening of periodontal instruments is done using sharpening stones that may be hand held or rotary. Arkansas, or ceramic stones are used for this purpose.

Instrument sharpening methods

1. **Manual method**
   a. **Stationary stone method:** This is the most common method of instrument sharpening.
   b. **Rotary stone method:** This is faster than the stationary stone method but requires more *expertise*.
2. **Automated:** Several mechanical devices are available for sharpening periodontal instruments.

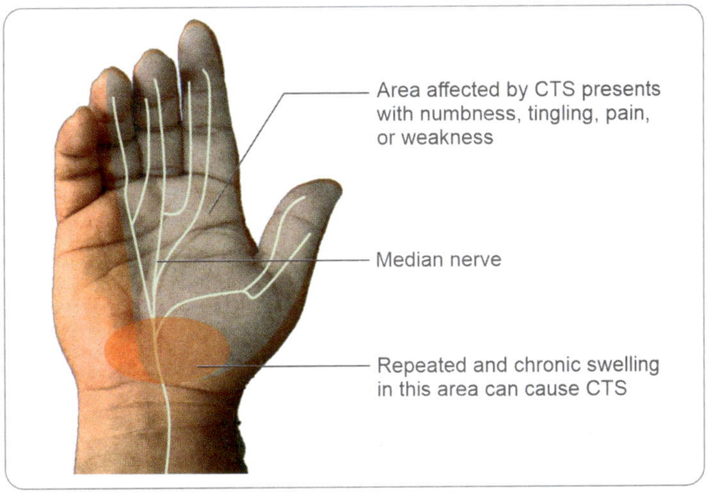

Fig. 14.18: Area of hand affected by carpal tunnel syndrome (*CTS*) (*blue shaded area*)

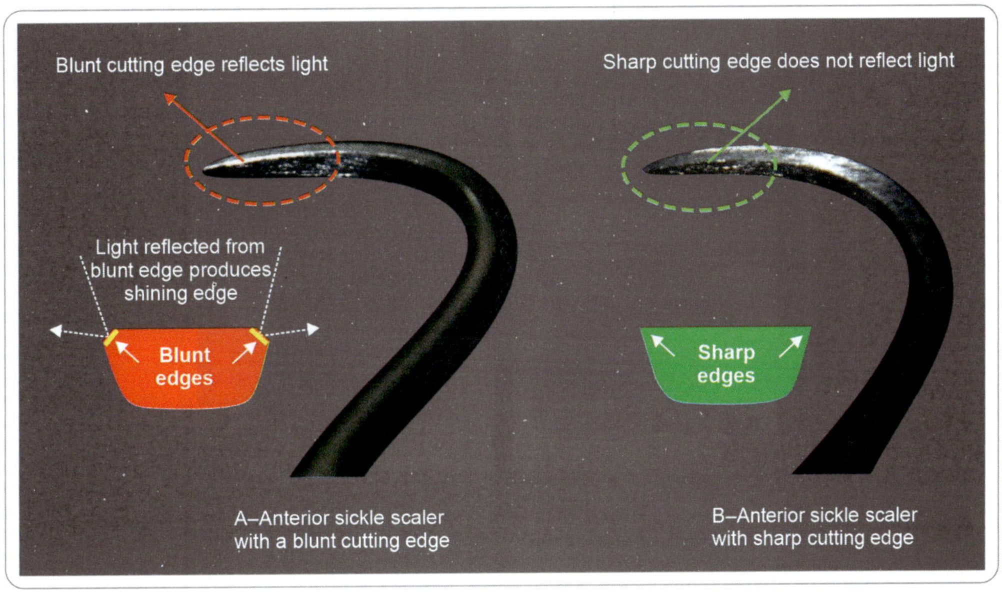

Fig. 14.19: Identification of sharp and blunt cutting edges

Sharpening with hand-held stone

1. Sharpening stone must be lubricated before sharpening.
2. Instrument is grasped with a firm grip in the ***non-dominating hand***, i.e. left hand for right-handed clinicians and vice-versa.
3. Instrument is held so that the terminal shank of the instrument is at 12 O′ clock position. The sharpening stone is held in the dominating hand in 1 O′ clock position and activated vertically (*moved*) in short to and fro motion with the ***entire*** arm making rhythmic strokes. (*left-handed clinicians should tilt the stone at 11 O′ clock position*).
4. Sharpening is ***started*** at the ***heel*** of the blade of the instrument.
5. To remove any flash of metal from the cutting edges, sharpening must be finished with a down stroke.
6. Only the ***lower*** cutting edge of a Gracey curette is sharpened.

◂ *How is an instrument sharpened using hand-held stone?*

◂ *Which cutting edge of the Gracey curette is sharpened?*

IV. Ensure a Firm Instrument Grip and a Supported, Steady Working Hand

Major factors affecting stability of the working hand and instruments are:

1. **Instrument grasp**
2. **Establishment of a fulcrum (*finger rest/palm rest*)**
3. **Instrument activation.**

◂ *Which factors affect stability of the working hand?*

Instrument Grasp

Which is the most commonly used instrument grasp?

What is modified pen grasp?

Why is modified pen grasp the preferred grasp for holding instruments?

- The most commonly used instrument grasp is ***modified pen grasp*** (Fig. 14.20). It is a modification of the way a pen is held when writing.
- To attain it, an instrument is first held in a pen grasp. Then, the middle finger is so positioned that side of its pad that is just adjacent to the fingernail rests on the instrument's shank. The first finger (*whose pad is resting on the instrument handle*) is then pulled back on the instrument handle so that the thumb lies between it and the middle finger.
- ***Modified pen grasp*** is the ***preferred*** instrument grasp because:
  i. A ***stable tripod*** is formed between fingers holding the instrument. This reduces uncontrolled rotation of the instrument during use.
  ii. It allows ***precise rolling*** of the instrument between the thumb, index and middle fingers.
  iii. It provides good tactile sensitivity.

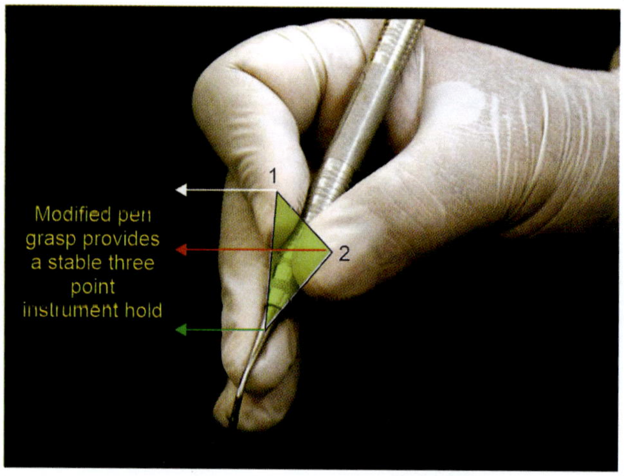

Fig. 14.20: The modified pen grasp

ALERT!

The ***palm and thumb*** grasp is a ***lesser*** commonly used grasp and is used only for sharpening instruments and holding three-way syringes.

Finger Rest—Palm Rest

The working hand should be stabilized and must ***not*** lift during instrumentation. To do this, a ***finger rest*** (*firmly resting fingers of the working hand on patient's face or teeth adjoining the areas where the instrument is being used*) is used.

Why is it important to establish a finger rest during SRP?

- The finger rest ***stabilizes*** the working hand and also serves as a ***fulcrum*** making the instrument easier to use (Fig. 14.21).
- Finger rest is most commonly established using the ***ring finger*** of the working hand.

How many types of rests can be made for SRP?

Finger rest or palm rest may be achieved in the following ways:

1. **Intra-oral rest**
   a. **Conventional:** Same arch—same side; rest is established on surfaces of teeth neighboring the area where work is to be done.

What is the difference between cross arch and opposite arch rests?

   b. **Cross arch:** Rest is established on one side of the arch to work on the other side of the same arch.
   c. **Opposite arch:** Rest is established on mandibular teeth to work on the maxillary teeth.
   d. **Finger on finger**: Index finger or thumb of non-operating hand is stabilized on teeth and finger rest is established over it. This improves the reach and the angle of approach of the instrument to certain areas.

2. **Extra-oral:** This is established by keeping fingers of the working hand on side of the patient's face. Extra oral rest can be:
   a. **Palm down**: Usually established on the left side of the patient's face (*by right-handed operator*) **(Fig. 14.22, diag. D,** red arrow).
   b. **Palm up:** Usually established on the right side of the patient's face (*by right-handed operator*) **(Fig. 14.22, diag. C,** green arrow).
3. **Reinforced:** Tip of the first finger or thumb of the non-operating hand is used to provide extra stability to the shank or handle of the instrument being used.

◂ *What are the usual places where palm up and palm down rests are established?*

◂ *What is reinforced finger rest?*

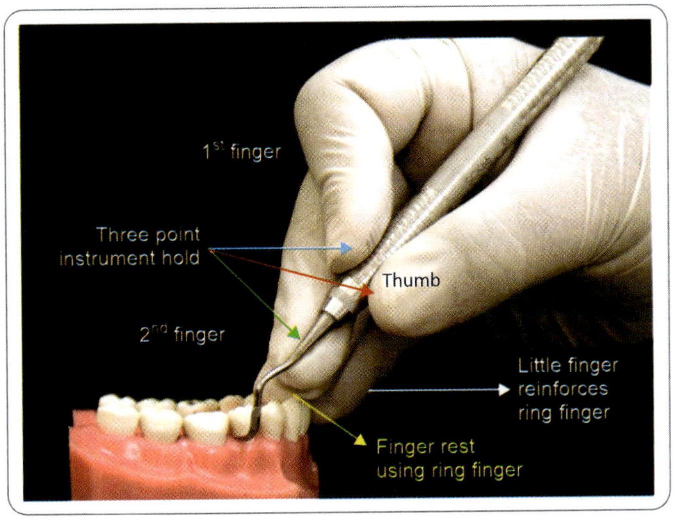

Fig. 14.21: Establishment of fulcrum/finger rest. The modified pen grasp allows good instrument grasp and stability during use. Finger rests allow establishment of fulcrum over which instrument movement can be done.

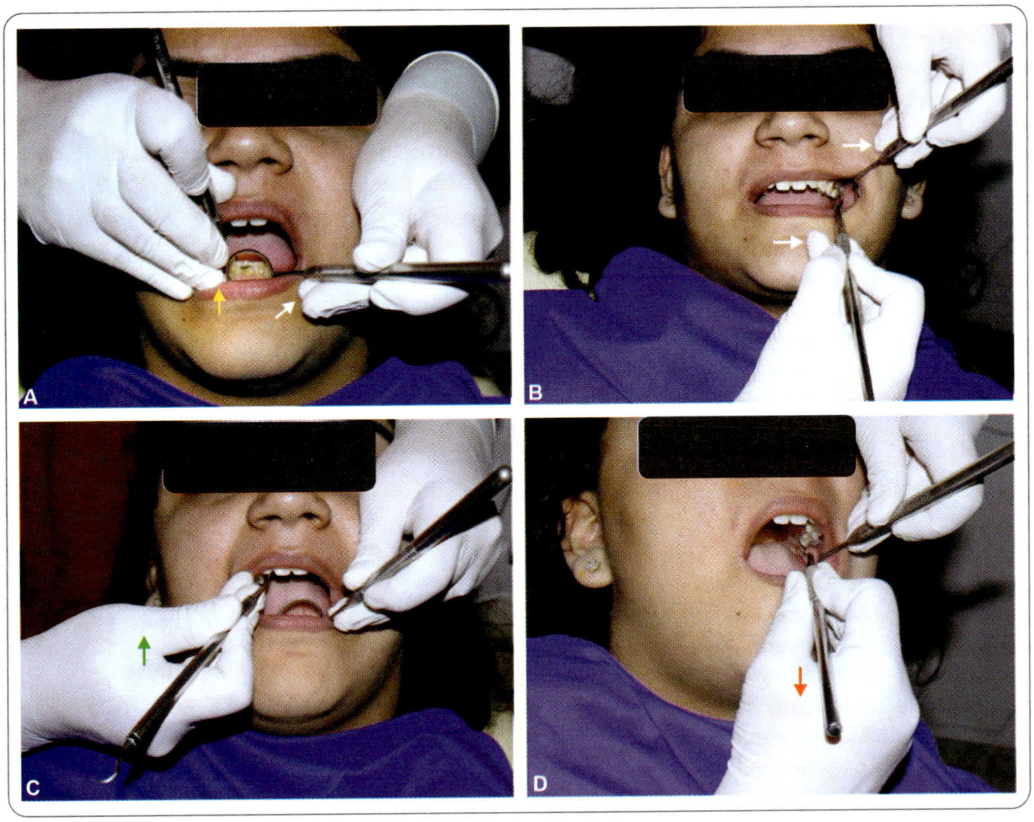

Fig. 14.22: Periodontal instrumentation using intra-oral finger rest (*diag. A, yellow arrow*), extra-oral finger rest (*diag. A and B, white arrows*), palm-up position (*diag. C, green arrow*) and palm-down position (*diag. D, red arrow*). Also note that clinician is holding instrument in modified pen grasp.

Instrument Activation

- **Adaptation**
- **Angulation**
- **Lateral pressure**
- **Strokes**

Adaptation: It is an act of adapting the working end of instrument on tooth surface.

- Good adaptation on different areas of tooth can be achieved by rolling handle of the instrument between index, middle finger and the thumb.

Which part of an instrument's blade must be adapted to the tooth surface during SRP and why? ▶

- ***Only*** the ***toe*** (*terminal end,* i.e. *lower 1/3rd of the working end*) of the blade of the instrument is used and is to be adapted **(Fig. 14.23, diag. A,** green marked area). If this is not done and middle part of the instrument is adapted to the tooth surface, the toe of the blade will project out, get lifted **(Fig. 14.23, diag. B)** and ***injure*** the adjacent gingiva and tooth surfaces during use causing pain and bleeding **(Fig. 14.23, diag. C)**.

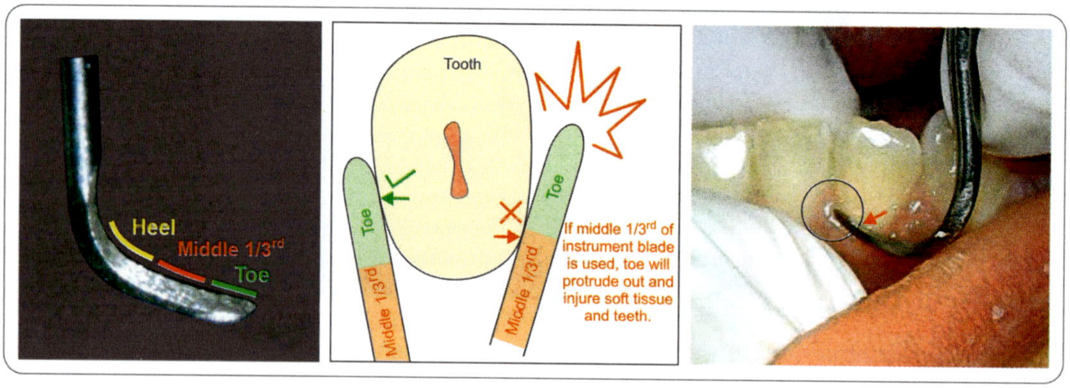

Fig. 14.23: Only the toe of the scaler or curette must be used for scaling and root planing (*diag. A and B green arrow*). If the middle part of the instrument blade is used, the toe will protrude out and injure gingiva and adjoining tooth during use (*diag. B and C, red arrow and black circle*).

Angulation: It refers to the angle at which face of blade of the instrument is brought in contact with tooth surface.

- Blade angle can be varied by tilting the lower shank away (*increases the tooth-blade angle*) or towards (*decreases the tooth-blade angle*) the tooth surface.

What is the insertion angle? ▶

- During insertion of a scaler or curette into the area of interest (*before activation*) face of the blade is maintained almost parallel to the tooth surface, i.e.; ***insertion angle is 0°*** **(Fig. 14.24, diag. A)**.

What is scaling and root planing angle? ▶

- Scaling and root planing angle should be between, ***45°–90°*** **(Fig. 14.24, diags A and B)**.

What is the preferred angle for removing hard calculus deposits? ▶

- If hard and tenacious calculus deposits are to be removed, instrument must be used at close to 90° angle.

Why is it important to ensure correct scaling angle before activating a scaler or curette during scaling? ▶

ALERT!

It is essential to establish correct tooth-blade angle for adequate scaling and root planing.

- A scaler or curette will ***not*** work properly if the tooth-blade angle is not between 45°–90°.
- If a smaller than 45° angle is made, instrument's blade will tend to glide over calculus and smoothen surface of the calculus.
- If greater than 90° angle is made, cutting edge of the instrument will lift away from the tooth surface and lateral surface of the blade will come in contact with the tooth surface. If instrument is activated at this faulty angulation, lateral surface of the blade will slip and glide over calculus and will not remove it. This way, the scaler will smoothen surface of the calculus.
- Such smoothened calculus is more difficult to detect and remove.

Name the types of strokes used for periodontal instrumentation. ▶

Lateral pressure and strokes: Pressure applied by the adapted blade of an instrument has not only to be adequate but it must also be ***varied*** continuously throughout the procedure. More lateral pressure is required for removing larger and tenacious calculus. Three types of strokes are used: ***exploratory, scaling and root planing stroke***.

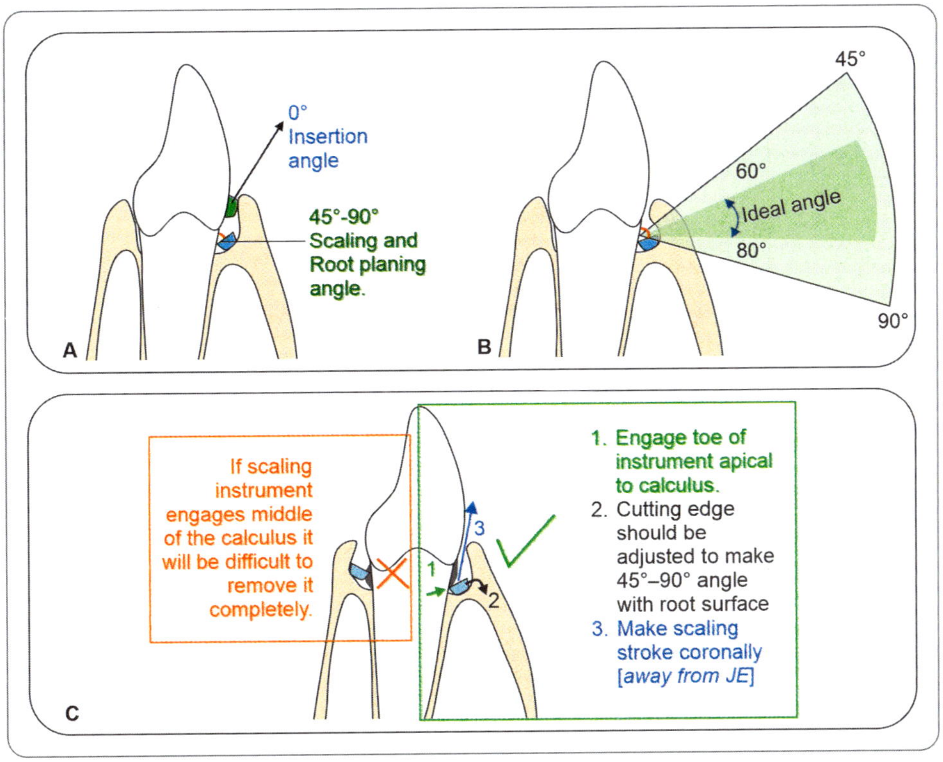

Fig. 14.24: For insertion, face of the blade of the instrument should be almost parallel to the tooth surface (*diag. A*). For scaling and root planing, face of the instrument should be at 45°–90° angle to the tooth surface (*diags A and B*), however, ideal scaling and root planing angle is between 60°–80° (*diag. B*). For scaling and root planing, instrument must be engaged apical to calculus, scaling angle attained and scaling stroke made coronally and away from the junctional epithelium (*diag. C*).

These strokes can be performed in ***horizontal, vertical*** or ***oblique*** directions. The pressure, direction, length and number of strokes required for SRP depend on nature of calculus, position of gingiva, dimensions of pocket, contour of the tooth surface, etc.

1. **Exploratory or assessment stroke:** This stroke is used to ***'feel'*** the working area. For this, the instrument is held lightly (*in a modified pen grasp*) and slowly moved across the tooth surface.

   ◄ *What is exploratory stroke?*

2. **Scaling stroke:** It is a ***'short'*** stroke made with a ***firm hand*** while applying adequate pressure and power **(Fig. 14.25)**.

   ◄ *How is a scaling stroke made?*

   - The wrist and the forearm must (*usually*) move as a single unit over the finger rest (*fulcrum*).
   - Instrument must not be operated using only the fingers alone, however flexing of the fingers to rotate the instrument for better adaptation is done.
   - For scaling, cutting edge of the toe/tip of the scaling instrument is adapted ***just apical*** to the border of the calculus **(Figs. 14.23 and 14.24, C)**. The scaling stroke is so directed that calculus after being dislodged must come out in a coronal direction and must not impact into the gingiva.

3. **Root planing stroke:** Root planing strokes are a series of short, even, overlapping shaving strokes made with a ***'light'*** hand (*without applying too much force*) **(Fig. 14.25, diag. A)**. As the root surface becomes smoother, the lateral pressure on the instrument used for root planing is progressively reduced. As curettes have short, delicate and flexible blades they are the best suited instruments for root planing.

   ◄ *What is the difference between scaling and root planing strokes?*

Instrument and Operator Hand Positions for Periodontics

Clinicians can work on a particular area in ***several*** different but correct and equally suitable work positions. There is ***no*** 'one and only' correct position for working on a particular area. The undermentioned guidelines are for a ***right-handed*** operator, i.e. clinician is seated on

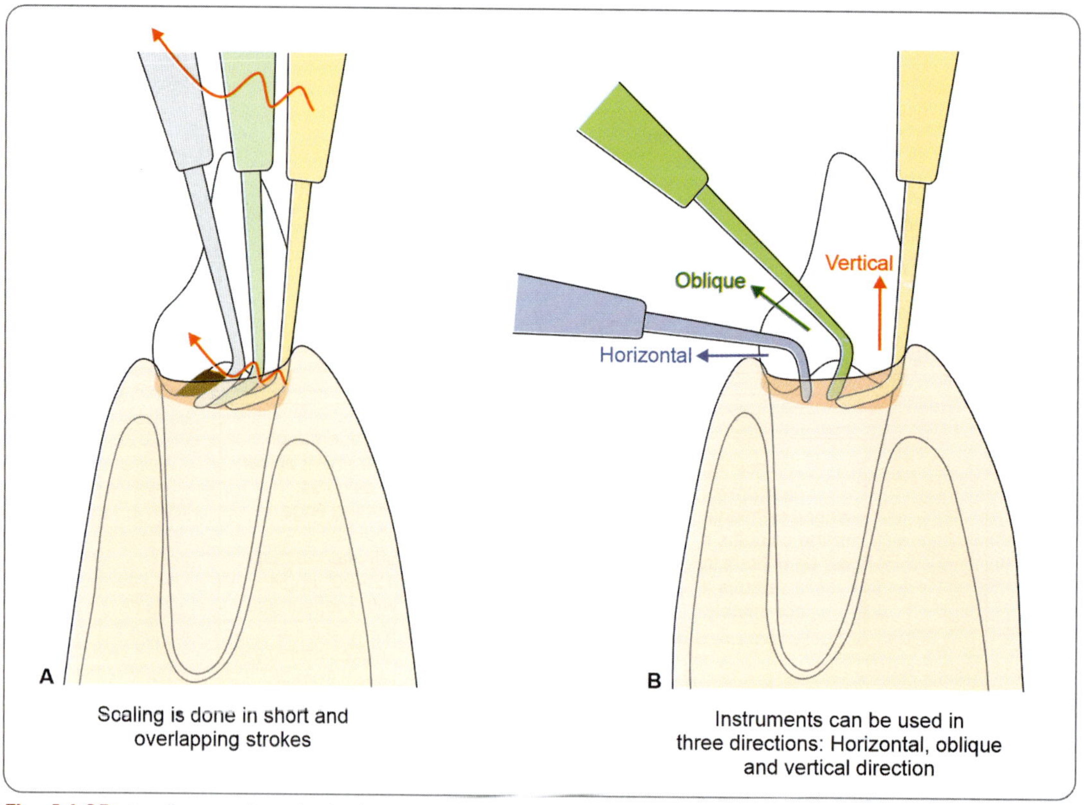

Fig. 14.25: Scaling and root planing must be done in a series of short and overlapping strokes with instruments used in horizontal, oblique or vertical direction during periodontal instrumentation.

patient's right side (Fig. 14.16). Clinician can make minor modifications in work positions according to their convenience and comfort.

1. Buccal Aspect of Right Maxillary Posterior Region (First Sextant)

a. **Patient's position:** Back of dental unit reclined at 30°. Patient's head facing straight or slightly to the left.
b. **Clinician's position:** 8 O' clock–9 O' clock position.
c. **Illumination:** Direct for all buccal and mesial surfaces of teeth. Indirect for distal surfaces of teeth (*easier if using a double surface mirror*).
d. **Visibility:** Direct for mesial and buccal surfaces. Indirect for distal surfaces of teeth (*easier if using a double surface mirror*).
e. **Retraction of cheek:** With mirror ***or*** first finger of non-working hand for pre-molars and mesial surface of first molar (*under direct illumination and visibility*).
f. **Hand position and Finger rest:** Palm down hand position, intra oral finger rest on right mandibular incisors-canine area.
g. **Instrument reinforcement:** If required handle and shank of instrument can be reinforced with thumb of non-working hand.

2. Palatal Aspect of Right Maxillary Posterior Region (First Sextant)

a. **Patient's position:** Back of dental unit reclined at 30°. Patient's head turned to the right and in chin-up position.
b. **Clinician's position:** 8 O' clock–9 O' clock position.
c. **Illumination:** Direct for all buccal and mesial surfaces of teeth. Indirect for distal surfaces of teeth.
d. **Visibility:** Direct for mesial and buccal surfaces. Indirect for distal surfaces of teeth.
e. **Retraction of tongue:** With mirror.

f. **Hand position and Finger rest:** Palm down hand position, intra oral finger rest established on mandibular incisor-canine region.

g. **Instrument reinforcement:** If required handle and shank of instrument can be reinforced with thumb or index finger of non-working hand.

3. *Buccal Aspect Maxillary Anterior Region (Second Sextant)*

a. **Patient's position:**

   i. Back of dental unit reclined at less than 30°. When working from the 8 O' clock–9 O' clock position, patient's head turned to the right for working on patient's left side's teeth and patient's head turned to the left for working on patient's right side's teeth.

   ii. Patient's head is in straight position if working from 12 O' clock position.

b. **Clinician's position:** 8 O' clock–9 O' clock position ***or*** 12 O' clock position.

c. **Illumination:** Direct.

d. **Visibility:** Direct.

e. **Retraction of upper lip:** Mirror ***or*** first finger of non-working hand.

f. **Hand position and Finger rest**

   i. If working from 8 O' clock–9 O' clock position, palm-down hand position, intra oral finger rest established on adjacent maxillary teeth's buccal surfaces or on mandibular incisors.

   ii. If working from 12 O' clock position, palm-up hand position, intra oral finger rest established on maxillary incisors-canine incisal surfaces or extra orally on right side of mandible.

g. **Instrument reinforcement:** When working from 8 O' clock–9 O' clock position, handle and or shank of instrument may be reinforced with thumb of non-working hand.

4. *Palatal Aspect Maxillary Anterior Region (Second Sextant)*

a. **Patient's position:** Back of dental unit reclined at 30°. Patient's head facing straight or turned to the left or right as convenient and in chin up position.

b. **Clinician's position:** 10 O' clock position ***or*** 12 O' clock position.

c. **Illumination:** Indirect.

d. **Visibility:** Indirect.

e. **Retraction of lips and tongue:** Not required.

f. **Hand position and Finger rest:** Palm up hand position, intra oral finger rest established on occlusal surfaces of right maxillary teeth.

5. *Buccal Aspect of Left Maxillary Posterior Region (Third Sextant)*

a. **Patient's position:** Back of dental unit reclined at 30°. Patient's head turned to the right and in chin up position.

b. **Clinician's position:** 8 O' clock–9 O' clock position.

c. **Illumination:** Direct for all buccal and mesial surfaces of teeth and indirect for distal surfaces (*easier if using a double surface mirror*).

d. **Visibility:** Direct for mesial and buccal surfaces and indirect for distal surfaces of teeth (*easier if using a double surface mirror*).

e. **Retraction of cheek:** Mirror or with first finger of non-working hand.

f. **Hand position and Finger rest:** Palm-down hand position, intra oral opposite arch finger rest established on left mandibular incisors and premolars.

g. **Instrument reinforcement:** Handle or shank of instrument may be reinforced with thumb or index finger of non-working hand.

6. *Palatal Aspect of Left Maxillary Posterior Region (Third Sextant)*

a. **Patient's position:** Back of dental unit reclined at 30°. Patient's head facing straight or turned slightly to the left and in chin up position.

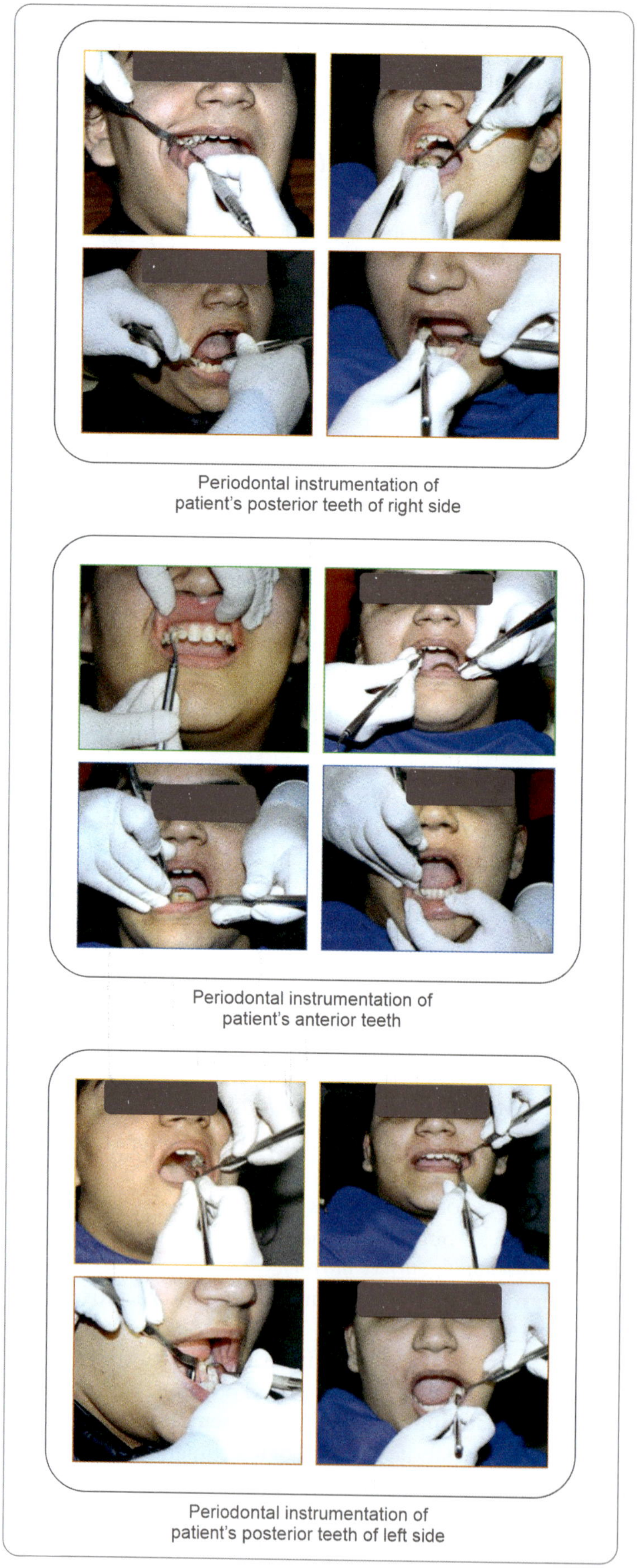

Fig. 14.26: Operator hand and instrument positions for periodontal instrumentation of different areas of the mouth

b. **Clinician's position:** 8 O' clock–9 O' clock position.
c. **Illumination:** Direct for all buccal and mesial surfaces of teeth and indirect for distal surfaces.
d. **Visibility:** Direct for mesial and buccal surfaces and indirect for distal surfaces of teeth.
e. **Retraction of cheek:** Not required.
f. **Hand position and Finger rest:** Palm down hand position, intra oral opposite arch finger rest established on mandibular incisors ***or*** left canine and 1st pre-molar region ***or*** on the right side of the patient's lower face.
g. **Instrument reinforcement:** Handle and shank of instrument may be reinforced with thumb or index finger of non-working hand.

7. *Buccal Aspect of Left Mandibular Posterior Region (Fourth Sextant)*

a. **Patient's position:** Back of dental unit reclined at around 30°. Patient's head turned to the right.
b. **Clinician's position:** 8 O' clock–9 O' clock position.
c. **Illumination:** Direct for all buccal and mesial surfaces and indirect for distal surfaces of teeth (*easier if using a double surface mirror*).
d. **Visibility:** Direct for mesial and buccal surfaces and indirect for distal surfaces of teeth (*easier if using a double surface mirror*).
e. **Retraction of cheek:** With a mirror.
f. **Hand position and Finger rest:** Palm-down hand position, intra oral same arch finger rest established on mandibular left canine or premolars.

8. *Lingual Aspect of Left Mandibular Posterior Region (Fourth Sextant)*

a. **Patient's position:** Back of dental unit reclined at around 30°. Patient's head facing straight or turned slightly to the left.
b. **Clinician's position:** 8 O' clock–9 O' clock position.
c. **Illumination:** Direct for all buccal and mesial surfaces and indirect for distal surfaces of teeth, (*easier if using a double surface mirror*).
d. **Visibility:** Direct for mesial and buccal surfaces and indirect for distal surfaces of teeth, (*easier if using a double surface mirror*).
e. **Retraction of tongue:** With a mirror.
f. **Hand position and Finger rest:** Palm-down hand position, intra oral same arch finger rest established on mandibular left canine and premolars.

9. *Buccal Aspect of Mandibular Anterior Region (Fifth Sextant)*

a. **Patient's position:** Back of dental unit reclined at around 30°–40° Patient's head facing straight.
b. **Clinician's position:** 8 O' clock–9 O' clock position (*dental unit's back may be slightly straightened for easier access*) ***or*** 12 O' clock position.
c. **Illumination:** Direct.
d. **Visibility:** Direct.
e. **Retraction of lower lip:** Index finger or thumb of non-working hand.
f. **Hand position and Finger rest:**
   i. If working from the 8 O' clock–9 O' clock position, palm-down hand position with intra oral finger rest established on mandibular anteriors or left canine or premolars.
   ii. When working from 12 O' clock position, palm-up hand position with same arch intra oral finger rest established on facial and/or incisal surfaces of mandibular anterior teeth or occlusal surfaces of right mandibular premolars.

10. *Lingual Aspect of Mandibular Anterior Region (Fifth Sextant)*

a. **Patient's position:** Back of dental unit reclined at around 30° and patient's head facing straight and in chin down position.
b. **Clinician's position:** 8 O' clock–9 O' clock position ***or*** 12 O' clock position.
c. **Illumination:** Indirect.
d. **Visibility:** Indirect when working from 8 O' clock–9 O' clock position; direct and indirect when working from 12 O' clock position
e. **Retraction of tongue:** With mirror.
f. **Hand position and Finger rest:**
   i. If working from 8 O' clock–9 O' clock position, palm-down hand position with intra oral same arch finger rest established on mandibular anteriors or left canine and premolars.
   ii. When working from 12 O' clock position, palm-down hand position with same arch intra oral finger rest established on facial or incisal surfaces of mandibular anterior teeth or occlusal surfaces of right mandibular premolars.

11. *Buccal Aspect of Right Mandibular Posterior Region (Sixth Sextant)*

a. **Patient's position:** Back of dental unit reclined at around 30° and patient's head facing straight or turned slightly to the left.
b. **Clinician's position:** 8 O' clock–9 O' clock position.
c. **Illumination:** Direct for all buccal and mesial surfaces of teeth and indirect for distal surfaces, (*easier if using a double surface mirror*).
d. **Visibility:** Direct for mesial and buccal surfaces and indirect for distal surfaces (*easier if using a double surface mirror*).
e. **Retraction of cheek:** Mirror ***or*** first finger of non-working hand.
f. **Hand position and Finger rest:** Palm-down hand position, same arch intra oral finger rest established on buccal or incisal surfaces of mandibular incisors or right canine.

12. *Lingual Aspect of Right Mandibular Posterior Region's (Sixth Sextant)*

a. **Patient's position:** Back of dental unit reclined at around 30° and patient's head facing straight or turned slightly to the right.
b. **Clinician's position:** 8 O' clock–9 O' clock position.
c. **Illumination:** Indirect (*easier if using a double surface mirror*). Direct if tongue retraction is adequate (*only for pre-molar region*).
d. **Visibility:** Indirect, (*easier if using a double surface mirror*). Direct if tongue retraction is adequate (*only for pre-molar region*).
e. **Retraction of tongue:** With mirror.
f. **Hand position and Finger rest:** Palm-down hand position, same arch intra oral finger rest established on buccal or incisal surfaces of mandibular incisors or left canine.

Review Questions

1. Classify periodontal instruments. What are the parts of periodontal instrument?
2. What is the difference between a periodontal probe and a dental explorer?
3. Which instruments are used for scaling and root planing? Describe a sickle scaler.
4. What is a dental mirror? What are its uses?
5. How are curettes different from scalers? How are universal curettes different from Gracey curettes?
6. Name some commonly used periodontal surgical instruments.
7. What are ultrasonic scalers?
8. What are the advantages, disadvantages and precautions that must be taken during use of ultrasonic scalers?

9. What is the difference between splatter and aerosol?
10. Why must tips of ultrasonic scalers be blunt rather than sharp as is the case with hand operated scalers and curettes?
11. What are the principles of periodontal instrumentation?
12. What is the difference between direct vision and indirect vision and direct illumination and indirect illumination?
13. How can the sharpness of a periodontal instrument blade be evaluated? Write a note on periodontal instrument sharpening.
14. Write note on the modified pen grasp.
15. Why is establishment of a fulcrum, finger rest and palm rest important during periodontal instrumentation?
16. Write a note on adaptation and angulation of scaling instruments. Why is maintaining a correct tooth-instrument blade angle important?
17. What are the different strokes used for periodontal instrumentation? Why is application of adequate lateral pressure on the instrument important?

Chapter

15

Mechanical and Chemotherapeutic Control of Plaque

Plaque forms on teeth and other oral surfaces within hours of its removal. Therefore, plaque must be removed frequently and repeatedly. Plaque can be controlled by removing it ***physically*** and by using ***chemical*** plaque control agents (*mouth-wash*). Effectiveness of plaque control can be assessed in two ways:

How can plaque deposits be identified? ▶

1. **Plain visual inspection of teeth for plaque deposits plaque:** As plaque is almost of the same colour as the teeth, it is ***difficult*** to see and identify plaque in this manner.
2. **Visual inspection after disclosing (*staining*) plaque:** After staining, plaque deposits can be identified easily. Showing disclosed plaque is a very effective tool for educating and motivating an individual for improving plaque control (Fig. 15.1).

CLINICAL UTILITY AND SHORT ANSWER

What are plaque disclosing solutions?

Plaque disclosing solutions contain dyes or colouring agents. They colour plaque (*and also calculus, food debris and soft tissue surfaces*). Commonly used disclosing agents are: Erythrosin (*FDC Red No. 3/ no. 28*), basic fuschin, FDC red no. 3 and FDC green no. 3 (*two tone dye-stains older plaque blue and younger plaque pink*), etc.

What is plaque control? ▶

Definition: Physical removal of oral plaque biofilm and using medicaments to prevent its formation on teeth and other oral surfaces is called plaque control.

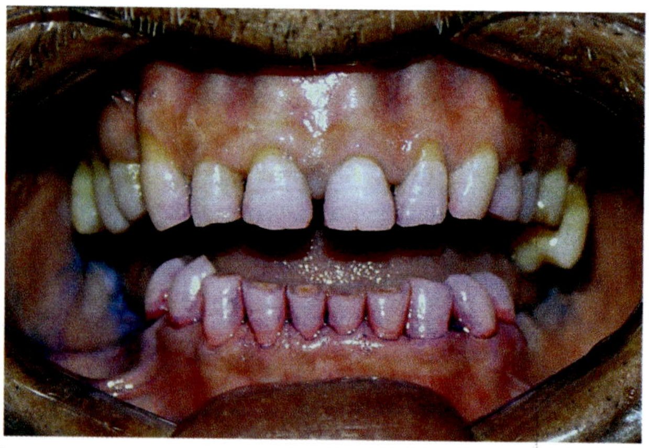

Fig. 15.1: Disclosed plaque (*lower arch*)

Name some devices used for physical removal of plaque. ▶

COMMONLY USED DEVICES FOR PHYSICAL PLAQUE CONTROL

Plaque can be removed physically with tooth brush, interdental cleansing aids, dental floss, oral irrigation devices, etc.

Tooth Brush and Tooth Brushing Techniques

A tooth brush is a simple but very ***effective*** device for plaque control. Tooth brushes have been used since many centuries. Earlier (*early part of the 20th century*) only natural materials (*hair of animals, e.g. pigs, horses, etc.*) were used for making tooth brushes. Nowadays, man-made synthetic materials are used (*plastic handles and nylon bristles*).

- Tooth brushes of varying sizes and designs, different lengths, hardness and arrangement of bristles are available. Of the many commercially available tooth brush designs, ***no*** design has been proven to be markedly superior to others, i.e. as such, all tooth brush designs are almost ***equally effective*** in removing plaque and preventing plaque induced periodontal disease (*gingivitis and periodontitis*).
- It has also been shown that a tooth brush of particular model and make, ***that a patient likes*** (*because of its color, shape, size, ease of use, etc.*) is ***more likely*** to be used properly by that patient (*for effective plaque control*). Clinicians therefore often leave the choice of tooth brush to the patient provided that the tooth brush head is not very large.

◂ *Is it a must for a clinician to prescribe a particular design and make of tooth brush to the patient for its effective use by the patient?*

ALERT!

Many other alternate 'devices' (*to tooth brushes*) are also commonly used for cleaning teeth.

- Although tooth brushes are widely used, they are still ***not*** available to, afforded and preferred by a vast majority of the population.
- As an alternate, people use stems, roots, bark and leaves of medicinal plants for cleaning teeth, e.g. neem, babool, etc.
- One of the most commonly used part of medicinal plants is its stem. Tender and thin twigs (*stems*) called chewsticks (*datun*), usually 6–8 inches in length, are chewed at one end till the chewed end becomes frayed and starts to resemble a brush.
- The frayed twig end is then vigorously rubbed horizontally on the surfaces of teeth to physically clean them. In addition to providing physical cleaning, juices from these plants are known to have astringent and anti-plaque properties.

Parts of Toothbrush

A tooth brush has three parts **(Fig. 15.2)**:

1. **Handle:** It is that part of the tooth brush with which it is held. A tooth brush's handle is flexible, can be of different shapes, diameters and is usually approximately 6 inches in size. Handle design should allow a firm and secure grip of the tooth brush.
2. **Shank:** The part of a tooth brush that connects the handle to the brush head is called shank. Shanks of tooth brushes may be straight or curved. Some shanks are made relatively more flexible to allow the brush head to flex (*bend*) during use.
3. **Head:** Working end of the tooth brush is called its head. It has tufts of bristles in it. To reduce the possibility of gingival injury and abrasion of teeth, 'rounded' bristles are preferred than flat cut or roughly cut bristles. Bristles of tooth brushes can be of different hardness (*firmness*). Hardness of bristles is dependent on:
   a. Material of which the bristle is made.
   b. Diameter (*thickness*) of the bristle (*larger the diameter, harder will be bristle and vice versa*).
   c. Length of the bristle outside the body of the brush head (*short bristles are harder and vice versa*).
   d. Temperature at which the tooth brush is used. Higher temperature reduces firmness of bristles and vice versa.

   Thicker and shorter bristles are therefore harder and less flexible while thinner and longer bristles are softer and more flexible. Plaque removing capacity of softer bristles is lesser than that of harder bristles.

◂ *Name the parts of a toothbrush.*

◂ *What type of tooth brush handle is preferred?*

◂ *Why bristles with rounded bristle ends preferred?*

◂ *On what factors does the hardness of tooth brush bristles depend on?*

◂ *Can tooth brushing be done with hot water?*

CLINICAL UTILITY AND SHORT ANSWER

What are the diameters of soft, medium and hard toothbrush bristles?

Average diameter of bristles of a soft tooth brush is 0.007 inch (*0.2 mm*), medium tooth brush is 0.012 inch (*0.3 mm*) and hard tooth brush is 0.014 inch (*0.4 mm*).

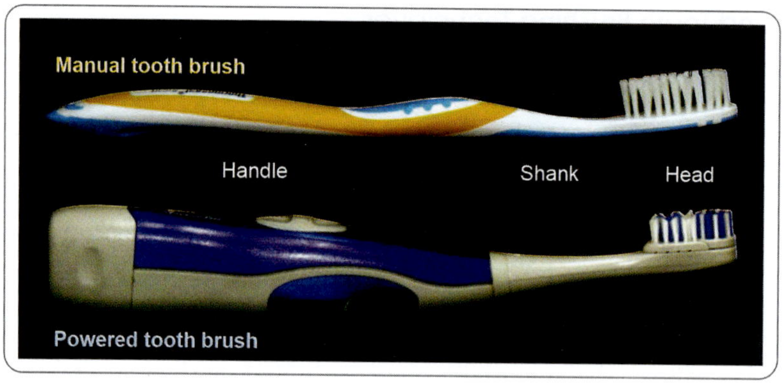

Fig. 15.2: Manual and powered tooth brush

Powered (Electrically Operated) Toothbrushes

Nowadays, powered tooth brushes are also available. Different powered tooth brushes differ in the type of movement of their heads; this movement may be circular, oscillating (*brush head rotates clockwise and counterclockwise alternately*), vibrating or combinations of these. Three types of powered tooth brushes are available:

What is the difference between a conventional electric and sonic tooth brush? ▶

1. **Powered conventional (*electric*) toothbrush**
   - It has a rotating or oscillating head that makes 2,500 to 7,500 strokes per minute and it relies on physical motion to clean teeth.
2. **Sonic tooth brush**
   - It also relies on physical motion to clean teeth but they vibrate at about 30,000 strokes per minute. As sonic toothbrushes move faster, they provide ***more*** mechanical cleaning power but may also cause more tooth abrasion.

How is an ultrasonic tooth brush different from a sonic tooth brush? ▶

3. **Ultrasonic tooth brush**
   - Ultrasonic tooth brushes ***do not*** rely on physical motion to clean teeth but produce ultrasonic waves at 20,000 Hz to remove plaque and kill bacteria.
   - Ultrasonic tooth brushes can clean teeth and pockets up to 5 mm (*by simply placing the brush on teeth*) but this cleaning efficiency is ***not*** 100%.

ALERT!

Tooth brush maintenance and its lifespan

When should a tooth brush be discarded? ▶

1. A tooth brush usually has 'useful lifespan' of a few ***weeks***. A toothbrush should be replaced once its bristles start to bend or start to get frayed at their ends (Fig. 15.3).
2. In general, tooth brushes with soft bristles have ***smaller*** lifespans whereas medium and hard tooth brushes have longer lifespans.
3. Physically or mentally challenged individuals are known to wear their tooth brushes faster.
4. A tooth brush ***harbors microorganisms***. It can therefore become a source of infection (e.g. *respiratory tract infections*) for its user. Patients with poor systemic health and low immunity are recommended to ***change*** their tooth brushes at ***shorter*** intervals and after every bout of respiratory tract infection.

Why must tooth brushes be stored in dry conditions? ▶

5. Tooth brushes must be washed under running tap water after every use and then ***dried*** in open air. If a tooth brush remains wet it will ***support growth of microorganisms on its surfaces***.
6. Tooth brushes should ***not*** be covered with covers (*even if they have holes*) as this will delay or even prevent complete drying.

How can tooth brushes act as a source of cross infection? ▶

7. To prevent cross infection, two individuals must never share tooth brushes and tooth brushes of two individuals must ***not contact*** each other during storage.

ALERT!

Studies have shown that:

Is tooth brushing with powered tooth brush better? ▶

- Most individuals will make up to ***300 strokes per minute when using a manual toothbrush***.
- Individuals using manual (*non-powered*) toothbrushes can maintain oral health and ***same degree*** of plaque control as individuals using as powered toothbrushes.

(*Contd.*)

(Contd.)

- Powered conventional (*electric*) tooth brushes are more likely to result in ***more abrasion*** of teeth than manual tooth brushes (Fig. 15.4).
- 'Poor' brushers, e.g. children, individuals with some handicap, old and sick individuals benefit more from using powered toothbrushes.
- Powered tooth brushes are not preferred by a vast majority of the population individuals as they are far more ***expensive*** than manual tooth brushes. Ultrasonic tooth brushes are more expensive than sonic tooth brushes.

◂ *What are the disadvantages of powered tooth brushes?*

◂ *Who can benefit more from use of powered tooth brush?*

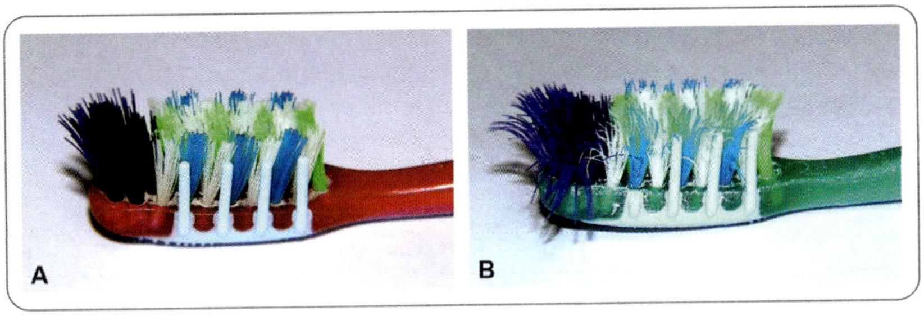

Fig. 15.3: Tooth brushes should be changed once their bristles get bent or damaged at their ends (*A*). Many individuals however continue to use tooth brushes much beyond their useful lifespan (*B*) due to ignorance and economic reasons. Damaged tooth brushes do not remove plaque effectively and injure gingiva during use.

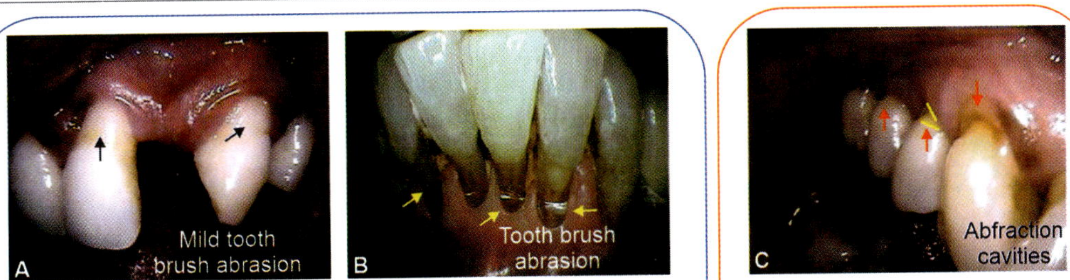

Gingival recession and mild abrasion in cervical areas of teeth due to tooth brushing. Note that surface is smooth and shining [*polished*]

Gingival recession and abrasion cavities in cervical areas of teeth due to tooth brushing. Note saucer shaped cavities have smooth and shinning surface and do not have well-defined margins

Gingival recession and abfraction cavities in cervical areas of teeth due to increased occlusal forces. Note wedgeshaped [*yellow marked area*] cavities well defined margins and unpolished surface.

Fig. 15.4: Vigorous tooth brushing using a hard tooth brush and relatively more abrasive tooth pastes or tooth powders can cause gingival recession and abrasion of teeth (*diag. A and B, arrows*). Such abrasions are usually found on buccal cervical areas of teeth (*roots*). As abrasion worsens, saucer shaped (*rounded*) cavities with polished surfaces form (*diag. B, yellow arrows*). Tooth brush abrasions must be differentiated from abfraction cavities that occur due to increased occlusal forces (*e.g. bruxism*). Abfraction cavities have relatively more well-defined margins, are wedge shaped (*Fig. C, yellow marked area*) and have unpolished and 'gritty' surfaces (*Fig. C, red arrows*).

CLINICAL UTILITY AND SHORT ANSWER

Is vigorous tooth brushing with hard tooth brushes more effective in removing plaque?

◂ *Why must hard tooth brushes not be used?*

No.

- It has been repeatedly found that individuals tend to do more harm when using hard tooth brushes vigorously.
- Brushing vigorously in a horizontal direction and use of very abrasive dentifrices (*tooth pastes*) can cause recession of gingiva and abrasions on surfaces of teeth (*especially buccal surface and cervical region, such surfaces are shining (polished)*) (Fig. 15.4).
- Brushing with a worn-out tooth brush (***that** has bent and frayed bristles*) (Fig. 15.3) is likely to cause more gingival injury and abrasion of teeth.

DENTIFRICES (*TOOTH PASTES AND TOOTH POWDERS*)

What is the composition of a tooth paste? ▶

A dentifrice is used for cleaning teeth (*as an abrasive cleaning agent*) after applying it on a toothbrush or some other applicator. Dentifrices contain detergents (*soaps*), abrasives, anti-plaque agents (*e.g. triclosan, etc.*), anti-caries agents (*e.g. sodium fluoride, etc.*), anti-tooth hypersensitivity agents (*e.g. stannous fluoride, potassium nitrate, etc.*), anti-calculus agents (*e.g. pyrophosphates*), water, humectants, flavoring, sweetening and colouring agents and preservatives.

ALERT!

How much tooth paste should be used every time for tooth brushing? ▶

- Abrasion of teeth occurs more because of abrasives in dentifrices rather than bristles of tooth brushes. ***More*** abrasion occurs on the ***maxillary*** more than on the mandibular teeth.
- As tooth powders are coarser, they are abrasive than tooth pastes.
- Only a small amount of tooth paste almost the size of a ***large pea*** is required for tooth brushing. If large amount of tooth paste is used, it will cause excessive foaming in the mouth; this reduces plaque removing capacity of a tooth brush.
- Excessive pressure while tooth brushing (*hard brushing*) can cause gingival abrasion and injury (*gingival ablations*) and increases abrasion of teeth (**Fig. 15.4**).
- Pressing too hard on a tooth brush while tooth brushing also causes bristles of the tooth brush bristles to over-bend. This brings sides of the bristles of the tooth brush in contact with the tooth brush (*rather than tips of the bristles*). This reduces plaque removing capacity of the tooth brush.

TOOTH BRUSHING METHODS

1. Scrub Technique

What is the scrub toothbrushing technique? ▶

In this method, teeth are brushed by moving the toothbrush over surfaces of teeth in a horizontal but random fashion. It is the simplest and most commonly used method of tooth brushing.

2. Modified Stillman Method (*Paul Stillman 1932*)

In which direction are the bristles placed in the modified Stillman method? ▶

How are teeth cleaning strokes made in the modified Stillman method? ▶

How are teeth cleaning strokes made on the occlusal surface in the modified Stillman method? ▶

How many teeth cleaning strokes are made with a tooth brush on a particular group of teeth in the modified Stillman method? ▶

- Toothbrush is placed on lateral surface of teeth in such a manner that it's bristles point in the ***apical*** direction (**Fig. 15.5, diag. A**) and half of its bristles rest on lateral surface teeth being brushed while the other half rest on the adjoining gingiva.
- For making a cleaning stroke, the tooth brush is moved coronally while ***simultaneously*** making short back and forth strokes (**Fig. 15.5, diag. A, 1 and 2**).
- For brushing occlusal surfaces, bristles of the toothbrush are positioned at right angles to the occlusal surface of posterior teeth. In this position, the brush is moved back and forth, ***without*** dislodging the bristles.
- Used this way, a tooth brush will cover 3–4 teeth at a time.
- After about 20 brushing strokes, the brush is lifted and placed over the next 3–4 teeth where tooth brushing sequence is repeated.

3. Modified Bass Technique (*Intrasulcular Method*) (*Charles Bass 1948*)

In which direction are the bristles placed in the modified Bass method? ▶

What makes the bristles enter and clean the sulcus when modified Bass method is used? ▶

How are the lingual surface of lower incisors cleaned in the modified Bass technique? ▶

How are the occlusal surfaces cleaned in the modified Bass technique? ▶

- Toothbrush head is positioned on the lateral surfaces of teeth in a manner that its bristles point in the ***apical*** direction and touch the lateral surface of teeth and gingiva making a 45° angle (**Fig. 15.5, diag. B**).
- Slight ***vibratory pressure*** exerted on bristle tips ***forces*** them ***into*** the ***interproximal embrasure*** and ***gingival sulcus*** and cleans these areas.
- The toothbrush is then moved back and forth making small vibratory movements ***without*** dislodging or lifting the bristles.
- On the lingual surface of lower teeth, if curve of the lower arch is too narrow, the brush is placed vertically with its bristles touching surfaces of teeth and moved out (*in the incisal direction*).
- For brushing occlusal surfaces, bristles of the toothbrush are positioned at right angles to the occlusal surface of posterior teeth. In this position the brush is moved back and forth, ***without*** dislodging the bristles.

- Used this way, a tooth brush will cover 3–4 teeth at a time. After about 20 brushing strokes, the brush is lifted and placed over the next 3-4 teeth where tooth brushing sequence is repeated.

◂ *How many tooth cleaning strokes are made with a tooth brush on a particular group of teeth in the modified Bass technique?*

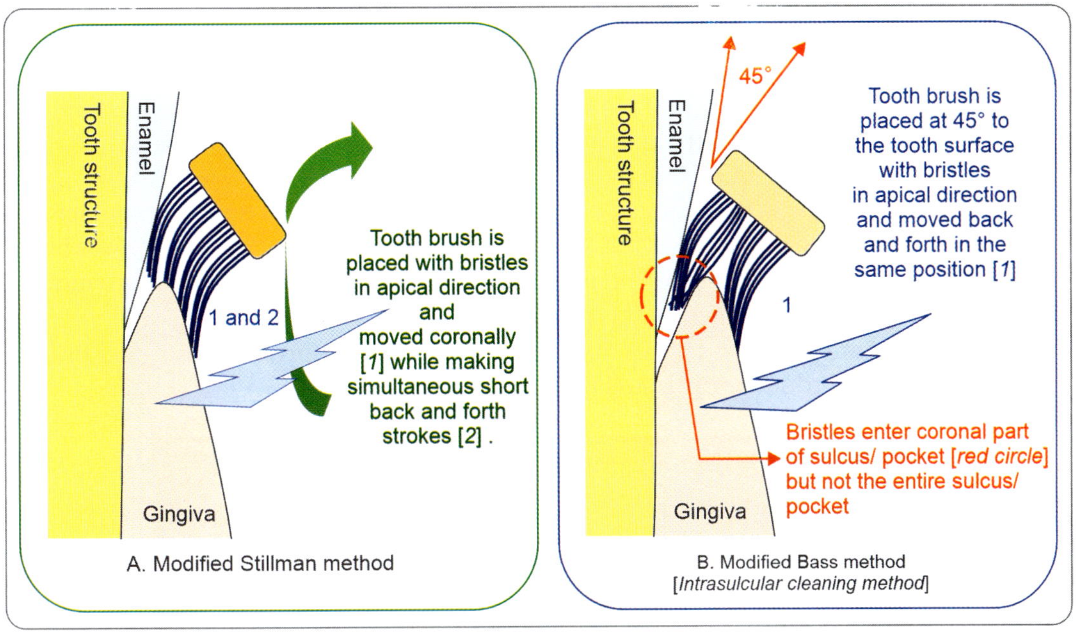

Fig. 15.5: Modified stillman and modified Bass method of tooth brushing

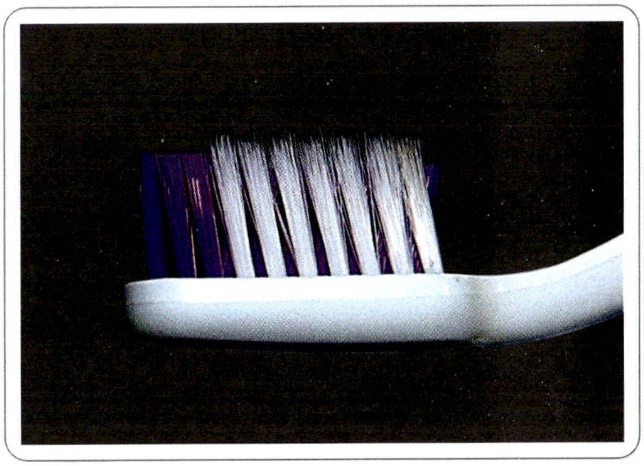

Fig. 15.6: Tooth brushes with extra fine and long bristles are designed to enter sulcus and perform intrasulcular cleaning (*to some extent*)

ALERT!

Patients must be taught to always brush their teeth ***sequentially*** by starting from posterior most teeth of one side of maxillary arch and continuing over to the other side. All surfaces of all teeth are brushed this way. After completing the maxillary arch, the same brushing sequence is repeated for the mandibular arch.

INTERDENTAL CLEANING AIDS

Interdental cleaning aids help in physically removing dental plaque from interdental areas that are otherwise inaccessible and hard to reach. Many interdental cleaning aids are available. Patient's dexterity and ability to use a particular interdental cleaning aid is one of the important factors in its selection for a particular patient. Commonly used interdental cleaning aids are: Dental floss, interdental brushes, wooden or plastic tips (*toothpicks*), conical rubber tips, etc. (Fig. 15.7).

◂ *What are interdental cleaning aids?*

◂ *Name some commonly used interdental aids.*

Dental Floss

What is dental floss? ▸

- Dental floss is available as a multifilament nylon yarn (*thread*) that may be twisted or non-twisted, waxed or un-waxed and thick or thin **(Fig. 15.7, diags A and B)**. It is used to clean interdental surfaces of teeth and interdental papilla.

How is a dental floss used? ▸

- To use, a floss thread 10–12 inches is taken and wrapped around the fingers, or tied in a loop.
- The floss is then stretched tightly between the thumb and forefinger of both hands and is slipped through the contact area of teeth with firm back-and-forth motion.
- The floss thread is then adapted to the proximal surface of the tooth being cleaned, apical to the contact point. It is then moved over proximal tooth surfaces up to the contact area and gently down into the sulcus again and over the interdental gingiva two or three times.
- After this, floss is removed in the opposite direction using firm sliding to and fro motion.
- The entire dentition is cleaned in this manner.
- Floss threaders are excellent devices that are used to pass floss thread easily under bridges and very tight interdental contacts **(Fig. 15.8)**.

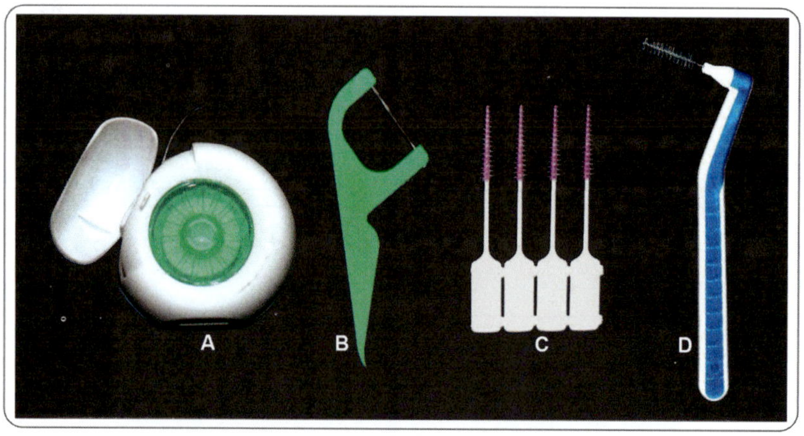

Fig. 15.7: Interdental cleaning aids. Floss (*A*), disposable flosser cum tooth pick with a pointed end that works as a tooth pick (*B*), conical rubber tips (*C*) and interproximal brush (*D*).

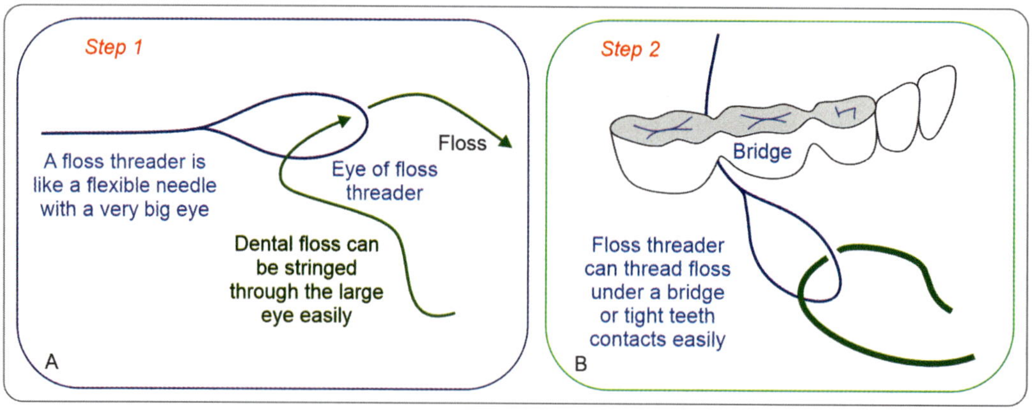

Fig. 15.8: Floss threader is used to thread floss under tight contacts and bridges. For this a 12 inches floss thread is first passed through the eye of the floss threader (*diag. A*). The floss threader with threaded floss is then passed under the tight interdental contact through the interdental space or under the bridge/appliance stiff end first (*diag. B*). Flossing is completed in the usual way and floss is then taken out.

ALERT!

1. All types of dental floss remove dental plaque equally well.
2. Floss must ***not*** be snapped past the contact point, rather it should only be slipped past it using a to and fro motion. Snapping the floss past the contact point will injure interdental gingiva.
3. Knitting yarn makes a very good ***substitute*** for floss. It can clean ***wide*** interdental spaces very effectively.

Interproximal Brush

- An interproximal toothbrush is a round mini toothbrush (*it looks like a small bottle brush*) that is used to clean ***interdental spaces, interdental surfaces*** (*proximal surfaces of adjoining teeth and interdental gingiva*) and ***furcation areas*** of multirooted teeth.
- It is inserted into the interdental space or furcation and moved to and fro horizontally using short in and out strokes.
- Interdental brushes are available in different shapes and sizes and are either made of twisted wire with nylon bristles inserted into it or only of a single small tuft of nylon bristles.

◄ *What is an interdental brush? How is it used?*

CLINICAL UTILITY AND SHORT ANSWER

In some situations, an interdental brush can clean the interdental space better than a dental floss.

If the proximal surface has a concavity in its surface, a floss thread will stretch over the edges of the concavity **(Fig. 15.9, diag. A, 2, red line)** without touching the depth of the concavity leaving such areas uncleaned. Interdental brushes can very efficiently clean such concavities in the proximal tooth surface **(Fig. 15.9, diag. B, 2, green line)**. Interdental brushes are also very efficient in cleaning tooth/implant abutments and under pontics of bridges.

◄ *Is floss suitable for cleaning all interdental spaces and surfaces?*

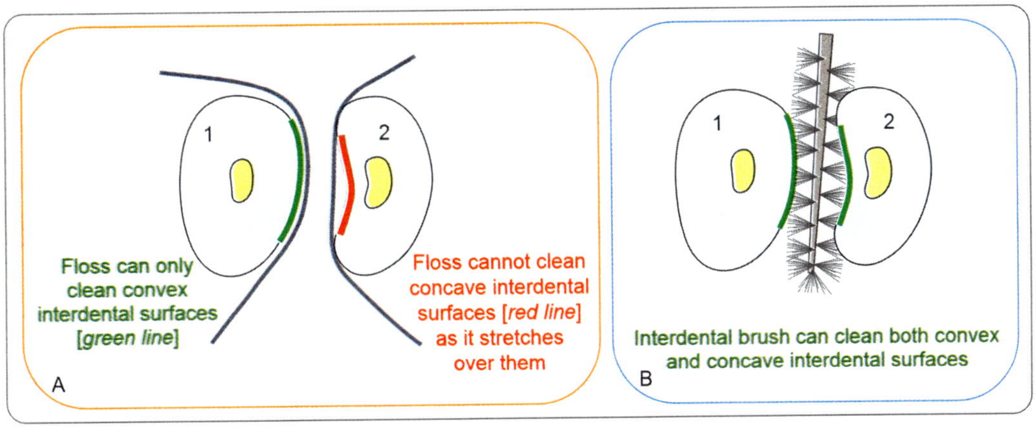

Fig. 15.9: A floss thread can clean convex interdental surfaces easily (*green marked area, diag. A, 1*) but as it does not make contact and stretches over concave surfaces (*red marked area, diag. A, 2*), it cannot clean depressions on root surfaces effectively. Multitufted interdental brushes can clean both convex and concave surfaces (*green marked areas diag. B, 1 and 2*).

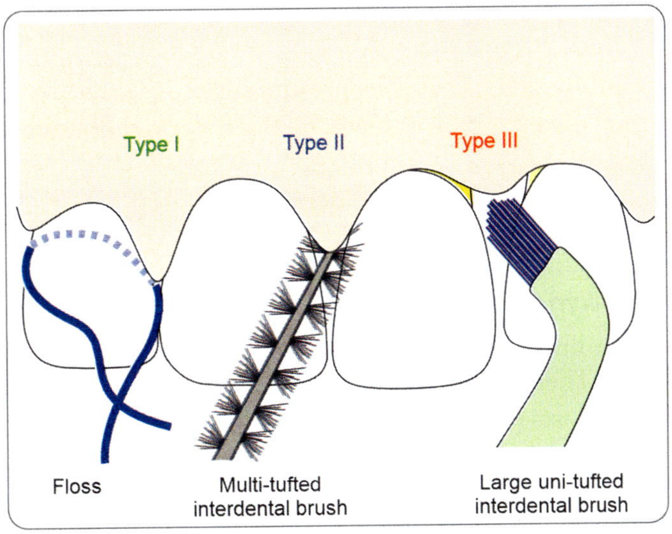

Fig. 15.10: Different interdental aids are recommended for interdental spaces of different sizes. For type-I interdental spaces, floss is recommended. As type-II spaces are slightly wider and have moderate papillary recession, a multi-tufted interdental brush is recommended. For still wider type-III interdental spaces, as there is complete loss of interdental papilla, a large uni-tufted interdental brush is recommended.

Wooden or Plastic Tips (*Toothpicks*) and Conical Rubber Tips

Are toothpicks effective plaque control devices? ▶

- A tooth-pick made of wood or plastic, small conical tips made of wood or plastic that can be mounted at a right angle on a handle, and small conical rubber tips attached to ends of toothbrush handles or individually mounted on plastic handles are available.
- All these are ***very effective*** in removing food debris, cleaning tooth furcations, interdental spaces, cervical area of teeth and gingival margins.

CHEMOTHERAPEUTIC PLAQUE CONTROL AND COMMONLY USED ANTIMICROBIAL AGENTS IN PERIODONTAL PRACTICE

Anti-plaque chemotherapeutic agents are used for controlling plaque. These act by: Stopping, slowing growth or killing microorganisms, preventing bacterial attachment to the oral cavity surfaces or by disrupting plaque's matrix leading to disintegration of plaque. Some commonly used chemical anti-plaque agents are described below.

Chemotherapeutic Plaque Control Agents (*Anti-plaque Mouth Washes*)

1. *Chlorhexidine*

What is chlorhexidine? ▶

- Chlorhexidine is a bisbiguanide and is available in ***three*** salt variations: Dihydrochloride, diacetate and digluconate.

Chlorhexidine is effective against which microorganisms? ▶

- It is a very effective anti-plaque agent that is active against bacteria (*both gram +ve and gram –ve, facultative anaerobes and aerobes*) and fungi. It is the 'gold standard' for comparing effectivity of other anti-plaque agents.

What concentration of chlorhexidine is used for plaque control? ▶

- If chlorhexidine is used in low concentration, it has a bacteriostatic effect but at high concentrations, chlorhexidine is bactericidal.
- 5–10 ml of chlorhexidine may be used in ***0.2% or 0.12% concentrations.***

How can effectivity of chlorhexidine be increased? ▶

- As chlorhexidine binds actively to oral sites, its ***effect lasts for up to 12 hours.***
- To maintain ***substantivity*** (*long duration antiplaque action*) of chlorhexidine, it must either be used before or 45 minutes ***after*** brushing with a toothpaste.

What are the other uses of chlorhexidine? ▶

- Chlorhexidine is also used for:
  - Pre-surgical preparation of skin and oral cavity and preventing infection after surgery.
  - As an irrigating solution during ultrasonic scaling, periodontal surgery, oral surgery, etc.
  - For treatment of aphthous ulcers, denture stomatitis, oral injuries caused by appliances, etc.

What are the side effects of chlorhexidine? ▶

- ***Adverse effects*** of prolonged use of chlorhexidine are:
  - Dark brown/grey discoloration of teeth, restorations and dorsum of tongue.
  - Alteration of taste.
  - Increased rate of shedding (*exfoliation*) of oral epithelium.
  - Increased formation of calculus.

2. *Quaternary Ammonium Compounds*

What are quaternary ammonium compounds? ▶

- Quaternary ammonium compounds (*e.g. cetylpyridinium chloride*) are used in 0.025 to 0.1% concentrations. Their mode of action is similar to that of chlorhexidine.
- After use, their effect lasts for up to 4–5 hours.
- On prolonged use, they cause brown staining of teeth and oral tissues.

3. *Essential Oils Containing Mouth Rinses*

What is the main benefit of using essential oil containing mouth washes for plaque control? ▶

- These contain contain eucalyptol, thymol, menthol and methyl salicylate.
- They are known to be safe and ***do not*** stain teeth or oral soft tissues or alter taste.
- They however contain alcohol which can ***increase*** severity of pre-existing ***xerostomia*** (*decreased salivary flow*).

4. *Triclosan*

- Triclosan is an anti-bacterial and anti-fungal agent commonly found in many consumer products, e.g. toothpastes, soaps, detergents, deodorants, etc.
- Additives like zinc citrate and gantrez are added to triclosan containing toothpastes to increase its effectivity in the mouth to 12 hours.
- It does not stain teeth and is not affected by tooth paste components. It causes taste alterations.

◂ *What is triclosan?*

5. *Povidone Iodine*

- Povidone-iodine is a broad-spectrum antiseptic that is effective against bacteria, fungi, viruses, protozoa.
- It is available as a 1% mouth rinse. Its effect lasts for an hour or so.
- Prolonged use of povidone iodine causes staining of teeth and oral tissues.

◂ *How long does the effect of povidone iodine last?*

6. *Hydrogen Peroxide*

- Hydrogen peroxide is a powerful antimicrobial agent.
- It works by releasing nascent oxygen that kills microorganisms (*especially anaerobic*) and loosens oral debris and plaque deposits. It is therefore commonly used to treat acute pericoronitis, NUG (*necrotizing ulcerative gingivitis*), etc.

◂ *What are the benefits of nacent oxygen released by hydrogen peroxide?*

Antimicrobials (*Antibiotics*) used in Periodontics

If host's immune system alone cannot control infection, antimicrobial medicines must be used to do this. A few commonly used drugs are discussed below.

Indications for use of antimicrobial chemotherapy in periodontal practice

1. Use as adjuncts to treat stage II, III and IV and grade B and C periodontitis and periodontal or periapical abscesses.
2. To reduce bacterial load and severe inflammation due to infection from deep pockets, furcations, tonsils etc when treating medically compromised patients.
3. After periodontal surgery.
4. For bio-modification of root surfaces, e.g. with tetracycline (*to improve chances of regeneration of periodontal tissues*).
5. To prevent spread of periodontal microbes from causing infections at other sites of body, e.g. ***prophylaxis*** for prevention of pneumonia, infective bacterial endocarditis, infections of artificial joints, etc.

◂ *Name the clinical situations in which antimicrobials used in periodontics?*

Commonly used Systemic (*Oral*) Antimicrobials

1. *Tetracyclines*

- They are ***broad spectrum*** and ***bacteriostatic*** antibiotics.
- In addition to killing microorganisms, tetracyclines also possess fibroblast stimulating, osteoclast inhibiting, anti-inflammatory and connective tissue protecting properties (*anti-collagenase, anti-proteolytic, etc. actions*).
- Commonly used tetracyclines for oral systemic use are: Tetracycline hydrochloride (*250 mg orally four times a day*), Doxycycline (*100 mg twice daily on the first day, then 100 mg orally every day*) and Minocycline (*100 mg orally twice daily*).
- One of the main benefits of tetracyclines is that their concentration in GCF (*gingival crevicular fluid in the periodontal pocket*) reaches ***2–10 times*** than that in blood. This increases their effectivity in the periodontal pocket (*where periodontitis causing microorganisms are present*) and makes them ideal antibiotics for periodontal use.
- **Side effects** of tetracyclines
  - They are usually minor and include diarrohea, nausea, oral candidiasis, photosensitivity, skin rashes, renal toxicity, etc.

◂ *Why are tetracyclines ideal for use in periodontics?*

◂ *How high is the concentration of tetracyclines in GCF as compared to that in blood?*

◂ *What are the side effects of tetracyclines?*

What are the contraindications of tetracyclines?

- **Contraindications of tetracyclines**
  - Tetracyclines cause ***permanent staining and discolouration of developing*** permanent teeth, they are therefore ***not*** prescribed to pregnant females, breast feeding mothers and children below 8 years of age.
  - Tetracyclines are broad spectrum antibiotics, their use kills many species of bacteria and this encourages fungal growth. Therefore, tetracyclines are not prescribed to patents in whom chances of fungal infection are already high, e.g. patients on long term immune suppressants, e.g. steroids, AIDS, etc. patients with renal disease, liver disease and uncontrolled diabetes, etc.

ALERT!

Tetracyclines must be taken an hour before or after meals and must not be consumed with antacids, iron supplements or with foods rich in calcium, e.g. milk products and wheat containing foods (*tetracycline becomes un-absorbable after it chelates calcium in these foods*).

2. *Metronidazole*

What is metronidazole used for?

- Metronidazole is effective against anaerobic organisms, e.g. *P. gingivalis* and is a bactericidal antimicrobial.
- It is therefore very useful for treating periodontal infections and periodontitis.

What is the dose of metronidazole?

- It is prescribed in doses of 200–400 mg orally three times a day for 7–10 days.
- It produces a strong metallic taste in the mouth.

What are the side effects of metronidazole?

- As metronidazole has disulfiram (*used in deaddiction of habitual alcohol consumers*) like action, patients must therefore not be allowed to consume alcohol when taking metronidazole.

3. *Ciprofloxacin*

What is ciprofloxacin?

- It is a bactericidal drug which is effective against gram –ve anaerobic and facultative periodontal pathogens.
- It is prescribed in doses of 250–500 mg orally twice daily for 7–10 days.

4. *Penicillins (Amoxicillin, Amoxicillin-clavulanate Potassium)*

Which penicillins are commonly used in periodontics?

- Amoxicillin is effective against G +ve and G –ve bacteria. Addition of clavulanate potassium increases amoxicillin's effectivity against penicillinase enzyme producing bacteria (*penicillinase makes amoxicillin in-effective*).
- It is therefore very useful to treat periodontal infections and severe hard to manage cases of periodontitis, e.g. stage III and IV and grade C periodontitis.
- Amoxicillin is recommended in 500 mg oral dose three times daily for one week. Amoxicillin-clavulanate potassium is recommended in 625 mg twice daily dose in adults.

5. *Clindamycin*

Why is clindamycin suited for use in periodontal infections?

- It is effective against anaerobic bacteria therefore; clindamycin can be used to treat periodontal infections (*which are primarily anaerobic*).
- It is given in a dose of 150–300 mg orally three times a day or twice a day for 7–10 days.

6. *Macrolides*

Can azithromycin be used to treat periodontal infections?

- The macrolide antibiotics (*e.g. azithromycin*) is effective against anaerobes and G –ve bacteria.
- It reaches high concentrations in periodontal tissues.
- It is therefore very effective in treating periodontal infections.
- It is prescribed as 500 mg once a day loading dose for the first day and the continued as 250 mg once a day for 5 days.

CLINICAL UTILITY AND SHORT ANSWER

Why is it preferred to use antibiotics in combinations?

Antimicrobials can be used together to produce a combined effect:

- Two or more antibiotics with overlapping antimicrobial spectra (*effective against same bacterial species*) can help reduce dose and duration of antibiotic therapy when compared to that of each one individually.
- This broadens antimicrobial range of treatment (*than when compared to that of each of these drugs individually*).
- Bactericidal 'antibiotics', e.g. amoxicillin, cephalosporin, etc. should however ***not*** be used along with bacteriostatic antibiotics, e.g. tetracycline, erythromycin, etc. as both do not support each other's mechanism of action (*i.e. are* ***antagonistic***). They may be given individually one after the other.

◂ *Why must bactericidal antibiotics not be used along with bacteriostatic antibiotics?*

CLINICAL UTILITY AND SHORT ANSWER

What is host modulatory therapy? What dose of tetracycline is used for host modulatory therapy?

Host modulatory therapy ***modifies host's response*** to infection in periodontal tissues and reduces periodontal destruction in periodontitis.

- For this effect, Doxycycline is prescribed in ***sub anti-microbial*** doses *20 mg twice daily orally* for ***3 months to 9 months*** (*normal* ***anti-microbial*** *adult dose is 100–200 mg per day*).
- NSAIDS, (*non-steroidal anti-inflammatory drugs*), bisphosphonate etc. have also been used for this purpose.
- Host modulation has ***not*** proved to be effective in significantly reducing periodontal destruction in periodontitis. Such therapy is therefore not commonly used and is ***not*** popular.

Local Drug Delivery (*of anti-microbial drugs*)

Local application of antimicrobials in periodontal pockets to reduce number of bacteria in them is called local drug delivery (*LDD*).

◂ *What is LDD?*

Rationale for LDD:

- ***High dose*** of a particular anti-microbial is deposited in a pocket and ***maintained locally for a long period of time*** without increasing the systemic concentration and toxicity of the drug. If the same local high concentration of the anti-microbial has to be produced by systemic route, a very high dose of the same will be needed.
- Drugs with ***high toxicity*** that cannot be used in high doses systemically can be used safely in high concentrations locally in periodontal pockets using LDD, e.g. chlorhexidine ***cannot*** be used orally (*systemically*) but can be safely used locally.
- To ensure prolonged availability of drug in high concentrations locally in the pockets, drugs used for LDD are used in combination with 'carriers', e.g. fibres, miniature tubes, strips or microspheres in a paste or gel to make a sustained release mechanism.

◂ *What is justification for use of LDD?*

◂ *Why can high efficacy drugs with high toxicity be used with LDD?*

◂ *How is longevity of drugs used in LDD increased?*

Some commercially available antimicrobial formulations for local delivery are:

1. *Tetracycline Containing Fibers*

- Ethylene or vinyl acetate copolymer fibres are impregnated with tetracycline (*12.7 mg tetracycline per 9 inches*) **(Fig. 15.11, diag. A)**.
- They when inserted into a pocket slowly release tetracycline in the periodontal pocket for more than 10 days.

◂ *What are tetracycline fibers?*

2. *Chlorhexidine Gluconate Impregnated 'Chip'*

- A thin biodegradable chip (*4 × 5 mm*) made of hydrolyzed gelatin matrix containing 2.5 mg of chlorhexidine gluconate is available. It can be inserted in more than 5 mm pockets **(Fig. 15.11, diag. B)**.
- Used this way very high chlorhexidine concentrations are attained and maintained for 7–10 days.

◂ *What is chlorhexidine chip?*

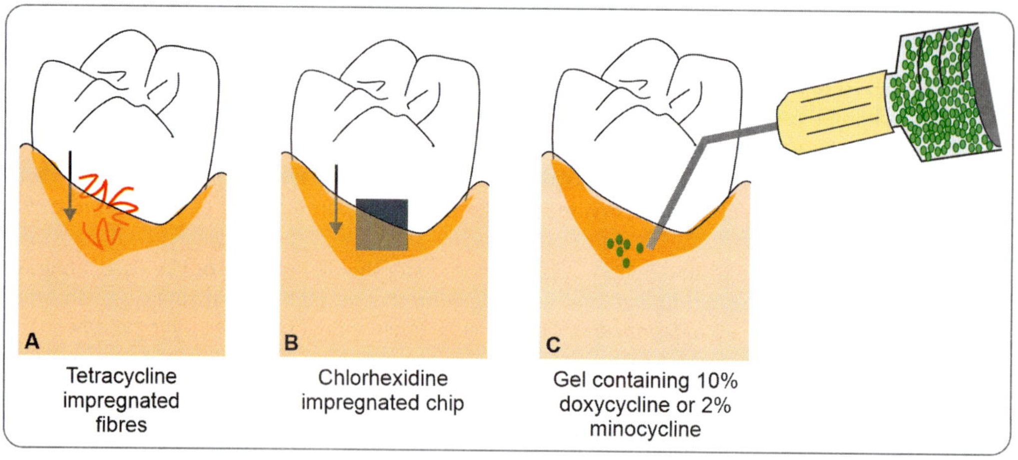

Fig. 15.11: Local drug delivery deposits antimicrobials directly into pockets. This is helpful in reducing probing pocket depth (*PD*) for a short while and till the time PD cannot be reduced surgically

3. *Subgingival Doxycycline*

- Doxycycline 10% is available in the local drug delivery mode in a ***gel***. This gel is directly injected into a pocket (Fig. 15.11, diag. C).

4. *Subgingival Minocycline*

- Minocycline 2% is infused in bioresorbable ***microspheres*** suspended in a gel base. This gel is directly injected into a pocket (Fig. 15.11, diag. C).

Review Questions

1. What is 'plaque control'?
2. Write a note on powered (*electrically operated*) toothbrushes.
3. Write a note on tooth brushing methods.
4. Why must interdental cleaning aids be used?
5. Write a note on importance of dental floss and interproximal brush in plaque control.
6. What are antimicrobial chemotherapeutic agents? Write a note on chlorhexidine.
7. Write on role of antibiotics in periodontics. Name some commonly used systemic (*oral*) antimicrobials in periodontal practice.
8. Write a note on locally delivered antimicrobial agents for treatment of periodontitis.
9. Write on host modulation.

Chapter

16

Scaling, Root Planing and Other Fundamentals of Periodontal Surgery

Calculus provides a rough surface for deposition of plaque. It is also rich in endotoxins (*which cause and maintain periodontitis*). Although plaque can be controlled by physical and chemical means, calculus has to be removed. Procedures done for removing calculus and diseased (*necrotic*) cementum are called scaling and root planing (*SRP*). Despite being immensely useful treatments, they are often under-estimated and under utilized. SRP is also amongst the most ***difficult*** dental procedures to perform and master.

SCALING AND ROOT PLANING (*SRP*)

Scaling: It is the process of removing calculus from both supra and subgingival areas of the tooth.

Root planing: It is a ***continuation*** of scaling and is performed to ***intentionally*** remove embedded ***calculocementum*** (*calculus embedded in cementum*) and diseased (*necrotic*) cementum from a tooth's root to produce a hard, clean and smooth 'glass' like root surface.

◂ *What is root planing? How is it different from scaling?*

All principles of scaling ***equally*** apply to root planing.

ALERT!

- Accidental and un-intentional removal of cementum also occurs during scaling.
- As cementum is removed both during scaling and root planing, the two procedures only ***differ*** in the ***intent*** of removing diseased cementum, i.e. in scaling, diseased cementum gets removed unintentionally (*accidentally*) whereas in root planing it is removed intentionally.

CLINICAL UTILITY AND SHORT ANSWER

What is the difference between calculocementum and diseased (*necrotic*) cementum?

Calculocementum: Calculus embedded deep in cementum is called calculocementum.

Diseased (*necrotic*) cementum: When cementum gets exposed due to periodontitis or gingival recession due to tooth position, etc. plaque and calculus deposit on it. Thereafter, byproducts and toxins of microbes (*especially endotoxins*) are deposited on its surface and get absorbed into it.

- These toxins absorbed into cementum continuously seep out of the root surface and cause an immune-inflammatory reaction in the surrounding periodontal tissues. This maintains inflammatory periodontal disease (*gingivitis and periodontitis*) in adjacent periodontal tissues.
- Calculocementum and absorbed toxins are relatively ***superficial***, therefore ***significant*** quantity of tooth structure (*cementum or dentin*) is ***not*** required to be removed during root planing.

◂ *What is calculocementum?*

◂ *What is necrotic or diseased cementum?*

◂ *Is calculocementum deep seated or superficially present in root structure?*

◂ *Does a significant quantity of cementum and/or dentine need to be removed to produce a 'clean' root surface during scaling and root planing?*

ALERT!

- ***Healthy*** tooth structure (*cementum, dentine and enamel*) also gets un-intentionally removed both during scaling and root planing.
- Cementum and dentine being relatively softer (*48–52% calcified*) than enamel (*98% calcified*), get damaged the most during SRP; on the other hand, enamel being very hard is usually only scratched (*but may get removed if there are enamel defects like hypo-calcification and malformation*).

Rationale of Scaling and Root Planing

(Why is it essential to perform SRP?)

What does SRP attain? ▸

SRP must be done at least every six months. In patients with increased susceptibility to periodontitis, SRP can be done every one to four months also. This is so because:

- Calculus and diseased (*necrotic*) cementum provide a rough surface for plaque deposition and maintain plaque and toxins of microorganisms in close contact with gingiva. This allows plaque microorganisms and their toxins to cause gingivitis and periodontitis.
- Therefore, when calculus and diseased (*necrotic*) cementum is removed, gingivitis and periodontitis get treated and periodontal health is attained. SRP is therefore an important and indispensable part of periodontal therapy.

How to do Scaling and Root Planing (*SRP*)

Why must SRP be preferably completed in a single sitting? ▸

If possible, SRP should be completed (*entire mouth*) in a ***single*** appointment. This reduces the possibility of re-colonization of treated sites by the microorganisms from untreated sites. If SRP cannot be completed in a single visit, then it must be completed in the minimum number of visits and ***shortest*** possible time.

Step 1: Identify Calculus and Areas of Diseased Cementum

Careful physical and ***mental*** charting of position of calculus and diseased cementum on the root surface is the most important step in SRP. Identification of both supra-gingival calculus and sub-gingival calculus that is just apical to the gingival margin is relatively easy. It is relatively ***difficult*** to identify sub-gingival calculus in difficult to reach areas that are wet with saliva and blood and are poorly illuminated. Calculus can be identified by:

How can presence of calculus on tooth's root be identified? ▸

1. **Visual examination (Fig. 16.1, diags A and B)**
2. **Tactile exploration**
    - Exploring the root surface with a dental ***explorer*** is the most commonly used method of detection of calculus. For this, the explorer is held lightly in a modified pen grasp and inserted to the base of the pocket.
    - Using ***light*** exploratory strokes, the explorer tip is moved back and forth on the tooth surface to identify rough (*calculus*) and softer (*diseased/necrotic cementum*) areas on the root surface.

How is calculus identified using an explorer? ▸

Can radiographs be used for identification of calculus? ▸

3. **Radiographs**
    - Identification of calculus in radiographs is ***by chance*** and this is ***not*** a routine and foolproof way of calculus identification.
    - Only large supra and sub-gingival calculus deposits can be identified in some radiographs.
    - Interdental calculus appears as ***spurs*** while calculus on buccal and lingual surfaces appears like horizontal ***bands*** **(Fig. 16.1, diag. D, white arrows).**
    - Radiographic identification of interdental calculus can be done more commonly than calculus on buccal or lingual surfaces of teeth.

ALERT!

Base of pocket is located 0.2–1.0 mm apical to the apical most extent of calculus.

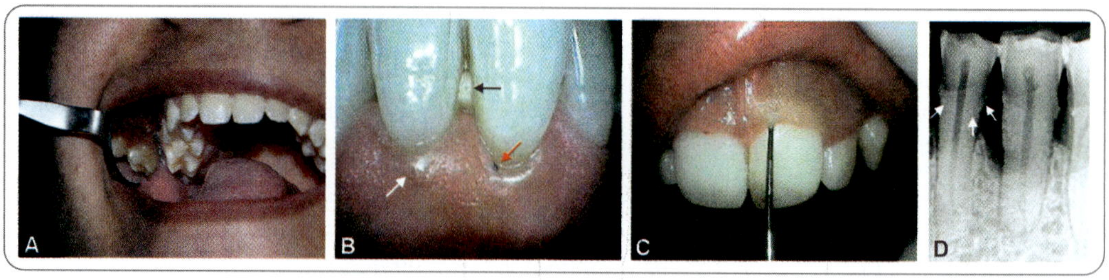

Fig. 16.1: Calculus can be identified by visual examination (*diag. A and B*), during periodontal instrumentation (*diag. C*) and in a radiograph (*diag. D*). In diag. B note bulge in free gingiva (*white arrow*) suggesting presence of calculus under it, red arrow in diag. B however points to impacted food while black arrow points to supragingival calculus.

Step 2: Scaling and Root Planing with a Hand Instrument (Scaler or a Curette)

(also see Chapter 14, 'Periodontal Instruments and Principles of Periodontal Instrumentation')

1. The patient and clinician must be seated in such a way that good accessibility, visibility and illumination of the area of work is present.
2. Instruments are held in a firm modified pen grasp. Finger or palm rest is established (Figs 14.20, 14.21, 14.22, and 14.26).
3. The ***correct*** cutting edge of the instrument is moved apical to the ***apical*** most extent of the calculus or base of the pocket (*instrument is inserted with its blade parallel to the root surface, i.e. at 0 angle*) and adapted at an angle of 45°–90° to the tooth surface (Figs 14.6, 14.7, 14.23, and 14.24).
4. The instrument is now pressed against the tooth surface and pulled coronally to remove calculus or root plane (Fig. 14.25). Only toe of the instrument, i.e. few ***terminal*** millimeters of blade of the instrument is used for SRP (Fig. 14.23). Controlled, overlapping and short scaling strokes are made to remove calculus and/or root plane the root surface. Lateral pressure and adaptation of the instrument blade are continuously ***adjusted*** by ***rolling*** the instrument handle between the thumb and fingers.

◂ *How is SRP done using a scalers and curettes?*

◂ *Where must the cutting edge of the scaler or curette be located for initiation of calculus removal?*

◂ *Which part of the instrument is used for scaling and root planing?*

ALERT!

It is preferable to remove large deposits of calculus in small pieces! (*Fig. 14. 25*)

- To remove large chunks of calculus all at once, the clinician has to exert greater force and pressure on the instrument.
- This reduces tactile sensitivity of the clinician and therefore his/her control on the instrument.
- In such situations, there is a high risk of injury to periodontal tissues and clinician's fingers and wrist.

Step 2b: Scaling and Root Planing with an Ultrasonic Scaler

(also see Chapter 14, 'Periodontal Instruments and Principles of Periodontal Instrumentation', section on ultrasonic scaling)

1. The patient and the clinician must be seated in such a way that good accessibility, visibility and illumination of the area of work is present.
2. The right scaling tips must be selected for scaling specific areas (Fig. 14.15). Special root planing tips are also available and these are made of steel or are diamond coated.
3. The ultrasonic scaler's handpiece is then held in the modified pen grasp and finger and/or palm rest are established. Unit is switched on, flow of irrigant is adjusted and the working ultrasonic scaling tip is applied to the tooth surface to be scaled. Scaling tip is worked in short, overlapping and light strokes.
4. ***Side*** of the scaling tip (*scaling insert*) rather than the pointed end of the scaling tip must be used for scaling (Fig. 16.2).

◂ *How is SRP done using ultrasonic scalers?*

◂ *Which part of the ultrasonic scaler insert is used for scaling?*

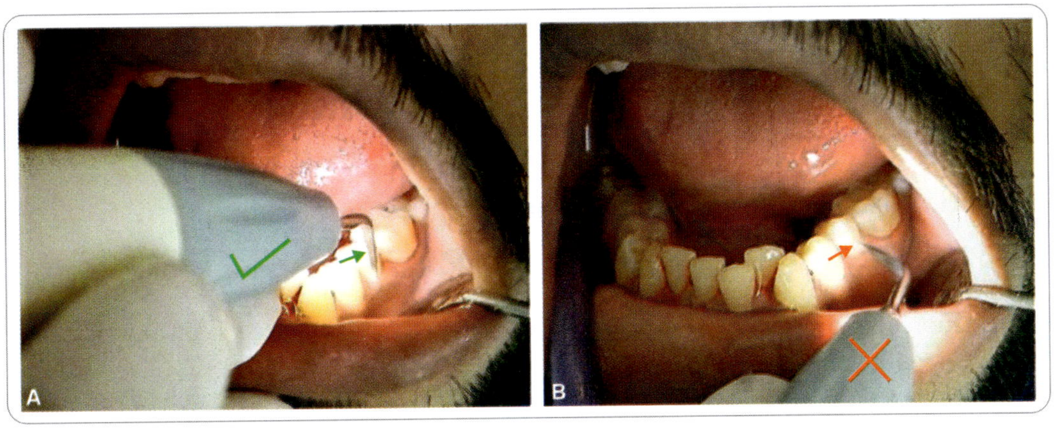

Fig. 16.2: Side of the ultrasonic scaling tip (*insert*) must be used for ultrasonic scaling (*green arrow, diag. A*). If only the pointed end of the scaling insert is used (*red arrow, diag. B*), it will cause damage to tooth structure due to localization of energy.

Why must ultrasonic scaler's power setting be kept at the lowest effective power setting during ultrasonic scaling? ▶

5. Aerosol and splatter produced during ultrasonic scaling **(Fig. 14.14)** are suctioned off with high vacuum suction tip that is placed near the working scaling tip.
6. Ultrasonic scaling is done using the lowest possible power setting (*power control knob on the ultrasonic scaler*). If high power settings are used, damage to tooth structure and surrounding periodontal tissues is possible.

Is finishing with hand instruments essential after ultrasonic scaling? ▶

7. Ultrasonic scaling tips may smoothen (*and not remove*) small tenacious calculus deposits. All root surfaces ***must*** therefore be thoroughly checked and if required, such left back calculus deposits must be removed with hand instruments (e.g. *curettes*) after ultrasonic scaling. In other words, ultrasonically scaled root surfaces must be 'finished' with hand instruments.

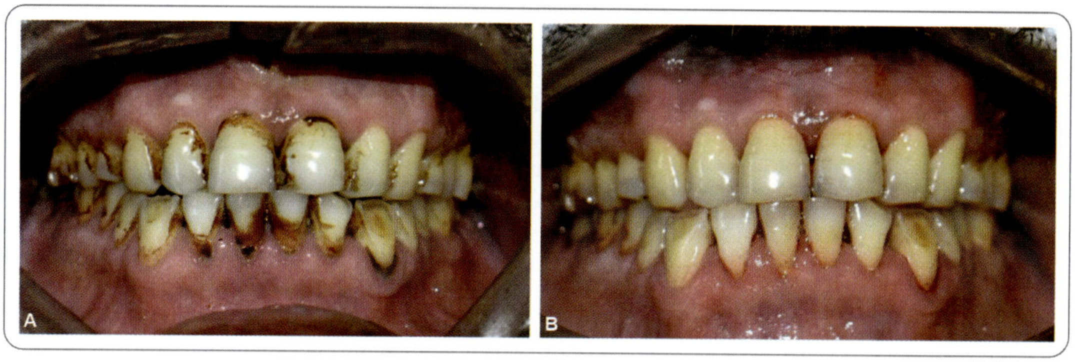

Fig. 16.3: Results after single appointment for scaling and root planing. Subgingival calculus inadvertently left back after the 1st appointment is likely to become exposed after a few days (*because of shrinking of gingiva after scaling*). Such calculus is removed during the subsequent scaling and root planing appointment.

ALERT!

Special benefits of ultrasonic scaling over hand scaling

(*also see Chapter 14, 'Periodontal Instruments and Principles of Periodontal Instrumentation', section on ultrasonic scaling*)

Why can narrow furcations be cleaned better with ultrasonic scaling? ▶

- In some cases, furcations of multi-rooted teeth are very narrow. Therefore, these cannot be cleaned thoroughly even with curettes as it may be difficult to insert or move the curette blade in the furcation. Thin ultrasonic scaling tips can be ideal for cleaning such narrow furcations or other closely placed roots.
- As endotoxins are weakly adsorbed on the root (*to diseased cementum*), they can be easily removed with ultrasonic scalers.

How does ultrasonic scaling provide microbial control? ▶

- Ultrasonic scaling itself can kill and ***reduce*** bacteria in deep pockets and furcations. Antimicrobials (*chemical plaque controlling agents like chlorhexidine*) can be added to the irrigating liquid for ultrasonic scaling for additional clinical benefit.

FUNDAMENTALS OF PERIODONTAL SURGERY

Phase II therapy or the Surgical phase must start only after successful completion of phase-I (*etiotrophic phase*) treatment.

Aims and Objectives of Periodontal Surgery

Why must periodontal surgery be done? ▶

Periodontal surgery is done with the following objectives:

1. Stopping and controlling ongoing gingivitis and periodontitis.
2. Correction of anatomic or morphologic periodontal tissue defects or conditions that:
   a. Contribute to periodontitis.
   b. Interfere with prosthetic replacements.
3. Improvement of prognosis (*of individual teeth and entire dentition*).
4. Improvement of smile.
5. Placing dental implants for replacement of lost teeth, etc.

Two Basic Types of Periodontal Surgery are done to Achieve the above Objectives

1. **Pocket reducing surgery**
   - Periodontal pockets are treated by reducing pocket depth (*PD*).
   - To reduce pocket depth, the pocket wall is either ***completely removed*** (*by gingivectomy*) or pocket depth is reduced to less than 3 mm by ***partial excision of coronal part of the pocket wall*** (*by flap surgery*).
   - If regenerative materials are used during the flap surgery, periodontal tissues can ***regenerate*** and move ***coronally*** to cover exposed root (*recession area caused by periodontitis*). This will also result in reduction of pocket depth.
   - Three surgical procedures can be done for reducing PD:
     a. Curettage
     b. Gingivectomy and Gingivoplasty
     c. Periodontal flap surgery (*including bone surgery*)
2. **Surgery for correction of morphologic and anatomic deficiencies**:
   a. Mucogingival surgery
   b. Surgery for aesthetic enhancement of teeth and smile
   c. Pre-prosthetic surgery
   d. Dental implant placing surgery.

How many types of periodontal surgery are there?

ALERT!

Need of periodontal surgery (*phase-II treatment*) is finally decided only after completion and then re-assessment of results of phase-I treatment.
- Many a times, improvement in periodontal health after phase I treatment is so great that need for corrective periodontal surgery is ***no longer*** there (*although it was believed that surgery would be needed at time of formulation of treatment plan*).
- Therefore, we must wait for this improvement in periodontal health to take place for 1–3 months after completion of phase-I treatment (*scaling root planing, etc.*), before deciding on need for phase-II, i.e. surgical treatment.

How long must a clinician wait for deciding need for surgical therapy after completing phase I therapy?

Source of Healing Cells after Periodontal Treatment affects Outcome of Healing of Periodontal Wounds

Periodontal treatment removes etiologic and contributing factors that cause periodontal disease; thereafter, healing is its natural outcome. Adequate periodontal treatment also creates the right conditions for regeneration of periodontal tissues lost due to periodontal disease. As all periodontal tissues are ***specialized*** tissues, their regeneration can only occur from cells originating from the same type of tissue. Outcome of healing is therefore dependent on local conditions and ***source*** of healing cells that first populate and dominate healing in a periodontal wound **(Fig. 16.4)**. The possible sources of healing cells in a periodontal wound are:

Why is outcome of healing dependent on source of healing cells?

1. *Gingival and Oral Epithelium*

If healing cells of a periodontal wound come from gingival and oral epithelium it will lead to re-establishment of base of sulcus on root surface either at the ***same*** level (*similar to the level base of sulcus before treatment*) or slightly coronal to it with formation of a long or normal length junctional epithelium. There is ***no*** regeneration of cementum, bone or periodontal ligament on the exposed root surface.

What happens if healing cells of a periodontal wound come from gingival and oral epithelium?

2. *Gingival Connective Tissue*

If cells of gingival connective tissue dominate the healing process, it leads to resorption of root, remodeling of alveolar bone and formation of ***non-functionally*** arranged connective tissue fibers (*fibers are parallel to the root surface and not attached to the root, therefore they do not provide tooth support*).

What happens if healing cells of a periodontal wound come from gingival connective tissue?

What happens if healing cells of a periodontal wound come from alveolar bone?

3. Alveolar Bone

If cells of alveolar bone dominate healing, it leads to resorption and formation of new bone. This is accompanied by resorption of root. New bone formation occurs directly over root leading to ankylosis (*direct joining of root to bone without intervening PDL*).

4. Periodontal Ligament

What happens if healing cells of a periodontal wound come from PDL?

If healing cells come from PDL, ***regeneration*** of all ***periodontal tissues*** (*new attachment*) is possible. This is because the PDL has regenerative cells that can form ***all periodontal tissues***, i.e. fibroblasts that form connective tissue/PDL fibers, osteoblasts that form bone, cementoblasts that form cementum (*see Chapter 3, 'Periodontal ligament, Cementum and Alveolar bone' and section on 'Cellular and Extra Cellular Constituents of PDL'*).

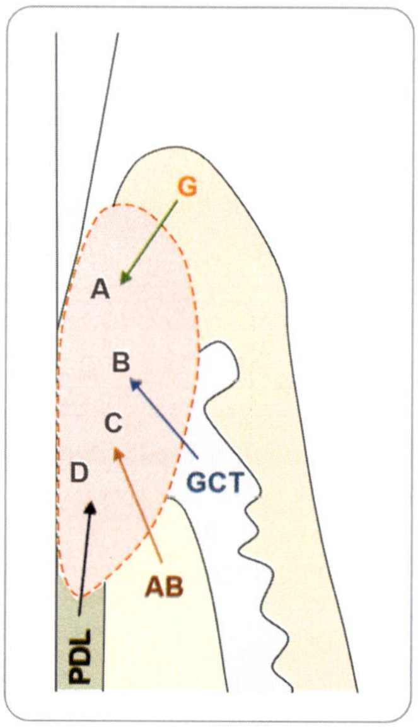

Fig. 16.4: Possible sources of healing cells in a periodontal wound: A: Gingival epithelial cells (*G*); B: Gingival connective tissue (*GCT*); C: Alveolar bone (*AB*) and D: Periodontal ligament (*PDL*).

Regeneration and Repair—The Two Basic Healing Processes in a Periodontal Wound

Healing in a periodontal wound, can either occur by regeneration or repair or their combinations:

What are repair and regeneration?

1. **Regeneration:** Healing by regeneration is said to have occurred if, ***re-formation*** and ***functional restoration*** of all periodontal tissues that were previously lost due to periodontal disease takes place. For this, all periodontal tissues must regenerate in their ***original proportions*** and ***orientation*** (*as found in normal periodontium*) and must be ***fully functional***.
2. **Repair:** Healing by repair is said to have occurred if, healing results in ***re-formation*** of either ***some or all*** periodontal tissues but the healed tissues do not have the same morphology and functioning as that of normal periodontium. Repair is also called healing by scar formation. It stops further periodontal loss.

Healing by repair or regeneration in a periodontal wound can result in:

1. *No* structural and functional *increase* in quantity of periodontal tissues, i.e. periodontal tissues establish at their pre-treatment levels but are now healthy (*repair*).
2. Complete or partial physical restoration of ***some*** but ***not*** all of the lost periodontal tissues over surface of the tooth root that was denuded by periodontitis. The newly formed periodontal tissue components however may not function normally (*complete functional restoration is not attained*) (*repair*).
3. Complete or partial restoration of ***both*** structure and function of ***all*** periodontal tissues ***over area of the root previously denuded by periodontitis*** (*regeneration*).

Healing Outcomes after Periodontal Surgery

(also see Chapter 18, Page 327 and 328)

1. Reattachment

Re-joining of gingiva to areas of the root of a tooth (*that was not previously exposed to oral environment, i.e. pocket*) after its surgical or traumatic separation is called reattachment. In most cases of reattachment after periodontal therapy, a normal length junctional epithelium forms with base of the sulcus almost at the ***preoperative*** level **(Fig. 16.5, diag. 2)**. In some cases, base of the sulcus can shift coronally due to formation of a long junctional epithelium over the root. This is accompanied by close adaptation of gingival wall of the pocket to the tooth surface (*repair*) but other periodontal tissues do not regenerate.

◄ *What is reattachment?*

2. New Connective Tissue Attachment

In many cases, newly formed PDL fibers are found to be attached to newly formed cementum on the root. But these fibers are ***not*** attached to alveolar bone at their other end. This type of healing is called ***New Connective tissue attachment*** (*repair*). It does ***not*** restore form and function of periodontium completely **(Fig. 16.5, diag. 3)**.

◄ *What is new connective tissue attachment?*

3. New Attachment

Shifting of base of sulcus coronally by formation of all and fully functional periodontal tissues over a ***previously diseased*** and ***denuded root surface*** (*denuded by periodontitis*) is called new attachment **(Fig. 16.5, diag. 4)**. In general clinical use, the term 'periodontal regeneration' (*new attachment*) usually refers to ***partial*** regeneration (*in height and function*) of periodontal tissues after periodontal therapy.

◄ *What is new attachment?*

◄ *What is the difference between reattachment and new-attachment?*

4. Combinations of above

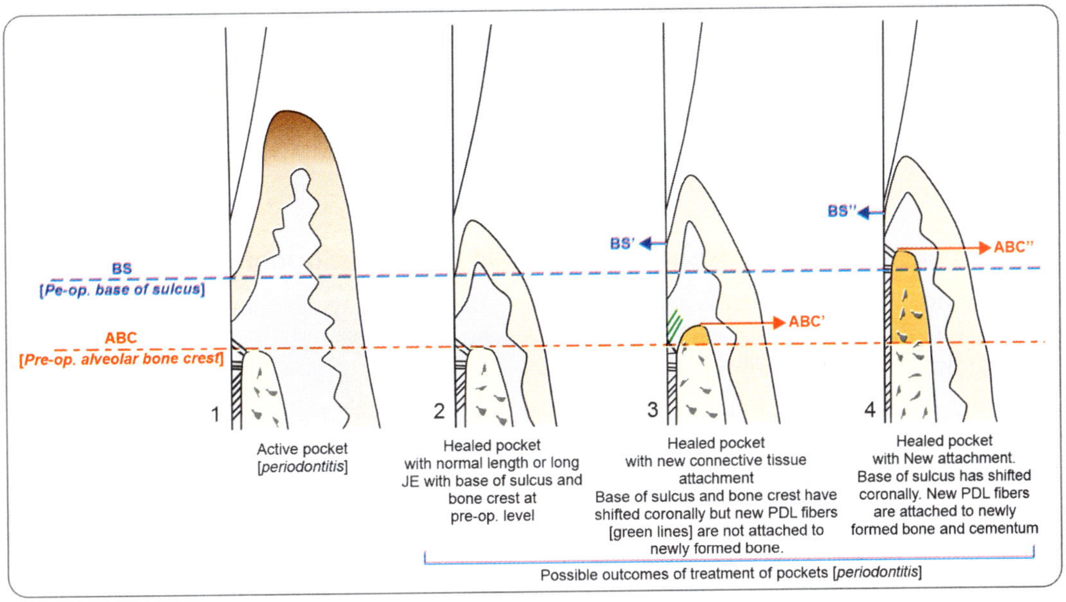

Fig. 16.5: Possible outcomes of surgical treatment of periodontitis

CLINICAL UTILITY AND SHORT ANSWER

What is close epithelial adaptation? How is it different from new attachment?

- Periodontal treatment leads to resolution of inflammation in the gingiva. This will cause firm adaptation of free gingiva to the tooth surface (Fig. 16.5, diags 2, 3 and 4 and Fig. 2.5). In many cases, adaptation of the free gingiva is so firm that a periodontal probe cannot be completely inserted into the sulcus down to its base, this results in recording of a smaller CAL reading (*which is less than actual*) (*CAL is distance between CE junction and tip of probe that has been inserted into sulcus/pocket for taking pocket depth; see Chapter 2, page 5 and 6*).
- In new attachment, reduction in CAL occurs due to regeneration of lost periodontal tissues.
- Inexperienced clinicians can wrongly interpret decrease in CAL due to firm epithelial adaptation as healing by new attachment.

CLINICAL UTILITY AND SHORT ANSWER

Why is healing of periodontal wounds a complex process and different from healing of other body wounds and tissues?

Healing of periodontal wounds is a complex process and different from healing of other body tissues because:

1. Many different types of cells and tissues have to coordinate and fine tune healing process so that all healing events occur in the ***correct sequence***.
2. The healing gingival flap is located over avascular tooth root that is contaminated with microorganisms and their products.
3. Healing occurs in an infected environment (*healing wound is exposed to microorganisms during the healing process*).

General Contraindications for Periodontal Surgery

In which situations is periodontal surgery contraindicated?

1. Uncooperative patients.
2. Incomplete phase I treatment.
3. Patients with uncontrolled systemic diseases or poor systemic health, e.g. severe and uncontrolled diabetes, recent heart surgery, etc.

Before Surgery, the Clinician must Ensure

1. **Informed consent of the patient for the surgery.**
2. **Premedication.** To reduce anxiety and stress (*anxiolytics like diazepam, etc.*) may be prescribed. For patients on long term corticosteroids, ***double*** dose of steroid one hour prior to surgery is usually needed. Patients with prosthetic heart valves and joints replacements may require prophylactic antibiotics (*as advised by the patient's physician*).
3. **Light diet at least half an hour prior to surgery.** This will help maintain normal blood glucose levels and prevent hypoglycemia in the patient during surgery.
4. **Sterilization of all instruments and disinfection of equipment.**
5. **Availability of emergency medicines.**

Precautions and Safety Measures to be taken during Periodontal Surgery

Name the safety measures and precautions that must be taken during periodontal surgery.

1. The clinician must frequently talk and observe the patient at all times for abnormal facial expressions, body movements, pallor and perspiration. This will help know if the patient is uncomfortable or is in pain.
2. Handle soft and hard tissue (*tooth and bone*) gently and carefully.
3. Ensure adequate blood supply to soft tissue flaps. For this, base (*apical end*) of the flap must be kept wider than the coronal end **(Fig. 17B.4, diag. 1 and 2)**. Very thin partial thickness flaps, narrow width flaps or free soft tissue grafts on very wide root recessions are likely to fail. Sutures should not be tied with too much tension as this will cause restriction of blood flow which may lead to tissue necrosis.
4. Re-assess and improve scaling and root planing during surgery.
5. Prevent and control excessive bleeding.
6. Ensure good wound closure with good approximation of flaps. Complete coverage of alveolar bone is desirable. Sutures must be placed to prevent dead space or excessive blood clot formation under the healing flaps.
7. Post operative instructions must be given and it must be confirmed that the patient has understood these properly.

Periodontal Packs (*Periodontal Dressings*)

What are periodontal packs? Why must they be used?

Wound dressings used to cover a periodontal wound are called periodontal packs **(Fig. 16.6, diag. A)**. They protect the healing wound from direct physical trauma and prevent undue pain and postoperative hemorrhage.

◂ What are the disadvantages of periodontal packs?

A periodontal pack also has its ***disadvantages***, these are:

1. A thick layer of plaque forms under the pack after 3–4 days. This causes increased inflammation in the healing tissue and may delay healing.
2. Sutures of the wound may get tangled in the pack and may make pack removal difficult and painful.
3. Overextended packs can irritate muco-buccal folds.
4. Some constituents of the packs (*e.g. eugenol in eugenol containing packs*) may cause chemical irritation to tissues. Non-eugenol packs are therefore preferred.

Method of Placing a Periodontal Pack

Commonly used periodontal packs come in two-paste systems. The two pastes (*base and catalyst*) are mixed, rolled into thin rolls and placed over the wound (*buccal and lingual/palatal*) under light adapting pressure. The pack is then gently pressed into interdental spaces (*with a round instrument*) for mechanical interlocking (**Fig. 16.6, diag. B**).

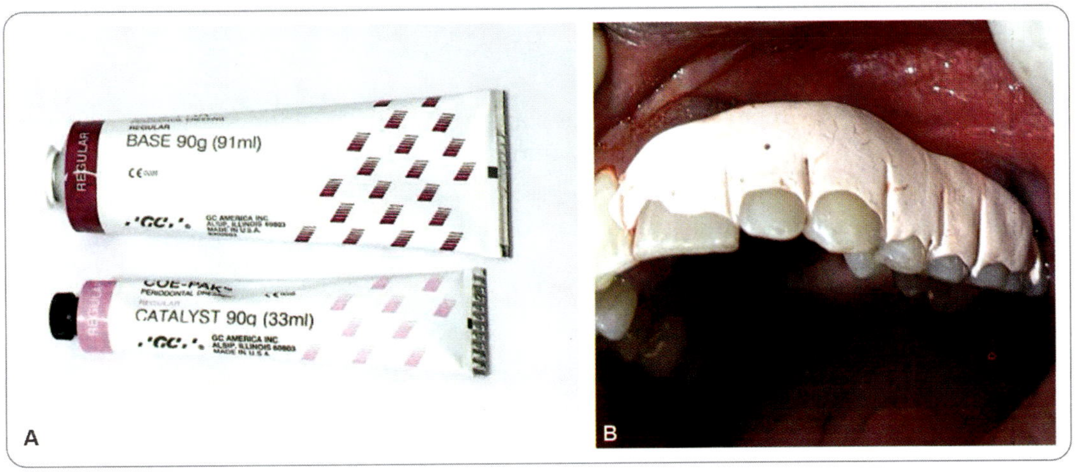

Fig. 16.6: Periodontal packs are commonly available in two paste systems: base and catalyst. The base and catalyst pastes are mixed and applied over the wound. Periodontal pack serves as a dressing over the periodontal wound.

Post-operative Instructions After Periodontal Surgery

◂ Which instructions must be given to a patient who has undergone periodontal surgery?

The following instructions are given to a patient who has undergone periodontal surgery:

1. Apply ice packs (*on the face over the operated area*) intermittently in 10-minute cycles for the first 30 minutes after surgery. This is done to reduce swelling.
2. Brush regularly as earlier but do not brush over the pack. Do not disturb the pack, if a small part of it breaks off, do not worry.
3. Take medicines as prescribed and do not smoke or consume alcohol for the next few days.
4. Small amount of blood oozing from the wound is normal, do not panic. If excessive bleeding is noticed, contact your doctor immediately.
5. Do not do excessive physical exertion for a few hours immediately after surgery.
6. Rinse with a mild antiseptic mouth wash (*e.g. chlorhexidine*) twice or thrice daily till regular tooth brushing is resumed.

Usual Possible Complications after Periodontal Surgery

◂ Which complications are usually seen after periodontal surgery?

1. Bleeding from some operated sites that may be spontaneous or after slight injury. This bleeding occurs from newly formed granulation tissue. It can be usually managed by pressure packs and cold packs.
2. Increased mobility is noticed in treated teeth for a few days after surgery. This occurs due to inflammation in periodontal ligament of operated teeth.

3. Teeth in the operated area may be become tender and hypersensitive for few days. Tooth hypersensitivity may persist for a long time after surgery and can be managed with desensitizing tooth pastes (*containing strontium chloride, potassium nitrate, etc.*)

Healing of Periodontal Wounds

Periodontal wounds may be ***excisional*** or ***incisional*** surgery wounds. ***Excisional wounds, e.g. gingivectomy wounds heal by secondary intention*** whereas ***incisional wounds, e.g. flap surgery wounds heal by primary intention*** at sites where wound edges meet and by secondary intention where there is gap between the wound edges.

Write the sequence of events during healing of excisional periodontal wound. ▸

Healing of Excisional Surgery Periodontal Wounds (Healing by Secondary Intention)

1. **0–5 hours**
   a. Blood clot and sero-fibrinous exudate cover the wound.
   b. Acute inflammation develops in the connective tissue.
   c. PMNs migrate into the clot and on the wound surface till a band of PMNs (*called polyband*) forms over the wound ***under*** the clot. This serves to protect the healing wound till epithelium forms over it.

What is a polyband? ▸

2. **5 hours to 1 day**
   a. Epithelial cells at the wound margins start rapid multiplication. New epithelial cells start to move across surface of the wound.
3. **2–3 days**
   a. Epithelial cells on wound surface start dividing.
   b. Acute inflammation starts subsiding and connective tissue under the wound surface starts to organize. A phase of chronic inflammation starts.
4. **4–10 days**
   a. Epithelium covers entire wound surface in ***4–7 days***.
   b. Proliferation of connective tissue starts and accelerates with time.
   c. Connective tissue in contact with tooth begins to proliferate in the occlusal direction; this will form the epithelial attachment.

After how many days does epithelium cover the entire wound after excisional surgery? ▸

5. **10–30 days**
   a. Healing tissue begins maturing. After ***21 days,*** epithelium covering the wound appears clinically normal.
   b. By ***28–30 days*** epithelial attachment and sulcus reforms.

After how many days does epithelial attachment reform after excisional surgery? ▸

Healing of Incisional Surgery Periodontal Wounds (Healing by Primary Intention)

1. **1st day**
   a. Blood clot forms between periodontal flap and underlying tissue.
   b. Acute inflammation starts in the connective tissue. Flap of gingiva becomes inflamed.
2. **2–4 days**
   a. Epithelial cells migrate across wound margin to contact surface of the tooth.
   b. Acute inflammation begins to recede and a phase of chronic inflammation starts.
   c. Some bone resorption activity is noticed in bone that was exposed during surgery.
3. **4–10 days**
   a. Fibrin clot starts undergoing resolution and is replaced by young connective tissue after 6–7 days.
   b. Healing tissues start to show revascularization.
   c. Sulcular epithelium and epithelial attachment reform.

After how many days does epithelial attachment reform after incisional surgery? ▸

4. **11–21 days**
   a. Inflammation gets resolved.
   b. New bone (*osteoid tissue*) formation starts.
   c. New collagen fiber bundles form.

5. **Beyond 21 days**
   a. Periodontal fibers reattach to the root surface.
   b. Bone remodeling is noticed.
   c. Epithelial attachment matures.

CLINICAL UTILITY AND SHORT ANSWER

Write the factors that affect rate of healing of periodontal wounds?

1. Wider the wound, slower the healing (*as epithelium has to travel longer distances*).
2. Infection in the wound delays healing.
3. Wounds with uneven wound margins show slower healing.
4. After flap adaptation, applying gentle pressure on the flap for a minute or so helps create a thinner clot under the flap and reduces dead space under flap. Minimal thickness of blood clot reduces infection under the flap. This fastens healing.
5. Maintenance of good oral hygiene improves healing.
6. Any calculus inadvertently left back during surgery will delay healing. Such calculus specks are usually noticed at the time of pack removal and must be removed when first noticed.

◂ *Why must wound margins be even?*

◂ *Why is it important to put slight finger pressure on the flap before suturing?*

ALERT!

To prevent injury to newly formed junctional epithelium, sulcular probing must only be done after 2–3 months of surgery.

◂ *Why should a healing periodontal wound not be probed immediately after surgery?*

Periodontal Splinting

Definition: A periodontal splint is any device or appliance that joins two or more teeth into a rigid unit for the purpose of providing support.

◂ *What is periodontal splint?*

Periodontitis, trauma from occlusion, bone pathologies cause loss of height of supporting alveolar bone that result in tooth mobility. Periodontal splints can be used to reduce tooth mobility in such cases.

Indications and Rationale of Periodontal Splinting

◂ *What are the benefits of splinting teeth?*

1. To provide ***rest*** and ***reduce*** traumatic occlusal force (*and hence TFO*) on mobile teeth by distributing occlusal load over all the splinted teeth.
2. To stabilize very mobile teeth for scaling and root planing and surgery.
3. To prevent ***pathologic migration*** of periodontally weak and mobile teeth.
4. If multiple dental implants are splinted together with a single fixed prosthesis (*that connects multiple implants*), it helps distribute occlusal loads equally amongst these implants. This allows:
   a. Immediate full arch loading (*within a week of dental implant placement*, i.e. *before osseointegration*).
   b. Success and long-term survival of short or thin dental implants in low alveolar bone volume or low bone density areas.
5. For prevention of supra-eruption of teeth that have lost their antagonists.
6. To retain teeth in their corrected positions after orthodontic treatment.
7. For stabilizing teeth for up to ***3–4 weeks*** after:
   a. Subluxation (*incomplete or partial dislocation of a tooth due to physical trauma*)
   b. Avulsion (*total dislodgement of tooth out of its socket after physical trauma*)
   c. Intentional re-implantation after planned extraction.

Contraindications of Periodontal Splinting

1. When sufficient number of non-mobile teeth are not present to splint mobile teeth (*there should be at least* ***two*** *firm teeth in the splint for each mobile tooth, if this precondition is not met, the firm teeth will also get mobile and also start to show features of secondary chronic TFO*).
2. If mobile teeth have a poor or hopeless prognosis.
3. If patient does not maintain good oral hygiene.
4. If splinting will lead to occlusal interference.

◂ *Why must mobile teeth be splinted only with sufficient number of non-mobile teeth?*

◂ *How many firm teeth must be present for every mobile tooth for safe splinting?*

Some Things to be kept Mind before Splinting

1. A splint should be:
   a. Of simplest possible design
   b. Non-irritating
   c. Aesthetically satisfactory
2. Extensive tooth preparation must be avoided to place a splint.
3. The splint's design should permit good plaque control and scaling.

Types of Dental Splints

How many types of dental splints are there? ▸

Splints are classified according to:

1. **Duration of use**
   a. Temporary (*used for less than 6 months*)
   b. Provisional (*used for 6 months to 12 months*)
   c. Permanent (*used for periods longer than 12 months,* i.e. *indefinitely*)
2. **Location of splint**
   a. Extracoronal
   b. Intracoronal
3. **Type of material**
   a. Dead soft steel wire (*orthodontic ligature wire*)
   b. Composite
   c. Reinforced composite or acrylic with wires or fibers, etc.

Which type of splint is the most commonly used? ▸

Extra-coronal (*external*) splints constructed with composite resin, ligature wires, nightguards or an interim fixed prosthesis are most ***commonly*** used.

Extra-coronal Splinting with Composite Resin

The technique is very similar to the one used for making composite restorations **(Fig. 16.7)**.

1. Composite resin is applied on the interdental surfaces and adjoining facial and lingual surfaces of adjoining teeth to be splinted and cured. Composite resin may be applied on unprepared tooth surfaces or small class III cavities may be cut into these for better retention and increasing bulk of composite. However, this type of splinting does not last long as composite often fractures at the interdental joints.
2. To increase the strength of composite resin, it is reinforced with fibers, steel wire or mesh, etc. Of these, fiber ribbons (*of different materials*) are the most commonly employed as they are ***high strength*** and ***aesthetic*** and composite resin bonds well with them.
3. Fiber ribbon is ***usually*** placed on the ***lingual*** surfaces of teeth or sometimes on buccal surface when adequate space is not present between surfaces of mandibular and maxillary teeth, e.g. presence of deep bite when splinting maxillary teeth, etc.

How is splinting done using fiber reinforced composite resin? ▸

4. To make a fiber reinforced composite resin splint:
   a. Surfaces of teeth to be splinted are lightly abraded with a diamond stone and acid etched.
   b. Bonding agent and a layer of composite is applied on the prepared surfaces.
   c. 2–3 mm wide fiber ribbon (*most commonly used*) of adequate length (*equal to total width of teeth to be splinted*) is adapted on uncured composite placed on teeth.
   d. Composite splint is now light cured.
   e. As reinforcing fibers are not polishable, another layer of composite is now placed on the fiber splint, light cured and polished.
5. Such splints are successful in anterior teeth but may have a shorter life if used in posterior teeth (*due to high occlusal forces*).

What other material can be used in place of reinforcing fiber for splinting teeth? ▸

ALERT!

Instead of reinforcing fiber ribbon, a coaxial orthodontic wire can also be bonded onto lingual/palatal surfaces of teeth using composite for splinting teeth **(Fig. 16.8)**.

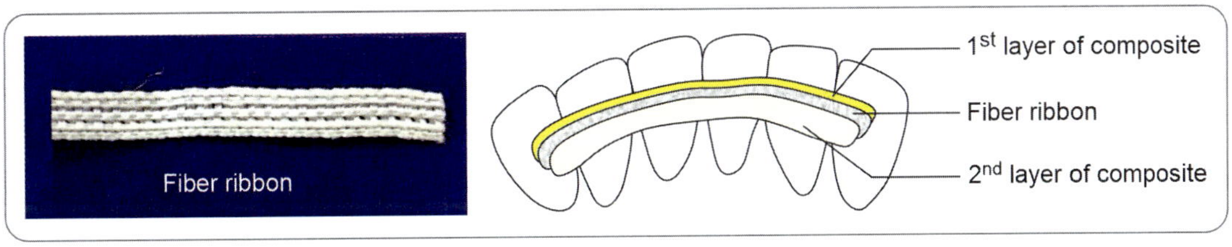

Fig. 16.7: Fiber ribbon reinforced composite bonded splint

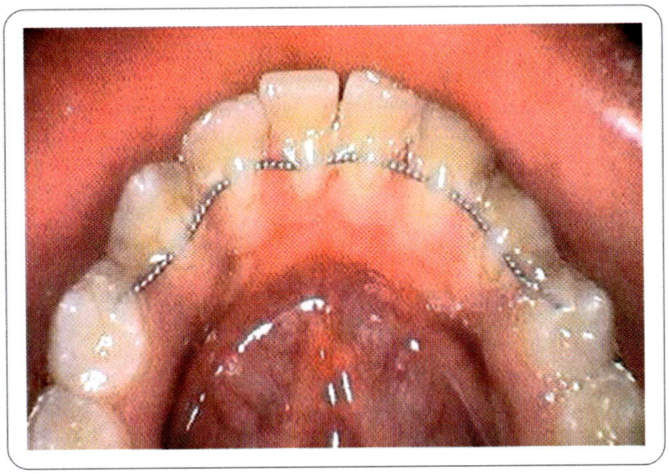

Fig. 16.8: A coaxial orthodontic wire used for splinting teeth

Extra-coronal Splinting with Dead Soft Steel Wire

It is one of the most commonly employed and economical method of splinting teeth. There are several ways of splinting teeth with a dead soft steel wire. Any of these methods is acceptable provided:

1. The wire crosses interdental surfaces of teeth ***apical*** to the ***interdental contact point*** (*so that the splint wire cannot be dislodged in the coronal direction*) and ***coronal*** to cingulum of anterior teeth (*so that the splint wire cannot be dislodged in the apical direction*). If needed, the wire is further stabilized with composite resin.
2. The wire ends do not injure soft tissues.

◂ *Where must the main splint wires be placed on the tooth surface?*

Method

1. A 12 inches length of dead soft stainless-steel wire of 0.007 inches to 0.010 inches thickness (e.g. *orthodontic ligature wire*) is taken.
2. The wire is doubled, bent around the group of teeth to be splint and its ends are loosely twisted together. This wire makes the main splint wire.
3. The main splint wire is then adapted to the surfaces of the teeth positioning it just apical to the interdental contact point but coronal to cingulum of teeth.
4. 4-inch pieces of the same steel wire are cut and bent to make hairpin restraints for the main splint wires. A hairpin wire is inserted interdentally from the buccal direction over (*coronal to*) the buccal and lingual main splint wires. When on the lingual side, the hairpin wire is bent ***around*** the lingual main splint wire and passed under it from the lingual side back to the buccal side to make it emerge apical to the buccal main splint wire. The two ends of the hairpin restraint wires are then held in a needle holder and twisted together.
5. After all hairpin restraint wires have been placed, all of these, except the last hair pin restraint wire, are tightened.
6. The main splint wires that were placed earlier are now tightened by twisting their ends with a needle holder while ensuring that the main buccal and lingual splint wires have not got dislodged from their positions.
7. The last hairpin restraint wire is now tightened.

◂ *How is splinting done with a dead soft steel wire?*

8. The twisted ends of the main splint wires and hairpin restraint wires are cut to about 4–5 mm length and bent into the interdental spaces ensuring that they do not cause injury to gingiva or the tongue.
9. If needed, composite may be applied over the splint wires to prevent them from dislodging.
10. As steel wires stretch during use, the splint might get loose with time; the hairpin restraint wires of the splint must therefore be checked and re-tightened periodically.

ALERT!

Does splinting teeth cure periodontitis? ▸

1. Periodontal splinting is done with the aim of ***temporarily*** reducing mobility of teeth; splinting will not treat or remove the cause of tooth mobility.
2. Splinting of the teeth does ***not*** prevent periodontitis induced attachment loss.
3. Splints with slight flexibility are more preferable for the splinting and management of traumatized teeth.

Review Questions

1. What is scaling and root planing? How is scaling different from root planing? What is the rationale of scaling and root planing?
2. Describe the technique for performing scaling and root planing.
3. What is calculocementum? What is necrotic or diseased cementum?
4. Write the shortcomings of ultrasonic scaler use.
5. What are the aims of periodontal surgery?
6. Why and for how long should a clinician wait after completion of phase I treatment before deciding on the need for phase II treatment?
7. Describe outcomes of periodontal wound healing. What are the factors that can delay and enhance the rate of periodontal healing?
8. Which post-operative patient instructions are given to a patient after periodontal surgery?
9. What are the general contraindications and complications of periodontal surgery?
10. What are periodontal dressings? Write the advantages and disadvantages of these.
11. Discuss the steps and precautions that when taken during periodontal surgery will improve its outcome.
12. What is periodontal splinting? What are its indications, contraindications and limitations?
13. What are the different types of splints used for periodontal splinting?
14. Describe the technique of extra-coronal splinting with composite resin using reinforcing fiber ribbon or dead soft steel wire.

Chapter 17

Surgical Treatment of Gingivitis and Periodontitis: Pocket Reducing Surgery

Gingival enlargement and increase in probing depth (*PD*) occur in gingivitis and periodontitis. Therefore, treatment of gingivitis and periodontitis requires ***reduction*** of probing depth (*PD*) to less than 3 mm and correction of contours of gingiva to normal contours.

Surgical treatment of gingivitis and periodontitis is done by curettage, gingivectomy and gingivoplasty that are discussed in Chapter 17A or by periodontal flap surgery that is discussed in Chapter 17B.

POCKET REDUCING SURGERY—BASIC SURGICAL PROCEDURES AND CONCEPTS

◂ *How are pockets treated?*

One of the basic goals of treatment of gingivitis and periodontitis is ***reduction of pocket depth to less than 3mm*** (*according to the 2018 classification of periodontal diseases*). A pocket has two walls—gingival soft tissue wall and tooth surface; periodontal pockets can therefore be treated by either:

◂ *How does pocket depth reduce with periodontal treatment?*

1. **Reducing length of the gingival pocket wall [*thereby reducing pocket depth* (*PD*)]**
   This can happen due to:
   a. Shrinking of gingival pocket wall as a result of resolution of inflammation after scaling and root planing.
   b. Shrinking of gingival pocket wall as a result of resolution of inflammation ***and*** surgical excision of coronal part of the gingival pocket wall (*e.g. flap surgery*).
   c. Removing a part or entire gingival wall of the pocket (*e.g. gingivoplasty and gingivectomy*).
   d. 'Elimination' of gingival wall of the pocket by shifting it apically and converting it to attached gingiva while maintaining base of pocket at the same level (*e.g. apically displaced flap*).
2. **Periodontal tissue regeneration**
   a. Pocket depth can also be reduced if base of the pocket is shifted coronally after regeneration of periodontal tissues that were lost due to periodontitis (*e.g. flap surgery and guided tissue regeneration*). Periodontal regeneration is usually partial (*in terms of volume of periodontal tissues regenerated and their relative proportions, orientation, and their functional inter-relationships*).
3. **Extraction of the tooth or its root** (*hemisection in mandibular molars and root resection in maxillary molars*) **to remove tooth side of the pocket.**

Pocket Reducing Surgery is Broadly Divided into the following Categories

◂ *Enumerate the surgical procedures used to reduce pockets.*

1. **Based on resection or regeneration potential of the procedure:**
   a. Resective procedures (*e.g. gingivectomy, undisplaced flap and apically displaced flap*).
   b. Regenerative procedures (*e.g. modified Widman flap surgery*).

2. **Based on reach and extent of procedure**
   a. Gingival surgical procedures (*restricted to gingiva*) (*gingivectomy and curettage*).
   b. Surgical procedures allowing access to alveolar bone (*flap surgery*).

The above Periodontal Surgical Procedures can also be Grouped as

What are access and non-access providing procedures? ▶

1. **Access providing or assess improving procedures**, e.g. gingivectomy and periodontal flap surgery.
   - These procedures provide easy access and visibility to diseased root surface and alveolar bone that are not otherwise visible (*because they are covered by gingiva*).
2. **Non access providing procedures**, e.g. curettage.

CLINICAL UTILITY AND SHORT ANSWER

What are the objectives of periodontal access providing surgery?

Periodontal access surgery has two main objectives:

What is the primary objective of access providing periodontal surgical procedures? ▶

1. **Primary objective:** To obtain access to and visibility of:
   i. Relatively inaccessible and hidden areas of teeth for thorough instrumentation (*for improving already done SRP to remove any calculus left back inadvertently during phase I treatment*).
   ii. Alveolar bone.

Gingivectomy, gingivoplasty can fulfill the 1st objective only (alveolar bone is not exposed during gingivectomy or gingivoplasty) whereas and flap surgery can fulfill both these objectives.

2. **Secondary objective:** To cause reduction in probing depth (*PD*) by:
   i. Resection of gingiva.
   ii. Regeneration of periodontal tissues and correction of alveolar bone defects.

Why can gingivectomy not be used for periodontal regeneration? ▶

Only flap surgery can fulfill both these objectives. Gingivectomy and gingivoplasty being gingival surgical procedures ***do not*** *involve exposure of alveolar bone; therefore, no bone resection or periodontal regenerative procedures are possible with gingivectomy or gingivoplasty.*

CLINICAL UTILITY AND SHORT ANSWER

How do 'access providing surgical procedures' (*periodontal flap surgery*) improve outcome of periodontal treatment?

What is the benefit of raising a flap for periodontal treatment? ▶

- Access providing procedures like flap surgery are done by surgically raising a gingival flap. Raising a flap provides improved access and visibility to tooth surfaces in deep pockets and root furcation areas that were earlier covered (*by gingiva*).
- If such areas are treated without raising a flap, restricted access and visibility will be there; this will make it very difficult to completely remove calculus and necrosed cementum from these root surfaces (*by scaling and root planing*). This compromises results of treatment.
- Access providing procedures thus improve clinical outcomes of periodontal treatment.

CLINICAL UTILITY AND SHORT ANSWER

What is the basis of choice between flap or gingivectomy for treating periodontitis? ▶

What is the difference between pocket elimination (*gingivectomy*) and pocket reduction surgery (*periodontal flap surgery*) for treatment of pockets? Which is better of the two?

According to the recent 2018 classification of periodontal diseases, probing depth of up to 3 mm is considered healthy and maintainable in a healthy state (*in a previously treated case of periodontitis, up to 4 mm pocket depth with no bleeding on probing is considered 'clinically healthy'*).

Pockets that are deeper than 3–4 mm, can be treated by two types of surgery: Pocket elimination surgery or pocket reduction surgery. Choice of procedure is based on:

1. **Procedure that will result in a shallower sulcus depth after treatment is preferred:**
   - Pocket ***reduction*** surgery (*periodontal flaps*) reduces the depth of a pocket and converts it into a healthy sulcus that can be up to 4 mm. If this presently healthy, up to 4 mm deep sulcus, is not maintained, it will reconvert into a pocket and periodontitis will recur.
   - Pocket ***elimination*** therapy (*gingivectomy*) eliminates the entire soft tissue pocket wall bringing the PD to 0 mm, i.e. there is no sulcus left to maintain in the immediate post-treatment period (*although after some time and despite excellent maintenance by the patient and the clinician, a very small sulcus will always re-form in all such cases*). Thus, there is a **greater** likelihood of maintenance of gingival health after pocket elimination surgery.

   Therefore, if there is a choice and if indicated, ***pocket elimination is better than pocket reduction***.

(*Contd.*)

(Contd.)

2. **Ease of performing the surgery:**
   - Pocket eliminating surgery (*gingivectomy*) is relatively ***easier*** to perform than pocket reducing surgery (*periodontal flaps*).
3. **Aesthetic concerns:**
   - Pocket maintaining surgery may be preferred over pocket elimination in anterior areas as pocket eliminating surgery (*gingivectomy*) will expose roots and open up interdental spaces that may appear as unappealing black triangles between teeth (Fig. 17.1, diag. A). This risk is lower in pocket reducing surgery (*flaps*).

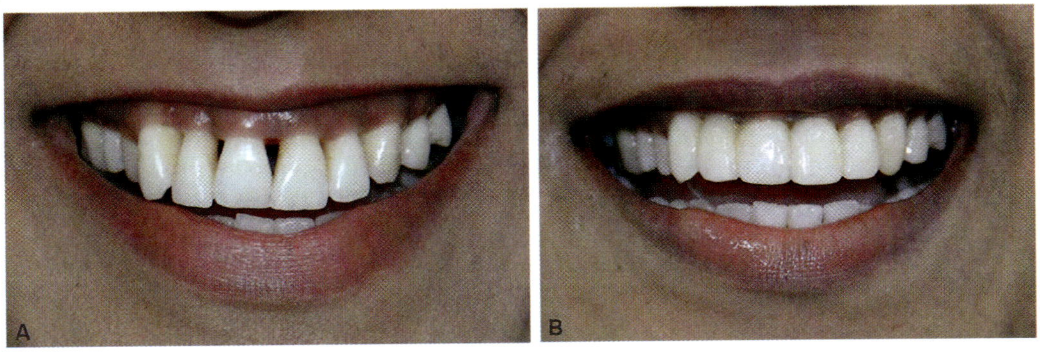

Fig. 17.1: Periodontal surgery can lead to opening of interdental spaces (*diag. A, black triangles between teeth*) and gingival recession. This is more likely after pocket eliminating surgery (*gingivectomy*). The patient later received laminates to improve her smile (*diag. B, note carefully reconstructed interdental embrasures*).

How to Choose between Pocket Elimination (*Gingivectomy*) and Pocket Reduction Surgery (*Periodontal Flap Surgery*)) for Surgical Reduction of Pockets in a Particular Patient

Selection of technique for pocket reduction is based on the following:

1. **General considerations:**
   i. If a patient is not likely to comply with instructions after treatment and patient is not performing adequate plaque control, gingivectomy is preferred over flaps.
   ii. If response of periodontium to phase-I treatment done earlier, and outcome of past periodontal treatments is not adequate, gingivectomy is preferred over flaps.
   iii. Systemic health concerns and age of patient. If systemic health concerns are present, gingivectomy is preferred over flaps.
   iv. If aesthetic concerns are present and possible future aesthetic complications are expected after surgery, gingivectomy is ***not*** preferred and flap surgery can be performed in such areas.

◂ *Which technique of pocket reduction is preferred in a patient who is not expected to perform adequate plaque control in the future?*

◂ *Which technique of pocket reduction is preferred in areas with esthetic concerns?*

2. **Specific local considerations:**
   i. **Condition of soft tissue (*gingival*) pocket wall:**
      - Degree of inflammation or fibrosis and anatomical characteristics of the gingival pocket wall are major factors in deciding choice of surgical procedure.
      - If fibrosis is present in the pocket wall, such pockets are best managed by excision (*gingivectomy—pocket elimination*) or flap surgery (*pocket reduction surgery*) whereas inflamed pocket walls can be easily treated by conservative means (*root planing and curettage*).

◂ *Which technique of pocket reduction is preferred in fibrotic pockets?*

   ii. **Condition of and access to the entire root surface (*hard tissue pocket wall*):**
      - Flap surgery can provide better adequate access and reach to difficult areas on the root as compared to gingival curettage and ENAP.
      - If access to entire root surface for plaque control and surgical debridement is not present, gingivectomy is preferred over flap surgery.

Which technique of pocket treatment is contraindicated if there is inadequate attached gingiva? ▶

Which technique of pocket treatment is contraindicated if there is need for bone surgery? ▶

iii. **Topography and condition of alveolar bone:**
   - If any kind of alveolar bone surgery is required, gingivectomy is contraindicated as it does not allow exposure of alveolar bone. Flap surgery has to be done in such cases.

iv. **Inadequate attached gingiva:**
   - If attached gingiva is already inadequate, any surgery that further reduces width of attached gingiva, e.g. gingivectomy and undisplaced flap are contraindicated and cannot be done.

v. **Type of healing desired versus one which is practically possible:**
   - Regeneration of lost periodontal tissues is desired but may not possible in all cases.
   - If there is any possibility of periodontal tissue regeneration, flap surgery is performed (*gingivectomy is contraindicated*).
   - If regeneration is not desired or expected, gingivectomy becomes indicated.

How does PD affect selection of technique surgical reduction? ▶

3. **Likelihood of reducing pocket depth (*PD*) to less than 4 mm after treatment**
   - According to the 2018 classification, PD has to be ideally maintained at less than 3 mm for all sites. As a relaxation to this rule, PD of up to 4 mm without any BOP (*bleeding on probing*) is considered normal at sites that have received periodontal treatment for periodontitis.
   - If pocket reducing surgery (*periodontal flap surgery e.g. modified Widman flap surgery*) is performed on deep pockets (*e.g. PD more than 6 mm*) the resulting PD after healing may remain more than 4 mm (*due to technique and limitation of the selected flap surgery procedure, e.g. modified Widman flap surgery*).
   - Pocket reducing surgery (*periodontal flap surgery, e.g. modified Widman flap surgery*) therefore becomes contraindicated. Pocket reducing surgery e.g. undisplaced flap, that can result in greater PD reduction can be performed in such cases.
   - In such cases pocket elimination (*gingivectomy*) is also preferred.

When must Pockets (*Gingivitis and Periodontitis*) be Surgically Treated?

When is surgical treatment of a pocket indicated? ▶

Surgical treatment of pockets is required in the following situations (*according to the 2018 classification of periodontal diseases*):

1. Pockets that have a depth of ***more than 3 mm*** are always at risk of progression of gingivitis or periodontitis; they are therefore to be treated urgently to reduce pocket depth to less than 3 mm. As an exception to this, in a previously successfully treated and now stable periodontitis patient, sites with PD up to 4 mm but with no BOP (*bleeding on probing*) are considered healthy and are not treated surgically to reduce pocket depth. If, however, BOP is present it means that plaque induced gingival inflammation has started again and there is risk of recurrent periodontitis. In these cases such pocket depths are surgically reduced to less than 3 mm.
2. Conservative treatment by SRP or curettage may not reduce pocket depth to 3 mm in all cases (*usually in fibrotic pockets more than 5 mm*). However, SRP must be done as a phase I therapy in all cases; thereafter if required, further PD reduction can be achieved by surgical pocket reduction (*flap surgery or gingivectomy*) **(Fig. 17.2)**.

Critical Probing Depth

What is critical pocket depth for surgical treatment of pockets? ▶

Decision on whether periodontal surgery is required for treatment of pockets or not is dependent on concept of critical probing depth (*5 mm*).

- Pockets ***less*** than 5 mm deep are ***likely*** to be effectively treated and probing depth (*PD*) reduced to less than 3 mm by scaling and root planing (*considered to be healthy PD according 2018 classification*).
- However, pockets that are ***5 mm or more*** in depth are ***less likely*** to be fully treated (*PD cannot be brought down to less than 3 mm*) only by scaling and root planing, they will require periodontal surgery to reduce their depth to less than 3 mm **(Fig. 17.2)**.

<u>In any case, if pockets less than 5 mm cannot be reduced to less than 3 mm by SRP, pocket reducing surgery must be done to bring the PD to less than 3 mm.</u>

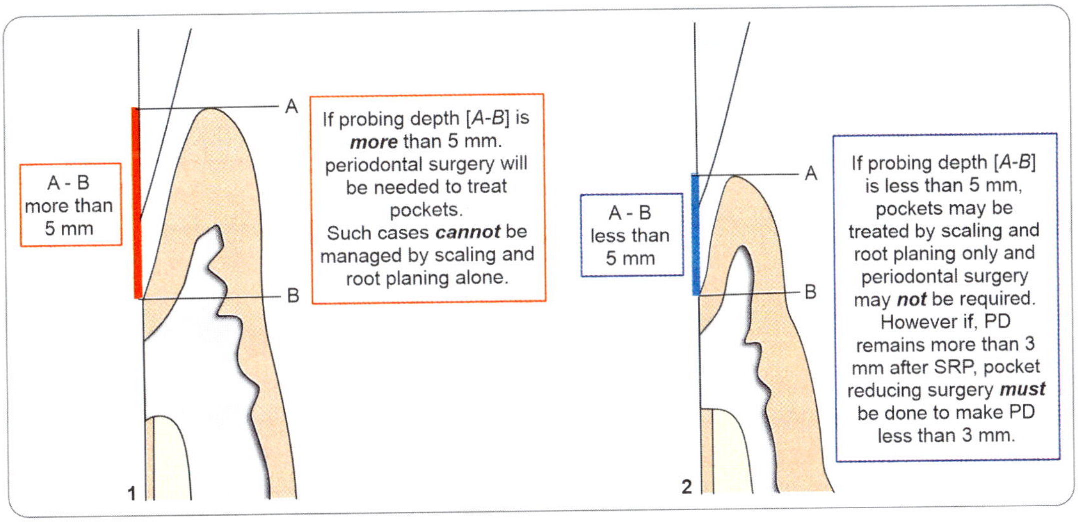

Fig. 17.2: Critical probing depth. Probing depth of more than 5 mm (*A-B, diag. 1*) is an indication for surgical treatment. If pockets are less than 5 mm deep (*A–B, diag. 2*), they can usually be treated by scaling and root planing only.

What is the Difference between Treatment of Pockets and Pocket Maintenance?

Treatment of pockets (*for treating gingivitis and periodontitis*) refers to reduction of pocket depth by treatment. This can be done either by pocket reduction or pocket elimination procedures, e.g. scaling and root planing, gingivectomy, flap surgery, etc.

◂ *What is pocket maintenance?*

Pocket maintenance refers to maintaining pockets in a disease-free state ***after*** treatment by repeated, regular periodic checkups and scaling and root planing procedures every 3–6 months (*or earlier, after every 2 months in case the disease is very severe and there are uncontrollable severe systemic risk factors, e.g. diabetes, genetic disorders, etc.*).

After treatment (*after pocket reduction surgery*) a well-maintained pocket shows:

- No clinical features of gingivitis, i.e. redness, swelling of gingiva, bleeding on probing (BOP), etc.
- Probing depth (PD) less than 3 mm.
- No increase in pocket depth and further loss of attachment and mobility.

Pocket reduction by gingival surgical procedures, i.e. curettage, gingivectomy and gingivoplasty is discussed in Chapter 17A, page 294.

Pocket reduction by periodontal flap surgery is discussed in Chapter 17B, page 303.

Review Questions

1. Name basic surgical procedures used to treat periodontal pockets.
2. What are access providing surgical procedures? Why is there a need of access providing surgery for mechanically cleansing the root surface?
3. Compare pocket reduction with pocket elimination.
4. For treatment of periodontitis, discuss the factors on which the selection of technique of surgical pocket therapy is based.
5. What is pocket maintenance?
6. What are the possible sources of healing cells in a periodontal wound? What is periodontal regeneration? Name surgical procedures for periodontal regeneration.
7. What is critical pocket depth for periodontal surgery?

Chapter

17A

Curettage, Gingivectomy and Gingivoplasty

When periodontal surgery for ***reduction*** or ***elimination of pockets*** and ***correction of abnormal gingival contours*** is ***limited*** to the gingiva (*alveolar bone is not exposed*) such procedures are called ***gingival surgical procedures.*** These include curettage, gingivectomy and gingivoplasty.

CURETTAGE

What is curettage? ▸

Definition: Removal of superficial layers of tissue by scraping or scooping with a periodontal curette is called curettage. In periodontics, the term curettage is also applicable to procedures that remove superficial layers of tissue using BP blades, LASER, etc.

How many types of curettage are there? ▸

Types of Curettage

1. *Gingival Curettage*

What is the difference between gingival and subgingival curettage? ▸

In this, lining of the gingival wall of the pocket containing sulcular epithelium and underlying connective tissue is curetted ***without*** elevating a flap (Fig. 17A.1, black line).

2. *Subgingival Curettage*

In this, curettage is carried further apically to remove the junctional epithelium along with sulcular epithelium and underlying connective tissue ***without*** elevating a flap (Fig. 17A.1, blue line).

Why are gingival and subgingival curettage not recommended to be done? ▸

Both the gingival and subgingival curettage are ***closed procedures*** (*no flap elevation is done*). However, both these procedures are ***not*** recommended to be done these days because:

- Both curettage and subgingival curettage do ***not*** provide any additional benefit over scaling and root planing (*results are similar to these obtained with scaling and root planing*).
- Both these procedures do ***not*** result in 'new attachment', i.e. regeneration of new periodontal tissues over root surfaces which were previously exposed by periodontitis.

3. *Curettage of Gingival Flap during Flap Surgery*

Is curettage recommended during flap surgery? ▸

Curettage is routinely done during flap surgery to remove granulation tissue attached to the flap (*gingival wall of the pocket*) and to thin the flap.

Indications of Curettage

1. *Gingival and Sub-gingival Curettage*

Although ***not recommended*** any more, some clinicians still perform gingival and subgingival curettage for the following indications:

i. Treatment of shallow suprabony pockets (*3–4 mm PD*) (*it is now proven that scaling and root planing are better alternatives to curettage*).
ii. Treatment of shallow infrabony pockets (*it is now known that infrabony pockets **cannot** be effectively treated by curettage*).

iii. As a compromise or maintenance procedure, especially in patients with recurrent periodontitis who cannot get periodontal surgery done due to systemic contraindications or other reasons (*scaling and root planing are better options as they produce the same results*).

◂ *In which situations can curettage be still recommended?*

2. *Curettage of Gingival Flap during Flap Surgery*

This is routinely performed and recomended

i. To remove bleeding granulation tissue attached to the flap that obstructs vision (*i.e. curettage is done for practical utility reasons rather than biologic reasons*).
ii. To thin the flap.

◂ *What is attained by curettage during flap surgery?*

Procedure of Curettage

1. *Gingival and Sub-gingival Curettage*

◂ *How is gingival curettage done?*

Gingival and sub-gingival curettage are ***no longer recommended***, however, for sake of academic interest, the steps in these procedures are:

i. Attain adequate anesthesia.
ii. Check and improve SRP done during phase I, if required.
iii. Suitable curette (*gracey curettes are preferred over universal curettes*) is inserted into the pocket and its cutting edge is adapted to the soft tissue wall of the pocket.
iv. After the cutting-edge bites into the pocket lining, it is pulled out coronally. Applying finger pressure on the gingiva from outside improves the bite of the curette.
v. A number of vertical and oblique overlapping strokes are used to remove the epithelial lining of the soft tissue wall of the pocket (Fig. 17A.1, black line).
vi. If sub-gingival curettage is to be done, curettage is extended apically to also 'completely' scoop out the junctional epithelium and the immediate underlying connective tissue (*coronal to the alveolar bone crest*), along with the pocket epithelium (Fig. 17A.1, blue line).
vii. The pocket is then irrigated with saline. After this, finger pressure is put on the curetted gingiva for a few minutes. This will ensure minimal clot formation.
viii. Sutures may be placed if necessary.
ix. Periodontal dressings (*packs*) may or may not be placed for few days.
x. After one week, teeth are re-checked for any remnant calculus or diseased cementum areas that may have been inadvertently left behind during the curettage. If any are found, these are removed with a curette.
xi. Polishing is done to ensure easier maintenance. It is done very gently and with utmost care to prevent injury to the underlying healing junctional epithelium.

◂ *How is subgingival curettage done?*

2. *Curettage of Gingival Flap during Flap Surgery*

i. This is done after raising a flap during flap surgery.
ii. For this, cutting edge of a suitable curette is adapted to the gingival wall of the pocket and pulled out coronally.
iii. Applying finger pressure on the gingiva from outside improves the 'bite' of the curette into the gingival pocket wall.
iv. Curettage is carried out till all the desired granulation tissue is removed.

◂ *How is curettage done during flap surgery?*

Other Ways of doing Curettage

1. *Curettage using LASER*

- In addition to removing superficial tissue, LASER energy:
  - Kills bacteria present in the pocket; this reduces inflammation and decreases pocket depth (*PD*) in shallow inflammatory pockets.
  - Increases speed of healing of periodontal wounds
  - Improves results of surgery done to treat periodontitis.
- Curettage done using LASER causes no or little bleeding during surgery (*LASER energy causes sealing of bleeding capillaries*).
- Diode and Nd:YAG lasers are commonly used for curettage (*diode laser is more commonly used*).
- This procedure is therefore ***recommended and routinely done***.

◂ *What are the benefits of doing curettage with LASER?*

◂ *Why is LASER curettage successful and recommended?*

◂ *Which LASERs are commonly used for periodontal curettage?*

2. Excisional New Attachment Procedure (ENAP)

What is ENAP?

- ENAP is curettage performed with a surgical blade **(Fig. 17A.1, red line)**. It is a modification of the gingival/sub-gingival curettage technique.
- In this, sulcular epithelium is excised by an incision extending from the crest of the free gingiva to the bottom of the junctional epithelium.

Why is ENAP not recommended?

- Results produced by ENAP are similar to those produced by scaling and root planing.
- This procedure is therefore ***not recommended***.

3. Curettage using Ultrasonic Scalers

- Some pocket epithelium can be removed with ultrasonic scalers.

What is inadvertent curettage?

- During ultrasonic (*and manual*) scaling and root planing some unintended and unplanned curettage can occur (*inadvertent curettage*).
- Results attributed to ultrasonic curettage are more because of the effects of scaling and root planing rather than the curettage itself.
- This procedure is therefore ***not recommended***.

CLINICAL UTILITY AND SHORT ANSWER

What is granulation tissue?

Is granulation tissue a diseased tissue?

- Granulation tissue is ***not*** an infected but a ***normal,*** healing fibrous connective tissue that replaces fibrin clot during wound healing.
- It is rich in new capillaries, light red or dark pink in color, soft to touch, moist and has a granular appearance.
- High vascularity of granulation tissue helps maintain suitable oxygen levels required for rapidly dividing cells, provide nutrients, remove waste products and transport immune cells to the healing wound area.
- It also has fibroblasts, macrophages and WBCs (*mainly neutrophils*).
- Microorganisms are also present in granulation tissue. These microorganisms are ***secondary*** invaders and are killed by the host immunity during the process of healing.

ALERT!

Can curettage remove pocket's epithelium completely?

No. Curettage done by any procedure, closed or open, cannot result in complete removal of pocket's epithelial lining.

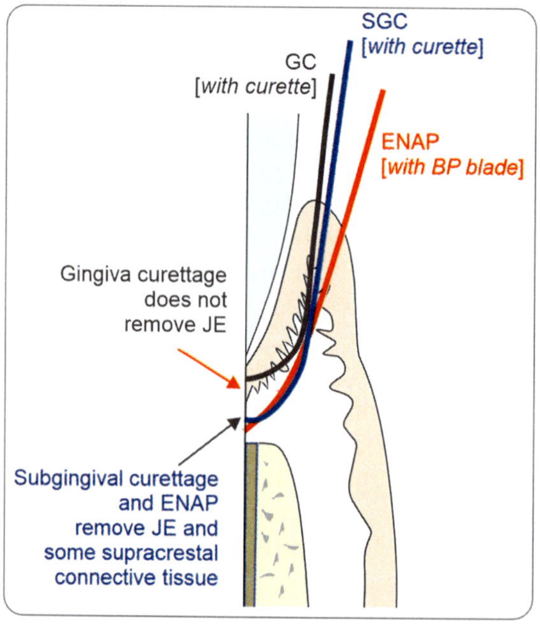

Fig. 17A.1: Extent of reach of incisions and tissue removal with incicions of gingival curettage (GC), sub-gingival curettage (SGC) and excisional new attachment procedure (ENAP).

GINGIVECTOMY

Definition: Gingivectomy is excision of gingiva. It is a gingival surgical procedure (*surgical procedure restricted to the gingiva only, i.e. not extending to the underlying bone*).

◂ *What is gingivectomy?*

Prerequisites of Gingivectomy

(*Ensure that the following Conditions are met before Planning Gingivectomy*)

1. Completed scaling and root planing (*SRP*) and other urgent treatments (*phase I*).
2. Presence of adequate attached gingiva and its likelihood of remaining adequate after gingivectomy is done (*see Chapter 2, 'Gingiva', pages 10–13, Figs 2.8, 2.9 and 2.10*).
3. No isolated deep pockets are present, i.e. depth of the pocket must be almost similar across the surgical field (*if depths of pocket are at different levels, gingivectomy will lead asymmetric gingival contour post-operatively*).

◂ *What conditions must be fulfilled before planning gingivectomy?*

Indications of Gingivectomy

Gingivectomy is done for:

1. Excision of gingival enlargements and correction (*reshaping*) of abnormal gingival contours to produce normal contours of the gingiva (*scalloped, knife edge and deflecting contour*).
2. Elimination of ***suprabony pockets*** and treatment of chronic suprabony gingival and periodontal abscesses.
3. Exposure of grade II, III or IV furcations.

◂ *When is gingivectomy recommended?*

◂ *Which of the two: Supra bony and infrabony pockets can be treated by gingivectomy?*

Contraindications of Gingivectomy

Gingivectomy is not done if:

1. Infrabony pockets are present **(Fig. 10.6, diag. B)**.
2. There is any need for alveolar bone surgery (*bone removing or bone grafting*).
3. Attached gingiva is inadequate, e.g. if base of pocket extends apical to the muco-gingival junction **(Fig. 2.10)**.
4. Attached gingiva is likely to become inadequate after gingivectomy.
5. Gingivectomy will result in extensive root exposure in the anterior teeth (*this will become unaesthetic*).
6. Keratinized gingiva (*free + attached gingiva;* **Figs 2.12 and 19.1** *and pages 10 and 336*) is needed for future mucogingival surgery, e.g. apically displaced flap (*gingivectomy removes free + attached gingiva*) (*see Chapter 19, 'Mucogingival Therapy', section on Apically Displaced Flap for Increasing Width of Attached Gingiva, page 338*).

◂ *When must gingivectomy not be done?*

ALERT!

Of all the surgical procedures for pocket treatment, gingivectomy is the easiest, simplest and surest way of pocket elimination.

Instruments used for Performing Gingivectomy (*and Gingivoplasty*)

1. Periodontal probes, explorers, mouth mirrors and tweezer.
2. Pocket markers—Crane-Kaplan or Goldman-Fox (*right and left*).
3. Gingivectomy knives—Kirkland, Waerhaug, Maryland, Orban, etc. and BP handle with scalpel blades #11, 12, 12D and 15.
4. Scalers, curettes and ultrasonic scalers.
5. Large burs/coarse grit diamond stones (*may be required in some procedures*).
6. Other special equipment, e.g. LASER, electrosurgical unit, etc. (*may be required in some procedures*).

◂ *Which instruments are used for gingivectomy?*

Procedure of Gingivectomy

1. **Follow aseptic technique**
2. **Attain anesthesia**

◂ *How is gingivectomy done?*

3. **Mark depth of the pocket—create bleeding points.**

A series of bleeding points marking the depth of the pocket, are made at short distances all along the surgical site on the surface of gingiva (*pocket wall*) **(Fig. 17A.2, diags E and H)**. There are two ways of doing this:

How are bleeding points marked with a pocket marker? ▶

i. **With a pocket marker:**

- Straight end of a pocket marker is inserted into the pocket up to depth of the pocket **(Fig. 17A.2, diag. A, 1)**.
- Then, the outer arm of the pocket marker that has a sharp and inward bent tip is pressed and inserted into the gingiva (*pocket wall*) to create injury and a bleeding point **(Fig. 17A.2, diag. A, 2 and D, 5)**.

In which cases is making bleeding points not possible with a pocket marker? ▶

Important: A pocket marker can however ***only*** be used if gingiva is flaccid and straight end of the pocket marker can be easily inserted into the pocket. Such gingiva is usually found in drug induced and idiopathic gingival enlargements. In cases where gingiva is not severely enlarged or is relatively firmer, pocket markers ***cannot*** be used because its straight end ***cannot*** be inserted into the pocket without tearing the gingiva. In such cases probes are used for pocket marking and creating bleeding points.

How are bleeding points marked with a periodontal probe? ▶

ii. **With a periodontal probe:**

- A probe is inserted up to depth of the pocket and the reading is noted **(Fig. 17A.2, diag. B, 1)**.
- It is then taken out and placed up to the same marking (*from the gingival crest*) on the outer wall of the pocket **(Fig. 17A.2, diag. C, 2)**.
- Then without displacing or moving the tip of the probe, the body of the probe is rotated to position its tip at right angles to the gingiva **(Fig. 17A.2, diag. C, 3)**.
- The probe tip is now inserted into the gingiva to create injury and a bleeding point **(Fig. 17A.2, diags C′, 4; D, 5; H and I, black arrows)**.

4. **Excision of gingival pocket wall**

This is done in the following steps:

i. **External bevel incisions:**

What is external bevel incision? ▶

- External bevel incisions are started ***1mm apical*** and ***parallel*** to an ***imaginary*** line joining the bleeding points and are directed ***coronally*** to end between the base of the pocket and the underlying crest of the alveolar bone **(Fig. 17A.2, diags D, 6, F, G and I**; *dotted lines represent imaginary line joining bleeding points, solid lines represent line of external bevel incision and white arrow in* **Fig. 17A.2., diag. I** *shows direction and orientation of external bevel incision at that particular point*).

What is the beveling angle made by the external bevel incision? ▶

- This way the external bevel incision makes a beveling angle of approximately 125°–130° to the tooth's long axis. This results in a sloping (*beveled*) gingival wound that will heal to produce a deflecting gingival contour **(Fig. 17A.2, diag. J, white arrows)**.

Which instruments are used for making an external bevel incision? ▶

- External bevel incisions are made either with Kirkland **(Fig. 14.12, diag. D)** gingivectomy knives or with BP blades #11, 12, 12 D or 15 mounted on BP handles. BP blades are sharper than gingivectomy knives therefore, incisions made with these are neater and require lesser force.

Why is precise placement of external bevel incision important? ▶

It is important to place the external bevel incision precisely as faulty incision placement and angulation may result in exposure of the alveolar bone or may not result in complete pocket wall excision.

How is external bevel incision made? ▶

- External bevel incisions can be made in the following ways:

What is a continuous incision? ▶

a. **Continuous incision:**
   – It is started from the distal surface of the posterior most tooth and is carried continuously in the anterior direction till the last tooth is reached in the surgical area **(Fig. 17A.2, diags F, solid blue line)**.

What is a discontinuous incision? ▶

b. **Discontinuous incision:**
   – The discontinuous incision is a combination of series of small interrupted incisions across the surgical field **(Fig. 17A.2, diag. G, solid blue line)**.

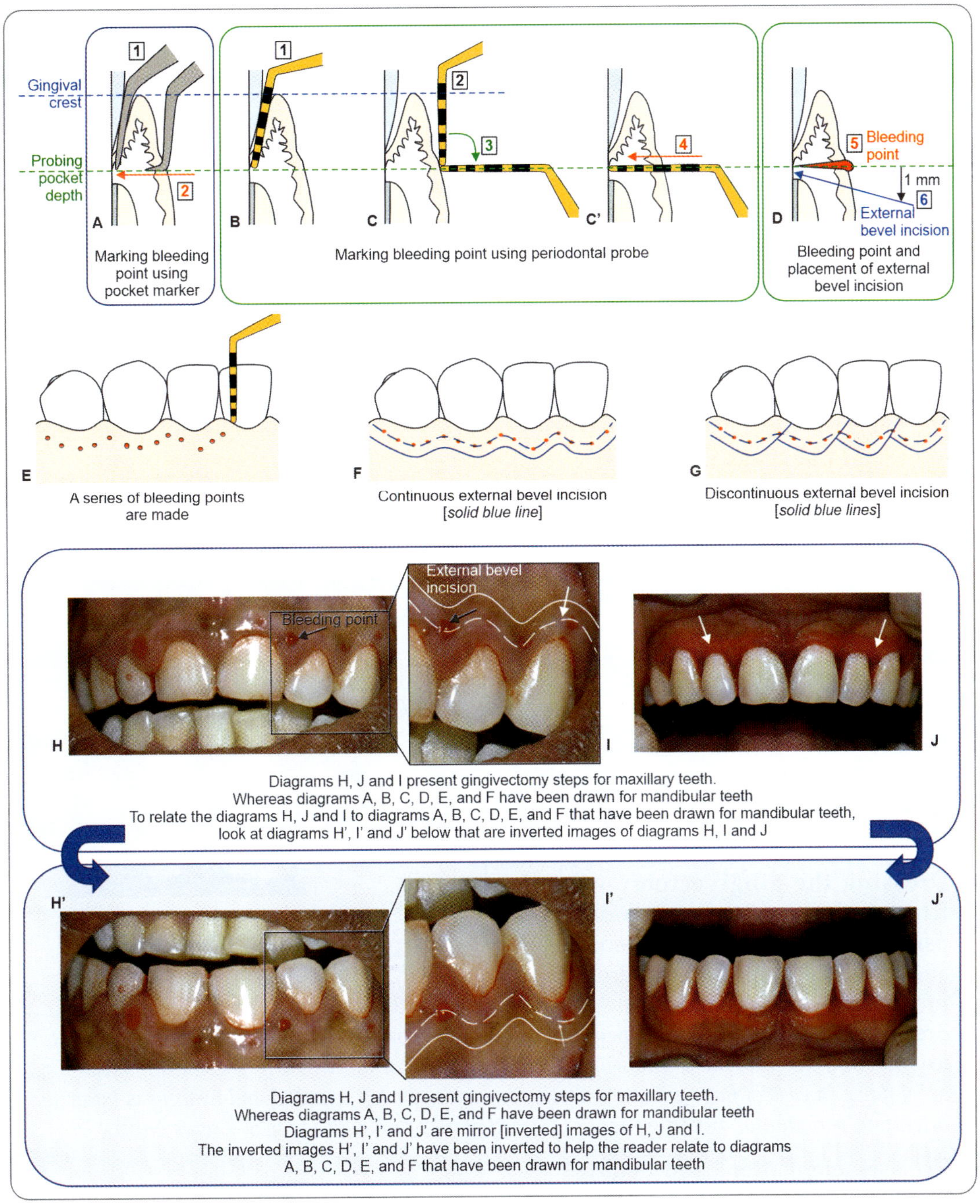

Fig. 17A.2: Marking bleeding points using a pocket marker and periodontal probe, placement of external bevel incision and beveled gingiva after completion of gingivectomy.

- It is also started from the distal surface of the posterior most tooth but is ***ended*** at the ***distal surface of the next anterior tooth.***
- The next incision is started at the point where the previous incision crosses the interdental papilla and it is ended at the distal surface of the next anterior tooth.
- Such interrupted incisions are repeated across each tooth till the last tooth in the surgical field is reached (Fig. 17A.2, diag. G, solid blue line).

◂ *How is a discontinuous incision made?*

c. **Combination incision:** Continuous and discontinuous incisions are usually given in combination as per requirements and convenience of the clinician.

- External bevel incisions are made both on the buccal and lingual/palatal side and these two are connected by a distal incision across the distal surface of the last tooth.

ii. **Interdental incisions:**

What is an interdental incision?

- The interdental incision connects the buccal with lingual or palatal external bevel incisions and separates the interdental papilla from the underlying bone crest.

Which instruments are used for making an interdental incision?

- Orban's or Waerhaug's interdental knives or BP blades are used to make this incision (Fig. 14.12, diag. C).
- This incision can be made from the buccal to the lingual/palatal side or vice-versa.

How is incised gingiva removed?

5. **Removal of the incised gingiva (pocket wall):** Scalers and curettes are used to detach the incised gingiva (pocket wall) from the tooth and the underlying bone.

How are gingival contours refined during gingivectomy?

6. **Refining the gingival contours and appraisal of the field of operation:**
   i. Confirm complete excision of gingival wall of pocket using a probe.
   ii. If any pocket depth remains after the first incision, the gingiva making the wall of the pocket, is excised and gingival contours are refined using scissors and tissue nippers (Fig. 14.12, diags E, F and G).
   iii. Granulation tissue and gingival tissue tags are removed. Tooth surfaces are examined for any remaining calculus deposits. If calculus is found, it is removed.

Which gingivectomy knife is used for contouring of gingiva during gingivectomy?

7. **Final correction of contour of gingiva:** If the desired deflecting contour of gingiva has not been attained with the above steps, contour of the gingiva is beveled and ***further improved*** by trimming 'extra' tissue with curved scissors or scrapping gingival surface using kirkland gingivectomy knives (Fig. 17A.3). Coarse grit diamond stones mounted in a handpiece can also be used for this purpose.

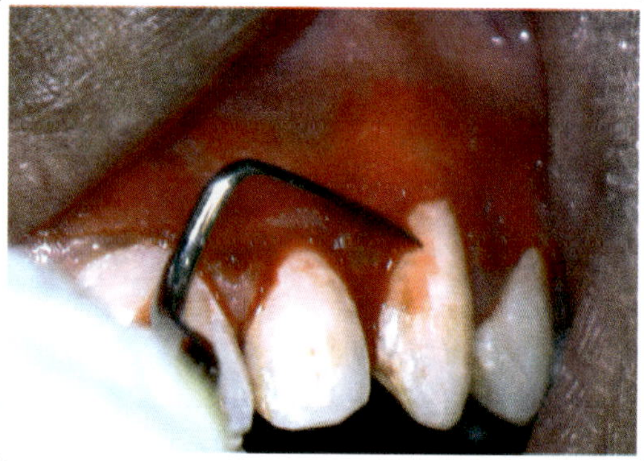

Fig. 17A.3: Beveling of gingiva with a kirkland knife to produce deflecting contour

Why is periodontal pack placed for a longer time after gingivectomy?

8. **Dressing the gingivectomy wound:** Exposed healing gingival connective tissue after gingivectomy bleeds easily and can be very painful. Therefore, to protect the healing gingivectomy wound and make the patient comfortable, a periodontal dressing (*periodontal pack*) is placed on the wound for 10–14 days (Fig. 16.6) (*gingivectomy wounds heal by secondary intention, therefore, periodontal dressing should be placed for up to 14 days; in case of flaps since connective tissue is not left exposed and healing is by primary intention, periodontal dressings are not needed at all or are placed for 5–7 days only).*

9. **Re-assessment after 7 and 14 days**
   i. Root surfaces are re-checked for calculus left behind unintentionally during the surgery and if found, it is removed.
   ii. After 14 days, polishing of teeth is done carefully to prevent injury to the gingiva.

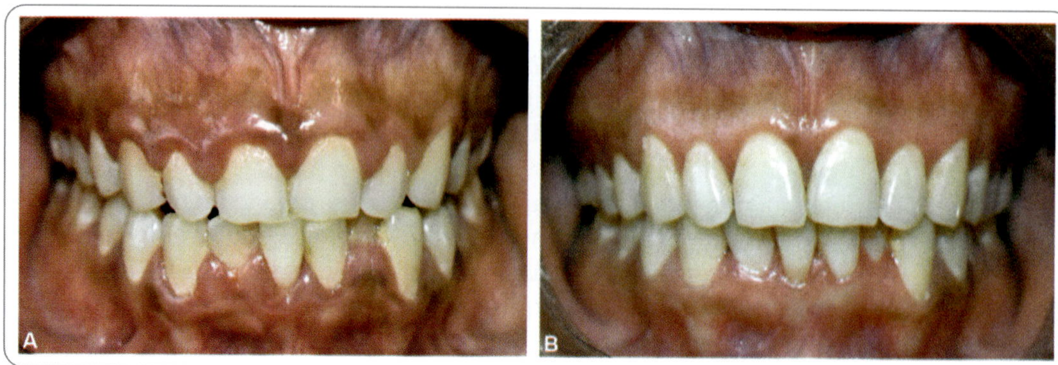

Fig. 17A.4: Result after gingivectomy (*preoperative view, diag. A and 3-week postoperative view, diag. B*)

CLINICAL UTILITY AND SHORT ANSWER

Gingivectomy can also be done using electrosurgery and LASERs

Both these modalities allow a bleeding free surgical field (*due to coagulation of blood and sealing of bleeding capillaries by the electrosurgery or LASER*).

- Electrosurgery is a very efficient way of excising and reshaping gingiva.
- However, if electrosurgical tips touch the underlying bone or tooth surface, they can cause bone resorption and damage the root surface.
- Use of electrosurgical units produces a strong unpleasant smell of burning tissue and these may not be usable in patients with cardiac pacemakers.
- LASERs can also be used for gingivectomy and gingivoplasty; however, it cuts and reshapes slower than electrosurgery.
- Results after gingivectomy using electrosurgery or LASERs is similar to that of gingivectomy done using scalpels.

◂ *What are the advantages and disadvantages of doing gingivectomy using electrosurgery and LASER?*

CLINICAL UTILITY AND SHORT ANSWER

Write the main advantages and disadvantages of gingivectomy over flap surgery when used for treatment of periodontitis.

Advantages of gingivectomy

- The main advantage of gingivectomy over flap surgery is—gingivectomy eliminates pockets whereas flap surgery leaves back treated pockets of reduced depth.
- If excellent plaque control is not practiced by the patient, such treated pockets left back after flap surgery can again lead to recurrent gingivitis or recurrent periodontitis.
- On the other hand, as no pockets are left after a gingivectomy, the chances of recurrent gingivitis or periodontitis are lesser.

◂ *In which situations is gingivectomy preferred over flap surgery?*

Disadvantages of Gingivectomy

a. Healing of gingivectomy wounds takes longer than flap surgery wounds as gingivectomy wounds heal by ***secondary*** intention (*flap wounds heal by primary intention*).
b. Gingivectomy results in ***loss*** of keratinized tissue (*pocket wall and part of attached gingiva*). This also increases chances of future muco-gingival problems.
c. Excision of gingiva in gingivectomy results in root exposure and open interdental spaces (*black triangles; Fig. 17.1 diag. A*). These can look unattractive especially in the anterior region.

◂ *What are the main drawbacks of gingivectomy?*

CLINICAL UTILITY AND SHORT ANSWER

What is internal bevel gingivectomy?

The ***Undisplaced flap*** is called internal bevel gingivectomy (*see Chapter 17B and Fig. 17B.8, pages 310 and 311*). This is so because the undisplaced flap (*like gingivectomy*) also excises gingival pocket wall; for this it uses an internal bevel incision to excise gingiva (*soft tissue wall of pocket*) (*an external bevel incision is used in gingivectomy*).

GINGIVOPLASTY

- Gingivoplasty is very similar to gingivectomy.
- Difference between gingivectomy and gingivoplasty lies in the ***intent*** of the clinician:
  - If clinician wants to ***eliminate*** the pocket completely, ***gingivectomy*** is done.
  - If clinician only wants to ***correct gingival contours***, ***reshape gingiva*** and reduce pockets but does not plan to eliminate pockets completely (*a shallow pocket depth is left after surgery, i.e. some probing depth remains*), the procedure is called ***gingivoplasty***.

◂ *What is the difference between gingivectomy and gingivoplasty?*

Indications of Gingivoplasty

1. To re-contour and reshape enlarged and fibrotic (*no or very little clinically identifiable features of inflammation*) gingiva with rolled and blunt contours, e.g. gingival enlargements, etc.
2. For crown-lengthening (*to expose tooth structure to place crowns over teeth*).
3. For cosmetic reasons:
   i. To expose more anatomic crowns of teeth in patients with 'gummy' smiles.

◂ *When is gingivoplasty recommended?*

ii. To create bilateral symmetry of gingival contours by excising 'extra' gingiva over a group of teeth or an isolated tooth.
iii. Correction of gingival craters resulting after healing of necrotizing ulcerative gingivitis (*NUG*).

Review Questions

1. What are gingival surgical procedures?
2. What is curettage? What is inadvertent curettage? What is the difference between gingival and sub-gingival curettage?
3. Does the curettage procedure also involve scaling and root planing?
4. What is the method of performing gingival and sub-gingival curettage?
5. Is it justifiable to perform gingival/sub-gingival curettage?
6. What is ENAP?
7. What is gingivectomy? What are its pre-requisites, indications and contra-indications?
8. What is the procedure of gingivectomy?
9. What are the advantages of gingivectomy over flaps?
10. What is gingivoplasty? What is the difference between gingivectomy and gingivoplasty?
11. What are the indications of performing gingivoplasty?
12. What is an internal bevel gingivectomy?

Chapter

17B

Periodontal Flap Surgery

Periodontal flap surgery can be done for many indications. However, it is usually done to treat advanced periodontitis in cases where more than 3 mm PD (*probing depth*) is present (*still remains*) even after phase I treatment. In such cases periodontal flaps provide the clinician an opportunity to reduce pocket depth, scale and root plane the root surface under better visibility and attempt periodontal regeneration. A gingival flap is also raised for correction of muco-gingival problems, wisdom tooth removal, apicoectomy, etc.

Definition: A periodontal flap is a surgically raised part of gingiva and/or alveolar mucosa that provides improved visibility of and access to roots of teeth and underlying bone. It also makes available a gingival unit that can be displaced coronally, apically or laterally to correct mucogingival complications.

◂ *What is a flap?*

Periodontal flaps are ***'conservative'*** procedures (*unlike gingivectomy which is radical*) as they maintain and/or add to the width of keratinized gingiva that is already present (*keratinized gingiva = free gingiva + attached gingiva; Fig. 2.12 and 19.1 and pages 10 and 336*).

CLASSIFICATION OF PERIODONTAL FLAPS

Periodontal flaps can be classified according to:

I. **Thickness of flap (*exposure/no exposure of bone after flap reflection*)**

   a. **Full thickness or Muco-periosteal flap:** In these flaps, ***entire*** soft tissue covering the alveolar bone, i.e. epithelium, gingival connective tissue and underlying periosteum are raised by ***blunt dissection*** to expose underlying alveolar bone using a muco-periosteal elevator (Fig. 17B.1, diag. A). Full thickness flaps are raised when any type of bone surgery (*resective or regenerative*) has to be done.

   ◂ *What is a full thickness flap?*

   b. **Partial thickness or Spilt thickness or Mucosal flap:** If epithelium and only a ***part*** of the underlying connective tissue is raised leaving the alveolar bone ***covered*** by the remaining connective tissue and periosteum, such a flap is called partial thickness flap (Fig. 17B.1, diag. B). Partial-thickness flaps are raised by ***sharp dissection*** with BP blades (*usually # 15 and 11*). Partial thickness flaps are raised for correction of mucogingival defects, e.g. root recession coverage, deepening of the vestibule, etc.

   ◂ *What is a partial thickness flap?*

II. **Final placement position of flap after surgery**

   ◂ *What is the difference between displaced and non-displaced flaps?*

   a. **Non-displaced flaps:** When flap is positioned back at its ***original*** location after surgery.

   b. **Displaced flaps:** When flap is positioned at a location which is different from its original location.

      - Displaced flaps can be of three types:

        i. **Coronally displaced flaps:** When flap is positioned coronal to its original position.

        ii. **Apically displaced flaps:** When flap is positioned apical to its original position.

        iii. **Laterally (*horizontally*) displaced flaps:** When flap is positioned mesial or distal (*lateral*) to its original position.

        ◂ *What is the difference between coronally displaced, apically displaced and laterally displaced flaps?*

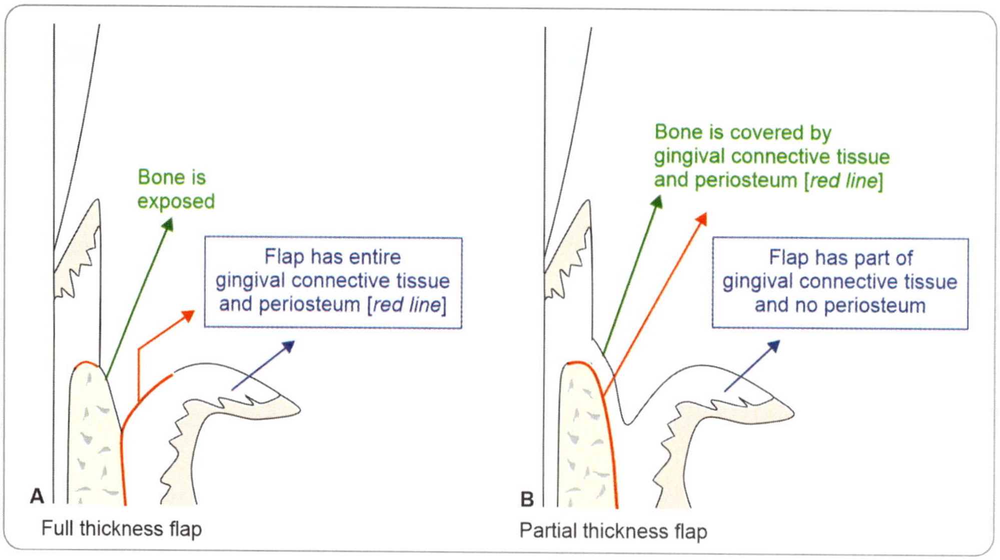

Fig. 17B.1: Full and partial thickness periodontal flaps

Which incisions are essential if a flap has to be displaced?

- Both full and partial thickness flaps can be displaced.
- To displace a flap, ***vertical releasing incisions*** are required and the flap has to be raised ***apical*** to mucogingival junction, i.e. into the alveolar mucosa.

III. Management of interdental papilla during incision

What is the difference between papilla splitting and papilla conserving flaps?

a. **Papilla splitting or conventional flap:** When horizontal incisions used to raise a flap incises and ***splits*** interdental papilla into two buccal and lingual/palatal parts (*that get incorporated into buccal and lingual/palatal flaps respectively*).

b. **Papilla preservation flaps:** When horizontal incisions are designed in such a way that interdental papilla is preserved and the ***entire*** interdental papilla is incorporated into either buccal or lingual/palatal flaps.

ALERT!

Other less commonly used terms to describe types of flaps are:

1. **Gingival flap:** When flap reflection is ***restricted*** to ***attached gingiva.***
2. **Mucogingival flap:** When flap is reflected beyond (*apical*) to mucogingival junction.
3. **Envelope flap:** When flap is raised using horizontal incisions only (*no vertical incisions are used*).
4. **Trap door flap**: When flap is raised using both horizontal (*at buccal end*) and vertical incisions (*on sides of flap*). A trap door flap can either be a mucogingival or a gingival flap.

INCISIONS USED DURING PERIODONTAL FLAPS

Name the incisions used for elevating flaps.

1. **Horizontal Incision:** This incision is made in the horizontal direction **(Fig. 17B.2, yellow line)**. There are ***three*** types of horizontal incisions:
   a. **Internal bevel incision** or **Reverse bevel incision**
   b. **Sulcular incision** or **Crevicular incision**
   c. **Interdental incision**
2. **Vertical incision:** These are made in the vertical direction at sides of the flap **(Fig. 17B.2, green dotted line)**.

1. Horizontal Incisions

a. *Internal Bevel Incision* (*also called reverse or inverse bevel incision*)

- It is the ***first*** incision to be given **(Fig. 17B.3., diag. A)**.
- It is made with a #11 or 15 BP blade.
- The internal bevel incision is made at variable distance from the crest of the free gingiva (e.g. *0.5–1.0 mm for modified Widman flap but more for undisplaced flap depending on depth of pocket*) with the blade held almost parallel to the long axis of the tooth and directed to end at or just lateral to crest of the alveolar bone **(Fig. 17B.3, diags A and 17B.5, diag. A)**.

How far away from the gingival crest is the internal bevel incision given?

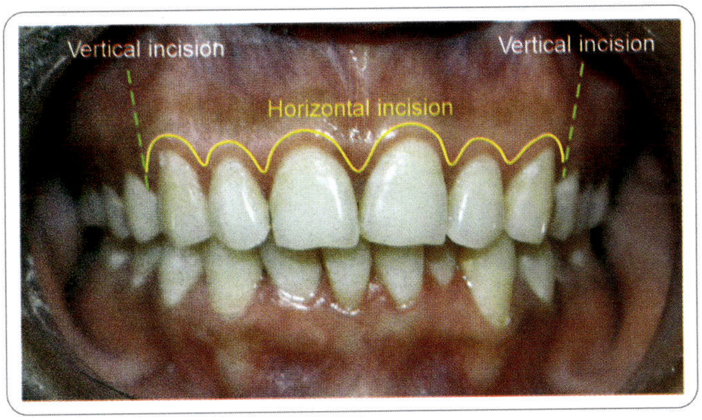

Fig. 17B.2: Horizontal and vertical incisions used for periodontal flap surgery

- This way it produces a ***bevel*** (*slanting/sloping surface*) on the tooth facing side of the gingiva.
- The internal bevel incision separates the epithelial lining of the pocket (*sulcular epithelium*) from the gingival flap and ***thins*** it. This helps re-create the 'knife' edge deflecting contour of gingiva.
- The flap is elevated from wound made by this incision.
- Partial thickness flaps can also be elevated using internal bevel incision. In this case, the incision is not extended down to the alveolar bone but is continued over the surface of the alveolar bone and ended lateral to the surface of alveolar bone.

◄ *What does the internal bevel incision achieve?*

◄ *Can partial thickness flaps also be elevated using internal bevel incision?*

b. *Sulcular Incision* (*also called crevicular incision*)

- Sulcular incision is the ***second*** incision (Fig. 17B.3, diags B and B′ and 17B.5, diag. B).
- It is made through the gingival sulcus using #12, 11 or 15 BP blades ***after*** inverse bevel incision.
- It starts from base of sulcus and ends at or near the crest of underlying alveolar bone.
- Sulcular incision along with internal bevel incision, accomplishes separation of gingival collar, i.e. the pocket wall containing inflamed and granulomatous tissue, from the underlying tooth and the bone (Figs 17B.5, diag. B and 17B.6, diag. B).
- Separation and subsequent removal of the gingival collar allows thinning of the flap, reduces bleeding (*as granulation tissue in the pocket lining is also removed with the gingival collar*) and contributes to the reduction of probing pocket depth (*PD*) (Fig. 17B.6, diags B, C and D).
- It is important to remember that periodontal regeneration can only be attempted if pocket lining (*contained in the gingival collar*) is completely removed.
- In some cases, flap can be raised using sulcular incision only (Fig. 17B.3, diag. B′).

◄ *Where does the sulcular incision start from?*

◄ *What does the sulcular incision accomplish?*

◄ *What does removing collar of gingiva separated after horizontal incisions for flap surgery accomplish?*

c. *Interdental Incision*

- Interdental incision is the ***third*** incision.
- It is made after internal bevel and sulcular incisions (Fig. 17B.3, diag. C and diag. 17B. 5, diag. C).
- It is usually made with an interdental knife, e.g. Orban's knife or # 11 or 12 BP blades.
- Interdental incision is made at ***right angles*** to teeth in the ***interdental regions*** just coronal to the crest of alveolar bone and ***through the wound*** made by internal bevel incisions given earlier (*it connects facial and lingual/palatal incisons*).
- The interdental incision is extended from the interdental area to the facial and lingual radicular surfaces of teeth (***through the wound*** *made by internal bevel incisions given earlier*) to allow easy separation of gingival collar from the teeth and bone.

◄ *Why is interdental incision called the third incision?*

◄ *Which instruments are used for making interdental incisions?*

◄ *How is the interdental incision made?*

2. Vertical Incisions

- Vertical incisions are called ***releasing incisions*** because they help raising a flap easily by releasing tension in the flap.

◄ *Why are vertical incisions called releasing incisions?*

How many vertical incisions are given to raise a flap? ▸

- None ***or*** one ***or*** two vertical incisions that may or may not extended beyond the mucogingival junction, may be given at the boundary of the flap to allow ***easier flap handling.***

What is an envelope flap? ▸

If only one vertical incision is planned, where must it be given and why? ▸

- Vertical incisions are ***avoided*** on the palatal aspects (*because they are difficult to manage on the palatal side*). When ***no*** vertical incisions are used the flap is called ***'envelope flap'.***

Why must vertical incision be extended beyond mucogingival junction for displacing flaps? ▸

- Flaps ***cannot*** be displaced if vertical incisions end in attached gingiva as attached gingiva is not movable or stretchable. Therefore, if a flap has to be displaced coronally, apically or laterally, it is necessary to ***extend*** vertical incisions apical to mucogingival junction and into the alveolar mucosa. For the same reason flap displacement is ***not*** possible on the palatal side as there is no alveolar mucosa.

If a single vertical incision is planned, where must it be given and why? ▸

- If only one vertical incision has to be given, it is given on the anterior end of the flap (*as this will not cut off blood supply coming from the distal end*).

ALERT!

Important points to remember with regard to vertical incisions:

Why must base of flap be broader than its coronal part? ▸

1. When two vertical incisions are used, it must be ensured that the apical end (*base*) of the flap is ***broader*** than its coronal end (Fig. 17B.4, diag. 1). This ensures adequate blood supply to the flap (*blood vessels supplying the gingiva run **vertically** from the apical side*) (*see Chapter 2, 'Gingiva', and Fig. 2.14*).

Why must a vertical incision not be given in the interdental papilla? ▸

2. Interdental papilla must ***not*** be split by a vertical incision, i.e. the interdental papilla should either be fully included in or fully excluded from the flap (Fig. 17B.4, diag. 3). If interdental papilla is split, it shrinks during healing and the interdental space becomes ***unaesthetic*** due to recession of interdental papilla.
3. Vertical incisions must ***not*** be made on bone or root prominences (Fig. 17B.4, diag. 4).

What is the ideal location for a vertical incision? ▸

4. Vertical incisions are ***best placed*** in between the interdental papilla root prominence.

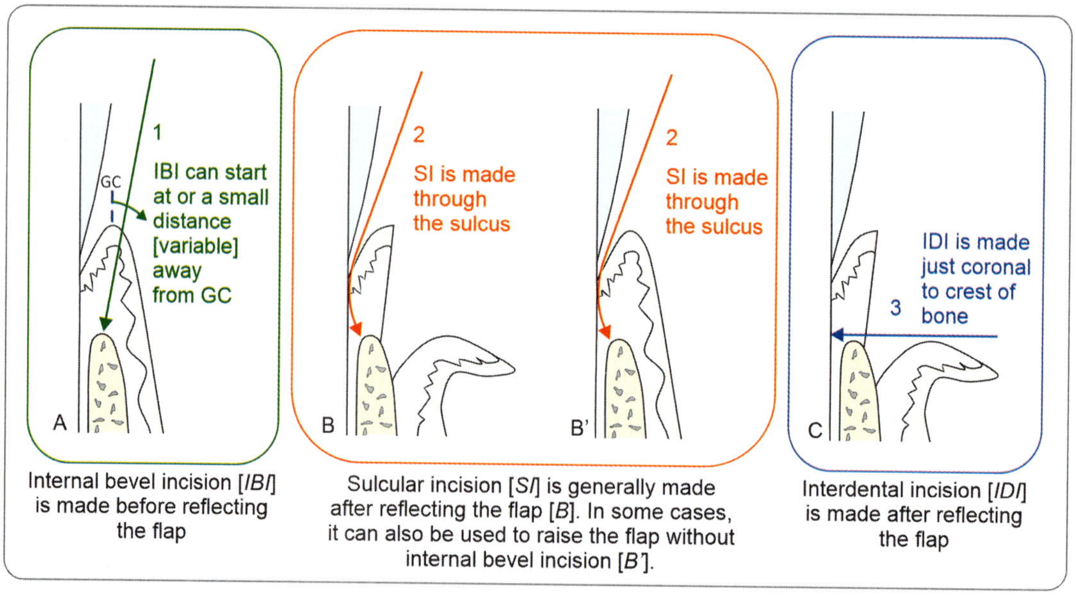

Fig. 17B.3: Incisions for periodontal flap surgery

CONVENTIONAL (*PAPILLA SPLITTING*) PERIODONTAL FLAPS

What are papilla splitting flaps? ▸

Conventional or papilla splitting flap design raises buccal and lingual/palatal flap as ***separate*** flaps and ***splits*** the interdental papilla into two halves by ***horizontal*** incisions. Two most commonly performed papilla splitting flap procedures are Modified Widman flap and Undisplaced flap. They are described below.

Modified Widman Flap (*MWF*)

Modified Widman Flap' (*Ramfjord and Nissle, 1974*) is a modification of 'Widman Flap' (*Widman, 1918*).

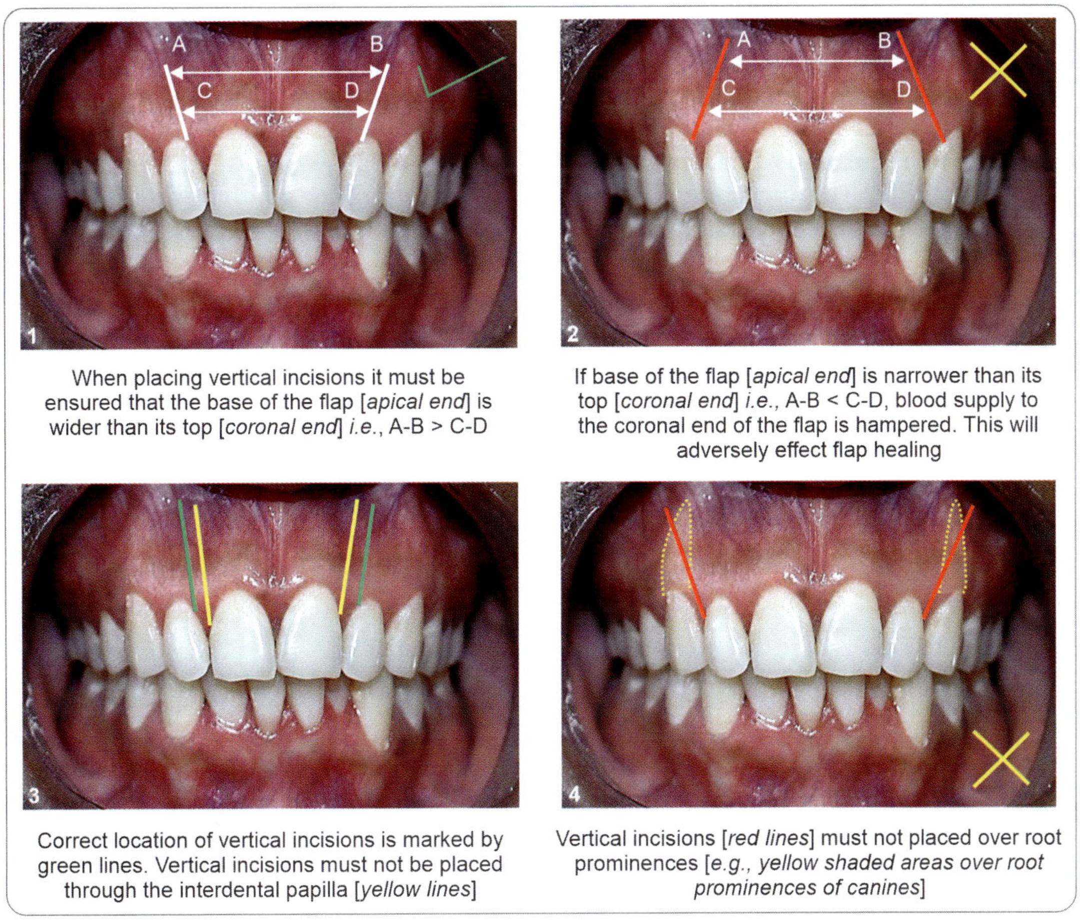

When placing vertical incisions it must be ensured that the base of the flap [*apical end*] is wider than its top [*coronal end*] *i.e.*, A-B > C-D

If base of the flap [*apical end*] is narrower than its top [*coronal end*] *i.e.*, A-B < C-D, blood supply to the coronal end of the flap is hampered. This will adversely effect flap healing

Correct location of vertical incisions is marked by green lines. Vertical incisions must not be placed through the interdental papilla [*yellow lines*]

Vertical incisions [*red lines*] must not placed over root prominences [*e.g., yellow shaded areas over root prominences of canines*]

Fig. 17B.4: Correct and incorrect vertical releasing incisions

Indications of MWF

MWF is indicated for:

1. Treatment of ***both*** supra and infra bony periodontal pockets (*true pockets*).
   - Ideally only pockets ***deeper*** than ***5 mm*** are treated by flap surgery (*critical pocket depth for periodontal surgery is 5 mm*) (*see Chapter 17 and Fig. 17.2, page 293*).
   - 3–5 mm pockets are ***preferably*** treated by scaling and root planing, however, if 3–5 mm deep true pockets do not reduce to less than 3 mm after scaling and root planing, flap surgery can be done.

◂ *Ideally, how deep pockets must be treated by flap surgery?*

2. Correction of alveolar bone defects by bone grafting and resective bone surgery.
3. Treatment of furcation defects.
4. Periodontal regeneration surgery.

Contraindications of MWF

MWF is contraindicated if:

1. Phase-I treatment has ***not*** been carried out.
2. There are gingival (*false*) pockets (*gingivectomy or gingivoplasty is indicated here*).
3. There are shallow periodontal (*true*) pockets less than 5 mm (*scaling and root planing must be tried first*).
4. Mucogingival complications are present.

Incisions for MWF

Three horizontal incisions—internal bevel, sulcular and interdental incision (described above pages 304–306) are used for MWF. Vertical incisions are used only if required.

◂ *How many incisions are used to raise MWF?*

Technique of MWF

1. Attain adequate anesthesia.
2. First incision, the ***internal bevel incision***, is made at distance of ***0.5–1.0 mm*** from the crest of the free gingiva with the blade held parallel to the long axis of the tooth and directed at the crest of the underlying alveolar bone **(Figs 17B.5, diag. A, 17B.6, diag. A and 17B.7)**. This incision follows scalloped contour of the gingiva and is extended interdentally to allow maximum interdental papillary tissue to be included in the flap.
3. Vertical incisions (*releasing incisions*) are best ***avoided***, but if given, must extend 2–3 mm apical to the gingival margin. MWF surgery can be easily done without vertical incisions (*a flap raised without vertical releasing incision is an 'envelope flap'*).
4. A ***full thickness flap*** is raised with a muco-periosteal elevator using blunt dissection ***through*** the wound made by the first incision (*internal bevel incision*) to expose only ***2–3 mm*** of alveolar bone margin.
5. Second incision or the ***sulcular*** incision is now made through the sulcus (*pocket*) till the ***crest*** of the alveolar bone with a #12 or 11 BP blade **(Figs 17B.5, diag. B and 17B.7)**.
   At some sites, where marginal gingiva is ***thin*** or there is a ***shallow pocket*** (*very small PD*), the MWF can be raised using ***sulcular incision only*** (*i.e. no internal bevel incision is needed, Fig. 17B.3, diag. B*).
6. Third incision or the ***interdental incision*** is then made using Orban's interdental knife and #11 or 12 BP blades **(Figs 17B.5, diag. C and 17B.7)**. This incision separates interdental papilla from underlying interdental bone. The interdental incision is also extended to the facial and lingual radicular surfaces of teeth to separate a collar of gingiva from underlying crest of alveolar bone and tooth surface.
7. Collar of gingiva separated from underlying crest of alveolar bone and tooth surface by the three horizontal incisions is now removed using scalers and curettes **(Figs 17B.6, diags B and C and 17B.7)**.
8. After flap elevation and removal of collar of gingiva, the exposed roots of teeth are checked for presence of any calculus or necrotic cementum. If required, scaling and root planing are re-done (*under **direct vision**, and **good access** to these areas due to elevation of flap*).
9. Any tissue tags or granulation tissue obstructing good vision of the root surface are also removed.
10. Bone architecture is corrected (*osteoplasty or ostectomy*) only if it is grossly defective or if it interferes with proper flap closure (*see Chapter 18, pages 309–311*).

How is the internal bevel incision designed for a MWF?

From where is the full thickness flap raised for MWF?

How much bone is ideally exposed after flap reflection during MWF surgery?

Can MWF be raised using only sulcular incision?

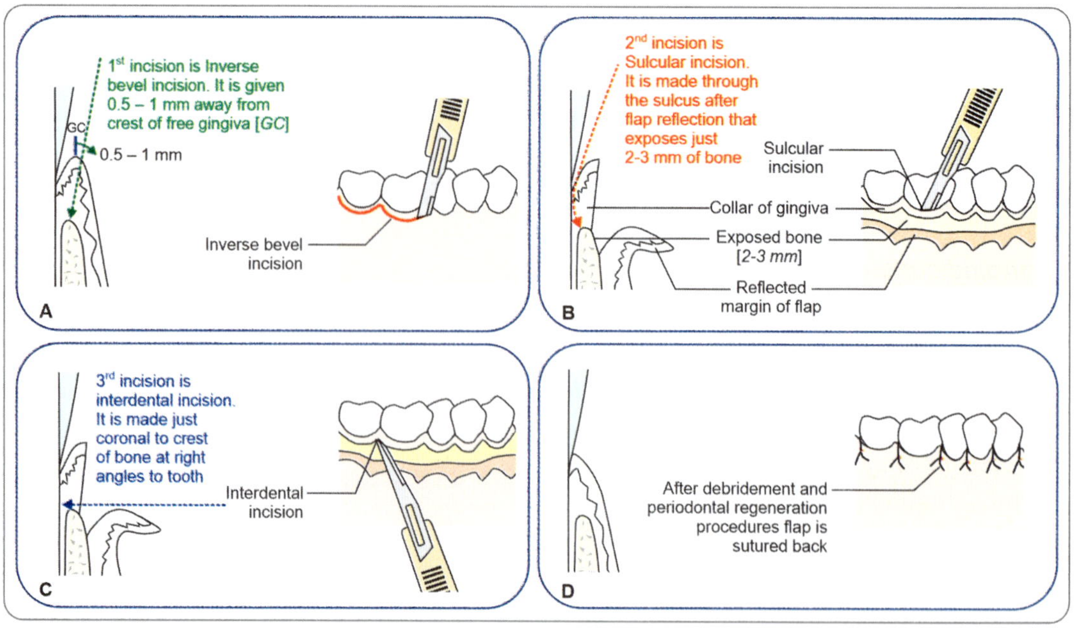

Fig. 17B.5: Basic steps of Modified Widman flap

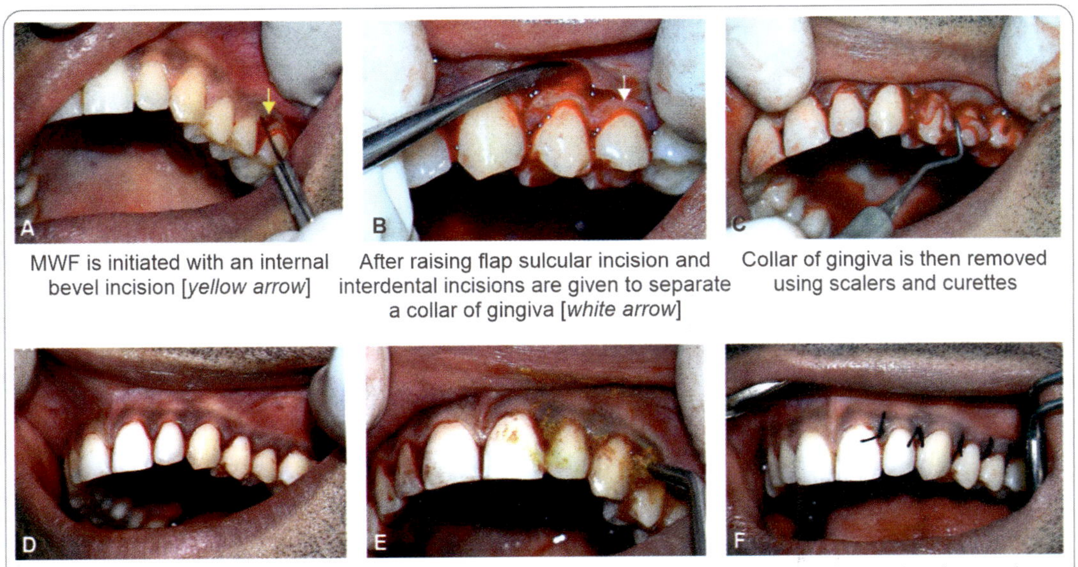

A. MWF is initiated with an internal bevel incision [*yellow arrow*]

B. After raising flap sulcular incision and interdental incisions are given to separate a collar of gingiva [*white arrow*]

C. Collar of gingiva is then removed using scalers and curettes

D. The flap is debrided, irrigated and root planing is improved if required

E. If required, periodontal regenerative procedures [bone grafting, GTR etc.] are done

F. Flap is then sutured securely

Fig. 17B.6: Modified Widman Flap

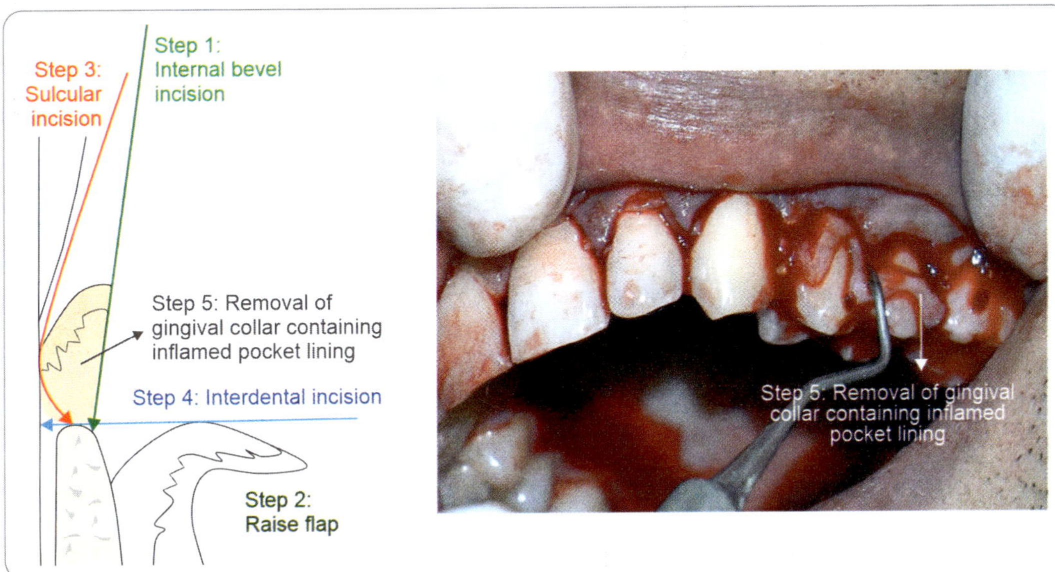

Fig. 17B.7: Steps in removal of collar of gingiva containing diseased (*inflammed*) pocket lining during flap surgery. Removal of gingival collar causes reduction in pocket depth and thinning of marginal gingiva these are the chief goals of modified widman and undisplaced flap surgery.

11. Surgical area is thoroughly irrigated with normal saline to flush out any debris in the surgical site.
12. Periodontal regenerative procedures (*e.g. GTR membrane placement and bone grafting*) if planned are now completed **(Fig. 17B.6, diag. E)** (*also see Chapter 18, 'Resective Bone Surgery and Regeneration of Periodontal Tissues', and Fig. 18.10, pages 330–331*).
13. Flaps are put back, wound is sutured and periodontal dressing is applied **(Fig. 17B.5, diag. D and Fig. 17B.6, diag. D)**. Sutures are removed after one week. At this time, roots of teeth are re-checked and, if any calculus that has been unintentionally left behind during earlier treatments is noticed, scaling and root planing is re-done.
14. Polishing of teeth may be done very carefully to ensure easier plaque control. Utmost care must be taken to prevent injury to the newly formed junctional epithelium.

Undisplaced Flap (UF) (*Internal Bevel Gingivectomy*)

The undisplaced flap is one of the ***most popular*** periodontal flap procedures for treatment of periodontal pockets (*periodontitis*).

What is the main advantage of undisplaced flap? ▸

- While MWF reduces PD (*probing depth*) to some extent and converts pockets into shallower sulci (*that must be maintained*), the UF ***almost eliminates*** pockets (*this decreases chances of recurrent periodontitis*) and brings PD down to almost 1 mm level.

Why is the undisplaced flap called internal bevel gingivectomy? ▸

- As the UF reduces pocket depth (*PD*) considerably, just as gingivectomy does, the ***UF is also called internal bevel gingivectomy***.

Pre-conditions for Undisplaced Flap

What must be ensured before planning an undisplaced flap? ▸

1. Presence of an ***adequate*** width of attached gingiva that is ***not*** likely to become inadequate in future must be ensured before UF.
2. ***No*** plan for ***extensive*** guided regeneration procedures (*GTR*) however, minor bone regeneration with bone grafting especially in infrabony defects can be done.

Indications and Contraindications of Undisplaced Flap

Are indications and contraindications of UF similar to those of MWF? ▸

- UF is not suited for performing extensive periodontal regeneration procedures.
- ***All other indications and contraindications of UF*** are the ***same as those of MWF*** (*see Section on modified Widman flap, page 307*).

Technique of Undisplaced Flap

How is UF done? ▸

1. Attain adequate anesthesia.
2. Pocket measurement and ***marking of bleeding points*** on the gingiva is done as is done during gingivectomy **(Fig. 17B.8)** (*also see Chapter 17A, pages 298 and 299*).
3. First incision, the internal bevel incision, is made just like it is made in the MWF but with ***some modifications***:

   From where is the internal bevel incision started in UF? ▸

   a. The incision is initiated *from* the bleeding point on the gingiva to a point located ***lateral and apical*** to crest of alveolar bone **(Fig. 17B.9, diag. E)** (*in gingivectomy this incision is initiated 1 mm apical to bleeding point and is directed in the coronal direction;* **Figs 17A.2 diag. F and G, page 299 and 17B.8, diag. F**). The incision is continued along an imaginary line connecting the bleeding points, across the length of the surgical site **(Fig. 17B.9, diag. C)**. As depth of the pocket and hence location of the bleeding point with respect to the crest of the gingiva will be variable across the length of the intended flap, the level of initiation of the incision on the gingiva can also be varied at different sites **(Fig. 17B.9, diags A and B)**.

   Where does internal bevel incision end in UF? ▸

   b. Ending point of the internal bevel incision on the lateral surface of the bone is also variable and depends on the thickness of the gingiva.

      How does thickness of gingiva affect the ending point of internal bevel incision in undisplaced flap? ▸

      i. If gingiva is ***thin***, the end point of the internal bevel incision is kept ***closer*** to the alveolar crest.
      ii. On the other hand, if gingiva is ***thicker***, the internal bevel incision is ended relatively more ***apically*** with respect to the alveolar crest.
      iii. However, in any case, the end point of the incision must always be ***apical*** to the bleeding point (*existing depth of the pocket*) and the crest of the alveolar bone.

   The internal bevel incision this way almost eliminates the pocket and thins the gingiva.

Which incisions are made after internal bevel incision in UF? ▸

4. Sulcular and interdental incisions are made and surgery is ***continued*** hereafter just as it is done in the MWF (*see Section on MWF on page 294*).

ALERT!

The internal bevel incision can be scalloped or straight.

When is the internal bevel incision kept straight? ▸

- If the flap has to be displaced to a coronal or apical position, the internal bevel incision maybe kept straight.
- If, however the flap has to re-placed at its original position, the internal bevel incision has to be scalloped.

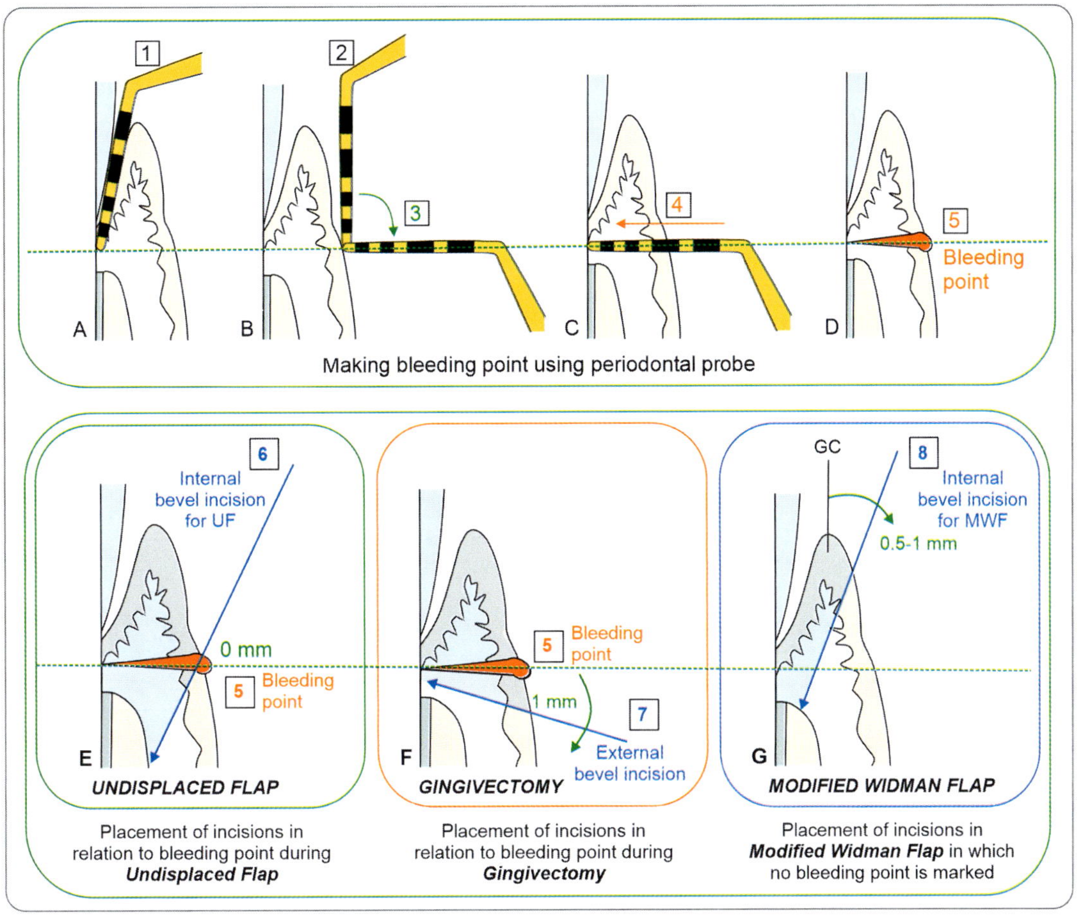

Fig. 17B.8: Marking of base of pocket by bleeding point (*diags A–F, BP*) and placement of incisions in relation to bleeding point. Making of bleeding point is shown in diagrams A–D. During undisplaced flap, an internal bevel incision is made at the level of the bleeding point (*diag. E, 6*). For comparison, in gingivectomy, the external bevel incision is made 1 mm apical to the bleeding point (*diag. F, 7*). A bleeding point is not required during modified widman flap (*diag. G*) and in this case an internal bevel incision (*diag. F, 8*) is made 0.5–1 mm buccal to the gingival crest (*diag. F, GC*). Blue shaded area (*diags E, F and G*) marks the gingival tissue that will be excised during the respective procedure (*diag. E undisplaced flap, F gingivectomy and G modified Widman flap*).

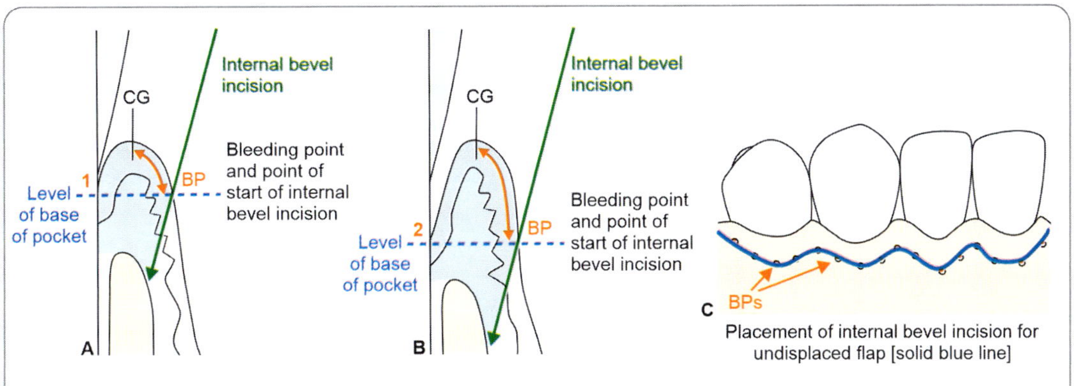

Internal bevel incision is started from a bleeding point [*BP*] that is made at the level of the base of the pocket [*diags. A, B and C*] and continued across the surgical site [*diag. C*]. In shallower pockets [*diag. A, 1*], bleeding point [*BP*] is located more coronally than when compared to that in deeper pockets [*diag. B 2*], therefore distance between crest of gingiva [*CG*] and bleeding point/point of starting of internal bevel incision [*red double arrows*] is smaller in shallower pockets [*diag. A, red double arrows*] and larger in deeper pockets [*diag. B, red double arrows*]. This allows reduction of PD/elimination of both shallow and deep pockets with undisplaced flap surgery

Fig. 17B.9: Diagrammatic representation of how variation in point of start of internal bevel incision can lead to reduction in probing depth/elimination of both shallow and deep pockets during undisplaced flap surgery.

CLINICAL UTILITY AND SHORT ANSWER

What is the justification behind eliminating the pocket (*with UF or gingivectomy*) instead of maintaining it (*with MWF like pocket reducing/maintaining surgery procedures*)?

Pocket maintenance procedures like the MWF convert a pocket (*diseased sulcus*) into a sulcus (*healthy*).

- A clinician using due to gingival recession pocket maintenance procedures wants to maintain gingival tissue to prevent tooth surface exposure due to gingival recession and hopes that the MWF and other treatments will result in periodontal regeneration.
- It is also expected by the clinician that the sulcus that results after surgery will be maintained by the patient in a disease-free state (*with good home care and periodic SRP as advised*).
- However, it is well known that periodontal regeneration does not occur usually and pocket converted to a sulcus is not well maintained by the patient thereby resulting in recurrent periodontitis and periodontal loss.

What is the advantage of UF? ▸

- For this reason, several clinicians do not leave things to chance and eliminate the pocket (*with gingivectomy or UF*) so that the chance of recurrent periodontitis is brought to bare minimum. This ensures long term success in most clinical situations.

What are the chief disadvantages of UF? ▸

- Obviously, pocket eliminating procedures like the UF and gingivectomy expose roots of teeth that may look unaesthetic and make them sensitive to hot and cold foods.
- Another disadvantage with pocket elimination procedures is that such procedures cause loss of keratinized gingiva (*free gingiva and a part of attached gingiva*).
- Keratinized gingiva is conserved with pocket maintenance procedures like modified Widman flap.

ALERT!

Some points of importance regarding suturing of flaps:

Why must flaps be coapted before suturing? ▸

1. Before suturing, flap must be coapted, i.e. flap tissue must be lightly pressed against the underlying roots of teeth and bone for a few seconds. This will ensure ***minimal*** clot formation under the flap (*thick clots delay healing and are likely to get infected*).
2. Minimal and gentle handling of the flaps is recommended.
3. Suture needles should be held (*with a needle holder*) just short of the midpoint but nearer to the needle swage (*point where the thread is inserted into the needle body*).

Where must the suturing needle pierce gingiva to prevent tearing of gingiva? ▸

4. To prevent suture thread from tearing through the flap, suture needle should enter gingival tissue at right angles and at least ***2–3 mm from the edge*** of the flap on both buccal and lingual/palatal flaps. The suture needle should perforate the interdental papilla just apical to its base **(Fig. 17B.10)**.
5. If possible, primary closure of the wound must be attempted (*no space must be there between flap wound margins*).

(*Contd.*)

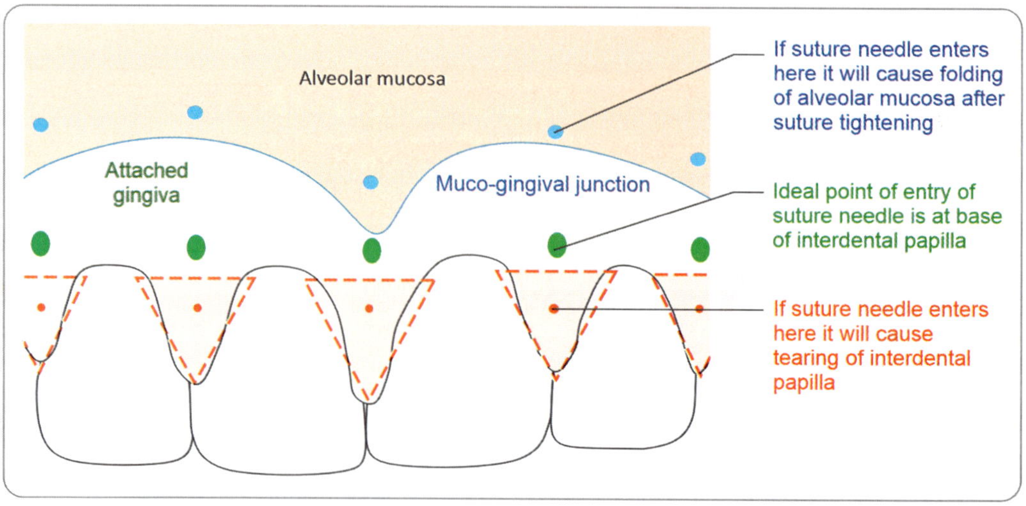

Fig. 17B.10: Ideal point of entry of suture needle is marked by green dots at the base of triangle of interdental papillae (*red dotted triangles*). If suture needle is pierced in the center of the interdental papillae (*red dots*), there are increased chances of tearing the interdental papillae while suturing. If needle entry points are more apical i.e. in the alveolar mucosa (*blue dots*), it will cause folding and crumpling of alveolar mucosa when sutures are tightened. Flap closing sutures starting in alveolar mucosa are therefore generally discouraged when attached mucosa is present.

(*Contd.*)

6. Gingival wound edges should slightly evert after suturing and suture tension must be so adjusted that there is ***no*** blanching of gingiva. The suture knot must be placed on one side of the approximated wound margins.
7. Sutures are generally placed in each interproximal space and distal to the last operated tooth, they should be evenly spaced.
8. Single interrupted sutures, one placed in every interdental space is the most commonly used suturing scheme.
9. Non-resorbable sutures are usually used for suturing periodontal wounds; they are removed 5–7 days after the surgery.
10. While suturing, the needle must be passed from more mobile to the lesser mobile flap, i.e. from buccal (*more mobile*) to a palatal flap (*lesser mobile*) flap. This prevents tissue tearing and undue tissue stretching.
11. Cutting needles facilitate tissue penetration but may cause ***larger*** needle entry wounds and may also cause gingival tearing especially if gingival flap is inflamed. Reverse cutting needles are better as these allow easy penetration but prevent tearing of gingival tissue. Round needles are difficult to insert but offer the best protection against tearing (**Fig. 17B. 11**).

◂ *Which type of suture needle must be used if gingival flap is inflamed and friable?*

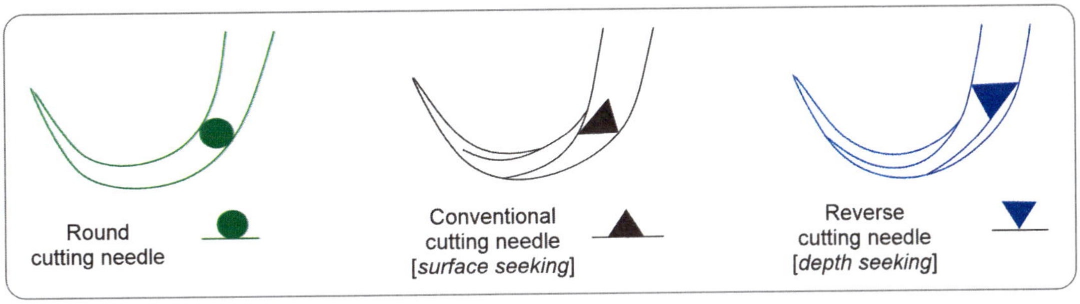

Fig. 17B.11: Round, conventional cutting and reverse cutting suture needles. Round suture needles have no cutting edge. Conventional cutting needles have a cutting edge inside their curvature (*cutting edge is directed towards the wound edge*), i.e. these are surface seeking needles; therefore, they have a tendency to tear through gingiva. Reverse cutting needles are depth seeking as there is a cutting edge outside their curvature; these therefore offer better protection against tearing gingiva while suturing. Round and reverse cutting needles are preferred for suturing gingiva and oral mucosa.

MODIFICATIONS IN FLAP PROCEDURE FOR SPECIFIC NEEDS AND AREAS

Papilla Preservation Flap (*Takei 1985*)

Preserving an intact interdental papilla during flap surgery, i.e. preventing its cutting into buccal and lingual/palatal halves is beneficial for many reasons. Splitting of papilla causes shrinkage of papilla after healing (*this results in empty interdental spaces post operatively*). A preserved papilla is also useful if bone grafts have to be used in interdental bone defects (*because the bone graft now does not lie just under the incision wound and therefore is relatively more protected*).

◂ *Why is it beneficial to maintain an intact interdental papilla during flap surgery?*

The papilla preservation flap technique preserves the entire interdental papilla in one piece instead of splitting it into two by horizontal incision (*internal bevel incision as used in conventional papilla splitting techniques like the MWF and UF*). In this regard it is important to remember that:

- Papilla preservation flap ***cannot*** be done if interdental papilla is very small/thin (*as in narrow interdental spaces*). In such cases the papilla tears during the process of lifting it when a papilla raising flap is being raised.
- Preserving the papilla is ***unnecessary*** if the surgical sites lie in the non-aesthetic zones and especially if no periodontal regeneration (*e.g. bone grafting*) has to be carried out.
- In addition to regular periodontal surgical instruments, availability of good set of micro surgical instruments and magnification (*loupe or operative microscope*) are ***preferable***.

◂ *Can a papilla preservation flap be done in all cases?*

Surgical Technique of Papilla Preservation Flap

The preserved papilla flap is raised using semilunar, sulcular and papilla undermining dissection (**Fig. 17B.12**). The steps in raising a preserved papilla are:

Can a preserved papilla be incorporated into either buccal or palatal/ lingual flaps?

1. Making the semilunar incision (*SLI*) and merging it with sulcular incision
   - The semilunar incision allows incorporation of the interdental papilla into ***either*** the buccal or lingual/palatal flaps.
   - It must ***only*** be made in the ***keratinized gingiva*** (*marginal gingiva and attached gingiva*).

What are the basic preconditions of designing a SLI?

   - If a bone defect is present, the semilunar incision must be-placed ***3 mm away*** from its boundary.
   - To reduce chances of shrinkage of the interdental papilla, the SLI must be placed at least ***5 mm away*** from the center of the interdental papilla.
   - SLI (Fig. 17B.12, diags A and B, red line) is made with # 11 or 12 BP blade held at right angles to the gingival surface. It is initiated from line angle of a tooth bordering the interdental space (Fig. 17B.12, diags A and B, red arrows). The incision line first goes apically towards the base of the interdental papilla, is curved across the interdental papilla and is then dipped coronally to end at the line angle of the other tooth bordering the interdental space (Fig. 17B.12, diag. A, 1 and blue arrow).
   - At this point the SLI (Fig. 17B.12, diags A and B, red line) is merged with sulcular/ internal bevel incisions all around the teeth on both sides of the preserved papilla (Fig. 17B.12, diag. B, SLI red line *merging with green and blue SI lines and red arrows*). The entire interdental papilla has now been incorporated into either the buccal or palatal flap as per design.

How is the interdental papilla freed form the underlying alveolar bone?

2. The interdental papilla is now freed from the underlying interdental bone using undermining sharp dissection that is done using BP blades # 11, 12 or 15, orban's knife and curettes inserted through the wound created by interdental semilunar incision. (Fig. 17B.12, diag. A, 2, black arrow).

How is the flap raised during preserved papilla flap surgery?

3. Raising of full thickness flap is initiated through the interdental semilunar incision and continued through the sulcular/internal bevel incisions.

   The preserved interdental papilla is ***gently pushed*** out of the interdental space with a round end instrument and raised along with the flap. Tissue tags and granulation tissue under the papilla are removed.
4. Flap surgery is now continued as in conventional flaps (*see pages 308 and 309*).
5. During closure the interdental papilla is pushed back into the same interdental space and sutured.

MODIFICATIONS IN TECHNIQUE FOR FLAP SURGERY ON THE PALATE

The following necessitate modifications in design of flaps on the palatal side.

Where must the palatal flap edge be located after suturing?

- After completion of surgery, the coronal edge of the palatal flap has to be located ***on*** (*covering*) the root-bone junction (*crest of alveolar bone*). As the entire palatal tissue is ***attached*** (*to underlying bone*) and is ***non-elastic***, it therefore ***cannot*** be coronally or apically displaced. Placement and designing of the internal bevel incision is therefore very important.

Which factors have a bearing on the design of flap incisions for palatal flap surgery?

- Placement and design of internal bevel incision is also dependent on thickness of palatal gingiva, whether vault of the palate is high or low and presence or absence of bone defects.

Why are vertical incisions not preferred on the palate?

- Vertical incisions are usually not made on the palatal side as there is a possibility of cutting the anterior palatine artery (*this causes massive bleeding*).

What is the drawback of using an internal bevel incision only to thin the palatal flap?

- Adequate thinning of very thick palatal flaps may not be possible with an internal bevel incision (*technique modification like the 'ledge-wedge technique described below solves this problem*).

What is the drawback of a thick palatal flap?

- As palatal flap is relatively thicker and if it not thinned effectively by the internal bevel incision, its edges will remain slightly lifted after suturing. This will result in a ***thicker*** and ***rounded*** contour of crest of palatal gingiva after healing (*instead of knife edge deflecting contour*). Such thick flaps not only take longer to heal but also are prone to recurrent gingival inflammation (*gingivitis*).

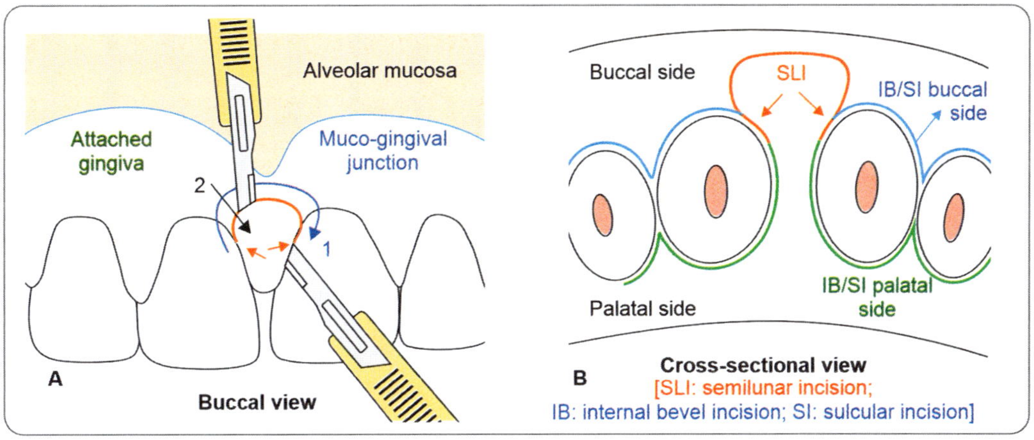

Fig. 17B.12: Incisions for papilla preservation flap. Semilunar incision is made first (*diag. A, 1 and blue arrow*). This is followed by interdental incision (*diag. A, 2 and black arrow*). Semi-lunar incision (*SLI, diag. A and B, red line*) is continued and merged with sulcular/interdental incisions on buccal and palatal sides (*SI, IB diag. A and B, red arrows*).

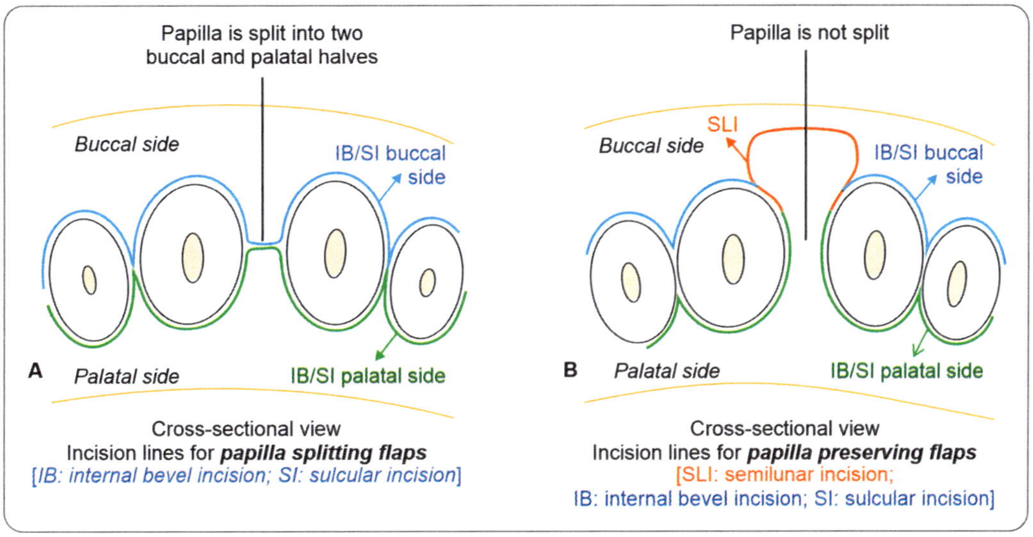

Fig. 17B.13: Cross sectional diagrams comparing incisions for papilla splitting flap (*modified widman flap, undisplaced flap, etc.*) (*diag. A*) and preserved papilla flap with the entire papilla incorporated into the *palatal* flap (*diag. B*).

Ledge-Wedge Procedure

The ledge-wedge procedure (Fig. 17B. 14, diags B and C) is an excellent technique to thin very thick gingiva adequately during flap surgery (*instead of the conventional internal bevel incision only approach;* Fig. 17B.14, diag. A). Steps of this procedure are:

◂ *In which situation is the ledge-wedge procedure done?*

◂ *How is the ledge-wedge procedure done?*

- An incision is first made at right angles to the gingiva for excising the gingival pocket wall (Fig. 17B.14, diag. B, 1 and green arrow). The gingival tissue coronal to the incision line is excised resulting in a flat ledge like wound in the palatal flap (Fig. 17B.14, diag. B, blue shaded area, 2 and red arrow).
- Then an internal bevel incision that starts in the flat ledge like wound and ends on the lateral surface of the palatal bone is made (Fig. 17B.14, diag. C, 3 and black arrow). A sulcular incision is then made through the sulcus to the crest of the palatal bone (Fig. 17B.14, diag. C, 4 and green arrow).
- These incisions separate a triangular wedge of palatal connective tissue from the underside of the palatal flap (Fig. 17B.14, diag. C, blue shaded area). This wedge of palatal connective tissue is removed using sharp dissection and curettes (Fig. 17B.14, diag. C, blue shaded area, 5 and red arrow).
- Thinned palatal flap is then sutured.

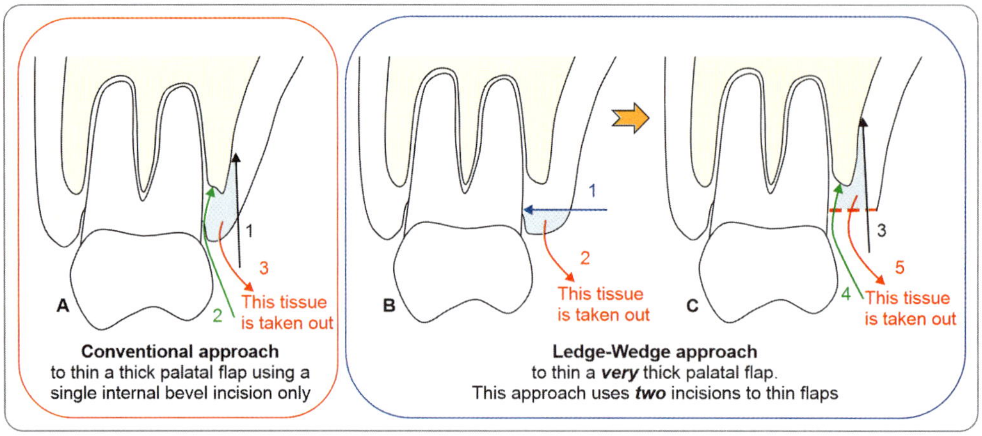

Fig. 17B.14: Steps in conventional internal bevel incision only approach (*diag. A*) and ledge–wedge technique to thin thick palatal flaps (*diags B and C*)

ALERT!

Although the ledge-wedge technique was originally designed for treating thick palatal flaps, it can ***also*** be used to thin buccal and lingual flaps when treating relatively thicker and firmer gingival enlargements.

FLAP MODIFICATIONS FOR THE RETRO-MOLAR (*BEHIND THE MOLAR/DISTAL MOLAR*) AREAS

Distal Wedge Procedure

What is the distal wedge procedure? ▶

This procedure is used to reduce a deep pocket distal to the last molar. Steps of this procedure are:

How is the distal wedge procedure done? ▶

1. Two distally ***converging*** or ***parallel*** incisions are made a few millimeters apart with a #12 BP blade in the gingival tissue distal to the last molar up to the underlying bone (Fig. 17B.15).
2. The wedge of gingival tissue thus outlined is dissected out and the wound margins are sutured.
3. Retro molar pockets (*pockets distal to last molars*) can also be reduced with a horizontal gingivectomy incision made distal to the last molar (Fig. 17B.16). Sutures are not required in such a case but this will leave an exposed gingival wound that will eventually heal with secondary intention.

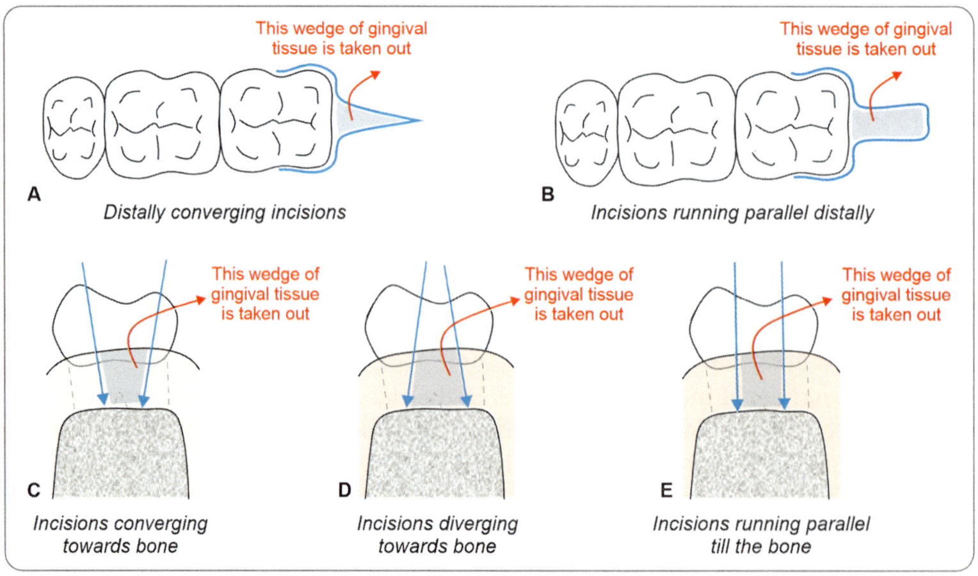

Fig. 17B.15: Incisions for removing gingival tissue distal to last molars (*distal wedge*) can be converging distally (*A*) or run parallel distally (*B*). These incisions can be converging (*C*), diverging (*D*) or parallel till the bone (*E*). Distal wedge of gingiva is removed and wound is sutured.

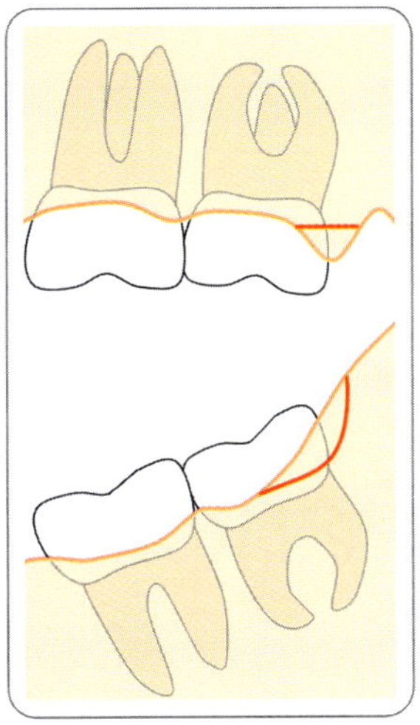

Fig. 17B.16: Retro molar pockets (*pockets distal to last molars*) can also be reduced with a horizontal gingivectomy incision (*red lines*)

Some points of importance for distal molar surgery for pocket reduction:

- As a general rule, ***deeper*** pockets require ***greater*** volume of gingival tissue to be excised. Therefore, incisions are made slightly farther apart in such cases; vice versa is also true.
- These incisions are preferably made in the ***keratinized*** tissue only. The incisions must therefore be ***inclined*** into areas having the greatest width of attached gingiva.

◂ *What modification must be done in the distal wedge procedure in case of deeper pockets?*

FLAP MODIFICATIONS FOR PERIODONTAL REGENERATIVE (*RECONSTRUCTIVE*) SURGERY

It is important to ensure ***primary closure*** over bone grafts, GTR membranes, etc. Modified widman flap and wherever possible, papilla preservation flap are suited for this purpose. In some cases, coronal displacement of flaps must be done to ensure primary closure (*palatal flaps cannot be displaced*).

REVIEW QUESTIONS

1. Define periodontal flap. Write the objectives and goals of periodontal flap surgery.
2. Classify periodontal flaps. Describe the terms gingival flap, mucogingival flap, envelope flap and trap door flap.
3. Describe the incisions used for elevating different types of periodontal flaps.
4. What are the indications and contraindications of modified Widman flap (MWF)? Describe the procedure of MWF in detail.
5. What are the pre-conditions for performing an undisplaced flap? Describe the procedure of performing undisplaced flap.
6. What is the preserved papilla flap? Write indications and contraindications of preserved papilla flap?
7. Write the procedure of performing the preserved papilla flap.
8. What modifications are required in the flap technique for palatal areas?
9. What modifications in the flap technique are required for retromolar areas?
10. What are the recommended periodontal flap procedures for regenerative (*reconstructive*) periodontal surgery? Describe any one in detail.

Chapter

18

Resective Bone Surgery and Regeneration of Periodontal Tissues

Why must bulky alveolar bone contours be corrected? ▶

A knife-edge deflecting contour of gingiva is required for maintenance of health of gingiva (*see Chapter 2, 'Gingiva' pages 19–20 and Fig. 2.19*). Gingiva follows contours of the underlying alveolar bone. Therefore, if contours of alveolar bone are bulky, overlying gingiva will certainly be rounded, bulbous and non-deflecting. Such abnormal contours of marginal gingiva result in increased plaque accumulation near gingival margins and result in start and worsening of gingivitis or periodontitis.

Why must angular bone loss and pit or crater like defects in interdental bone be corrected? ▶

Angular bone loss, pit or crater like defects, etc. may be present in interdental alveolar bone at some oral sites. Sulci (*or pockets*) overlying such defects have greater PD (*probing depth*) as compared to that present at adjoining areas where there are no such defects. Due to greater PD, such sites have increased risk of periodontitis.

Do alveolar bone defects self-correct? ▶

It is therefore essential to correct all bone defects to reattain normal gingival contours and PD of less than 3 mm. Alveolar bone defects ***do not self-correct*** automatically. They need to be surgically corrected during a periodontal flap surgery. Correction of bone defects (*re-shaping of alveolar bone*) is either done by removing bone, i.e. resection (*osteoplasty and ostectomy*) or by new bone formation in bone defects (*bone grafting*).

ALVEOLAR BONE ANATOMY IN HEALTH AND PERIODONTAL DISEASE

Architecture of Alveolar Bone

What is the normal position of interdental bone with respect to buccal and lingual/palatal bone? ▶

The following terms are used to describe alveolar bone crest line.

1. *Normal or Positive Architecture*

When crest of interdental bone is ***coronal*** to buccal or lingual/palatal alveolar bone (Fig. 18.1, diag. A, green arrows).

In which areas is flat architecture of alveolar bone seen? ▶

2. *Flat Architecture*

When crest of buccal and lingual or palatal alveolar bone is at the ***same*** level as that of interdental bone (Fig. 18.1, diag. B, blue arrows). This is more commonly seen in anterior teeth.

In which cases is flat architecture of alveolar bone seen? ▶

3. *Reverse or Negative Architecture*

When crest of interdental bone is ***apical*** to buccal or lingual/palatal alveolar bone (Fig. 18.1, diag. C, red arrows). This is may be seen in stage III and IV periodontitis (*moderate or severe periodontitis*) and after necrotizing ulcerative periodontitis (*NUG*), etc.

Bone Defects Occurring in Periodontal Disease

(*Resulting from Periodontitis and Traumatic Occlusion*)

How many types of bone defects are found in periodontal disease? ▶

There are several types of alveolar bone defects and these occur due to periodontitis and traumatic occlusion. Such defects (*alveolar bone loss*), may be present in relation to several teeth (*generalized*) or restricted to one or two teeth (*localized*).

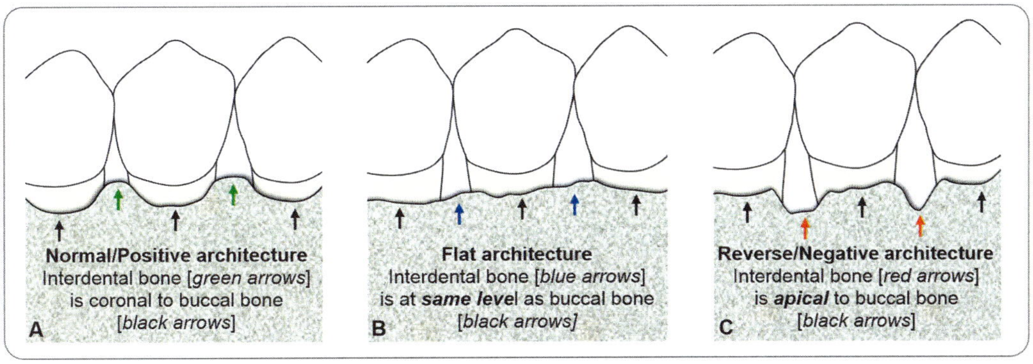

Fig. 18.1: Normal/positive (A), flat (B) and reverse/negative (C) architecture of alveolar bone

Different types of alveolar bone defects are:

1. Reduced Height of Alveolar Bone

(Apical Shift of Crest of Bone in Relation to CEJ) (also see Chapter 3, 'Periodontal Ligament, Cementum and Alveolar Bone', pages 41 and 42, Figs 3.11, 3.12 and 3.13)

This could be of *two* types:

i. **Horizontal bone loss:** When resorbed alveolar bone crest is parallel to the imaginary line joining two CE junctions of two adjacent teeth, bone loss is said to be horizontal **(Fig. 18.3, diags A and B)** (*also see Chapter 10, 'Plaque Induced Gingivitis and Periodontitis', page 143 and Fig. 10.6*). This is most ***common***. Horizontal bone loss results in ***suprabony*** alveolar bone defects.

ii. **Vertical or angular bone loss:** When resorbed alveolar bone crest is at an angle to the imaginary line joining two CE junctions of two adjacent teeth, bone loss is said to be vertical or angular **(Fig. 18.3, diag. C)** (*also see Chapter 10, 'Plaque Induced Gingivitis and Periodontitis', page 143 and Fig. 10.6*). Angular bone loss results in ***intrabony*** or ***infrabony*** alveolar bone defects.

◂ *What is the difference between horizontal and vertical bone loss?*

◂ *What are suprabony bone defects?*

◂ *What are infrabony or intrabony bone defects?*

2. Interproximal Crater

Interproximal bone crater is a ***pit*** like bone defect (*loss*) in the interdental bone septum and is usually found in the posterior regions.

◂ *Where is interproximal crater usually found?*

3. Funnel-shaped Defect

It appears like an extreme widening of the periodontal ligament space at the coronal aspect (*opening*) of the tooth socket that may be present all around a tooth or localized to one surface of the tooth. It is also called a ***one-walled*** angular defect **(Fig. 18.3, diag. C, red arrows)**. Funnelling is commonly seen in teeth with TFO (*trauma from occlusion*).

◂ *In which teeth is funnelling commonly seen?*

4. Hemiseptal Defect

Partial bone loss on the mesial or distal side of an interdental bone septum is called a hemiseptal defect **(Fig. 18.3, diag. D, red arrow)**. Hemiseptal defects can form only in a ***thick*** interdental septum of posterior teeth.

◂ *What is the precondition to formation of hemiseptal defects?*

5. Bullous Contours

When alveolar bone thickens (*hypertrophies*) to bear increased occlusal loads (*e.g. TFO*), it can become thick and bulbous. Bullous alveolar bone contours can be of two types:

i. **Lipping:** When thickening of the alveolar ***bone margin*** produces a 'shelf like' bulging extension of the alveolar bone crest. Lipping often occurs after healing of osseous craters and vertical (*angular*) defects.

ii. **Exostoses:** These are ***outgrowths*** of bone arising from the surface of the alveolar bone and they may or may not involve the bone crest **(Fig. 18.3A)**.

◂ *What is the lipping? How is it different from bone exostosis?*

6. Ledges

When a thick crest of the alveolar bone gets resorbed evenly, it produces a flat plateau like alveolar bone crest surface called a ledge.

◂ *How are ledges formed?*

7. Combination of above Defects

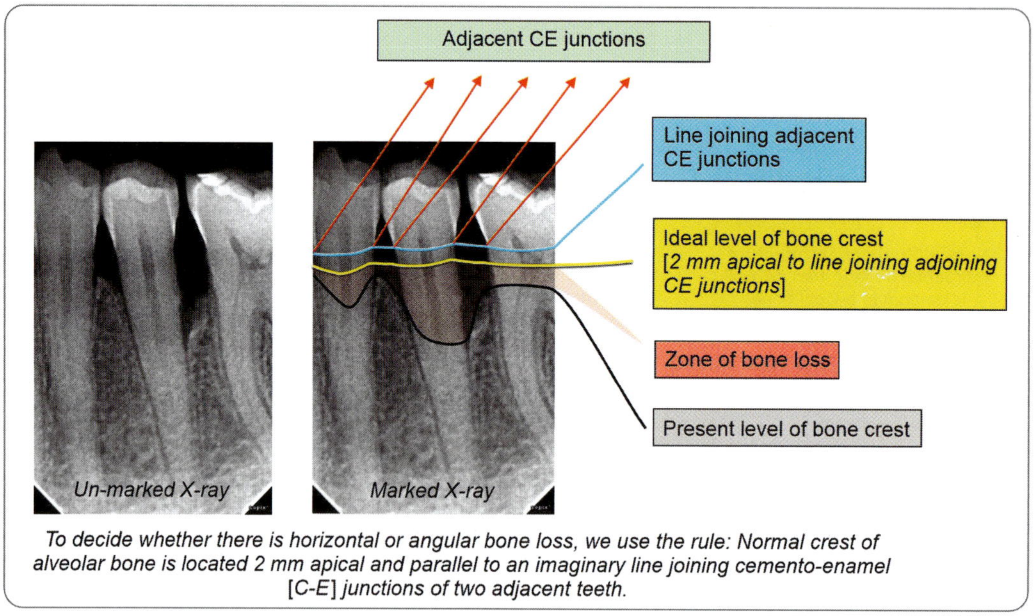

Fig. 18.2: Determining extent and type of bone loss

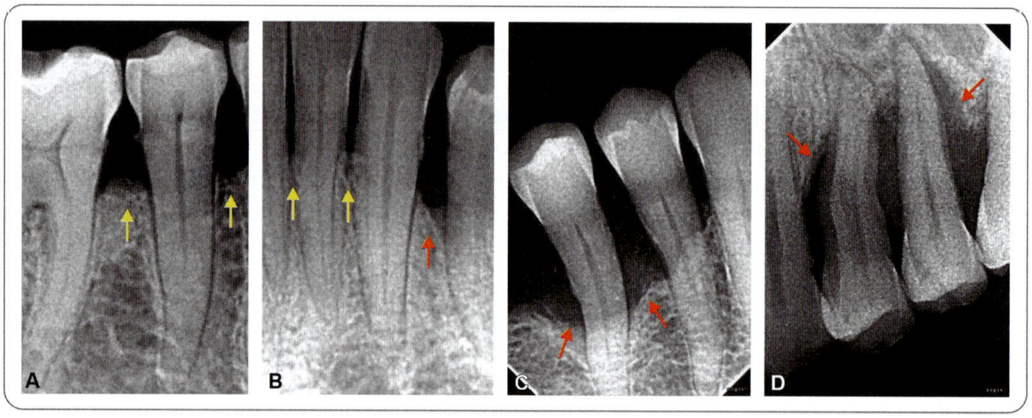

Fig. 18.3: Different types of bone defects. Horizontal or suprabony (*yellow arrows, diags A and B*), vertical bone or infrabony (*red arrow, diag. B*), funnel like (*red arrows, diag. C*) and hemiseptal (*diag. D red arrows*) bone defects.

Identification of Type of Bone Contours and Bone Defects

How can bone defects be diagnosed? ▸

This can be done by:

1. *Palpation of Gingiva*

Why is palpation of gingiva not the ideal way of diagnosing bone defects? ▸

This can give an idea about bone overgrowths, e.g. exostosis, ledges, etc. but ***not*** about bone defects like craters, vertical bone loss, etc.

2. *Gingival and Transgingival Probing*

What is bone sounding? ▸

This can help identify suprabony and infrabony defects. Trans-gingival probing is also called bone sounding and is ***done under local anaesthesia***. In this, a probe is inserted through the gingiva to 'feel' the bone crest and bone defect with the tip of the probe. Intrabony defects, furcations, dehiscence/fenestration in the bone, etc. can be identified in this may (*see Chapter 13, 'Planning and Initiating Periodontal Treatment', page 218 and Fig. 13.9*).

Which radiographs are suited for diagnosing bone defects? ▸

3. *Radiographic Examination*

Why are IOPA radiographs not ideal for diagnosis of bone defects? ▸

i. **IOPA radiographs:** They provide ***two-dimensional*** view of contours of the alveolar bone and some bone defects. Interdental horizontal bone loss, angular bone loss, craters in interdental bone, etc. can be identified in IOPA radiographs. However accurate dimensions of such defects ***cannot*** be known.

ii. **Orthopantomogram (*OPG*):** It is also a widely used radiograph. However, it is ***not*** the ideal radiograph for periodontal diagnosis (*see Chapter 13, 'Planning and Initiating Periodontal Treatment', page 216 and Fig. 13.3*).

iii. **CBCT (*cone beam computed tomography*):** It can provide accurate three-dimensional views of bone contours and defects. It is not commonly used due to high radiation exposure and cost (*see Chapter 13 pages 215–217 and Fig. 13.4, 13.5 and 13.6*).

◂ *Why CBCT is not routinely used for diagnosis of bone defects?*

4. Surgical Exposure of Bone

This is the ***best*** way to know type and dimensions of bone defect. However, this cannot always be done.

◂ *Which is the best way of diagnosing bone defects?*

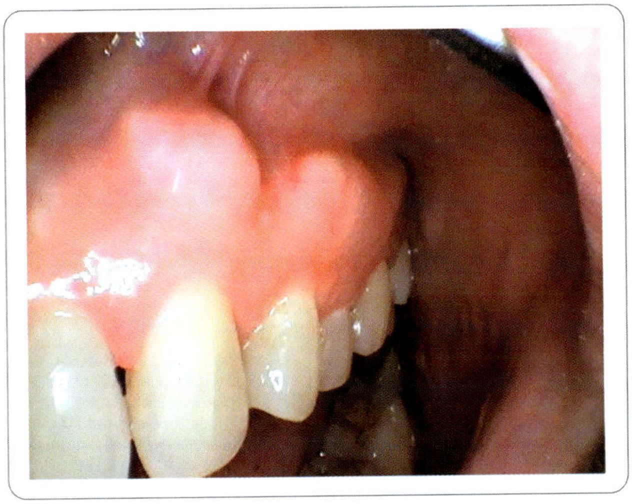

Fig. 18.3A: Bone exostosis in alveolar bone. Such bone out growths are seen as an attempt of the alveolar bone to strengthen (*buttress*) the bone.

CLINICAL UTILITY AND SHORT ANSWER

Why is it necessary to correct alveolar bone defects like lipping and ledge formation?

- As gingiva always follows the contour of alveolar bone, thickened bone contours like lipping and ledge formation are always covered by gingiva that has non-physiologic gingival contours. Such gingiva, even if presently healthy, has a greater chance of developing gingivitis and periodontitis in the future.
- Correction of such bone defects (*re-shaping of alveolar bone*) is done by removing bone, i.e. resection (*osteoplasty and ostectomy*).

CLINICAL UTILITY AND SHORT ANSWER

Why is it necessary to correct interdental bone loss (*angular, pit or crater like bone defects*)?

1. Gingiva overlying interdental angular bone loss, pit or crater defects **(Fig. 18.4, diag. B, red arrows)** has greater PD (*probing depth*) **(Fig. 18.4, diag. B, dark red shaded areas)** as compared to areas where there are no such defects **(Fig. 18.4, diag. A, green arrows and green shaded areas)**. Due to greater PD, such sites have increased risk of periodontitis.
2. As alveolar bone defects do not self-correct automatically, it is therefore essential to correct all bone defects to reattain normal gingival contours and PD of less than 3 mm.
3. If pocket reduction surgery (*gingivectomy or flap surgery*) is done but such defects are not corrected, these areas will continue to have deeper PD as compared to adjoining areas after healing **(Fig. 18.4, diag. C, red shaded areas)**. Due to greater PD, such sites will therefore continue to be at increased risk of future periodontitis (*despite pocket reduction surgery*). This will worsen the outcome of previous treatment.
4. Bone defects can ***only*** be corrected by periodontal flap surgery. Correction of bone defects (*re-shaping of alveolar bone*) is done by:
   i. Removing bone around such defects, i.e. bone resection (*osteoplasty and ostectomy*) **(Fig. 18.4, Option 1, diags D and E)**. Although this will lead to some gingival recession **(Fig. 18.4, diag. E)** but it will also result in healthier periodontium that is at lesser risk of future periodontitis.
   ii. New bone formation in bone defects, i.e. bone regeneration (*bone grafting*) **(Fig. 18.4, Option 2, diags F and G)**.

◂ *Do alveolar bone defects self-correct?*

◂ *What will happen if interdental bone defects are not corrected during pocket reduction surgery?*

◂ *How can alveolar bone defects be corrected?*

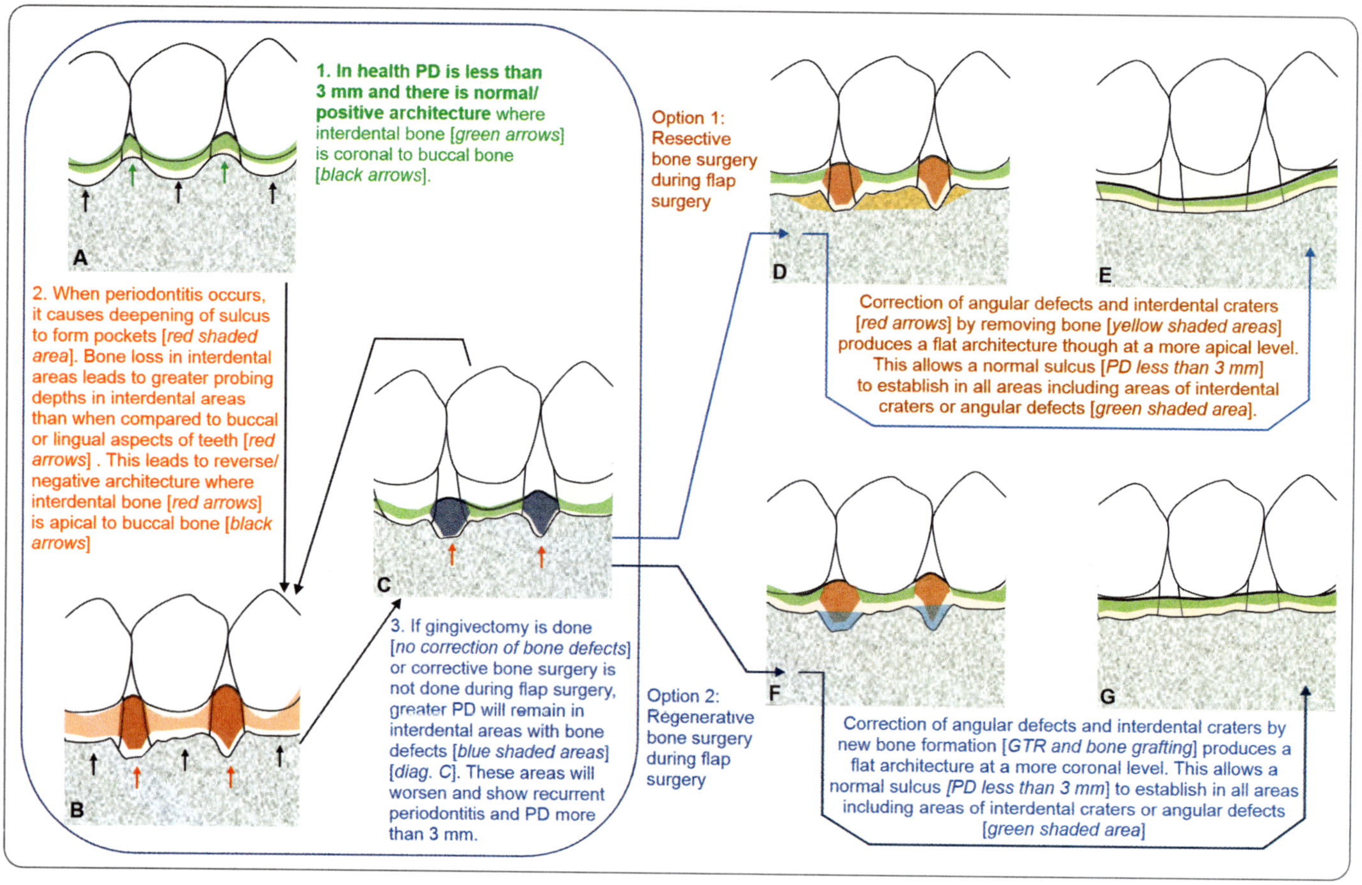

Fig. 18.4: Why and how interdental bone defects must be corrected

ALERT!

Why more bone loss is seen in interdental areas?

More bone loss is seen in interdental bone as compared to buccal and lingual or palatal bone because:

1. Interdental areas are non-self-cleansing areas, i.e. are not cleaned properly by natural physical cleaning mechanisms like scrubbing action of tongue and food during mastication, etc. This leads to initiation and worsening of periodontitis in the interdental areas. On the other hand, buccal and lingual or palatal areas are cleaned very well by natural cleaning mechanisms.

Why does interdental bone resorb faster? ▶

2. Interdental bone septum is composed primarily of cancellous bone overlaid by a thin coat of cortical bone (*crestal lamina*). The crestal lamina (*superficial cortical bone layer*) being more calcified resorbs slowly in periodontitis, but after it gets totally resorbed, the underlying cancellous layer being less calcified (*hence softer*), resorbs at a much faster rate. On the other hand, the buccal and lingual/palatal bone plates are made mostly of cortical bone (*which is harder than the cancellous bone*). They therefore resorb at a slower rate than the interdental septum.

ALERT!

- Periodontitis with ***less than 5 mm*** PD (*probing/pocket depth*) (*critical probing depth; see Chapter 17, 'Surgical Treatment of Gingivitis and Periodontitis', pages 292 and 293 and Fig. 17.2*) and minor bone loss is usually treated with ***SRP*** (*scaling and root planing*) alone. However, if PD does not reduce to less than 3 mm after SRP, pocket reduction must be carried out surgically (*flap surgery or gingivectomy or gingivoplasty*).
- Periodontitis presenting with ***more than 5 mm*** PD and moderate/severe horizontal and/or vertical bone loss or other bone defects before initial treatment (*phase I therapy—SRP, etc.*) has to be treated by flap surgery (*includes resective or regenerative bone surgery*) or by gingivectomy (*if no bone surgery is required*) to bring PD to less than 3 mm.

  If more than 3 mm PD remains few weeks after flap surgery, further pocket reduction must be done to bring PD to less than 3 mm (*by gingivectomy or gingivoplasty*).
- In general, one and two walled intrabony defects and horizontal bone loss ***do not*** show increase in bone height after bone grafting (*regenerative bone surgery*).

CLINICAL UTILITY AND SHORT ANSWER

Which type of bone defect is most and least likely to regenerate bone after bone grafting?

- Bone grafting regenerates bone only if the bone defect (*bone loss*) is ***three-walled***, i.e. it is pit like and is surrounded by bone walls on all sides (**Fig. 18.9, diag. A**).
- One-walled bone loss defects usually ***do not*** show bone regeneration (**Fig. 18.9, diag. C**).
- Horizontal height of bone (*around teeth*) usually ***cannot*** be increased.

RESECTIVE OSSEOUS SURGERY (*OSTEOPLASTY OR OSTECTOMY*)

Resective bone surgery (*removing bone to re-shape it and correct its contours*) can be done by osteoplasty or ostectomy. If re-shaping of alveolar bone is done by removing bone that does not support the tooth directly, it is called ***osteoplasty***. On the other hand, if ***tooth supporting*** bone is removed, it is called ***ostectomy***.

◂ *What is the difference between osteoplasty and ostectomy?*

Indications of Osteoplasty or Ostectomy (*Resective Osseous Surgery*)

◂ *When must resective osseous surgery be done?*

1. For correcting negative architecture of alveolar bone and converting it to flat or positive architecture.
2. For correction of intra-bony defect around a tooth with sufficient periodontal support.
3. To thin very thick alveolar bone margins, ledges, bone exostoses and correct inter-dental craters, widow's peaks, etc.
4. To widen furcation entrance for providing easy access to instruments and oral cleaning devices.
5. To perform clinical crown lengthening for restorative or prosthetic reasons, etc.

Contraindications of Osteoplasty or Ostectomy (*Resective Osseous Surgery*)

◂ *When must resective osseous surgery not be done?*

1. If anatomic structures, e.g. mental foramen, maxillary sinus, etc. are present within 5 mm of the bone defect.
2. In aesthetic regions if it will lead to root exposure and opening of interdental space.

ALERT!

◂ *Can resective osseous surgery be done in relation to single tooth?*

◂ *Why is it important to keep bone cool when bone cutting is being done?*

1. Resective osseous surgery is ***rarely*** indicated to be done only in relation to a single tooth rather it must be performed on a couple of adjoining teeth to produce physiologic contours of the bone.
2. To prevent overheating of bone, bone cutting if done with surgical burs must be done at ***slow speed*** and under ***constant irrigation with normal saline*** (*if bone temperature rises above 42°C during cutting, it will lead to bone cell death and local bone necrosis*).

Instruments commonly used in osseous surgery

Small tipped bone rongeurs, steel and coarse grit diamond bone cutting burs, Schluger and Sugarman bone files, ochsenbein bone chisels, etc.

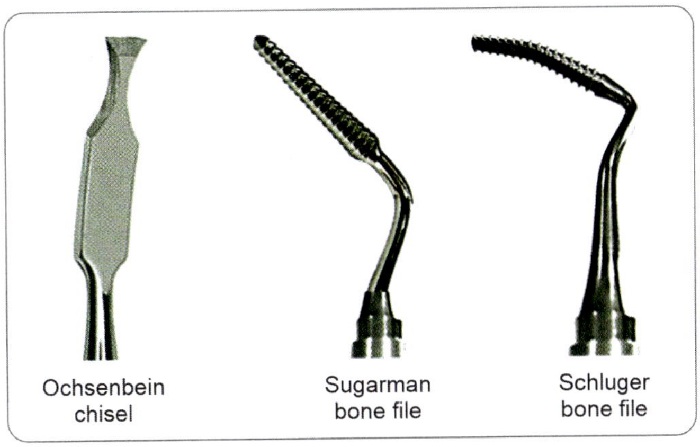

Fig. 18.4A: Commonly used hand instruments for bone recontouring

Basic Technique of Resective Osseous Surgery (*Bone Recontouring*)

Can osteoplasty or ostectomy be done without raising a flap? ▶

Both osteoplasty or ostectomy can only be done ***after*** raising a flap. After attaining adequate anaesthesia, a muco-periosteal (*full-thickness*) flap is raised at least one or two teeth beyond the area where osseous surgery is required. If significant amount of bone is trimmed at the crest, the flap will have to be displaced apically before suturing. To do this, the flap is raised beyond the muco-gingival junction after giving vertical incisions at both ends of the flap (*see Chapter 17B, 'Periodontal Flap Surgery', pages 305 and 306*).

Bone recontouring is very similar to wax carving of a denture. It is done to 'gradualize' (*blend*) alveolar bone contours and is started by removing non-tooth supporting bone (*osteoplasty*). Care must be taken to prevent unnecessary surgical trauma to bone covering tooth roots. Tooth supporting bone is removed (*ostectomy*) only if needed. Steps in osseous recontouring are:

What are the steps in osseous recontouring? ▶

Step 1: Vertical Grooving and Radicular Blending

Where is the bone reshaping started? ▶

This step is done primarily to remove non-tooth supporting bone (*osteoplasty*). Bone reshaping is started in the inter-radicular regions (*between roots of teeth*). For this, shallow vertical grooves are first cut in bone **(Fig. 18.6, diag. B)**. Radicular blending is then done, i.e. grooves are blended with surrounding bone (*gradualized*) by removing bone on the sides of the vertical groove. This gives prominence to radicular bone (*bone over roots*). If vertical grooving is minimal, radicular blending may not be required. Vertical grooving and radicular blending is ***not*** done ***if***:

What are the preconditions to performing radicular blending? ▶

1. Bone is thin, i.e. adequate volume of cancellous bone core is not present under the cortical bone plates.
2. Roots are closely placed.
3. Fenestrations are present on the root (*see chapter 3, 'Periodontal Ligament, Cementum and Alveolar Bone', page 44 and Fig. 3.16*).

Step 2: Flattening Interdental Bone

When must interdental bone septum be levelled? ▶

If crest of the interdental septum is very ***uneven*** or walls of bone defects are at a very different level, in such cases bone crest is levelled using rotating diamond stones, bone files or small hand chisels. Bone removal is done only till floor of the bone defect (*crater*) gets levelled and becomes the new (*just modified*) surface of interdental septum **(Fig. 18.6, diag. C)**.

Step 3: Gradualizing Marginal Bone

What is a widow's peak? ▶

This is done to remove the part of crestal (*marginal*) alveolar bone on the buccal and lingual or palatal surfaces of roots that rises coronal to level of interdental bone **(widow's peaks; Fig. 18.5 and Fig. 18.6, diags A, B and C)**. Care must be taken to prevent damage to tooth roots during bone removal and reshaping.

After the above three steps are completed, flap is sutured back in a way that it fully covers the bone crest but does not over extend too far coronally above the alveolar bone crest.

- Buccal and lingual flaps may either be displaced apically or coronally as the need maybe; palatal flaps however, ***cannot*** be displaced (*palatal flap is trimmed if required*).
- During the immediate post-operative period, interdental papilla shrinks and wide interdental spaces result after surgery.
- Buccal and lingual or palatal gingiva attains its normal contour around two weeks post-operatively while the interdental papillae re-grow to their physiologic form approximately after 3–4 weeks.

Recommendations for Treatment of Different Types of Bone Defects

What are the recommended options for treatment of different bone defects? ▶

- One-wall defects (*one remaining bone wall; Fig. 18.9*) must be managed by bone resection (*bone cutting to remove the one wall and flattening the defect up to its floor*).
- Two-wall defects (*two remaining bone walls*) are preferably treated by bone resection although bone grafting (*regeneration*) may be tried.
- Three-wall defects (*three remaining bone walls*) and interdental craters are preferably treated by bone grafting (*regeneration*).

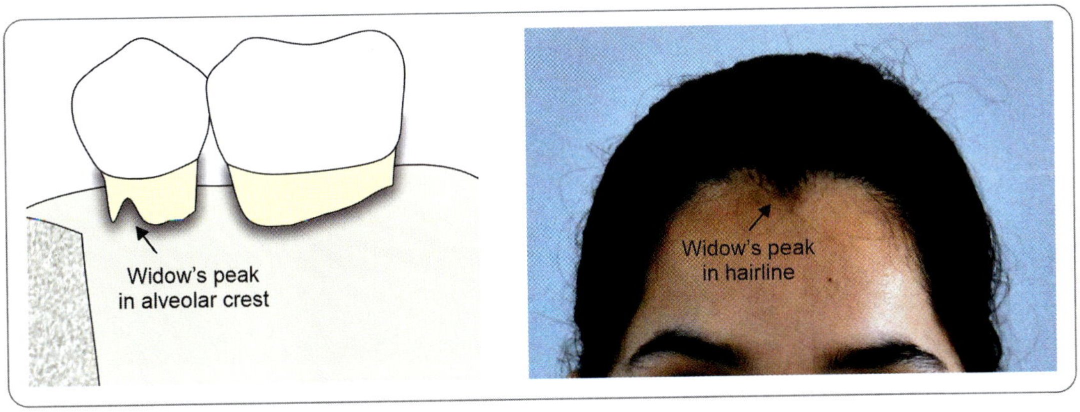

Fig. 18.5: Widow's peak in crestal alveolar bone (*this is a metaphor taken from widow's peak of hairline*).

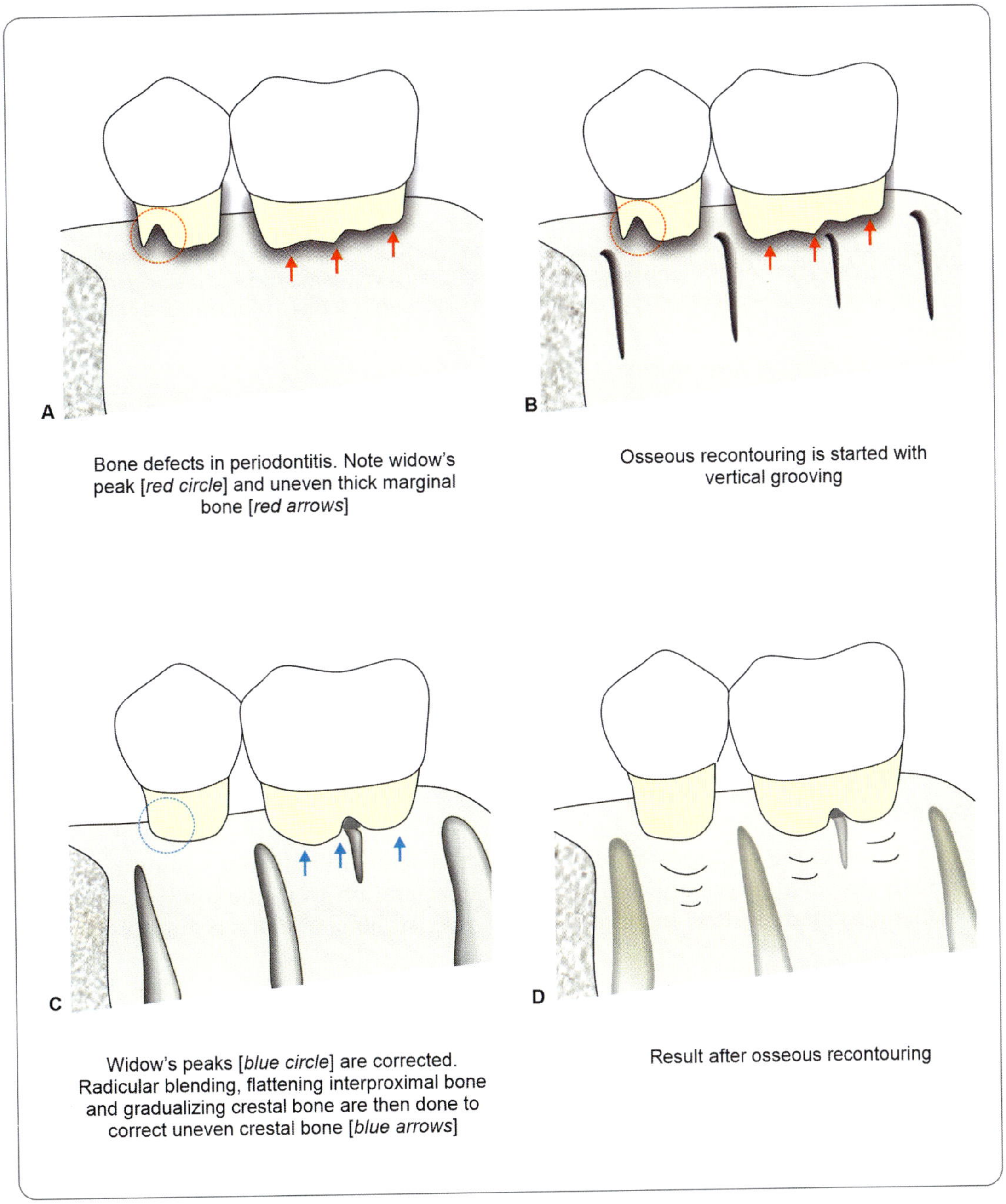

Fig. 18.6: Steps in osseous recontouring

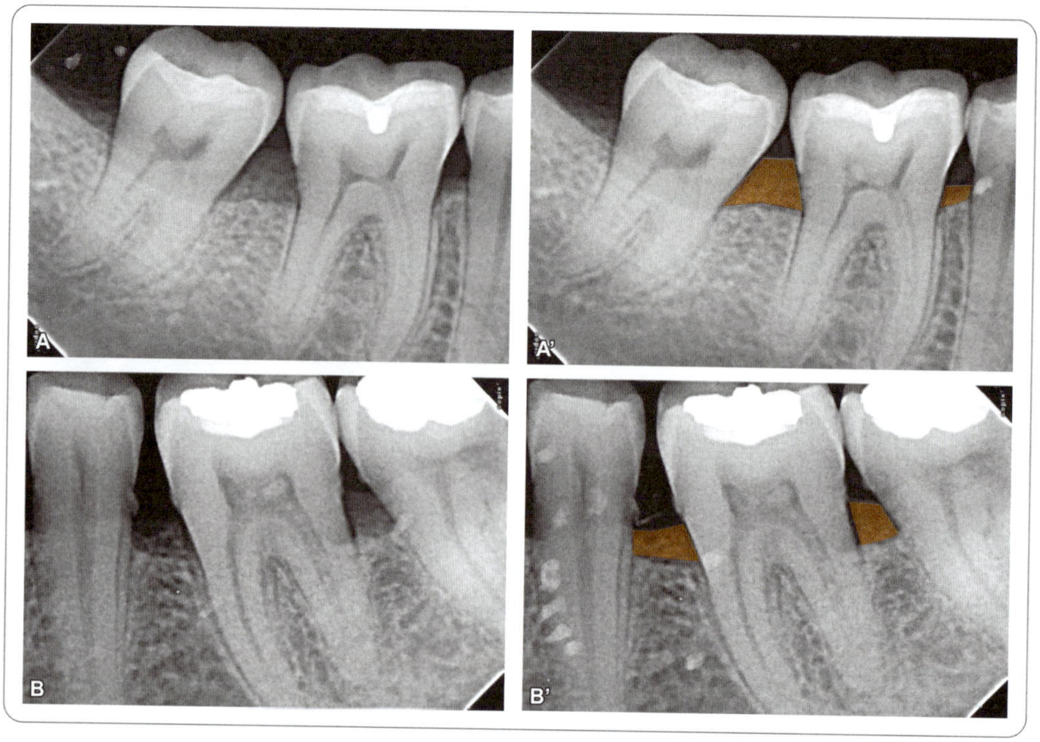

Fig. 18.7: Ostectomy (*flattening*) of interdental bone. Surface of interdental bone septum can become uneven due to unequal bone loss. Such areas appear hazy in radiographs (*red marked areas in diags A' and B'*). Selective removal of bone (*ostectomy at red marked areas in diags A' and B'*) to produce a levelled and even surface of interdental septum may be done in such areas.

CLINICAL UTILITY AND SHORT ANSWER

Is it always essential to perform bone recontouring during flap surgery?
No. Minor bone defects may not be corrected during periodontal flap surgery.

REGENERATIVE PERIODONTAL SURGERY

(Techniques for Regeneration of Lost Periodontal Support)

Surgical procedures to regenerate lost periodontal support are called regenerative periodontal surgical procedures. Materials like bone grafts and barrier membranes are used for regenerative periodontal surgery.

Terminology used in Periodontal Regeneration

(also see, 'Chapter 16, 'Scaling, Root Planing and Other Fundamentals of Periodontal Surgery' pages 280 and 281 and Fig. 16.5)

1. *Reattachment*

What is reattachment? ▶

The act of re-joining of periodontal tissues to the same area of root where they were previously attached after surgical or traumatic separation from the tooth is called re-attachment. No gain in attachment or height of alveolar bone or PDL occurs.

2. *New Attachment*

What is new attachment? ▶

When healing results in complete recovery of periodontal tissues in amount, form and function by formation of new alveolar bone and new connective attachment via collagen fibers (*PDL and gingival*) that are ***functionally*** (*physiologically*) oriented and inserted into new formed cementum over root surface ***previously*** denuded by periodontitis, i.e. root surface with gingival recession, is called new attachment.

How is new attachment different from reattachment? ▶

(New attachment is different from reattachment. In reattachment, healing occurs over a root surface that has been surgically exposed and which was already covered by periodontal tissues prior to its surgical exposure).

3. New Connective Tissue Attachment

Most of the time only partial regeneration of periodontal tissues occurs after periodontal regeneration is attempted (*despite best efforts at new attachment*). This may be characterized by new cementum formation only on a part of the exposed root, formation of new gingival and PDL fibers that are attached to new formed cementum but these may not be functionally oriented (*cannot provide support to the tooth*), etc. In many cases lost alveolar bone does not reform (*in height*) to completely restore the periodontal supporting apparatus. Such partial healing that only regenerates periodontal tissues partially (*both in form and hence function*) is called new connective tissue attachment.

◂ *What is new connective tissue attachment?*

◂ *How is new connective tissue attachment different from new attachment and reattachment?*

4. Bone Fill

Bringing about formation of new bone in treated periodontal defects is called bone fill.

◂ *What is bone fill?*

5. Guided Tissue Regeneration (GTR)

Procedures designed to allow or exclude particular cells of the periodontium from entering the healing periodontal surgical wound site are called GTR procedures. GTR is done to improve chances of periodontal tissue regeneration (*new attachment or new connective tissue attachment or bone fill*). A GTR membrane is designed to bar entry of epithelial cells and only allow cells originating from the PDL to colonize and populate the periodontal healing site. If bone graft has been used to fill a bone defect, GTR membranes also prevent the graft material from spilling out of the grafted site while also allowing healing cells to come only from the surrounding alveolar bone.

◂ *What is guided tissue regeneration (GTR)?*

6. Guided Bone Regeneration (GBR)

It is a collective name for procedures done to encourage formation of bone in a treated periodontal bone defect.

◂ *What is guided bone regeneration (GBR)?*

CLINICAL UTILITY AND SHORT ANSWER

Can new attachment be regularly attained with GTR procedures?

No. Though regeneration of periodontal tissues lost due to periodontitis (*new attachment*) is the goal of periodontal treatment, it still remains a mostly ***un-attained*** goal in most clinical situations (*despite best materials and techniques*). When it is said new attachment has occurred, we usually mean that the periodontium has ***partially*** regenerated in both form and function.

SOURCE OF HEALING CELLS THAT POPULATE A HEALING PERIODONTAL WOUND AFFECTS OUTCOME OF PERIODONTAL HEALING

(also see Chapter 16, 'Scaling, Root Planing and Other Fundamentals of Periodontal Surgery', page 281 and Fig. 16.5)

Periodontal flap surgery wounds can receive healing cells from **(Fig. 18.8)**: Gingival epithelium, gingival connective tissue, alveolar bone or periodontal ligament. Periodontal ligament has all the types of cells required for regeneration of all periodontal tissues, i.e. cementoblasts (*for cementum formation*), fibroblasts (*for formation of PDL fibers*) and osteoblasts (*for formation of alveolar bone*). Therefore, if only healing cells originating from the periodontal ligament populate and dominate the wound healing, regeneration of all periodontal tissues can occur. This fact is the basis of GTR therapy.

◂ *What are the sources of healing cells in a periodontal wound?*

GUIDED TISSUE REGENERATION (GTR) AND GUIDED BONE REGENERATION (GBR)

The primary goal of GTR is new attachment, i.e. regeneration of all periodontal tissues over root surface that was previously exposed due to periodontitis. In GBR the aim is to regenerate only lost bone in bone defects. Some important points with regards to GTR are:

- GTR techniques and materials are designed for ***preventing*** gingival epithelial cells from entering the healing periodontal wound site.

◂ *What is the difference between GTR and GBR?*

◂ *What is the main purpose of GTR tecniques?*

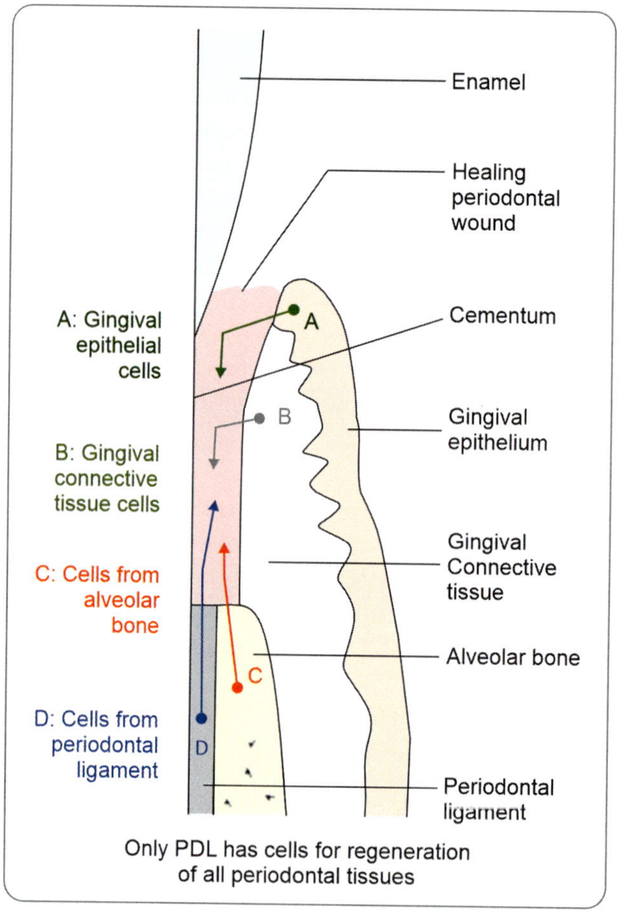

Fig. 18.8: There are four sources of healing cells in a healing periodontal wound: gingival epithelium, gingival connective tissue, alveolar bone and periodontal ligament. All formative and resorptive cells required for regeneration of periodontal tissues are present in the periodontal ligament.

What happens if cells of gingival epithelium enter the healing periodontal wound? ▶

- Gingival epithelial cells must not be allowed to enter (*populate*) the healing periodontal wound because gingival epithelium heals very fast. Therefore, if epithelial cells populate the healing wound, they will multiply rapidly and cover the tooth facing surface of the periodontal flap within 4–5 days post-operatively. Once the epithelium forms on the flap wound, it leads to establishment of base of sulcus at the same level as was present before the surgery.
- Epithelium then also acts like a separating layer between healing cementum and gingival connective tissue, alveolar bone and PDL thereby making union between these tissues and thus regeneration of lost periodontal tissues impossible.

How does a GTR membrane assist regeneration in a healing periodontal wound? ▶

- If, however a GTR membrane is placed between the flap and healing periodontal wound, the slower healing connective tissue healing cells get a chance to enter the healing site and cause desired periodontal tissue regeneration (Fig. 18.10).

In which type of bone defects is bone regeneration expected? ▶

- Better healing and regeneration can be expected in narrow and shallow bone defects than the deep and wide defects. This is because the bone graft is better retained in narrow and shallow bone defects and healing cells have a smaller distance to travel to the centre of the defect and the bone graft in it.
- As ***three-walled bone defects*** provide better protection, retain bone graft material better and healing occurs from three sides, they are most likely to ***show good results after GTR*** (Fig. 18.9, diag. A).

Which type of bone defects do not show periodontal tissue regeneration? ▶

- ***One- and two-walled bone defects*** and ***horizontal bone loss areas***, usually ***do not*** show periodontal regeneration or increase in bone height after GTR surgery (Fig. 18.9, diags B and C).

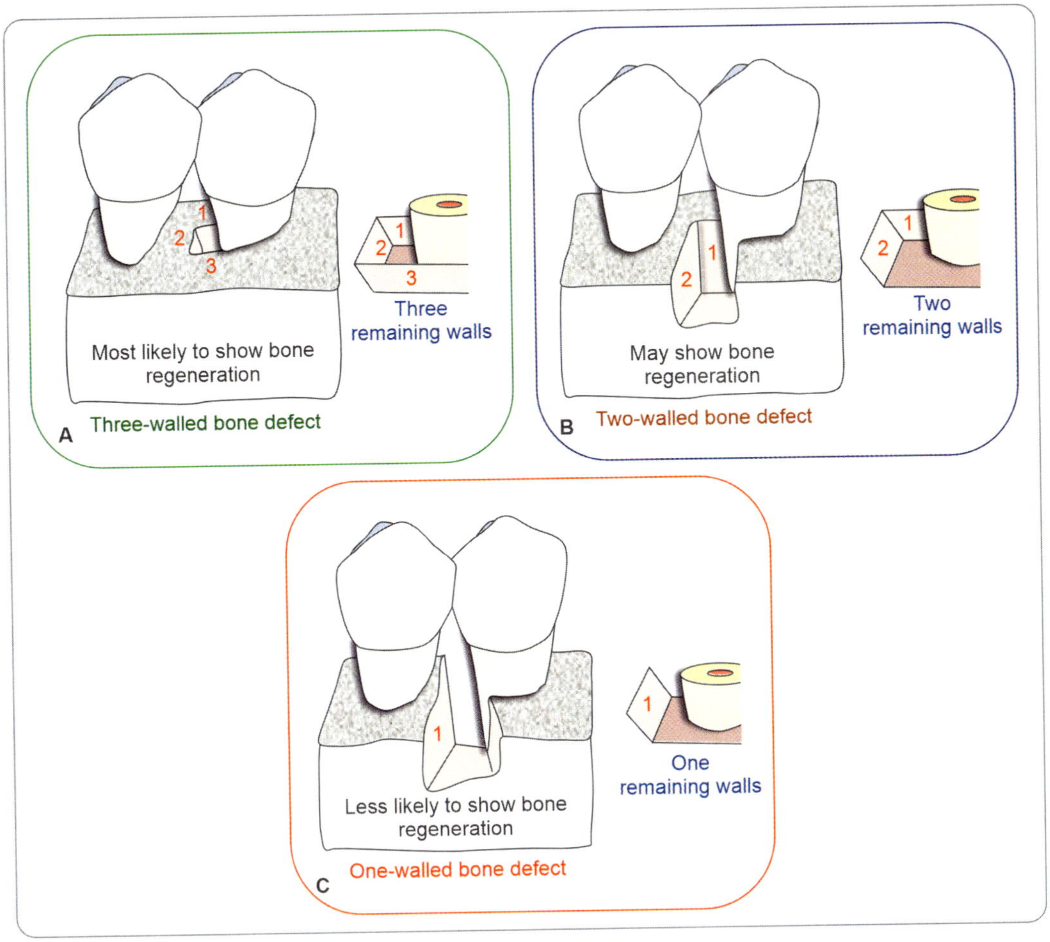

Fig. 18.9: Bone regeneration potential in different types of bone loss defects

Technique and Materials used in GTR/GBR

How are GTR and GBR done?

GTR and GBR are done ***during*** flap surgery. GTR membranes protect and help in creating a favourable environment (*in the wound*) for periodontal regeneration. For this, just before suturing the flap, at the end of periodontal flap surgery (*e.g. modified widman flap*), GTR materials, e.g. bone grafts, platelet rich fibrin, etc. are placed in the periodontal wound/defect. The GTR material may or may not be additionally covered with a GTR membrane. GTR membranes are made of many materials and may be ***resorbable*** or ***non-resorbable.***

Procedure for GTR

Can GTR and GBR be done if active periodontitis is present at that site?

Is chemical preparation of root surface needed for GTR?

1. GTR should ***not*** be done if active infection exists in the site (*GTR and GBR should only be done after completion of phase-I treatment; see Chapter 13, 'Planning and Initiating Periodontal Treatment', page 232*).
2. Chemical root surface bio-modification is generally ***not*** done as root surface bio-modifying agents (*e.g. citric acid at pH1, tetracycline, EDTA, etc.*) can cause death of cells in the wound.
3. For placing the GTR membrane, the osseous defect is carefully debrided and if required, the root planing is done again.
4. Bone graft and any other material selected for GTR is packed in the defect taking care not to overfill the defect.
5. A GTR membrane is selected and shaped by trimming so that it not only covers the defect properly but also extends at least 3–4 mm beyond the edges of the wound/defect. It is then placed over the periodontal defect that has just been filled with bone graft. The GTR membrane is immobilized and fixed in position using sling sutures (*around the tooth*). Care must be taken to ensure minimum salivary contamination of GTR membrane and surgical site.

What precautions must be taken when suturing flaps after GTR/GBR? ▶

6. The flap is then sutured taking care that the entire GTR membrane is covered by the flap. To ensure this, the flap maybe coronally displaced. It must also be ensured that suture threads do not pass over the GTR membranes as this may press on and cause collapse of the membrane thereby restricting the possibility of periodontal regeneration.
7. Antibiotics are prescribed usually for a week and patients are asked to refrain from tooth brushing to prevent disturbing the healing wound for a few days. For adequate plaque control, mouth wash, e.g. chlorhexidine *0.2% or 0.12%* may be prescribed for few weeks. Patients are also advised to avoid eating on the side of surgery for few days.

What is done if GTR membrane gets exposed? ▶

9. If the GTR membrane gets denuded (*this usually happens after 4–6 weeks*), it may be tugged out gently or a minor second surgery is done to remove it.
10. Non-resorbable membranes are removed as per manufacturer's recommendations a few weeks after surgery (*as per manufacturer's instructions*). If large membrane exposure, severe infection or inflammation develop, the membrane may be removed earlier than the suggested time.

For how long must the operative site not be probed after GTR surgery? ▶

11. The site must ***not*** be probed or unnecessarily debrided for at least one year after GTR (*as healing will be continuing*).

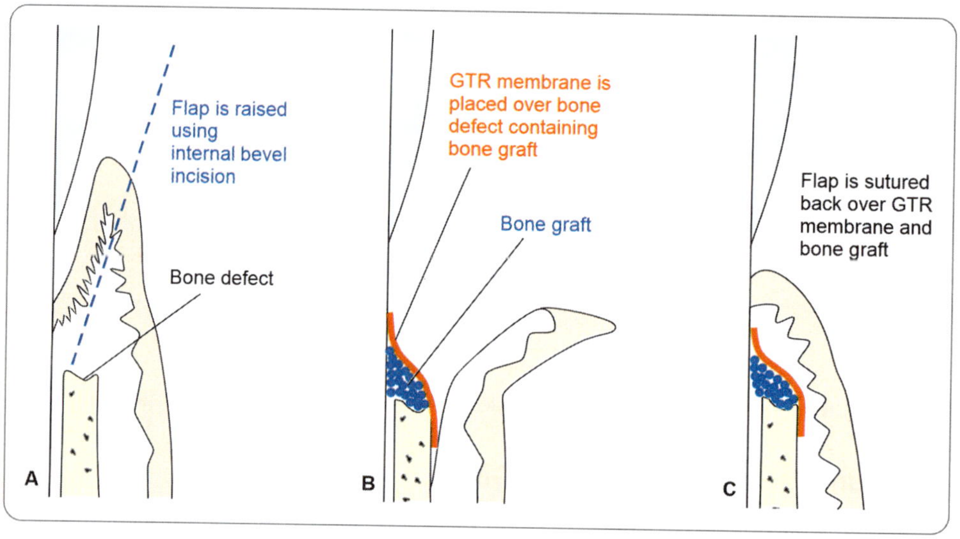

Fig. 18.10: Technique for GTR. A full thickness flap is raised (*diag. A*) and bone defect is thoroughly debrided. Bone graft is placed in the defect (*diag. B*) and GTR membrane is placed over it (*diag. B, red line*). Flap is then sutured back in place using interrupted sutures (*diag. C*).

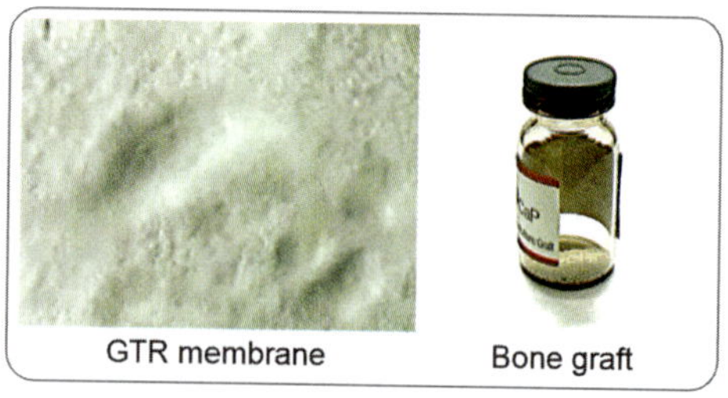

Fig. 18.11: Commercially available GTR membrane and bone graft.

BONE GRAFTS USED FOR GTR OR GBR

Bone grafting is done for regenerating bone (*lost due to periodontitis*). It is done by applying bone graft material (*natural or synthetic*) in bone defects during flap surgery.

Classification of Bone Grafts

I. Depending upon whether graft material is bone or its substitute bone grafts may be classified as:

1. *Natural Bone Grafts*

What are autografts, allografts and xenografts? ▶

i. **Autograft/autogenous graft:** When bone is transplanted from one site of body to another in the *same* individual.

ii. **Allograft/allogenic graft:** When bone is transplanted from one individual to a ***different*** individual.

iii. **Xenograft/heterograft:** When an individual receives bone from an animal source of ***different species*** (*e.g. bovine bone*).

2. *Non-bone Graft Materials*

These are man-made ***substitutes*** for natural bone graft material. They are also used as extenders and/or enhancers for autogenous bone graft when it is not available in sufficient quantity (*less bone graft is available for grafting into a large bone defect*). They may be:

i. **Natural**, e.g. cartilage, dentin chips, enamel matrix proteins, calcium phosphate biomaterials, coral derived materials, etc.

ii. **Synthetic**, e.g. bioactive glass, ceramics, etc.

◂ *Which natural non-bone materials can be used as bone grafts?*

II. Depending upon the reaction a bone graft material produces in the tissues bone grafts may be classified as:

1. *Osteogenic*

◂ *What is the difference between osteogenic, osteoconductive, osteoinductive and osteopromotive bone grafts?*

Graft material containing ***living*** bone forming cells which can ***form new bone*** is called osteogenic.

2. *Osteoconductive*

These materials ***promote*** new bone formation (*but do not by themselves cause new bone formation*) by the already present bone at the boundaries of the bone defect into which graft is placed. They do this by acting as a scaffold over which new bone is formed.

3. *Osteoinductive*

Bone graft materials that have the capacity to ***induce*** new bone formation in the ***soft tissue*** surrounding graft site are called osteoinductive. Such materials also act as a scaffold for new bone formation.

4. *Osteopromotive*

These graft materials are by themselves not osteoinductive, but when used along with other osteoinductive bone graft materials, promote osteoinductive capability of osteoinductive graft materials.

Bone Autograft (*Autogenous Graft*)

Autogenous bone grafts for periodontal use can be sourced from the following donor sites: Maxillary tuberosity, chin area, healing extraction wound, extra oral sites like iliac crest, bone marrow from areas that have abundant cancellous bone, e.g. maxillary tuberosity can also be used.

◂ *From where can bone autografts be sourced?*

The harvested bone is used after cutting it into small pieces and mixing it with patient's own blood or incorporating it into PRF.

Advantages of using bone autografts:

◂ *Why are bone autografts the best bone grafts?*

- It is the ***best*** possible bone graft.
- Due to their bone cells, mineral, collagen and matrix proteins, bone autografts have osteogenic, osteoinductive and osteoconductive properties.
  - Trabeculae of cancellous bone being used as graft material, act like a scaffold and facilitate bone growth.
- Since autogenous bone graft is taken from the same individual, there is ***no risk*** of rejection or disease transmission associated with their use.

Disadvantages of bone autografts:

◂ *Why can't bone autografts be used always and in all situations?*

- Limited supply.
- Need of additional operative site (*donor site*).

- Increased operative time, blood loss and more pain due to two surgical sites (*recipient and donor sites*).
- If large autografts are harvested there is risk of deformity and weakening of donor bone site.

CLINICAL UTILITY AND SHORT ANSWER

How can maximum vitality of the harvested autogenous bone graft be retained?

For this, the following must be ensured:

Why must harvesting of bone graft be done under profuse normal saline irrigation, with trephines or burs in good condition and these being run at slower speeds?

1. During harvesting of bone graft, temperature of the bone graft site must not be allowed to exceed 42°C. To ensure this, only trephines that are in good condition should be used (*trephines or burs should not be blunt*) and bone harvesting should be under constant and abundant normal saline irrigation. If bone temperature increases more than 42°C it will cause bone cell death which leads to lower bone regenerating potential of the bone graft.
2. Harvested bone graft should be kept wrapped in a gauze piece wetted with normal saline (*to prevent it from drying; drying causes bone cell death*) at around 32°C (*normal body temperature*) and used within 30 minutes of it being harvested.
3. Autografts must ***not*** be stored in any antibiotic solution or in a chemical disinfectant (*as this will cause bone cell death*).
4. Bone graft must be placed on recipient bone bed that has been well-decorticated (*cortical bone removed or perforated many times to expose spongy bone*). This allows blood supply and healing components from the bone to reach the graft.
5. When suturing flaps over grafts, thick clot or dead space formation under the flap must be prevented (*thick clots and dead space will reduce chances of graft success*).

Bone Allografts (*Allogenic Bone Grafts*)

Why are bone allografts the most commonly used grafts?

These are the ***most commonly*** used bone grafts and are good ***alternatives*** to bone autografts.

- They are preferred (*most commonly used bone grafts*) because they are readily available in ***unlimited*** quantity (*in sealed sterile vials having a long shelf life*) and there is no need for another surgery at donor site.
- Bone allografts provide a biologic scaffolding over which the patient's own bone grows.
- Decalcified freeze-dried bone allograft (*DFDBA*) is the most commonly used type of bone allograft.
  - It is osteo-conductive and osteo-inductive.
  - The major disadvantage of allografts is that they do not have living bone cells that can contribute directly to bone formation (*osteogenesis*) (*unlike autografts in which bone cells are living*).
  - There is also a very small chance that a patient has an allergic reaction to DFDBA.

What is the major shortcoming of bone allografts?

Bone Xenograft (*Heterologous Bone Grafts*)

What are xeno bone grafts?

Xeno bone grafts are sourced from bovine animals (e.g. *cow*) and coral skeletons (*corals are sea animals*).

- Grafts made from coral skeleton can be resorbable or 'non-resorbable' (*slowly resorbable*).
- Xeno bone grafts sourced from bovine animals or corals show similar results as DFDBA grafts and are well tolerated by patients.

Alloplastic Bone Graft Materials (*Synthetic Bone Grafts*)

What are the major advantages of alloplastic bone grafts?

Alloplastic grafts are ***synthetic*** bone graft materials.

- They maybe 'resorbable' or 'non-resorbable', i.e. it may or may not be replaced by natural bone.
- They act as a scaffold on which natural bone forms.
- Blocks of alloplastic bone grafts can be manufactured to fit a particular size or shape of bone defects.
- Commonly used alloplastic grafts in periodontology are calcium phosphate (*hydroxyapatite and beta-tricalcium phosphate*), bio-active glasses and polymers.

CLINICAL UTILITY AND SHORT ANSWER

What is the most important advantage of natural bone grafts over alloplast (*synthetic*) bone graft materials?

- Allografts are ***natural*** graft materials while alloplastic grafts are ***synthetic*** man-made materials.
- Natural bone grafts (*autografts, allografts and bovine Xenografts*) have growth factors called bone morphogenetic proteins (*BMPs*) that induce formation of bone and cartilage. BMPs are not present in synthetic grafts.

CLINICAL UTILITY AND SHORT ANSWER

What are the most important qualities of a good bone graft material?

A good bone graft material should:

1. Have osseoinductive and osseoconductive properties.
2. Have high degree of porosity in it (*60–80%*) with pore sizes ranging from 250–500 μm (*similar to that of human bone*).
3. Be resorbable.
4. Have convenient handling and be available in block or powder form.
5. Should have no untoward host reactions.

GUIDED BONE REGENERATION (*GBR*) IN EDENTULOUS SPACES FOR INCREASING BONE VOLUME FOR IMPLANT PLACEMENT

(*See Chapter 22, 'Dental Implants'*)

Platelet-rich Fibrin (*PRF*) and its use in GTR (*Including Implants*)

Platelets are a rich source of growth factors and cytokines (*chemical message molecules from cells*). Platelet-rich-fibrin (*PRF*) is an autologous platelet concentrate (*obtained from patient's own blood*). It is used for providing high concentrations of growth factors (*e.g. vascular endothelial growth factor, epidermal growth factor, etc.*) for GTR. These growth factors play important roles in regulating inflammation, wound healing and tissue regeneration. ◂ *What is PRF?*

Preparation of PRF (*Choukroun's Method*)

1. 10 ml of blood is drawn from the patient's median antecubital vein and dispensed into a blood collection tube that does ***not*** have any added anticoagulant. ◂ *How is PRF prepared?*
2. The blood collection tube is then ***immediately*** centrifuged (*before the initiation of blood clotting*) at 3000 rpm for 10 minutes.
3. During centrifugation, blood coagulates and three layers can be identified in the blood sample in blood collection tube (**Fig. 18.12**):
   i. **Plasma:** It is all fluid layer that is devoid of platelets. It is therefore also called platelet poor plasma (*PPP*). ◂ *After centrifugation, blood separates into which three components?*
   ii. **Platelet-rich-fibrin (*PRF*) clot:** It is an off-white gel like fibrin clot having entrapped platelets, leucocytes and other blood molecules like growth factors, fibronectin, etc.
   iii. **RBCs:** RBCs collect together as a deep red third layer.
4. After discarding the plasma, PRF clot is taken out from the just centrifuged blood collection tube. Red blood cell layer attached to the PRF clot is cut off and also discarded.
5. The PRF clot is then put in a sterile container, shaped as per need (*e.g. into a thin membrane by squeezing it, etc.*) and left for another 10 minutes (*for clotting to complete and mature*).
6. After this it can be used after cutting it into different shapes and dimensions to suit surgical needs.
7. PRF in this prepared form has platelets, growth factors, cytokines and stem cells of the blood. ◂ *What does PRF contain?*

Can bone graft material ▸ be added to PRF?

8. When a bone grafting material is added to PRF it acts like a biocompatible natural expander and binding material for the bone graft and thus facilitates easier manipulation and placement of bone grafts.
9. Additionally, as the PRF-graft mixture has growth factors, cytokines and stem cells of the blood, in addition to the bone graft material itself, it favours healing and periodontal tissue regeneration. Such PRF-bone graft mixture can be used for: filling periodontal bone defects during GTR and GBR procedures, preserving width of extraction sockets (*alveolar bone*) for future implant placement, bone regeneration around dental implants, maxillary sinus floor augmentation, etc.
10. PRF clot shaped as membrane can also be used as a ***resorbable barrier membrane*** for *GTR or GBR*, covering perforation in the lining of the maxillary sinus during indirect or direct sinus lift surgeries for implant placement, covering palatal wounds after harvesting free gingival grafts, covering root surfaces under a flap during root coverage surgery, etc.

CLINICAL UTILITY AND SHORT ANSWER

What are the advantages of PRF?

1. It is practically free, simple to prepare and requires a commonly used lab centrifuge to prepare.
2. As it prepared from patient's own blood, it is fully biocompatible and carries no risk of cross infection or allergic reactions.
3. It can be used alone or after mixing with bone graft materials.
4. It increases rate of healing and regeneration.
5. It can also be used as a GTR membrane.

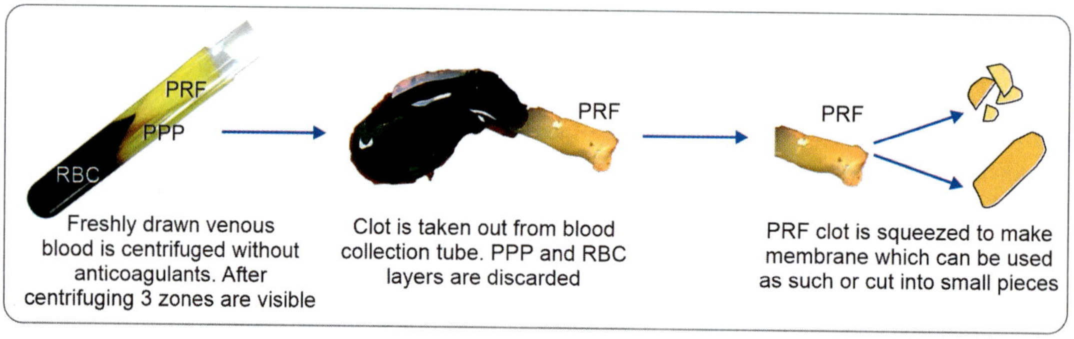

Fig. 18.12: Method of preparing Choukroun's platelet-rich fibrin (*PRF*).

HEALING AND REMODELING OF ALVEOLAR BONE

What are the phases ▸ in which bone healing and remodeling of take place?

Alveolar bone is continuously remodelled (*normal body function*). Bone is healed and remodelled (*resorbed and laid down*) by osteoclasts and osteoblasts under the influence of hormones (*parathyroid, thyroid growth, etc.*), vitamin D, cytokines, etc. This may take six months or more (*maturation of bone may take up to 2 years*). Phases in healing and remodeling of bone are:

1. *Origination*

It starts with initiation of organization of osteoclasts and osteoblasts (*basic multi-cellular unit*). This phase is activated by bone damage caused due to injury, mechanical stress or increased physiologic needs.

2. *Osteoclast Recruitment*

Pre-osteoclasts are activated to form mature osteoclasts that resorb bone.

3. *Resorption*

At a particular site, bone is resorbed by osteoclasts for about two weeks. After this, osteoclasts die. New osteoclasts are continuously activated till bone resorption goes on.

4. Osteoblast Recruitment

Osteoblasts are attracted to the site of bone resorption under influence of growth factors that are derived from bone and osteoclasts. Bone morphogenetic proteins (*BMPs*) induce new bone formation by stimulating proliferation and migration of osteoblasts to site of bone formation.

5. Osteoid Formation

Osteoblasts start laying down bone matrix by secreting osteoid to slowly fill the area from which bone has been resorbed (*resorption bay*).

6. Mineralization

When the osteoid layer is about 6 μm thick (*1 μm = 0.001 mm*), it starts to mineralize.

7. Mineral Maturation

Bone density increases with time for several months after start of mineralization.

8. Quiescence

After required bone mineral density is reached a phase of quiescence (*rest*) starts. At this time, some osteoblasts become lining cells over the surface of bone. These help regulate ongoing calcium release from bones. Some osteoblasts also become osteocytes which remain within bone and are connected by long cell processes that help them sense functional stresses on bone.

Review Questions

1. Write on different types of bone defects seen in periodontitis. How can osseous defects be diagnosed?
2. What are osteoplasty and ostectomy? What is the rationale of corrective osseous surgery?
3. What is positive, flat and negative architecture of alveolar bone? What is a 'widow's peak'?
4. Why must negative architecture of alveolar bone be corrected?
5. What are the indications and contraindications of resective osseous surgery? Describe the technique for recontouring alveolar bone.
6. What is regenerative periodontal treatment? What is the rationale for regenerative periodontal surgery?
7. What is new attachment? How is new attachment different from new connective tissue attachment?
8. What are the criteria for defect selection for attempting periodontal regeneration?
9. What are the possible sources of healing cells in a healing periodontal wound?
10. Describe the technique of GTR and GBR.
11. Write the factors that have a bearing on the outcome of GTR procedure.
12. Why is possibility for periodontal regeneration greater in three-walled infrabony pockets?
13. What is the difference between autograft, allograft and xenograft? What are the possible sources of bone autografts?
14. What is the difference between osteogenic, osteoconductive, osteoinductive and osteopromotive bone graft materials?
15. What steps must be taken to preserve the vitality and quality of harvested bone autografts? Write on the precautions that must be taken during transplantation of a bone graft material during GTR/GBR surgery.
16. What are advantages and disadvantages of bone allografts?
17. What is PRF? What are its uses and advantages in periodontics?
18. Write a note on remodeling of alveolar bone.

Chapter

19

Mucogingival Therapy

What is mucogingival therapy? ▶

All periodontal plastic surgical and non-surgical procedures meant for correction of supporting bone and soft tissue defects around natural teeth and implants and orthodontic tooth position correction for improving root coverage and reconstructing interdental papilla come under mucogingival therapy (*MGT*).

WHAT ARE MUCOGINGIVAL CONDITIONS (*COMPLICATIONS*)?

Which abnormalities of the periodontium come under the head mucogingival complications? ▶

How do mucogingival complications appear clinically? ▶

The following clinical presentations are mucogingival conditions:

- Gingival recession (*causing root exposure and open interdental spaces that appear as 'black triangles' between teeth during smiling*).
- Inadequate zone of attached gingiva (*see Chapter 2, 'Gingiva', section on attached gingiva, pages 10–13 and Fig. 2.10*).
- Reduced width or complete absence of only attached gingiva or entire keratinized gingival tissue (*width of keratinized gingiva includes free gingiva + attached gingiva*) **(Fig. 19.1)**.
- Base of pocket or probing pocket depth (*PD*) extending apical to the mucogingival junction.
- Thin gingiva.
- Absence of interdental papilla due to periodontitis, open tooth contacts, etc.

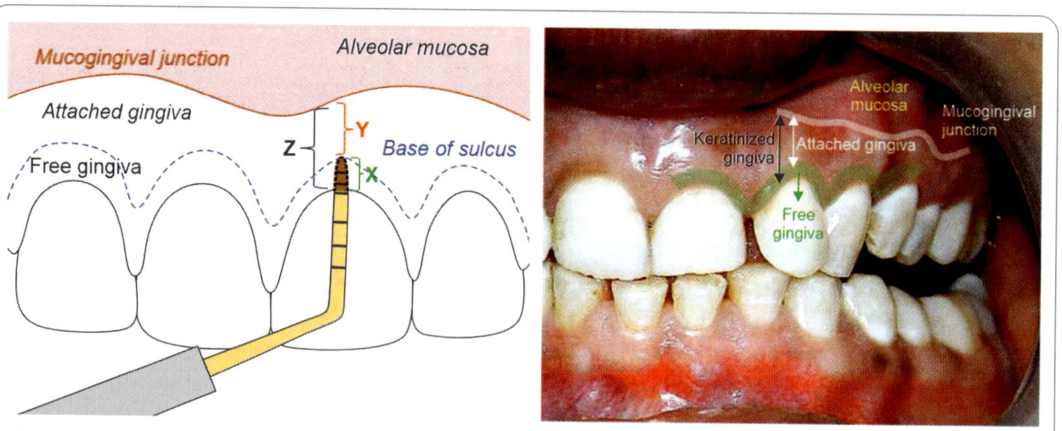

Both free gingiva [X] and attached gingiva [Y] are keratinized. Total width of the keratinized gingiva is X + Y = Z.

Fig. 19.1: Total width of the keratinized gingiva can be obtained by adding width of free and attached gingiva

Factors Contributing to Creation of Mucogingival Conditions (*Complications*)

Which local conditions predispose to mucogingival complications? ▶

1. Abnormal tooth position (*tooth protruding out of the curve of the arch*). This causes apical location of crest of gingiva margin (*gingival recession due to tooth position*) (*Fig. 2.20, diags 1 and 2, page 25*).

2. High frenal attachment and shallow vestibule. They lead to reduced width of attached gingiva.
3. Irregular alveolar ridge anatomy (*e.g. too thin, covered by loose flabby soft tissue, etc.*).
4. Thin gingiva (*thin gingival biotypes*).

WHAT IS MUCOGINGIVAL THERAPY (*MGT*)?

◂ What is mucogingival therapy?

MGT includes all periodontal plastic surgical procedures meant for correction of contour, position, volume of soft tissue and tooth supporting bone in relation to teeth and implants and also all non-surgical procedures meant for attaining these goals, e.g. correction of tooth position to improve root coverage and reconstruction of interdental papilla. Mucogingival therapy therefore includes the following:

◂ Mucogingival therapy includes which procedures?

- Procedures for increasing gingival thickness and width of attached gingiva
- Frenectomy and frenulotomy
- Procedures for improving aesthetics:
  - Root coverage in cases of gingival recession
  - Reconstruction of interdental papilla
  - Prevention of post-extraction ridge collapse (*by grafting in extraction sockets immediately after extraction*).
  - Gingivoplasty for correction of gummy smiles
- Increasing width and height of alveolar ridge for implant placement
- Crown lengthening for restorative reasons (*crown preparation and restorations*)
- Orthodontic correction of tooth position to improve gingival contours and gingival recession.
- Vestibular deepening procedures, etc.

INCREASING WIDTH OF ATTACHED GINGIVA

◂ Which preconditions must be met before attempting increase in width of attached gingiva?

Before planning increase in width of attached gingiva the following must be remembered and ensured:

1. An ***adequate*** zone of attached gingiva not only prevents gingival recession and but is also required for root coverage surgery in cases where gingival recession has already occurred **(Fig. 19.1 and 2.10)**.
2. Surgery for increasing width of attached gingiva must only be done on healthy gingiva (*no gingivitis or active periodontitis must be there*).
3. Other correctable causes of gingival recession like prominent root of the tooth (*orthodontic correction of tooth position*), etc. must be treated before attempting widening of attached gingiva.

Indications for increasing zone of attached gingiva

◂ In which situations is increasing width of attached gingiva indicated?

1. To create an adequate zone of attached gingiva by widening it.
2. For vestibule deepening.
3. As a first step of root coverage surgery for treatment of gingival recession (*after widening attached gingiva, coronally displaced flap is done later as a second stage surgery*).

Techniques of Increasing Width of Attached Gingiva

◂ How can the width of attached gingiva be increased?

1. **Vestibular extension procedures**
   a. Apically displaced (*repositioned*) partial thickness flap
   b. Denudation technique with or without periosteum retention (*not popular as it is not very successful*).
2. **Gingival grafts**
   a. Free gingival
   b. Connective tissue grafts.

Apically Displaced Flap for Increasing Width of Attached Gingiva

Indications for apically displaced flaps

What are the indications of apically displaced flap surgery?

1. Increasing width of attached gingiva.
2. Eliminating pockets (*by apical displacement of pocket wall; this retains keratinized gingiva instead of excising it as is done during gingivectomy and undisplaced flap surgery*).
3. Crown lengthening for correction of gummy smiles or prosthetic reasons (*by apical displacement of pocket wall; this retains keratinized gingiva instead of excising it as is done during gingivectomy and undisplaced flap surgery*).
4. Deepening vestibule while maintaining keratinized gingiva (*by apical displacement of pocket wall; this retains keratinized gingiva*).

Procedure

Why must vertical incisions be extended beyond mucogingival junction during apically displaced flap surgery?

What are the indications of raising a full or partial thickness during apically displaced flap surgery?

1. Ensure adequate asepsis and attain anaesthesia.
2. A full ***or*** partial thickness flap is raised using internal bevel incisions with ***two vertical incisions*** placed at both the boundaries of the planned flap. Vertical incisions must extend ***apical*** to the M-G junction to allow flaps to be raised beyond the mucogingival junction and subsequent apical displacement.
   a. Full thickness flap is preferred if:
      i. Gingiva is thin.
      ii. Bone has to be recontoured.
   b. Partial thickness flap is preferred if:
      i. Gingiva is thick.
      ii. There are no pockets.
      iii. Bone recontouring is not needed.
3. If a full thickness flap is reflected, a flap comprising the ***entire*** thickness of marginal and attached gingiva is displaced apically and sutured keeping the margin of the gingiva ***slightly coronal*** to or at the level of the crest of the alveolar bone. This will:
   a. Eliminate pockets
   b. Displaces the attached gingiva apically
   c. It also exposes the tooth root.
4. If a partial thickness flap is reflected, a flap comprising ***a part of the marginal and attached gingiva*** is shifted (*displaced*) apically and sutured to the underlying periosteum a few millimeters apically. This will widen the attached gingiva.

Gingival Denudation Procedure for Increasing Width of Attached Gingiva and Deepening of Vestibule

Why is gingival denudation procedure not very popular?

Gingival denudation procedure for increasing width of attached gingiva and deepening of vestibule is an easy but ***not*** a very successful procedure. This is so because the increase in width of attached gingiva attained with this surgical procedure is ***lost*** after a few months of this surgery.

Procedure

How is gingival denudation procedure done for increasing width of attached gingiva?

1. Attain adequate asepsis and anesthesia.
2. Pull out the lip/cheek to stretch the alveolar mucosa; this will clearly demarcate the mucogingival junction.
3. A stab incision is made in the mucogingival junction at one end of the surgical site while maintaining constant pull on the lip to keep alveolar mucosa stretched. This will produce a gaping wound (Fig. 19.2, diag. A).
4. Incision is extended along the mucogingival junction till the other end of the surgical site is reached (Fig. 19.2, diag. B).

5. Control bleeding from the site and put a periodontal pack in two stages:
   - The first installment of pack is put on the teeth to act like an anchor for the second installment (Fig. 19.2, diag. C, green shaded area).
   - The second instalment of the pack is directly put and spread over the wound (Fig. 19.2, diag. C, blue shaded area).
   - The second portion of pack acts like a wound extending and separating layer. This allows the thus extended wound to heal and deepens the vestibule by shifting the mucogingival junction apically.
6. In the above technique, the ***periosteum*** is exposed but is ***left intact*** covering the underlying bone.
7. ***Alternately***, some clinicians prefer removing the periosteum and exposing the alveolar bone (***complete denudation technique***) before applying the periodontal pack.
8. Gingival denudation procedure results in an increase in width of attached gingiva and deepening of the vestibule by shifting mucogingival junction apically. However, this increase in width of attached gingiva does ***not*** last very long as the ***mucogingival junction shifts coronally*** within a few weeks/months post operatively thus reducing the width of attached gingiva ***back to its original width***.

◂ *Why is periodontal pack used in two instalments during gingival denudation procedure?*

◂ *Which of the two: Periosteum or bone is left exposed in wound created during gingival denudation?*

◂ *Why is gingival denudation technique not very popular?*

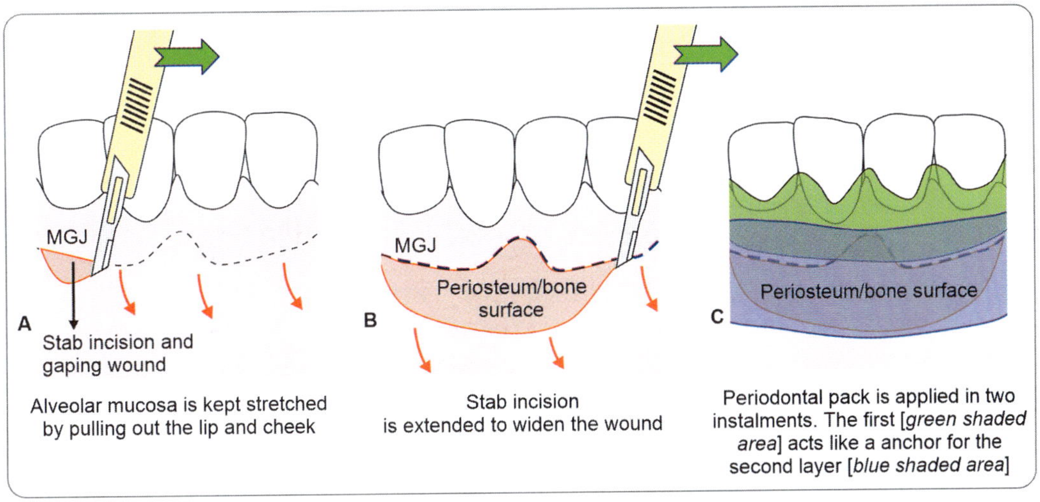

Fig. 19.2: Denudation procedure for increasing width of attached gingiva

Gingival Grafting for Increasing Width (and thickness) of Attached Gingiva

Living tissue transplanted to another site is called a graft. As attached gingiva is keratinized, donor graft tissue to increase width and thickness of attached gingiva must also be sourced from keratinized areas of the oral cavity.

◂ *What is a graft?*

CLINICAL UTILITY AND SHORT ANSWER

Why can only keratinized graft donor tissue be used to increase width of attached gingiva?

- Only keratinized gingiva can serve as graft donor tissue for increasing width of attached gingiva.
- Connective tissue underlying keratinized mucosa can ***also*** be used as donor tissue for FGG.
- This is because keratinized gingiva and connective tissue underlying keratinized gingiva have the ***genetic predisposition*** to get ***attached*** to the underlying periosteum to become attached gingiva. If non-keratinized mucosa is used a donor tissue, it will ***not*** become attached gingiva or keratinized.

◂ *Why non-keratinized gingiva cannot serve as donor tissue for increasing width and thickness of attached gingiva?*

Free Gingival Graft (FGG)

Free gingival graft is used alone or in combination with other procedures for increasing width and thickness of attached gingiva and covering exposed root surfaces in recession defects (*discussed later in this Chapter*).

- Donor tissue for FGG must be ***keratinized*** gingiva which can be harvested from: Palate (*entire hard palate is keratinized*) (Fig. 19.3), maxillary tuberosity, edentulous alveolar ridge, excised gingivectomy tissue (*keratinized gingiva*) can also be used for FGG.

◂ *What are the sources of keratinized gingiva for FGG?*

- After increasing the width and thickness of attached gingiva with FGG, a second stage coronally displaced flap surgery can be done after a few weeks to cover exposed roots (*treatment of gingival recession*).

By how much does a FGG shrink postoperatively? ▶

- FGGs ***shrink*** up to **50%** after healing (*usually by 6th week but up to 6 months*). Therefore, if possible, graft tissue of ***double*** the width of the desired increase in dimension of attached gingiva must be harvested and grafted to compensate for post-operative shrinkage.
- Free gingival grafts can be **(Fig. 19.3)**:
  - Thin (*less than 0.5 mm*)
  - Medium thickness (*0.5 mm–0.75 mm*)
  - Thick (*0.75 mm–1.25 mm*)
  - Full thickness (*more than 1.25 mm*).

What are the indications of FGG of different thicknesses? ▶

- Thick, medium and thin grafts are ***partial thickness*** grafts (*i.e. an intact layer of periosteum is left over bone at the donor site*).
- Thin and medium thickness grafts are more suited for increasing width and thickness of gingiva in anterior (*aesthetic*) zone.
- Thick and full thickness grafts are used for root coverage and filling soft tissue ridge defects.

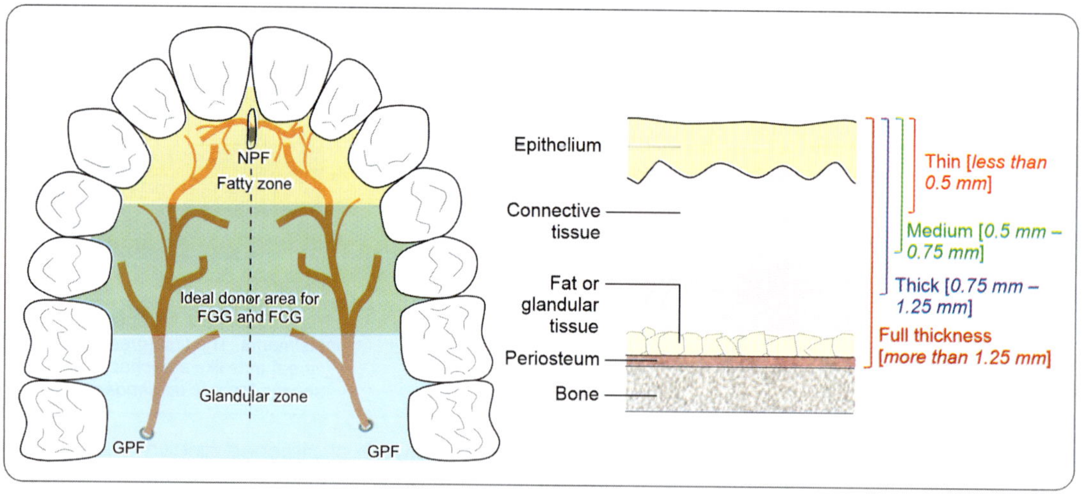

Fig. 19.3: Anatomical considerations and cross-sectional diagram of palatal gingiva showing the possible thicknesses of free gingival grafts. Entire hard palate is keratinized; therefore, it is an ideal site for obtaining donor soft tissue (*gingiva and underlying connective tissue*) for free gingival and free connective tissue grafts. The preferred area for obtaining donor tissue is between midline of palate and gingival crest opposite premolars (*green area*). This is because anterior palate has more fat tissue (*yellow area*) and posterior palate has many small glands (*blue area*). Location of greater palatine vessels and nerves emerging from greater palatine foramina (*GPF*) and nasopalatine vessels and nerves emerging from nasopalatine foramen (*NPF*) respectively is also shown.

CLINICAL UTILITY AND SHORT ANSWER

Why does FGG shrink during healing?

- FGGs show primary and secondary shrinkage during healing.
- Primary shrinkage occurs due to elastic fibers of the graft tissue.
- Secondary shrinkage occurs due to scar formation in-between graft tissue and recipient bed.

When is post operative shrinking of FGG completed? ▶

- FGGs can shrink almost ***50%***; shrinking is usually completed by the ***6th week*** post-operatively but may continue for up to 6 months.

Does a FGG placed directly over bone shrink more postoperatively? ▶

- FGG placed directly over bone, show ***lesser*** shrinking, i.e. ***25%***.
- FGG will shrink ***more*** if they are placed deeper into the vestibule for attempting greater vestibular deepening (*due to coronal push of muscles*).

Procedure of free gingival graft surgery

◂ *How is free gingival graft surgery done?*

Step 1: Preparation of the recipient site

1. Attain adequate anaesthesia while taking care that too much anesthetic solution is not injected into the recipient site as it will cause soft tissue to balloon out (*this makes local clinical landmarks, e.g. mucogingival junction invisible making recipient site surgery difficult*).
2. Clearly identify boundaries of recipient site and gently pull the lip and/or cheek opposite recipient site outwards. This will lift alveolar mucosa from the underlying bone and will help identify the mucogingival junction.
3. Keeping the lip and cheek pulled, a shallow stab incision is made at the mucogingival junction with a #15 BP blade at the distal or mesial end of the recipient site. This results in a gaping wound (Fig. 19.4, diag. A).
4. While keeping the blade almost parallel to the alveolus, the blade is drawn from the gaping wound to the other end of the surgical site along the mucogingival junction (Fig. 19.4, diag. B).
5. The wound is extended apically and alveolar mucosa is separated from the underlying periosteum using sharp dissection.
6. Muscle fibers and ***loose*** connective tissue fibers on the recipient site's periosteal bed are removed with scissors or tissue nippers; failure to do this will lead to a moving graft tissue and thus no increase in attached gingiva despite a successful FGG procedure.

◂ *Why is it important to completely remove muscle fibres and loose connective tissue form the recipient bed?*

7. Margin of the incised alveolar mucosa is now sutured at the apical boundary of the recipient site (*using mattress sutures*) (Fig. 19.4, diag. C).
8. Dimensions of the recipient site (*length and width*) are recorded. This can be done in two ways:
   a. An aluminium foil template (*tin foil template*) is made by diag. adapting and trimming a piece of aluminium foil over the recipient site (Fig. 19.4, diag. D). This template is used to transfer the exact shape and dimensions of the recipient site to the donor site for harvesting FGG of required size (Fig. 19.4, diag. E).
   b. Alternately a periodontal probe can also be used for recording the length and breadth of the recipient site.

◂ *How are the dimensions of the recipient site transferred to the donor site during free gingival graft surgery?*

9. The recipient site is now covered with a gauze piece moistened with normal saline. This helps attain hemostasis and prevents drying of the recipient site.

◂ *Why is recipient bed kept covered with moist gauze till grafting?*

Step 2: Harvesting, preparing and grafting donor tissue

1. Palate is the most ***common*** donor site. Harvesting of donor tissue is started after ensuring adequate anaesthesia.
2. Harvesting of donor tissue is started by transferring dimensions of the recipient site to the donor site.
   a. If an 'aluminium foil template' method was used, the aluminium foil that was cut and trimmed to the size of the recipient site (*step 1, # 8a, above*) is lightly wetted in normal saline and placed on the donor site. A shallow marking incision is then traced all along the margins of the foil (Fig. 19.4. diag. E). This will mark the dimensions of the recipient site on the donor site. The aluminium foil template is then removed and discarded.
   b. If dimensions of the recipient site were recorded with a probe (*step 1, # 8 b, above*), a bleeding point is first made by inserting the tip of a periodontal probe at one corner of the donor site. Then, using a periodontal probe placed horizontally over the donor site, length and breadth of the recipient site (*recorded earlier*) are marked with additional bleeding points relative to the first bleeding point. To mark the boundary of donor tissue to be harvested, the bleeding points are connected with a shallow 'marking incision' made using a # 11 or 15 BP blade.

◂ *How are dimensions of the to be intended FGG recorded and transferred to the donor site using an aluminium foil template?*

◂ *How are dimensions of the to be intended FGG recorded and transferred to the donor site using a periodontal probe?*

3. Harvesting of the gingival graft is started from one end of the donor site marking incision. A # 15 BP blade is inserted into the marking incision up to the desired graft thickness (*0.5–2.0 mm*) and graft of even thickness is harvested (*if donor site is on the palate, most clinicians prefer to start graft harvesting from the anterior-occlusal edge of the marked donor site.*) (Fig. 19.4, diag. F).

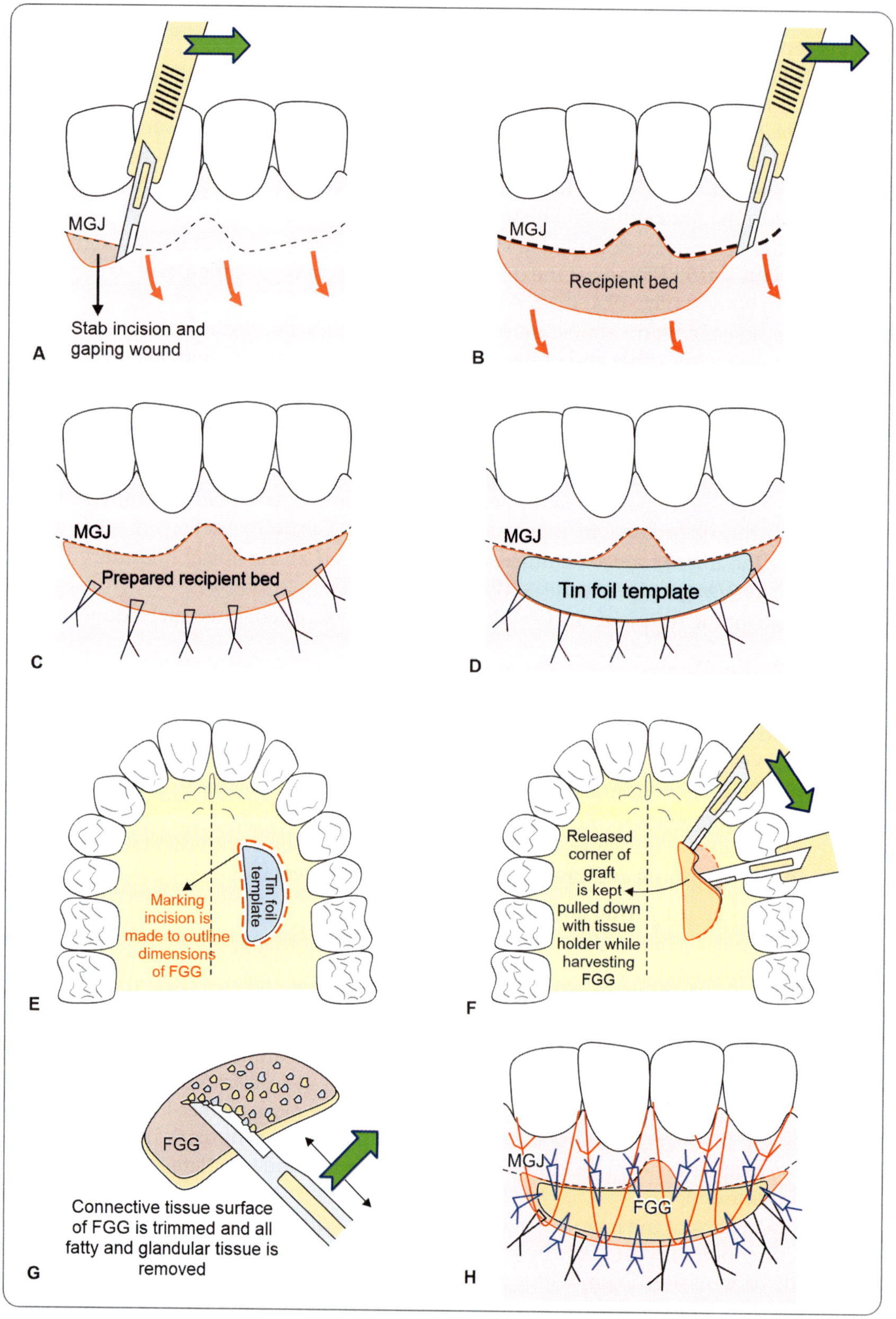

Fig. 19.4: Illustration of steps of free gingival tissue grafting

Why must the harvested graft be kept moist till it is grafted? ▶

4. After harvesting the FGG, it is placed on a saline moistened gauze piece (*do not dip graft in normal saline*) to prevent it from drying (*drying leads to cell death*).

When is a Hawley's retainer used to cover the donor site wound on the palate made? ▶

5. A periodontal pack is placed over the donor site wound facing area of a prefabricated modified Hawley's retainer (*made prior to the surgery*), this is then is fitted in mouth for one week. Although approximation of palatal wound's edges is usually not possible, still the wound may be sutured to help in hemorrhage control before fitting the Hawley's retainer.

6. The harvested graft's connective tissue surface (*undersurface*) is cleared of glandular or fatty tissue and trimmed to even thickness and size (Fig. 19.4, diag. G).
7. If a small graft has been harvested, the graft scan be stretched to increase its size by making small alternating incisions on opposite sides of the graft and then stretching it before grafting it on the recipient site (*Accordion technique*) (Fig. 19.5, diag. A). Alternately a small graft is cut into strips which are then grafted almost 1 mm apart on the recipient site (*Strip technique*) (Fig. 19.5, diag. B). Both these techniques can be used in combination also (Fig. 19.5, diag. C).
8. The free gingival graft is placed on the recipient site with its ***connective tissue side*** in contact with the periosteum and sutured to stabilize it securely. For adequate stabilization, grafts are first stabilized by placing horizontal graft stretching sutures at their mesial and distal ends. These sutures stretch grafts by 2–3 mm to open up the blood vessels in the FGG and counters primary contraction of FGG (Fig. 19.4, diag. H, blue lines). Graft is then adapted under light finger pressure to the underlying recipient bed. Further stabilization of the graft is done with multiple sling sutures around teeth (Fig. 19.4, diag. H, red lines). Sutures are removed after 1–2 weeks.
9. The graft and recipient site are ***not*** covered with a periodontal pack as it increases chances of graft movement (*graft movement leads to breaking of capillary connections developing between the recipient bed and graft tissue during the early healing phase thus leading to failure*).

◂ *What are the accordion and strip technique used for?*

◂ *How is the FGG stabilized on the recipient site?*

◂ *Why are the FGG and recipient site not covered with a periodontal pack?*

After allowing healing for two weeks, if the grafting procedure has been successful, widening of the attached gingiva is seen. ***Over the next 6 weeks and up to 6 months the graft will shrink by about 50%.***

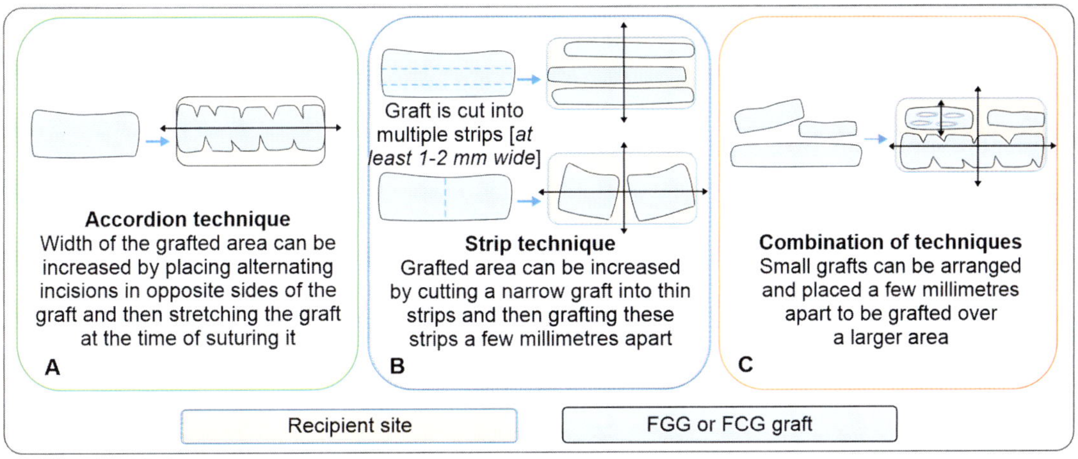

Fig. 19.5: Modifications for covering recipient site of larger area than that of harvested graft/s

CLINICAL UTILITY AND SHORT ANSWER

Why does FGG fail if it is not sutured properly (*stabilized securely*)?

It is very important to stabilize the FGG securely or it will fail. This is because:

1. Initially (*first few hours after grafting*), FGGs draw nutrition from the underlying recipient bed by diffusion only. Later, within the first few days of grafting FGG, new capillaries grow into it. To prevent breakage of these new capillaries providing blood supply to the FGG, the graft must not be physically disturbed during the initial healing phase. Immobilizing grafts using sutures is therefore very important for this reason.
2. Adequately placed sutures over the graft will also reduce dead space formation and size of clot formed under the graft. Both dead space (*area under FGG that is not in close contact with the underlying bed*) and large clots under FGG increase microbial growth (*infection*) and reduce diffusion of nutrients and ingrowth of capillaries into the FGG; they thus reduce chances of successful FGG.

◂ *Why is it very important to suture and stabilize the FGG properly?*

Stages of healing of a free gingival graft

- For the first few hours after grafting, the graft survives only on nutrition and hydration it receives from the recipient bed by diffusion.

◂ *How does the FGG receive its nutrition initially after placement?*

- The FGG's connective tissue undergoes disorganization and degeneration on the 1st day.

By when is revascularization of the FGG complete?

- New capillaries start to grow into the FGG by the 2nd day and by the 10th day revascularization is almost complete.
- Fibrous organization of the graft starts on 2nd day and continues for several days.

By when does new epithelium start to form in the FGG?

- Most of the epithelium of the FGG degenerates (*as it is farthest away from the source nutrition, i.e. recipient bed*). New epithelium starts to form by the 4th day.
- Upon healing, FGG appears bulbous and gets functionally integrated by the 3rd week. It however appears different from the surrounding tissues both in colour and physical characteristics, for many months.

Free Connective Tissue Graft (FCG)

Why is FCG preferred over FGG?

Experienced clinicians prefer FCG instead of FGG because a FCG provides the same benefits as the FGG but with ***lesser donor site complications***. Also, ***FCG donor sites heal faster*** than donor sites from where FGG has been harvested.

What are the indications of use of FCG?

- FCG is used for ***same indications*** and in a ***similar way*** as the FGG.

From which areas can a FCG be harvested?

- FCG donor tissue (*connective tissue*) must be harvested ***only*** from areas covered by ***attached*** and ***keratinized*** gingiva (*palate, edentulous alveolar ridges, etc.*).
- The connective tissue graft gets covered with epithelium after a few days of healing and then becomes keratinized gingiva.

How thick must the palatal tissue be for a FCG to be harvested from the palate?

- FCG should be at least 2–3 mm thick, therefore the ***palatal tissue from where the FCG has to be harvested should be at least 4 mm thick***.
- When compared to FGG, the color and surface characteristics of FCG resemble those of the surrounding gingiva more closely.

Harvesting FCG—The 'Trap door' technique

How is FCG harvested from the palate?

1. A horizontal incision extending to the underlying bone surface and as long as the length of the required graft tissue (*i.e. length of the recipient site*) is made ***perpendicular*** to the palatal bone (Fig. 19.6, diag. A, 1). This incision is given some distance away from the palatal gingival margin.
2. ***2 mm apical*** to the first incision, a shallow second incision as long as the first horizontal incision is made ***parallel*** to the palatal bone (Fig. 19.6, diag. B, 2). This second incision is then ***extended vertically*** (*following the curve of the palate*) towards the palatal midline to the desired width of the connective tissue to be used for grafting (Fig. 19.6, diag. B, 2). Thus, a flap of palatal tissue (*palatal epithelium and a small amount of sub-epithelial connective tissue*) is separated and can be raised as a trap door (*palatal bone is left covered with connective tissue*).
3. Through the wound of the first incision, connective tissue underlying the raised palatal tissue trap door flap (*that was left attached to palatal bone after step1*) is separated from the underlying palatal bone using a mucoperiosteal elevator and BP blades # 11 or 15 (Fig. 19.6, diag. C, 3) and is gently pulled out (Fig. 19.6, diags D and E). If required, the trap door can be raised fully after giving two vertical incisions at the mesial and distal boundaries first horizontal incision.
4. The palatal trap door flap is then sutured (Fig. 19.6, diag. F).
5. The FCG is grafted on the recipient just as the FGG.

CLINICAL UTILITY AND SHORT ANSWER

What are the reasons of failure of FGG or FCG?

1. Improper diagnosis and assessment of mucogingival condition.
2. Improper preparation of the recipient site.
3. Too thin graft or if graft is torn at several places.
4. Dehydration (*drying*) of the graft after harvesting.
5. Improper suturing leading to movement of graft on periosteal bed after grafting.
6. Too thick clot or dead space formation under the graft.
7. Smoking.

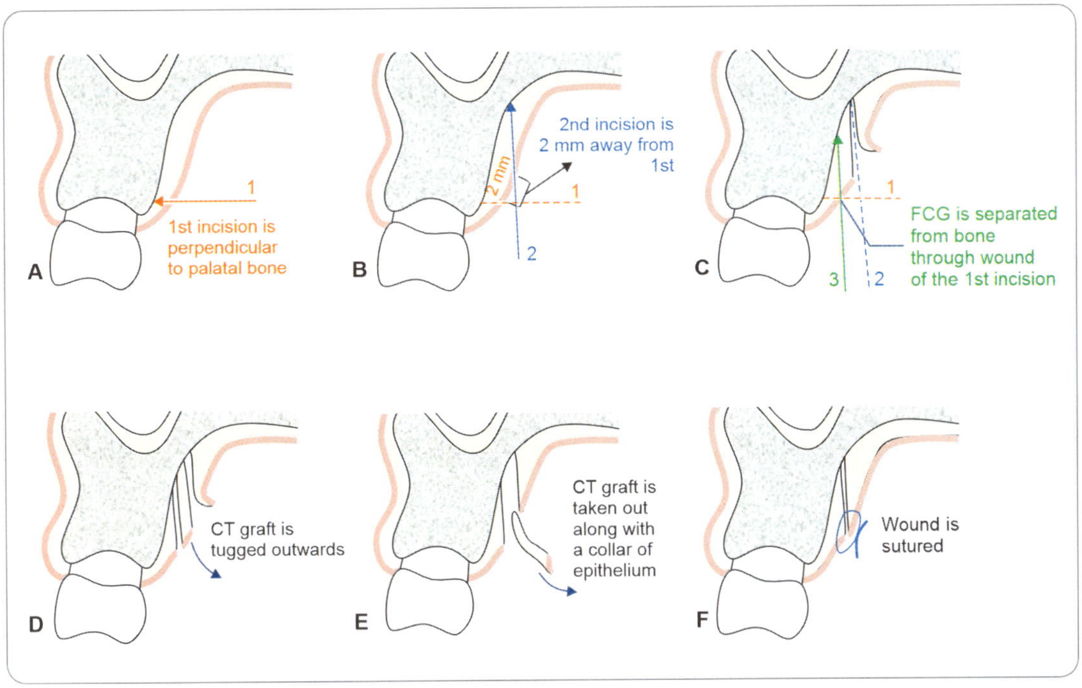

Fig. 19.6: Trap door technique of harvesting free connective tissue graft from the palate

GINGIVAL RECESSION AND ITS TREATMENT

Definition: Exposure of the anatomical root of a tooth due to shift of gingiva apical to the CE junction is called gingival recession.

◄ *What is gingival recession?*

Apparent, Hidden and Total Gingival Recession

- Apparent recession is the distance between CE junction and crest of gingiva (Fig. 19.7, green line).
- Hidden recession is distance between crest of gingiva and base of sulcus or pocket (*probing depth—PD*) (Fig. 19.7, blue line).
- Total gingival recession is sum of apparent and hidden recession (Fig. 19.7 red line).

◄ *What is the difference between apparent, hidden and total gingival recession?*

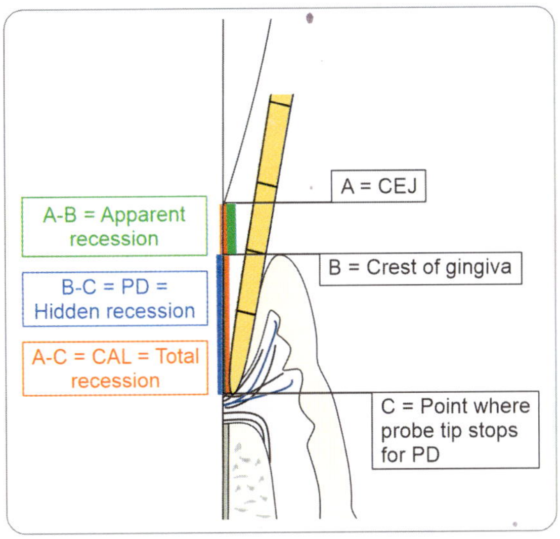

Fig. 19.7: Apparent, Hidden and Total gingival recession

Etiology of gingival recession

Several factors can cause gingival recession:

◄ *What are the causes of gingival recession?*

- Periodontitis (Fig. 19.8, diag. A, white arrow) and Stillman's defects (*see Chapter 10, 'Gingivitis and Periodontitis', page 147 and Fig. 10.9*).

- Root prominence due to tooth malposition that is natural or has been produced by orthodontic movement of a tooth (*root prominence causes thinning of overlying alveolar bone and marginal gingiva in the area of root prominence; this makes such areas more prone to recession*).
- Alveolar bone dehiscence on prominent root surface that is overlaid by thin gingiva (*thin gingival biotype*) (*see Chapter 3 page 44, Fig. 3.16*).
- Narrow or inadequate zone of attached gingiva. High frenal attachment leading to narrow width of attached gingiva and shallow vestibule.

What are abfraction cavities? ▸

- Abfraction cavities (*wedge shaped cavities in cervical area of tooth caused by chronic TFO*) (Fig. 19.8, diag. C, black arrow).

How can gingival recession caused by tooth brush abrasion be diagnosed? ▸

- Recurrent and chronic physical trauma to gingiva by vigorous tooth brushing, etc. (Fig. 19.8 diag. B, white arrow). In these cases, root surface coronal to receded gingiva is shining and smooth due to polishing effect of tooth brushing (Fig. 19.8, B, black arrow).
- Iatrogenic factors like violation of biologic width during restorative treatments, excessive keratinized tissue excision during periodontal surgery, orthodontic movement that results in prominent roots (*Fig. 21.11, page 373*), etc.

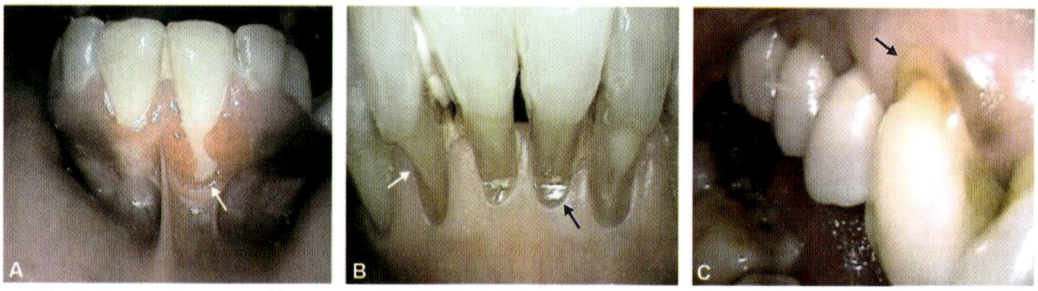

Gingival recession caused by prominence of root and periodontitis | Gingival recession caused by tooth brush abrasion | Gingival recession caused by abfraction cavities

Fig. 19.8: Common causes of gingival recession. Prominent tooth root and periodontitis (*diag. A*). Tooth brush abrasion, this is easily recognized by shining tooth surfaces produced by polishing effect of tooth brushing (*diag. B, black arrow*). Abfraction cavities (*wedge shaped class V non-caries cavities*) (*diag. C*)

Miller's Classification of Gingival Recession

In which type of Miller's recession defects is root coverage surgery likely to be the most effective? ▸

Miller's classification is useful for predicting possible extent of root coverage after root coverage surgery (Fig. 19.9). Root coverage surgery is most likely to be successful in class I and II defects. Class III and IV defects have poor prognosis.

Class I	Gingival recession is present only on facial surface and it does ***not*** extend up to the mucogingival junction. There is no loss of interdental bone or interdental papilla. The recession defect may be narrow or wide.
Class II	Similar to class I, but recession extends apical to the mucogingival junction.
Class III	A wide gingival recession defect extending up to or apical to the mucogingival junction is present. Both interdental papilla and interdental bone are apical to CEJ of adjoining teeth but are coronal to the apical extent of the gingival recession. There may be severe mal-positioning of teeth.
Class IV	Gingival recession extends up to or apical to the mucogingival junction. There is severe bone or soft-tissue loss around the entire tooth and the interdental bone crest is apical to crest of the receded gingival tissue. There may be severe mal-positioning of teeth. Class IV recession defects may arise from periodontitis or resective surgery.

Surgical Treatment of Gingival Recession

(Root Coverage Surgery)

Name some surgical techniques to cover exposed roots. ▸

Surgical root coverage can be done in several ways, these include: Coronally positioned flaps, free gingival graft, free connective tissue graft, sub-epithelially placed connective

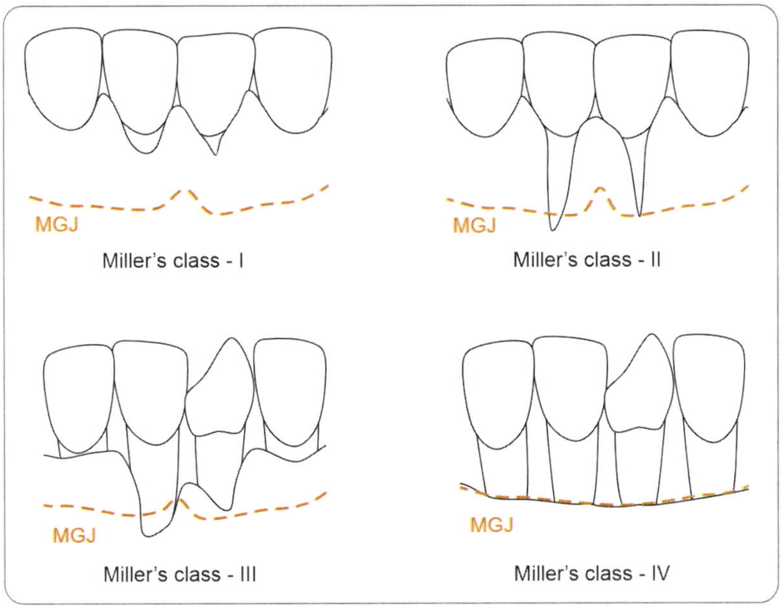

Fig. 19.9: Miller's Classification of gingival recession

tissue graft, laterally positioned flaps, etc. The following preconditions must be met before attempting root coverage surgery:

1. If indicated, orthodontic correction of tooth's prominent position in the arch must be done ***before*** attempting surgical correction of gingival recession over the prominent root.
2. Presence of an adequate zone of attached gingiva is a must. If attached gingiva is not adequate, width of attached gingiva must be increased surgically (*as described in earlier in this chapter*) ***before*** attempting root coverage surgery.

◂ *What are the preconditions for surgical correction of gingival recession?*

ALERT!

Important facts about *black triangles* between teeth due to receded interdental papilla

- Recession of interdental papilla is caused by periodontitis.
- If teeth are not in contact, i.e. there is no interdental contact, interdental papilla is rounded and lies about 2 mm coronal to interdental bone.
- Interdental papilla can fill up interdental space a ***maximum*** 5 mm coronal to the crest of the interdental bone but only if there is a ***good interdental contact*** between adjacent teeth.
- Therefore, if loss of height of interdental papilla has to be corrected, the first precondition to doing so is establishment of interdental contact point between adjoining teeth. After this is done, only then can the papilla be expected to fill up and grow into the interdental space but only up to a maximum height of 5 mm.
- Interdental papilla will recede further if resorption of interdental bone septum (*periodontitis*) worsens.

◂ *Where is the tip of interdental papilla located if there is no interdental contact between teeth?*

◂ *Where is the tip of interdental papilla located if there is good interdental contact between teeth?*

I. Root Coverage using Free Gingival Graft (FGG) and Free Connective Tissue Graft (FCG)

Technique for harvesting the FGG or FCG for root coverage is the same as described earlier in this chapter (Figs 19.4, 19.5 and 19.6). However, recipient site preparation and graft suturing need to be modified for root coverage. ***Thick/full thickness grafts*** (*1.5 mm–2.0 mm*) are ***preferred*** for root coverage (*thin and medium thickness grafts usually do not show good results when used for root coverage*).

◂ *Which of the four thin, medium, thick or full thickness grafts are preferred to cover exposed roots?*

Preparation of exposed root and recipient site, positioning and suturing of FGG and FCG for root coverage

Step 1—Preparation of the root surface

- Thorough root planing of exposed part of root is done.
- If required, prominence (*convexity*) of the root is reduced using rotary diamond stones and curettes. This is done to decrease lateral distance from graft bed to the center of the graft that lies over the avascular root surface. This increases supply of nutrients to the

◂ *Why is prominence of the root reduced before attempting root coverage surgery?*

graft's central region overlying the avascular tooth root (*during first few hours of grafting*) and decreases chances of necrosis of graft's central region (*if this happens, it will result in partial root coverage or total graft failure*).

Step 2—Preparation of the graft bed

- The recipient bed is prepared as described earlier in this chapter.

How far must recipient bed be extended beyond the exposed root surface for ensuring success of root coverage surgery using FGG or FCG? ▸

- It must be ensured that the recipient bed (*made by removing epithelium and exposing the underlying connective tissue*) extends at least ***4–6 mm on mesial, distal and apical sides of the exposed root.***
- While designing the recipient bed it must be kept in mind that the coronal margin of the graft can be placed ***maximum at the level*** of CE junctions of adjoining teeth.

Where must the coronal margin of the graft be placed in relation to CE junction? ▸

- However, if crest of gingiva on adjoining teeth is apical to CE junctions of those teeth, the graft must then be placed at level of adjoining gingiva on these teeth. ***In no case must the coronal margin of the graft be placed more coronal to the crest of free gingiva of adjoining teeth*** (*even if it means some part of the exposed root is left uncovered by the graft*).

Step 3—Adequate immobilization of graft with sutures

- This prevents movement of the graft in the initial few hours of healing. Graft movement breaks newly formed capillary connections between graft bed and graft thereby resulting in graft failure.

What is dead space? Why is it important to ensure there is no dead space under the graft? ▸

- Proper suturing technique also helps in closely adapting the graft to the graft bed. This reduces thickness of clot and dead space under the graft (*dead space is the area under the graft which is not in close contact with the underlying recipient bed, it reduces chances of graft survival; thick clot under a graft can get infected leading to graft failure*) **(Fig. 19.10, diag. B)**.

How can dead space and thick clot formation under a graft be prevented? ▸

  To ensure good physical contact between graft and recipient bed on the lateral sides of the exposed root, sutures must be placed in such a way that they pass over areas that are just lateral to the exposed root **(Fig. 19.10, diags A and C)**.

- In case an FCG is used, its chances of success can be increased if it is submerged under a gingival or mucosal flap raised on the sides of the exposed root (*this will allow nutrient diffusion to the FCG both from upper and lower surface of the FCG*).

When is FCG/FGG considered to be successful? ▸

Root coverage using FGG/FCG is said to be successful if root coverage occurs (*even if to a limited extent*) and the graft has a 'clinical attachment' to the earlier exposed root surface (*clinical attachment is very close adaptation of gingiva to root; it is not 'New attachment'; such a graft has a sulcus depth of 2 mm or less and there is no bleeding on probing*).

II. *Root Coverage using Laterally Sliding Flap*

What is a pedicle flap? Where is it used? ▸

The laterally sliding flap is a ***pedicle*** flap (*graft*) (*pedicle graft/flap is one that is attached to the base of the donor site*). It is used for treating ***isolated*** root recession. The technique for performing laterally sliding flap is as under:

Step 1—Exposed root is root planed.

Step 2—Gingival sulcus bordering the exposed root **(Fig. 19.11, diag. A, red shaded area)** is excised by making a V' shaped incision all along the border of the root (*1st incision*) using a # 15 BP blade **(Fig. 19.11, diag. A, red dashed arrow)**. This is done to expose gingival connective tissue all around the exposed root.

Is the pedicle flap partial or full thickness? ▸

Step 3—A scalloped and shallow ***inverse beveled*** incision not extending down to the bone is then made just a small distance away from the gingival margin (*2nd incision*). This incision starts from the 'V' shaped incision given earlier and ends at the boundary of the surgical site, i.e. boundary of the donor flap from where the third incision will start (*laterally sliding graft must be **double** the width of the recipient site*) **(Fig. 19.11, diag. B, blue dashed arrow)**. This incision allows raising of a partial thickness laterally sliding flap. If the gingiva is very thin, a full thickness laterally sliding flap can also be raised (*though this is not preferable*).

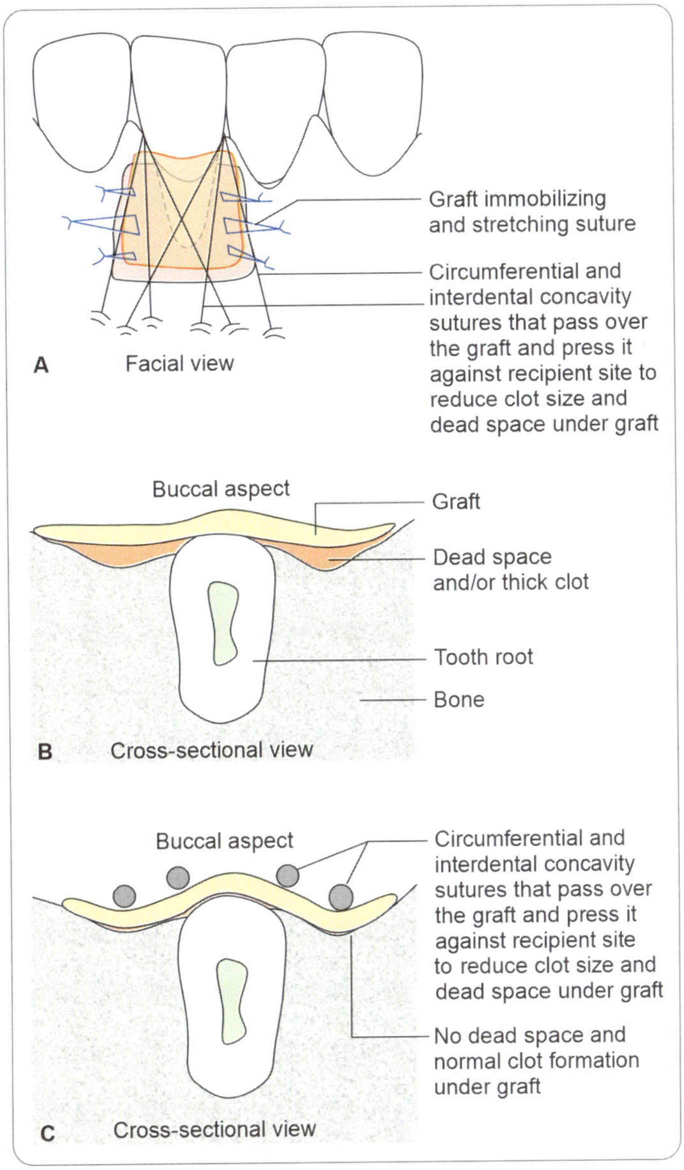

Fig. 19.10: Suturing technique for preventing dead space formation under free soft tissue grafts (*Holbrook and Ochsenbein technique*)

Step 4—A vertical incision (*3rd incision*) is started from the point where the horizontal incision ended. It is extended vertically, up to the muco-gingival junction at the boundary of the donor site almost parallel to the 1st incision **(Fig. 19.11, diag. B, green dashed arrow)**.

Step 5—If required, a small releasing incision (*4th incision*) is made at the end of this vertical incision **(Fig. 19.11, B, black dashed arrow)**.

Step 6—Sharp dissection is now carried out from the vertical incision (*3rd incision*) to the 'V' incision (*1st incision*) to raise a partial thickness flap **(Fig. 19.11, diag. C)**. As a general rule, the donor flap must be almost double the width of the recipient site and at least 3–4 times longer than its width. Its base (*apical end*) should be wider than its top (*coronal end*).

◂ *What must be the dimensions of the pedicle flap/graft in relation to the root surface to be covered?*

Step 7—The flap is now pulled coronally and laterally and sutured at the ***level*** of the adjacent interdental papillae with 5–0 suture thread using interrupted sutures **(Fig. 19.11, diag. D green arrow)**. A sling suture (*around the tooth*) may be required to pull the flap coronally and keep it in place. Aluminium foil is placed on the wound and it is then covered with periodontal pack for one week.

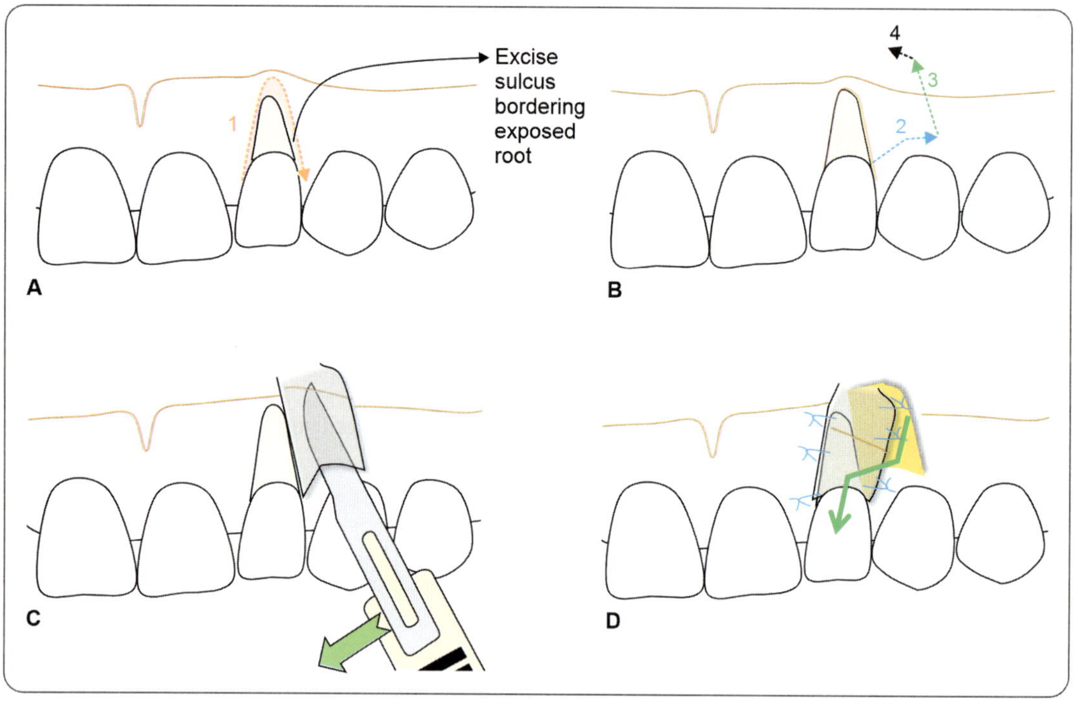

Fig. 19.11: Laterally sliding pedicle graft

CLINICAL UTILITY AND SHORT ANSWER

What is the difference between a free graft (*gingival/connective*) and a pedicle graft?

- Pedicle grafts are those grafts that remain physically connected (*in part*) to the donor site after placement at the recipient site. Pedicle grafts ***retain*** their blood supply through this connection.
- On the other hand, a free graft (*free gingival/connective tissue graft*) is one that after being harvested and placed at the donor site retains ***no*** physical connection with the site from where it was harvested (*donor site*).

ALERT!

How is the exposed root surface biomodified to improve chances of root coverage? ▸

- To increase chances of root coverage, some clinicians chemically prepare (*bio-modify*) the exposed root (*area of root recession*) after root planing but just prior root coverage surgery. Biomodification of root surfaces causes surface demineralization, detoxification and exposes root collagen fibers for initial linkage with the graft tissue's collagen.
- Root surfaces can be biomodified (*chemically prepared*) with super saturated solution of citric acid at pH 1.0, tetracycline hydrochloride, EDTA, etc. Either of these can be applied on the exposed root surface with a cotton pledget for 1–5 minutes.

III. *Root Coverage using a Coronally Displaced Flap*

If adequate amount of attached gingiva is present, gingiva can be displaced coronally to cover root recession using the coronally displaced flap technique for root coverage (Fig. 19.12).

How must the vertical incisions for coronally displaced flap designed? ▸

Step 1—After root planing, two ***parallel*** or ***slightly divergent*** vertical incisions (*1st incisions*) are made from gingival margin on mesial and distal sides of the exposed root beyond the muco-gingival junction (*into the alveolar mucosa*). Incisions are designed in such a way that they ***exclude*** interdental papillae on both sides of the recession defect.

Step 2—A horizontal internal bevel incision (*2nd incision*) that extends from vertical incision on the mesial side to the vertical incision on the distal side and from the crest of gingiva to the base of the sulcus at the apical most extent of the recession defect is made. This initiates a ***partial thickness flap***.

Step 3—Partial thickness flap is raised 3 mm beyond the apical most extent of the recession defect; after this the partial thickness flap is ***converted*** into a ***full thickness flap*** and flap is then raised ***apical to the muco-gingival junction***.

Step 4—Flap is pulled coronally and sutured at the level of gingival crests of neighbouring teeth. Flap is secured in its coronally advanced position by suturing first in the region of the interdental papillae. Vertical releasing incisions are sutured afterwards. Periodontal pack is placed. Sutures are removed after 7–10 days.

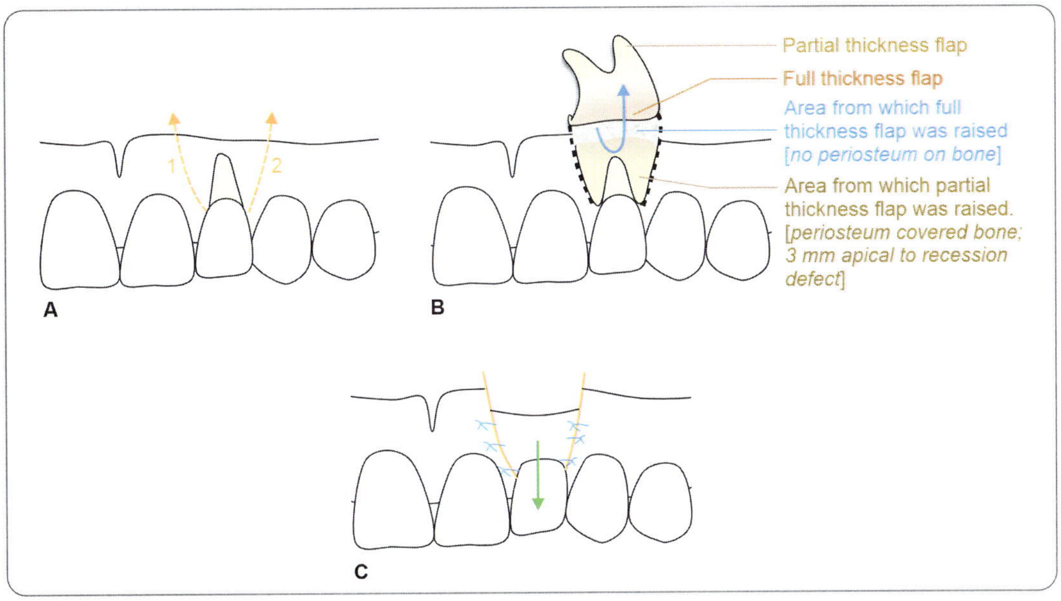

Fig. 19.12: Coronally displaced flap

ALERT!

Peak theory: We cannot increase height of gingival margin coronal to the height of marginal gingiva of adjacent teeth.

◂ *What is the peak theory?*

PREVENTION OF LOSS OF HEIGHT AND RECONSTRUCTION OF INTERDENTAL PAPILLAE

The interdental space is occupied by interdental papilla. If interdental space is not completely filled by it, a very unattractive 'black triangle' is seen between teeth.

◂ *How far can the papilla grow coronal to the alveolar bone?*

Etiology of empty interdental spaces and loss of height of interdental papilla:

1. **Open interdental contact:** Interdental papilla can grow only up to 5 mm coronal to interdental bone crest ***only if*** a tight interdental contact is present between two adjacent teeth. If interdental contact is not present the interdental papilla will ***not*** form rather interdental gingiva will curve 2 mm over the underlying alveolar bone.
2. **Periodontitis:** If loss of bone height is more than 5 mm, in such cases interdental space will remain partially empty even if the teeth have tight contacts.
3. **Aggressive flossing that causes continuous injury to the interdental papilla.**
4. **Iatrogenic causes:** Placing vertical incisions through or cutting of interdental papilla for raising flaps, etc. can lead loss of height of the interdental papilla.

◂ *If there no interdental contact what will be the shape of interdental papilla?*

◂ *If good interdental contact is present but more than 5 mm bone has been lost due to periodontitis, how far can the papilla grow coronal to the alveolar bone?*

Reconstruction of Interdental Papilla

Regeneration of interdental papillae is only attempted in the ***anterior/aesthetic*** region. One of the most successful ways of increasing papillary volume is placing sub-epithelial connective tissue grafts under the connective tissue of papilla (*Han and Takei 1996*) (Fig. 19.13).

◂ *In which areas is reconstruction of the papilla attempted?*

FRENECTOMY AND FRENULOTOMY

Frenectomy: Excision (*removal*) of frenum and its attachment to the underlying bone is called frenectomy.

Frenulotomy (*frenotomy*): Incision of the frenum to separate it from its attachment to the alveolar bone is called frenulotomy.

◂ *What is the difference between frenectomy and frenulotomy?*

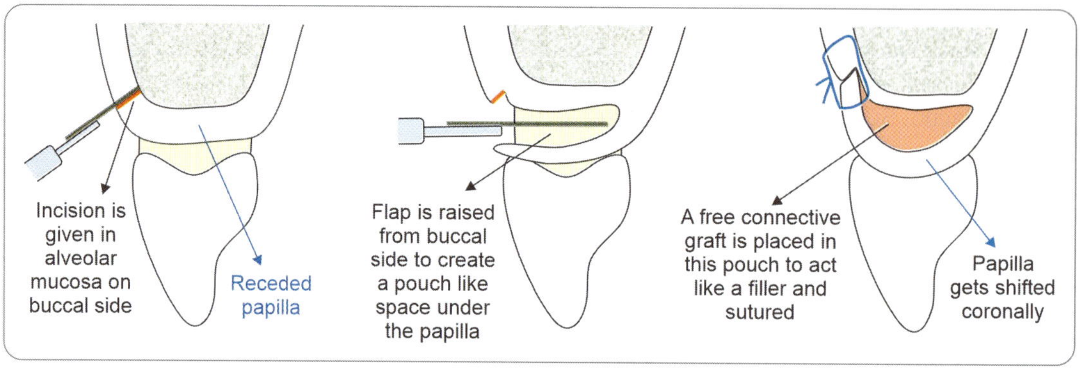

Fig. 19.13: Semilunar coronally repositioned papilla technique (*Han and Takei 1996*)

Both these procedures are performed if the high frenal attachment causes narrowing of attached gingiva, midline diastema between anterior teeth, etc.

Frenectomy

Step 1—After anesthesia, lip is stretched to extend the frenum. The extended frenum is grasped in a hemostat that is inserted up to depth of the vestibule.

How is the rhomboidal wound formed during frenectomy? ▶

Step 2—Using a # 15 BP blade, incisions are made along the upper and lower surface of the hemostat (*along frenal attachment to the lip and gingiva*) and the frenum grasped in the hemostat is removed. This makes a rhomboidal wound (*made by combination of triangular wound on the gingiva and triangular wound on the lip*).

Step 3—Fibrous attachment of the frenum to the bone is now removed by incising and blunt dissection.

Step 4—The wound in the lip is sutured while gingival wound is covered with periodontal pack. Periodontal pack prevents reunion/reformation of the frenum by acting like a separating medium between wound on the lip and gingiva.

Frenulotomy

How is the triangular wound formed during frenulotomy? ▶

Step 1—In frenulotomy only the frenum's attachment on gingiva is incised, i.e. the frenum is released only from its attachment to the gingiva. This makes a triangular wound on the gingiva.

Why is the triangular frenulotomy injured to produce scarring? ▶

Step 2—Then periosteum at the base of the frenum (*wound in area where frenum has been incised*) is injured (*scored*) with a knife (*this will cause scarring during healing that will prevent regrowth of frenum to original level*). Muscle fibers and tissue tags are removed.

Step 3—Wound margins on the lip (*at the edge of the gingival wound*) are sutured at the depth of the vestibule. Periodontal pack is applied for one to two weeks to prevent reunion of the frenum to the gingiva.

CROWN LENGTHENING

What is crown lengthening? ▶

What are the indications for crown lengthening? ▶

Increasing the length of clinical crown of a tooth surgically by either removing gingiva or both gingiva and alveolar bone together is called crown lengthening. It is done to:

1. Lengthen clinical crowns of anterior teeth for aesthetic reasons (Fig. 19.15).
2. Expose additional tooth structure to provide retention for restorative crowns.
   - At least 5 mm height of tooth structure coronal to base of sulcus (*clinical crown of tooth*) is required for adequate retention of cemented restorative crowns.
   - In case less than 5 mm tooth structure (*clinical crown*) is available, more tooth structure needs to be exposed. However, to increase available length of clinical crown, tooth preparation (*cutting*) cannot be extended apical to base of sulcus as doing this will cause breach of biologic width (*distance between crest of alveolar bone and base of gingival sulcus, it is occupied gingival connective tissue and JE*) (*see Chapter 7, 'Dental Calculus and Other Factors Contributing to Periodontal Disease' pages 95 and 96 and Figs 7.10 and 7.12*).

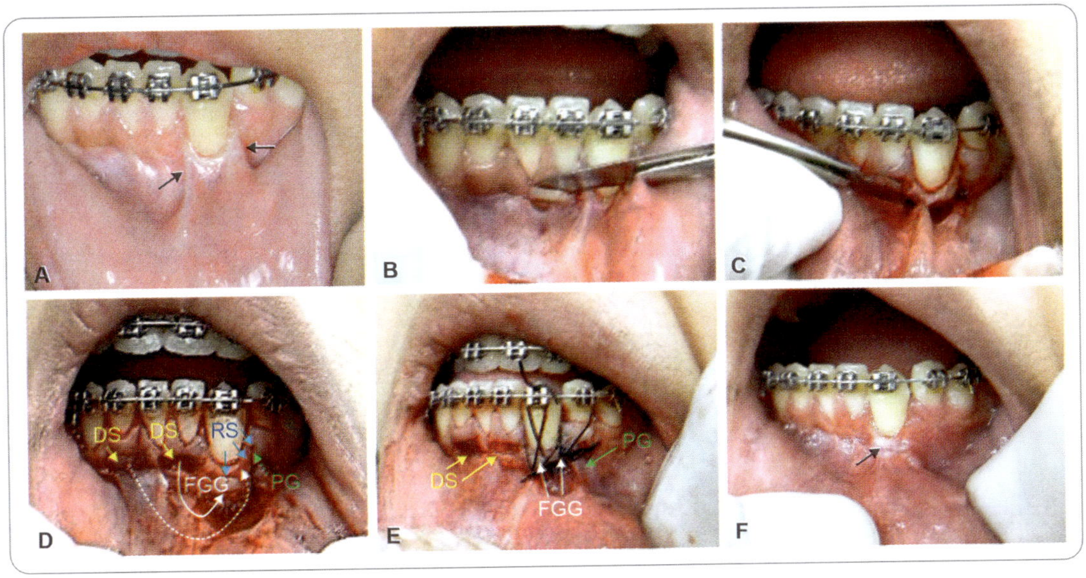

Fig. 19.14: MG surgery for increasing width of attached gingiva and correction of aberrant frenula with free gingival graft strips and pedicle graft. Diag. A: preoperative view showing high frenal attachments (*diag. A black arrows*) and inadequate attached gingiva on buccal aspect of left mandibular canine. Diags B and C: show harvesting of free gingival graft strip from adjoining attached gingiva (*diag. B*) and frenulotomy (*diag. C*). Diag. D: shows donor (*diag. D, DS, yellow arrows*) and recipient sites (*diag. D, RS, blue arrows*), one transplanted free gingival graft (*diag. D, FGG, white arrow*), plan of transfer of second free gingival graft strip (*diag. D, white dashed arrow*) and plan of transfer of pedicle graft (PG) at site of frenal attachment (*diag. D, green dashed arrow*). Diag. E: shows placement of transplanted free gingival grafts (*diag. E, FGG, white arrows and pedicle graft, PG, green arrow*) and graft holding sutures. Diag. F: shows healing of recipient and donor sites after six weeks; note that both free gingival grafts and lateral pedicle graft have united to the recipient bed and frenula have been successfully displaced apically but attached gingiva is still not adequate (*diag. F, blanching of gingiva on buccal aspect of canine, black arrow*), if attached gingiva remains inadequate after allowing graft to mature, a second stage MG surgery to further increase zone of attached gingiva will be needed.

How Crown Lengthening is Done

(see also, Chapter 21, 'Interdisciplinary Interrelationships and Supportive Periodontal Therapy', section on crown lengthening for prosthetic or restorative reasons, page 367, and diag. 21.6)

1. *Gingivectomy (Gingivoplasty) and/or Ostectomy*

◂ *How is crown lengthening done?*

This is one of the most commonly performed treatments for crown lengthening especially for posterior teeth (*also see Chapter 17A, 'Curettage, Gingivectomy and Gingivoplasty', section on prerequisites and contraindications of gingivectomy, page 297*). Crown lengthening for aesthetic reasons is done in anterior teeth in cases of 'gummy' smiles caused by gingival overgrowth and defective passive eruption (*when gingiva of anterior teeth has not receded naturally after eruption of the tooth*). In such cases, gingivectomy exposes additional tooth structure and makes the smile more attractive (Fig. 19.15). Gingivectomy is done ***only if*** an adequate zone of attached gingiva is present.

◂ *When is gingivectomy done for crown lengthening?*

2. *By Apically Displaced Flap*

A full thickness flap is raised and sutured at a more apical level to expose the required amount of tooth structure. If needed, crestal bone is also removed (Fig. 19.15). Apically displaced flap can be done even if an adequate zone of attached gingiva is ***not*** present.

◂ *What is the main advantage of apically displaced flap when it is used for crown lengthening?*

3. *Forced Eruption with Fiber Resection*

This procedure is done to expose fractured tooth roots for restoration with crowns. The fractured tooth's root is moved out of the socket using orthodontic force after incising alveolar crest and horizontal fibers of the periodontal ligament. Alveolar crest and horizontal

Why are alveolar crest and horizontal fibers incised during forced tooth eruption? ▶

fibers of the periodontal ligament are incised every week till completion of forced eruption because if this is not done, the crest of the alveolar bone will move coronally along with the tooth root. Forced eruption usually takes around 2–3 weeks to expose adequate amount of root (*tooth structure*) for placement of restorative crown.

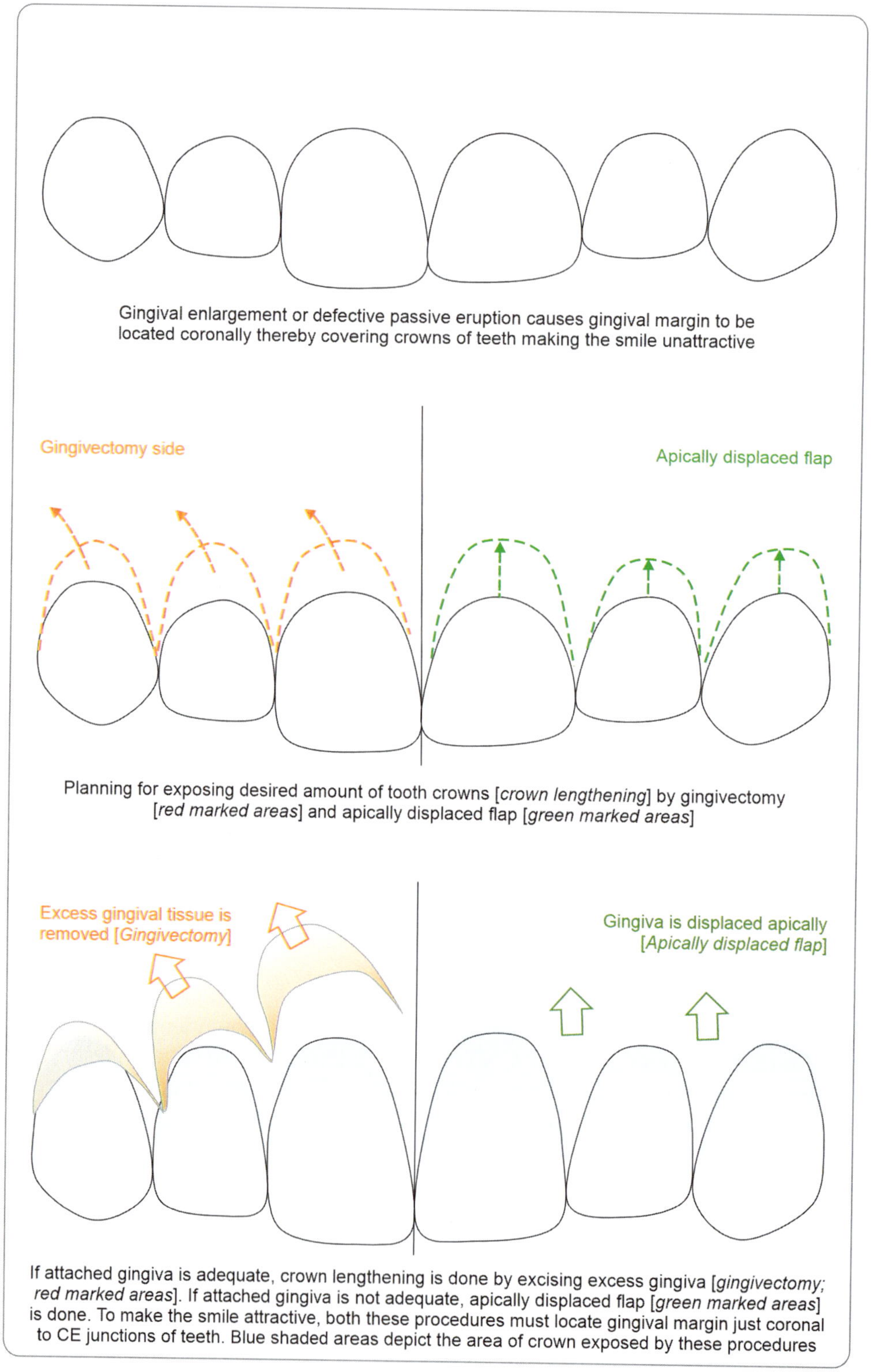

Fig. 19.15: Crown lengthening by gingivectomy (*left side*) or apically displaced flap surgery (*right side*) can make smiles more aesthetic. Diag. A shows line diagram of gummy smile. Diag. B shows planned gingivectomy (*red arrows and markings*) and apically displaced flap (*green arrows and markings*). Diag. C shows increase in length of clinical crowns (*blue marked areas*) after surgery; note change in aesthetics on the same line diagram of teeth when gingiva is drawn apically (*diag. A vs. diag C*).

DEPIGMENTATION (*REDUCTION OF BROWN COLOUR OF BUCCAL GINGIVA IN THE AESTHETIC ZONE*)

Although pigmentation of free and attached gingiva is a normal occurrence, however, in some cases the gingiva can be very darkly pigmented (Fig. 19.16, diag. A). Many individuals do not prefer such dark colour of the gingiva and seek correction of colour of the gingiva. It is important to remember that:

- For depigmentation of gingiva, entire gingival epithelium and part of the connective tissue under the epithelium have to be removed (*cells causing pigmentation, i.e. melanocytes and melanophages are present in the basal layer of the epithelium, see pages 15 and 16*).
- Pigmentation tends to ***recur*** after a few months of depigmentation surgery.

◂ *Why must gingival connective tissue be removed for depigmentation?*

Procedure for depigmenting gingiva

◂ *How is gingival depigmentation done?*

◂ *Which parts of the gingiva are worked on for depigmentation?*

1. **Scalpel method:** One of the most commonly used methods for depigmentation of gingiva is de-epithelization of gingiva (*keratinized gingiva, i.e. free gingiva + attached gingiva*) by gingival scrapping using a Kirkland's knife (*as is done in gingivectomy or gingivoplasty procedure*) (Fig. 19.16, diag. B) (*also see Chapter 17A, 'Curettage, Gingivectomy and Gingivoplasty', pages 297 to 301, section on procedure of gingivectomy*). After complete de-epithelization of gingiva, gingival wound is covered with a periodontal pack for about two weeks by which time gingiva will heal by secondary intention (Fig. 19.16, diag. C).
2. **Lasers:** Depigmentation can also be done using diode lasers.

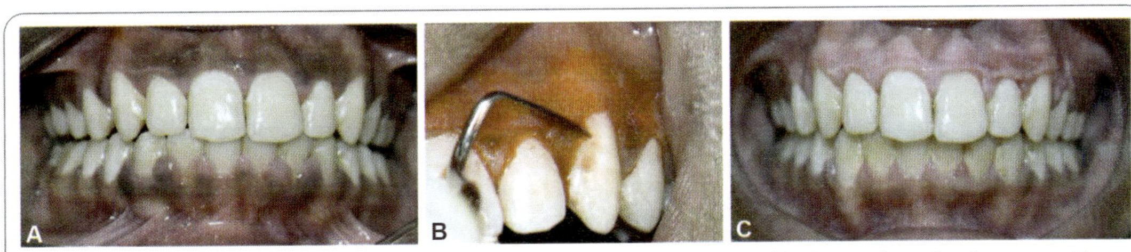

A Pre-operative view [*upper arch*] B Gingival scrapping C Post-operative view [*upper arch*]

Fig. 19.16: Gingival depigmentation using the gingival scrapping method with scalpel

REVIEW QUESTIONS

1. What are mucogingival complications/conditions? List the goals of mucogingival therapy.
2. How can width of attached gingiva be increased?
3. What is the difference between a free graft and a pedicle graft?
4. Write the procedure of performing a free gingival graft procedure. Discuss factors that can cause failure of free grafts.
5. What is free connective tissue graft? What are the advantages and dis-advantages of a connective tissue graft over a free gingival graft?
6. What is gingival recession? What are its causes?
7. Classify gingival recession. How does the type of defect affect the success of root coverage?
8. How can gingival recession be treated? Discuss root coverage using a free gingival graft.
9. Discuss root coverage using a free connective tissue graft.
10. What is pedicle or laterally sliding flap? Write technique of root coverage using laterally sliding pedicle graft.
11. Write the technique of root coverage with coronally displaced flap.
12. Write the differences between frenectomy and frenulotomy (*frenotomy*). Write the procedure for performing frenectomy and frenulotomy (*frenotomy*).
13. What is crown lengthening? How can it be done?
14. How can colour of heavily pigmented gingiva be surgically corrected?

Chapter

20

Furcation Involvement and its Management

What is bifurcation and trifurcation? ▸

A furcation is that area of multirooted teeth where roots of a tooth branch from the root trunk. If two roots arise from the root trunk, the furcation is called a bifurcation **(Fig. 20.1, diag. A)**. However, if there are three roots, the furcation is called a trifurcation **(Fig. 20.1, diag. B)**. Furcations of teeth are normally covered by periodontium.

What is etiological significance of furcations? ▸

As furcations of teeth have complex anatomy, they are ***difficult*** to clean; maintaining them in a disease-free state therefore remains a challenge for the patient. If periodontitis is present in the furcation area, many unique challenges related to diagnosis, assess, visibility and instrumentation of the area complicate its treatment.

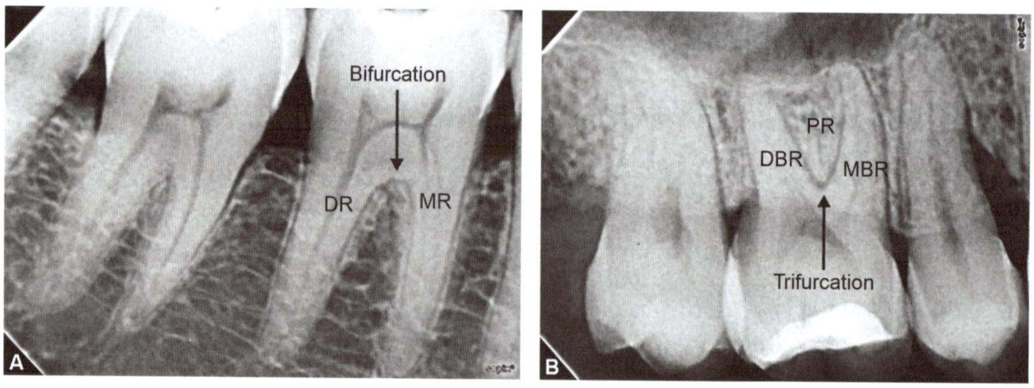

Fig. 20.1: Bifurcation made by mesial and distal roots in mandibular molars (*diag. A, MR and DR*) and trifurcation is made by distobuccal, palatal and mesiobuccal roots in maxillary molars (*diag. B, DBR, PR and MBR*)

CLINICAL UTILITY AND SHORT ANSWER

Describe the terms used in reference to furcation involvement.

Root trunk length: Distance from CE junction to furcation entrance of the tooth.

Furcation entrance: Point of entry to furcation.

Fornix: Roof of furcation.

Angle/degree of Separation: Angle between two roots in a multirooted tooth.

Coefficient of Separation: Length of root apical to furcation divided by distance from CE junction to the root tip.

DIAGNOSIS OF FURCATION INVOLVEMENT

What is furcation involvement? ▸

Furcation involvement is an event in advancing periodontitis. When furcation of a multirooted tooth gets involved with ongoing periodontitis, a diagnosis of furcation involvement is made. Furcation involvement can be diagnosed by:

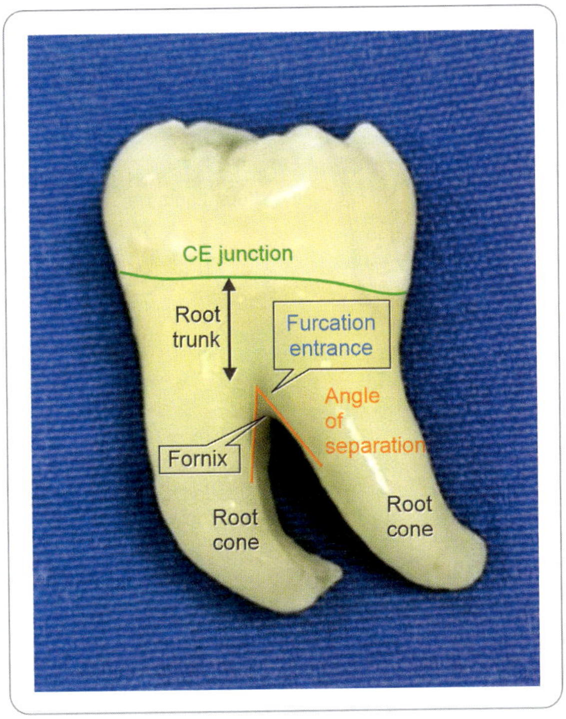

Fig. 20.2: Furcation landmarks and terminology

1. **Clinical oral examination:** Probing with straight and curved periodontal probes (*Naber's probe*) **(Fig. 20.3)**.
2. **Radiographic examination:** IOPA radiographs are best suited for this purpose **(Fig. 20.4)**. CBCT can also be used. OPGs are of little use as they do not provide necessary detail to make a good diagnosis.

◂ *How is furcation involvement diagnosed?*

ALERT!

Diagnosis of furcation involvement can be difficult and challenging.

Furcation involvement is difficult to detect because:

1. It is not be readily visible (*grade I, II and III*) due to presence of gingiva over the furcation.
2. Furcations may not show clearly in IOPA, Bitewing or OPG radiographs:
   - Grade I furcations may not show at all (*due to very minor bone loss*).
   - Radiographic image of grade II furcation may be superimposed by image of one of the two remaining bone plates or root of the tooth.
   - Radiographic image of furcation may be superimposed by image of one of the tooth's root, e.g. palatal root of maxillary molars. In such cases, a zone of fuzziness in the furcation area especially if it is accompanied by loss of bone height on the adjoining roots of the tooth, is suggestive of furcation involvement.
   - ***No radiographic image*** can be seen in cases of furcation involvement of ***maxillary premolars*** as image of their buccal and palatal roots superimpose the image of their furcation area.
   - Grade III and grade IV furcation involvement in ***mandibular molars appear most clearly*** in radiographs.
   - All furcations may be clearly seen in a CBCT scan.
3. Gingiva covering the furcation (*grade I, II and III*) also acts like an obstruction to insertion of probe; this makes diagnosis difficult.
4. Tortuous anatomy of osseous defects, narrow root divergence angles (*closely placed roots*), ridges in fornix area of furcation make insertion of probes into the depth of the furcation defect difficult. This may limit ability of making diagnosis and determination of the actual severity of furcation involvement.

◂ *Which furcations cannot be readily identified in radiographs?*

◂ *Which furcations cannot be seen at all radiographs?*

◂ *Which furcations cannot be seen most clearly in a radiograph?*

CLASSIFICATION OF FURCATION INVOLVEMENT

Glickman's classification **(1953)** is one of the most widely used and simplest classifications. It classifies furcation involvement into four grades:

◂ *Classify furcation involvement.*

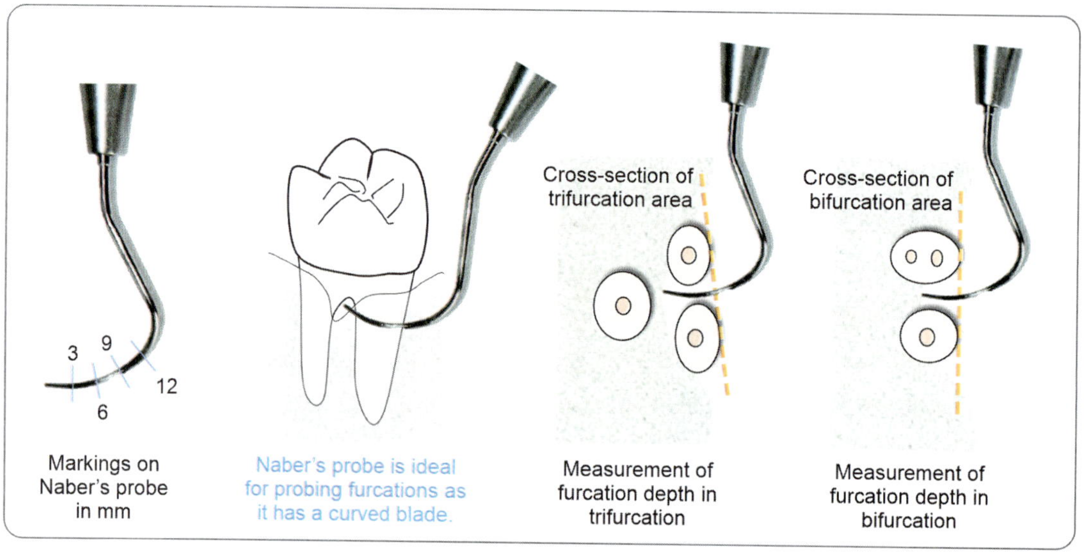

Fig. 20.3: Naber's probe is used for probing furcations

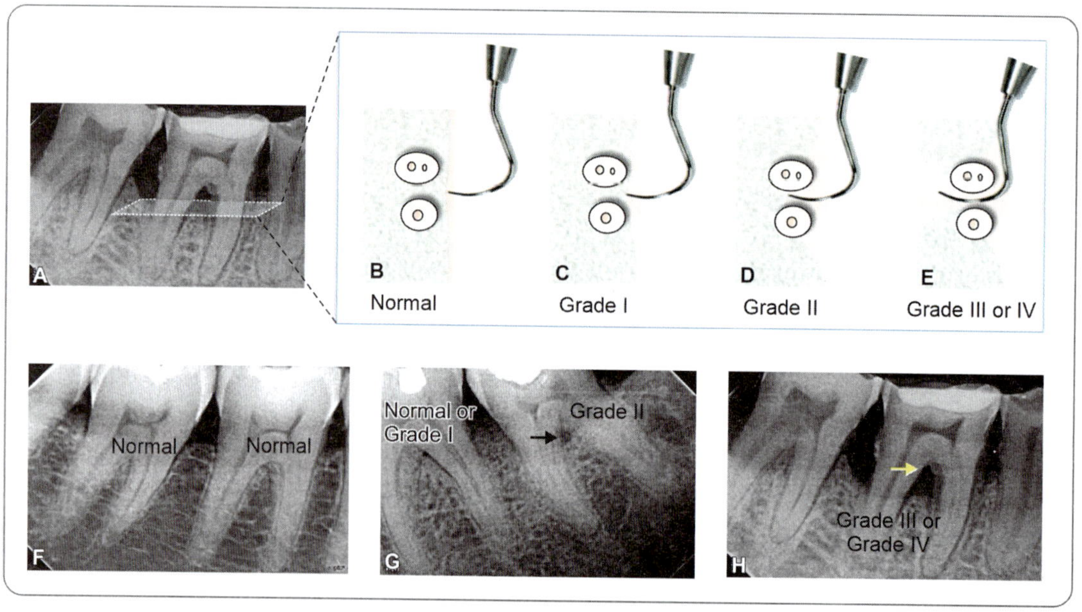

Fig. 20.4: Grading and radiographic diagnosis of furcation involvement. Slight fuzziness in furcation area of a tooth is indicative of grade II furcation involvement (*diag. G*). Grade III and IV furcation involvements look similar radiographically (*diag. H*); clinical examination is required to distinguish between the two. If furcation is not covered by gingiva such furcation is grade III, if it is exposed, furcation is grade IV.

How does a grade I furcation involvement appear on a radiograph? ▶

Grade I: There is only a minor periodontal defect in the furcation area and periodontal loss is usually ***restricted*** to the soft tissues. Bone defects if present, are suprabony and not easily detectable. ***No*** radiographic changes are present (Fig. 20.4, diags C and G).

How does a grade II furcation involvement appear on a radiograph? ▶

Grade II: Bone loss extends into the furcation up to a variable distance from one side but it does ***not*** cross to the other side of the tooth (Fig. 20.4, diags D and G). If more than one grade II furcation defects arising from different surfaces of the same tooth are present, they do not communicate with each other. Horizontal or vertical bone loss may be present.

Radiographic changes may or may not be there and they usually appear as slight fuzziness or radiolucency in the furcation area (Fig. 20.4, diag. G).

How does a grade III and IV furcation involvement appear on a radiograph? ▶

Grade III: Bone loss extends from one side of the tooth furcation to the other, i.e. there is a through-and-through bone loss that allows passage of a periodontal probe from one side to the other side (Fig. 20.4, diags E and H). However, the furcation area is covered by gingiva and is not exposed. Such defects are visible in radiographs as radiolucent areas (Fig. 20.4, diag. H).

Grade IV: These are similar to grade III furcation defects but here the furcation defects are ***exposed***, i.e. not covered by gingiva (*gingiva over furcation is receded and furcation is visible*). They appear as radiolucent areas in radiographs (Fig. 20.4, diags E and H).

◂ *What is the difference between grade III and IV furcation involvement*

ETIOLOGY OF FURCATION INVOLVEMENT

Etiopathogenesis of furcation involvement is the ***same*** as that of periodontitis (*because it is a progressive event in ongoing periodontitis*) (*see Chapter 10, 'Plaque Induced Gingivitis and Periodontitis', page 135*). Some ***additional*** factors that may contribute furcation involvement are:

◂ *What is the cause of furcation involvement?*

1. Tooth fractures in the furcation area.
2. Iatrogenic causes, e.g. perforation of the pulpal floor during RCT treatment, overhanging restorations, etc.
3. Trauma from occlusion.

CLINICAL UTILITY AND SHORT ANSWER

Which factors can affect the outcome of treatment of furcation defects (*furcation involvement*)?

1. **Soft tissue (*gingival*) anatomy:** Presence of adequate zone of attached gingiva improves prognosis and reduces rate of spread/worsening of periodontitis in the furcation.
2. **Position of tooth in the arch:** If a multirooted tooth is placed outside the arch, it increases chances of gingival recession. Such teeth are predisposed to early furcation involvement if periodontitis is present in the region (*more commonly seen on buccal side of maxillary and mandibular molars*).
3. **Root Trunk Length:** Multirooted teeth with shorter root trunks have greater chances of getting get furcation involvement early. However, when such teeth do have furcation involvement, its management is easier (*due to easier assess than when compared to that of teeth with longer root trunks where assess to the furcation can be very difficult*).
4. **Number of roots and angle of separation between two roots of a furcation:** Greater number of roots (*e.g. 3 versus 2*) in a multirooted tooth reduces angle of separation between the roots, i.e. roots are more closely placed. This makes diagnosis, instrument insertion and treatment difficult due to reduced assess. Prognosis of such teeth is relatively ***poorer***.
5. **Anatomy of furcation's fornix area:** Furcation area of the tooth may have ridges, concavities or other defects on the tooth surface that can further restrict access and make treatment more difficult. Accessory pulpal canals opening in the furcation area can channelize products of inflammation and infection from the infected pulp of the tooth into the furcation and cause periodontal destruction. Enamel projections into the furcation areas can be present. These features make the fornix area more prone to periodontitis.

◂ *How does the length of root trunk affect treatment of furcations?*

◂ *How does number of roots affect treatment of furcations?*

◂ *Which anatomical features in the fornix area of the furcation can contribute to periodontitis?*

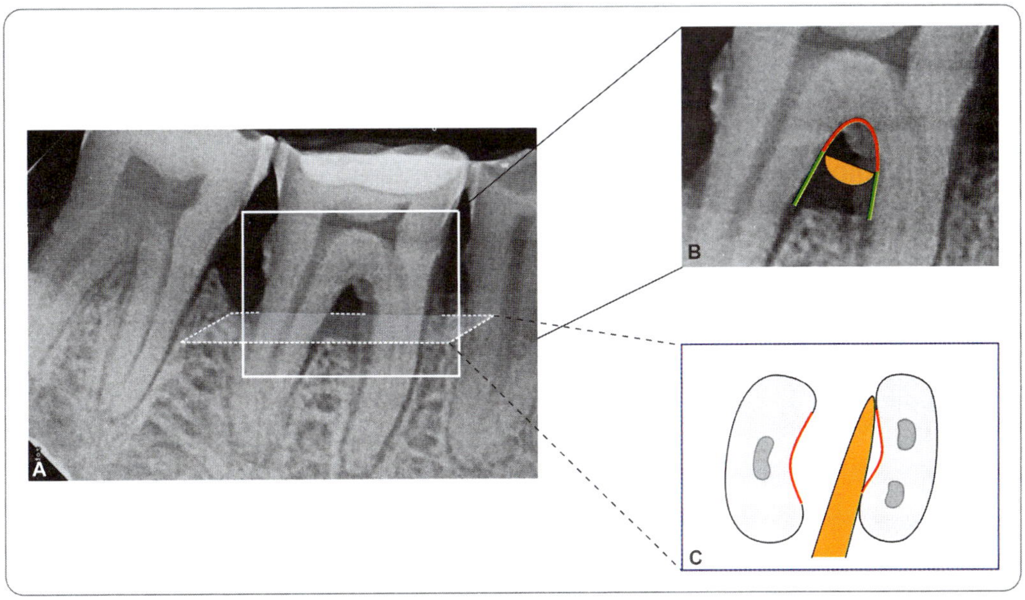

Fig. 20.5: Narrow furcations (*small angle of separation between roots*) restrict access into the furcation making it is difficult or even impossible to insert a scaler or curette for scaling and root planing (*diag. B, red marked area; orange half circle: curette cross section*). Some roots making a furcation have concave surfaces (*diag. C, red marked area on cross section of roots; orange area: cross section of scaler*) which are also difficult to scale and root plane.

ALERT!

81% of furcations are classified as narrow because they are less than 1 mm wide. As blades of most scalers and curettes are wider than 1 mm, these cannot be inserted into such furcations with narrow entrances. This makes scaling and root planing these areas difficult or even impossible.

TREATMENT OF FURCATION DEFECTS

How is furcation involvement treated? ▸

It includes SRP and surgery for reducing or eliminating pockets (*flap surgery or gingivectomy*) and making the furcation easily cleansable for easy plaque control by the patient.

1. Grade I furcations have no identifiable bone loss in the furcation area but have a pocket coronal to the furcation area of the tooth. They are treated by scaling and root planing, gingivectomy or flap surgery as indicated.

How are grade II furcations treated? ▸

2. Grade II furcations are also treated the same way as Grade I furcations. Because grade II furcations have bone loss, guided tissue regeneration (*GTR*) may be required (*see Chapter 18, Resective and Regenerative Bone Surgery for Periodontal Bone Defects; page 330 and Fig. 18.10*). If bone loss is extensive, a Grade II furcation can be converted to a Grade IV furcation by sacrificing some interradicular bone and exposing the furcation by removing gingiva covering the furcation (*tunnel preparation*).

Why are grade III converted to grade IV furcations? ▸

3. All grade III furcations are first managed by SRP. Flap surgery and GTR may be attempted. If GTR is not done or is not successful, gingivectomy is done to convert a grade III furcation into grade IV furcation (*expose the furcation area for easy cleaning by patient*) and then maintained as such. If all this is not successful, root amputation or hemisectioning may be done or the tooth may be extracted.
4. Grade IV furcations are managed like grade III furcations.

CLINICAL UTILITY AND SHORT ANSWER

What is 'tunnel preparation'?

Tunnel preparation can ***only*** be done ***in mandibular molars*** with ***widely separated*** roots and with short root trunks. Teeth with wide pulp chambers are ***not*** good candidates for this. Tunnel preparation is done as under:

1. Buccal and lingual flaps are raised.
2. Interradicular bone, i.e. bone in the furcation between two roots of a mandibular molar is removed to gain access to the other side (*access from buccal to lingual side*).
3. Flaps are then sutured in such a way that the furcation is left exposed.
4. After healing, tunnel preparation results in an exposed furcation that allows easy access from buccal to the lingual side thereby permitting easy cleanability.

How does a tooth benefit from tunnel preparation? ▸

Tooth Hemisection, Root Resection and Bicuspidization

Hemisection

In which teeth is tooth hemisection possible? ▸

- Hemisection (*splitting a tooth into two*) is done on ***mandibular*** molars and in cases where severe bone loss (*due to periodontitis*) is present in relation to ***only one*** of the roots of the mandibular molars.
- Hemisection is done only ***after*** successful endodontic treatment (*RCT*).

What is tooth hemisection? ▸

- The mandibular molar is cut labio-lingually, in the centre, into two halves.
- The tooth half with the untreatable root is extracted while the other is covered with a restorative crown shaped like a premolar.

Bicuspidization

In which teeth is bicuspidization done? ▸

- Some ***mandibular molars with furcation involvement*** have poor prognosis because both their mesial and distal roots are moderately diseased (*bone loss*) and furcation area ***cannot*** be treated in the conventional way (*as discussed above*).

What is tooth bicuspidization? ▸

- In such cases, the tooth is cut into two labio-lingually to ***eliminate*** the furcation and both tooth halves are retained, i.e. a molar tooth with furcation is converted into two small teeth almost of the size of premolars (*furcation is eliminated; this improves the prognosis*).

- Each of these tooth halves is then covered with a restorative crown of the shape of a premolar. This is called bicuspidization.

Root Resection

- Root resection is done on ***maxillary*** molars ***only*** if one of the two ***mesiobuccal*** or ***distobuccal*** root has severe bone loss due to periodontitis while the other two roots have good bone support (*palatal root cannot be resected as such a tooth will not be left with enough periodontal support*).
- Root resection is done only ***after*** successful endodontic treatment (*RCT*).
- The root with severe bone loss is cut (*amputated*) and extracted.
- The rest of the tooth with two remaining roots (*palatal and either mesiobuccal or distobuccal*) is retained as a maxillary molar after covering it with a restorative crown with a smaller occlusal table.

◂ *In which teeth is root resection possible?*

◂ *Which treatment must be done before root resection?*

◂ *Which modification is done in restorative crown of a tooth with resected root?*

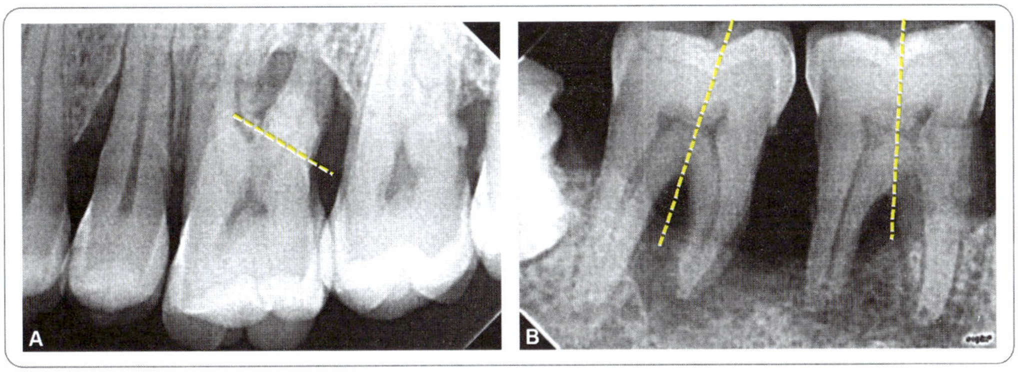

Fig. 20.6: Planned root resection (*diag. A*) and hemisection (*diag. B*). Root resection and hemisection are to be done after endodontic treatment (*RCT*).

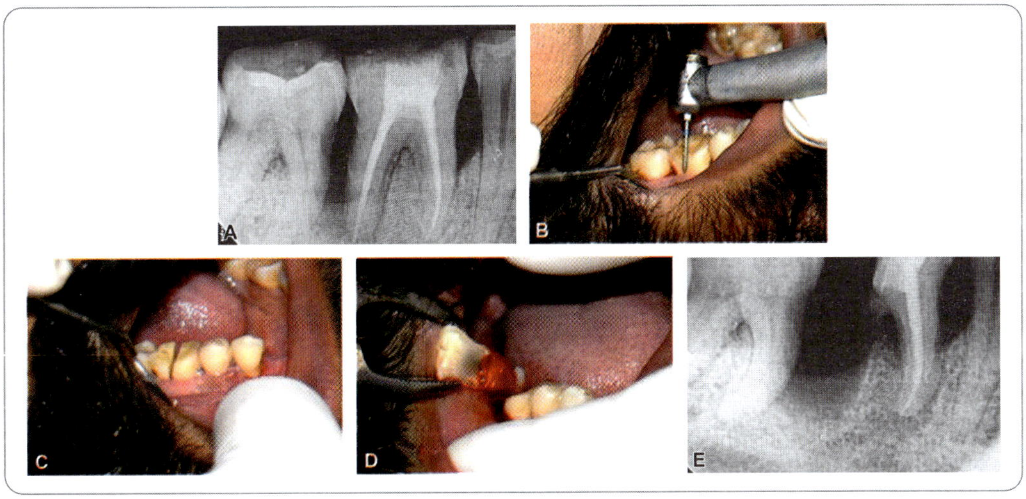

Fig. 20.7: Clinical steps for performing hemisection. Diag. A: Preoperative radiograph after endodontic treatment; Diags B and C: Tooth is cut into two mesial and distal pieces; Diag. D: Distal fragment is extracted and Diag. E: Postoperative radiograph.

CLINICAL UTILITY AND SHORT ANSWER

How does a diseased pulp contribute to furcation involvement?

Infection from the pulp chamber can reach the furcation and result in bone loss in the following ways:

- Pulpal infection can extend into the furcation area through accessory canals (*from the pulp*) opening into the furcation area (*endo–perio complication*).
- Perforation of floor of pulp chamber during endodontic treatment or insertion of retentive posts, etc. can result in furcation involvement.
- Tooth fractures lines passing through the furcations of multirooted teeth can lead to persistent furcation involvement.

◂ *How can infection from pulp chamber and root canals reach furcation area and cause bone loss?*

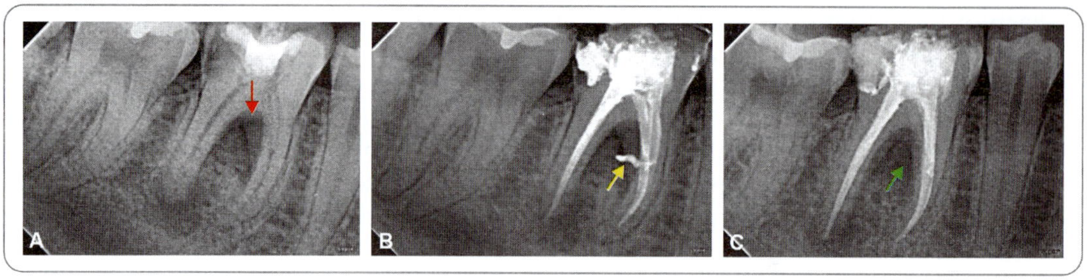

Fig. 20.8: Furcation involvement caused by pulpal infection (*diag. A, red arrow*). Accessory canals are not readily visible in routine radiographs. They are however, easily visualized after endodontic sealants are forced flowed into these during obturation. In diag. B (*yellow arow*), accessory canal in the mesial root of mandibular first molar that is responsible for furcation involvement is seen clearly (*yellow arow*). Note resolution of furcation involvement and improvement periapical bone resorption around distal root after five weeks of endodontic treatment. Endodontic sealer that had flowed out has also resorbed (*diag. C, green arrow*)

Review Questions

1. What is a furcation? Are they present in all teeth? What is furcation involvement?
2. What are the etiological, predisposing and contributing factors for furcation involvement?
3. How can furcation involvement (*defects*) be diagnosed?
4. What is root trunk length, furcation entrance, degree of separation and co-efficient of separation of a furcation?
5. Classify furcation involvement.
6. Name the factors that have an effect on management and prognosis of furcation defects. How can furcation defects be managed?
7. What is the difference between management of grade III and IV furcation defects?
8. What is tunnel preparation?
9. What is tooth hemisection, bicuspidization and root resection (*amputation*)? What are the indications and preconditions for doing these procedures?
10. Describe the procedure of performing hemisection and root resection.

Chapter

21

Interdisciplinary Interrelationships and Supportive Periodontal Therapy

It is important to understand that all dental specialties are interconnected and periodontal health is an important common denominator for success of dental treatment involving all other specialties of dentistry. Teeth having poor periodontal health are not good candidates for other dental treatments till their periodontal health improves (*e.g. are not fit to act as abutments for bridge work, etc.*). Clinicians must ensure that dental treatments are done in such a way that they do not increase the risk of periodontal disease in the dentition.

INTERDISCIPLINARY INTERRELATIONSHIPS

Interrelationships between Periodontics and Prosthodontics/Restorative Dentistry

(also see Chapter 7, 'Dental Calculus and Other Factors Contributing to Periodontal Disease' and section on iatrogenic factors contributing to periodontal disease, page 94)

Prosthodontic and restorative corrections, e.g. restorations, crowns and bridges have an effect on periodontal tissues as they can put additional occlusal loads on the periodontium. Additionally, as margins of restorations/prostheses lie close to the gingiva, they can increase plaque accumulation in its vicinity. The following points are important in this regard:

◂ *What are the disadvantages of wrongly designed crowns?*

1. If prosthetic crowns or restorations put excessive occlusal load over abutment teeth it can cause acute or chronic trauma from occlusion.
2. If margins of restorative crown or restoration are not well fitting, the gap between margin of the crown and the tooth preparation's margin becomes an ideal space for plaque accumulation. This results in periodontitis and caries. A similar effect is noticed if there are overhanging margins.

◂ *What happens if crowns are not well fitting?*

3. Fabricated crowns and prostheses must have normal tooth shape, form and size. Normal tooth contours deflect masticated food away from the gingival sulcus and remove plaque as food rubs past gingival surfaces. Faulty crown shapes result in food lodgment in the sulcus and increased plaque accumulation thereby leading to gingivitis and periodontitis. Large crowns have larger occlusal area, this will lead to more occlusal loads on the tooth which will cause trauma from occlusion.

◂ *What happens if crowns do not have normal shape and size?*

4. If adequate tooth structure is not available coronal to crest of alveolar bone, crown lengthening may be needed prior to tooth preparation. This can be done by excising gingiva and/or removing alveolar bone.
5. Crown cutting preparation margins on a tooth must be placed at least **3 *mm*** coronal to the underlying bone crest. This distance is called biologic width (*junctional epithelium 0.97 mm + gingival connective tissues 1.07 mm = biologic width 2.04 mm average*) **(Fig. 21.1)**. If this distance is not maintained, persistent gingival inflammation and attachment loss will occur **(Fig. 21.1)**.

◂ *How far away must crown cutting end from the crest of alveolar bone?*

6. Tooth preparation finish lines can be either supragingival (*i.e. coronal to gingival crest*), equigingival, i.e. at the level of the gingival crest or subgingival **(Fig. 21.2)**. Of these, supragingival finish lines (**Fig. 21.2, diag. A** are the easiest to clean while the

◂ *In relation to the gingival crest where can the crown cutting margins be placed?*

subgingivally placed finish lines are the most difficult to maintain (*due to inaccessibility to the area*) (**Fig. 21.2, diag. C**).

What is the disadvantage of under and overhanging crown and restoration surfaces? ▶

7. Crown and restoration surfaces should ideally be in the same plane as tooth surface near the tooth preparation margins (**Fig. 21.3, diag. A**). Higher plaque deposits are seen in cases where crown or restoration surface is either short (**Fig. 21.3, diag. B**) or project out of tooth surface, i.e. are overhanging (**Fig. 21.3, diag. C**) near tooth preparation margin.
8. Tight interproximal contacts between two teeth must be there to prevent food impaction in the interproximal region (*see Chapter 7, 'Dental Calculus and Other Factors Contributing to Periodontal Disease', pages 96 and 97 and Fig. 7.13*).

How many types of pontic designs are there? Which is the best suited for periodontal needs? ▶

9. Pontics of a bridge may be ridge lap, bullet shaped, sanitary etc. in design. Bullet (*for anterior teeth*) and sanitary pontics (*for posterior teeth*) are preferred as they allow easy cleaning under pontics (**Fig. 21.4, diags B and C**).
10. During crown cementation, cement that flows out must be carefully removed. If this is not done it can lead to periodontitis and peri-implantitis.
11. Dental materials can cause allergic reactions. If impression materials fragments remain stuck in the gingival sulcus, they can cause gingival inflammation.

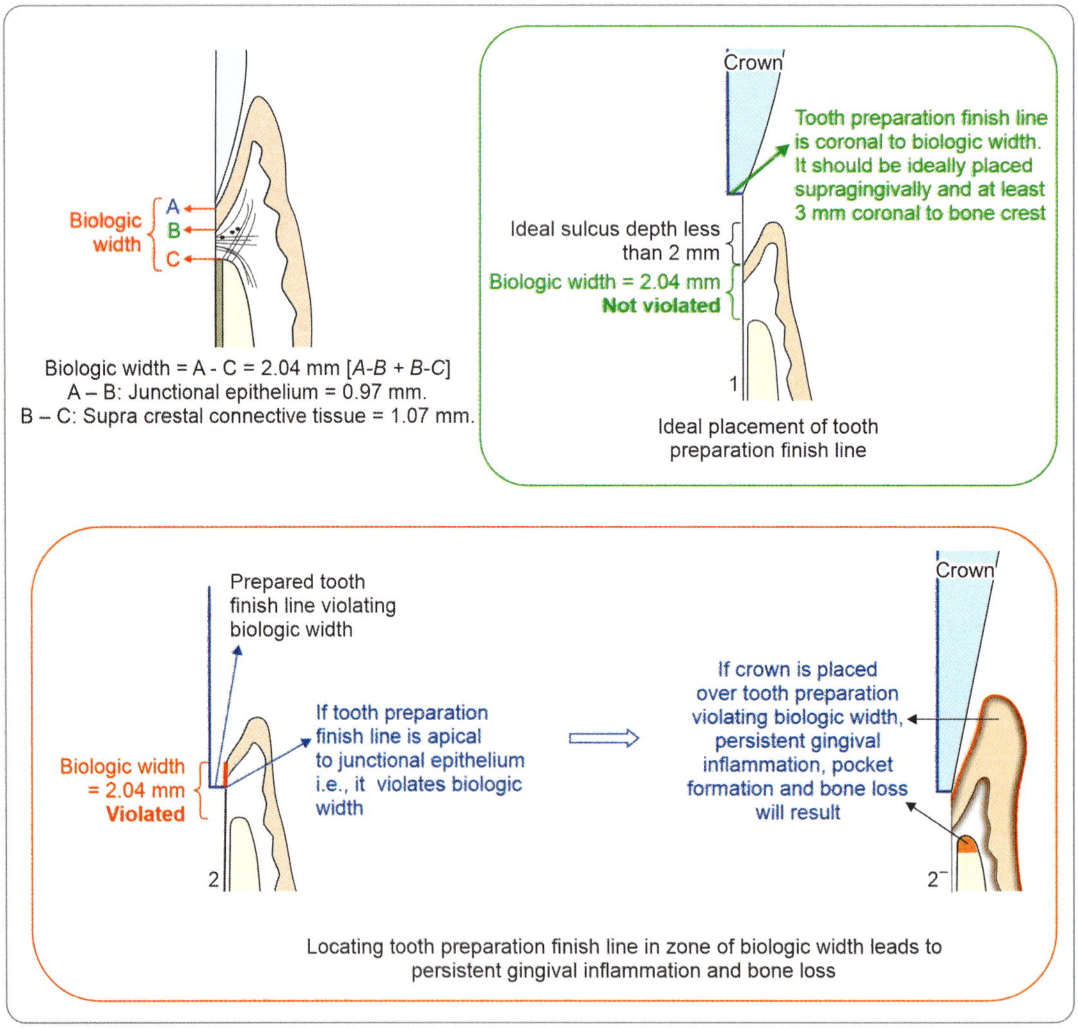

Fig. 21.1: Biologic width. It is the space between base of sulcus and crest of alveolar bone. It is occupied by supra-crestal tissues (*junctional epithelium and gingival connective tissue*). If biologic width (*diag. 1*) is violated by restorative procedures, it causes persistent gingival inflammation and bone loss (*diag. 2 and 2'*). Ideally, tooth preparation finish lines (*crown margins*) and restorations should *end* 3 mm coronal to crest of alveolar bone (*diag. 1*).

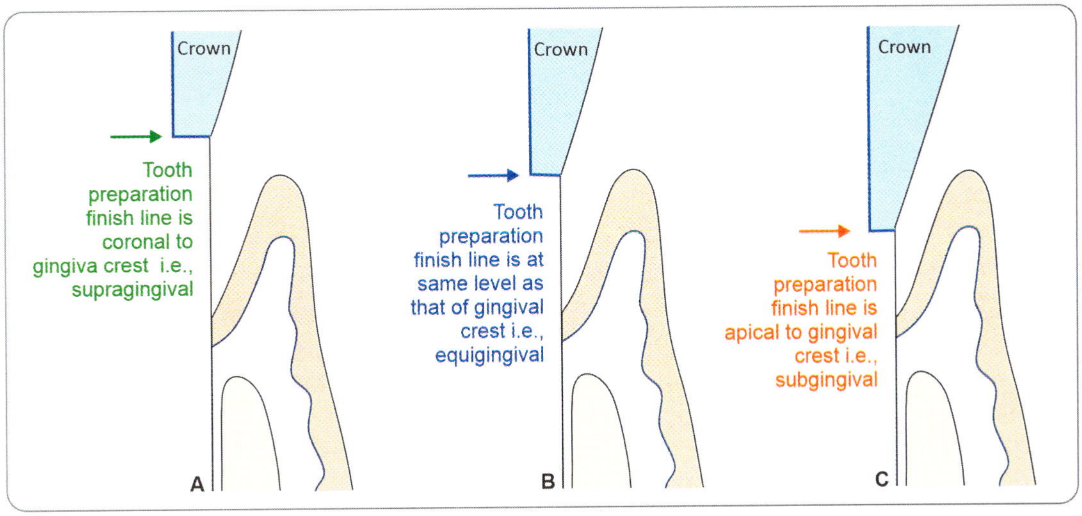

Fig. 21.2: Supragingival, equigingival and subgingival tooth finish lines. Supragingival (*diag. A*) and equigingival (*diag. B*) tooth preparation lines are ideal as they can be easily cleaned and maintained in a plaque free state.

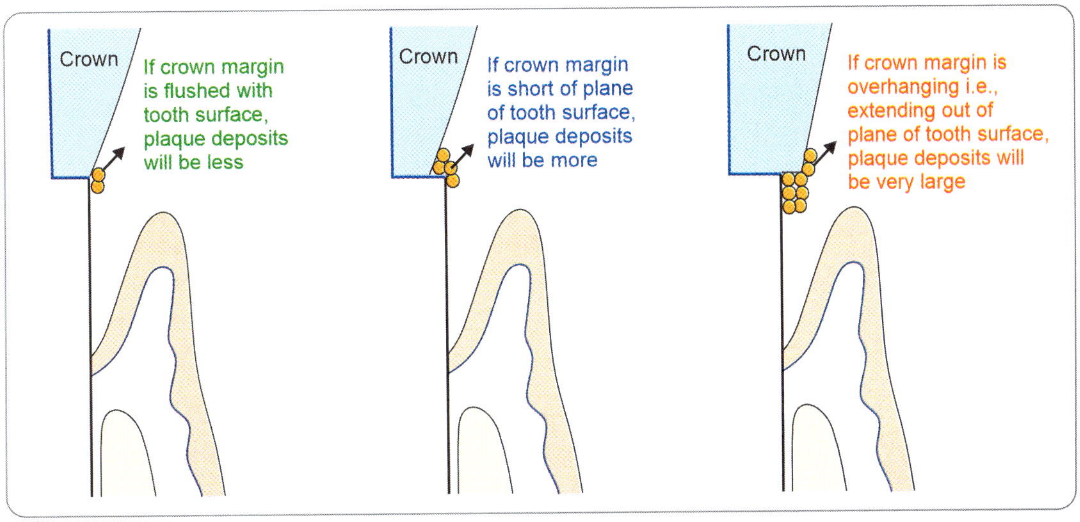

Fig. 21.3: Crown and restoration surfaces should ideally be in the same plane as tooth surface near the tooth preparation margins (*diag. A*). Higher plaque deposits are seen in cases where crown or restoration surface is short of tooth surface near tooth preparation margin (*diag. B*). Very high amount of plaque forms in relation to over-hanging crowns or restorations (*diag. C*).

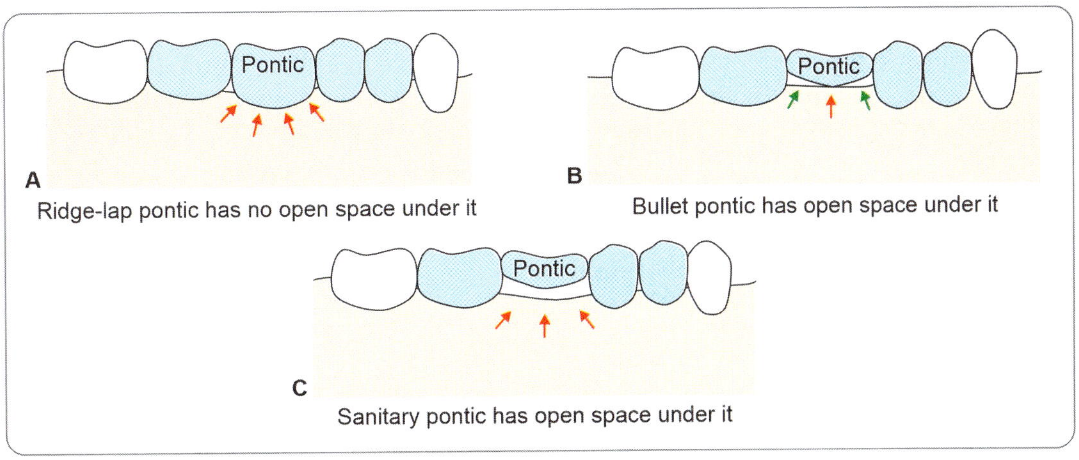

Fig. 21.4: Pontic design can be ridge lap (*A*), bullet (*B*) or sanitary (*C*). Sanitary pontics are the easiest to maintain while ridge lap pontics are the most difficult to clean.

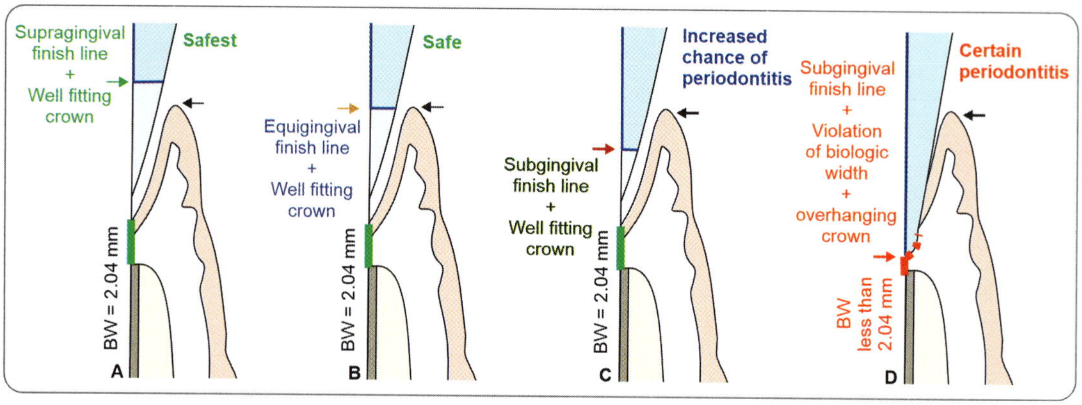

Fig. 21.5: Tooth preparation for restorations and crowns—safe practices

Crown Lengthening for Prosthetic or Restorative Reasons

What are the precautions and preconditions for performing crown lengthening? ▸

If sufficient tooth structure for crown retention is not present, crown lengthening is done. In this regard the following must be kept in mind:

1. Crown margins must end at least ***3 mm coronal*** to alveolar bone crest at that site. This will allow adequate space for supra-crestal tissues (*gingiva + biologic width*) (Figs 21.1, 21.1 and 21.5).
2. If width of supra-crestal tissues (*gingiva + supra-crestal space, i.e. biologic width*) is ***more than 5 mm*** and the ***width of attached gingiva is adequate***, crown lengthening can be done by gingivectomy (Fig. 21.6, diags A, A′ and A″).
3. If width of supra-crestal tissues (*gingiva + supra-crestal space, i.e. biologic width*) is ***less than 5 mm*** or ***width of attached gingiva is inadequate,*** flap surgery and ostectomy (*alveolar bone resection*) is done to expose adequate amount of tooth structure (Fig. 21.6, diags B, B′ and B″).

CLINICAL UTILITY AND SHORT ANSWER

Why is plaque control especially very important for teeth supporting prostheses and restorations?

More food debris and plaque collect under dental appliances, removable partial dentures and on natural surfaces of teeth adjoining them. Large amount of plaque is also found at junctions of crown margins and tooth preparation margins. If such areas are not cleaned regularly and maintained in a plaque free state, caries and periodontitis will result. Such areas can be cleaned with tooth brushes, interdental cleaners, floss, oral irrigation devices, etc. Floss threaders can be used to thread floss under pontics (*see Chapter 15 'Mechanical and Chemotherapeutic Control of Plaque', pages 268 Figs 15.7, 15.8, 15.8 and 15.9*).

Interrelationships between Periodontics and Endodontics (*'Endo–Perio Relationship'*)

Microorganisms in periodontal pockets can easily survive in a tooth's pulp (*infected pulp*) and vice versa. Therefore, there is a very close ***two-way*** relation between pulpal (*endodontic*) and periodontal health. In this regard, it is important to remember:

- Physical communication pathways are present between periodontium and pulp. These include accessory canals, apical foramen and dentinal tubules and non-physiological pathways like root fractures, perforations, etc.

Where are accessory canals most likely to be found? ▸

- Accessory canals are commonly found in middle/apical 1/3rd of roots of teeth and furcation areas of multirooted teeth.
- Microorganisms and their byproducts can easily travel from the periodontium to pulp and vice-versa via these pathways.
- This way microorganisms from an active pocket can reach and infect the pulp of a tooth and cause pulpitis (*infection of pulp*).
- An infected pulp can also produce and sustain periodontal infection and inflammation (*periodontal pocket*) via accessory canals and apical foramen.

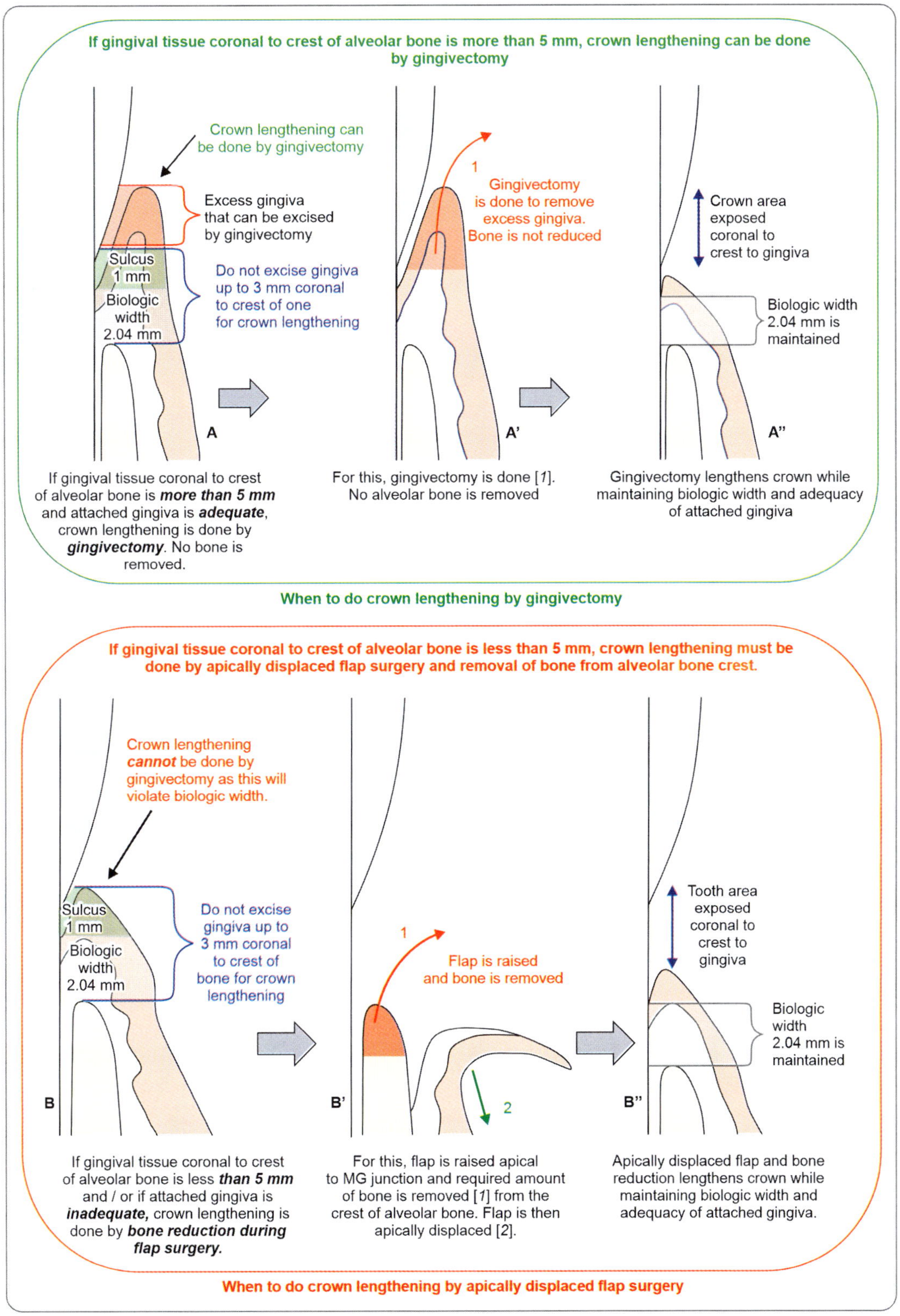

Fig. 21.6: Crown lengthening—deciding between gingivectomy (*diag. A*) and apically displaced flap surgery (*diag. B*).

ALERT!

Can accessory canals and non-physiologic pulp-periodontal tissue communications like root fractures and perforations be seen in radiographs?

Lateral canals are usually ***not*** visible in radiographs. They are most often identified after obturation when (*and if*) they get filled with radiopaque root canal sealers **(Fig. 21.8)**. Root fractures and perforations may be identifiable sometimes.

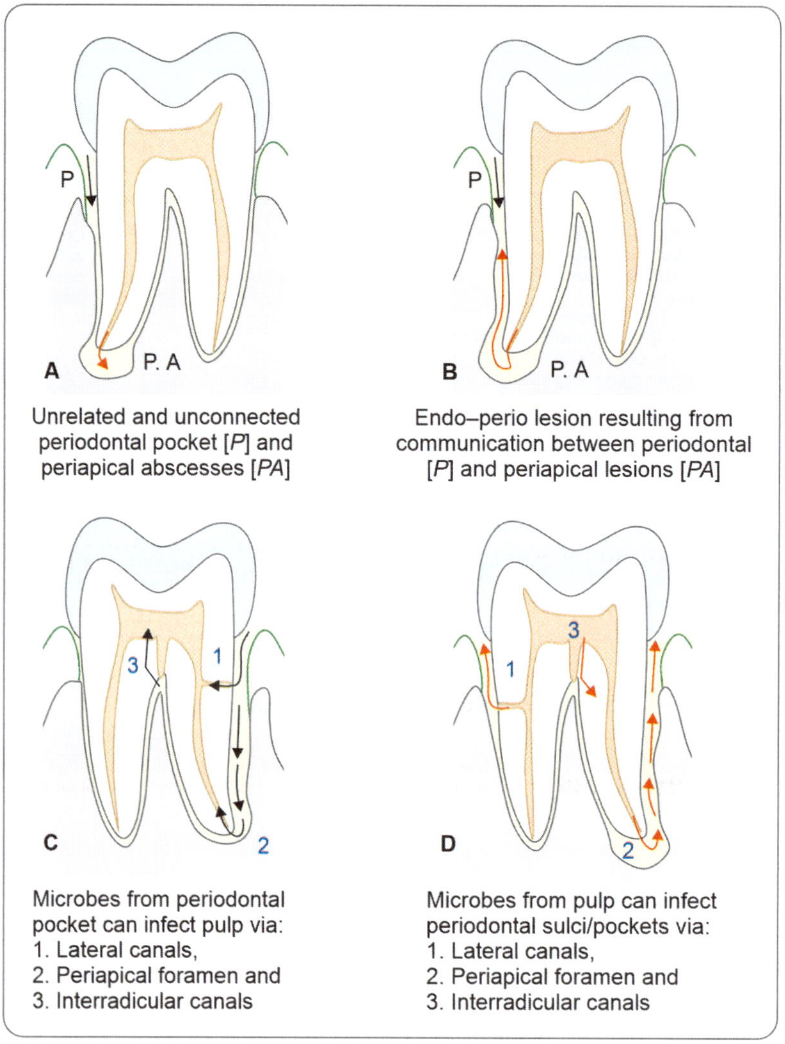

Fig. 21.7: Endo-perio lesions. Infected lesions in the periodontium and pulp can occur independent of each other. Microbes from a periodontal pocket can infect pulp and vice-versa via lateral canals, interradicular canals and apical foramen.

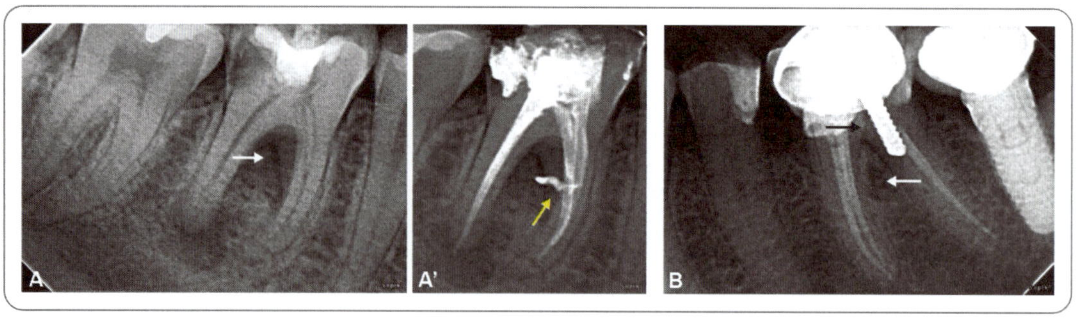

Fig. 21.8: Accessory canal and root fracture resulting in furcation involvement. Accessory canal in tooth # 46 due to necrosed pulp that was unseen in the preoperative radiograph (*diag. A*) is identified by root canal sealer leak into furcation area during obturation (*diag. A', yellow arrow*). Root fracture (*diag. B, black arrow*) and resulting furcation involvement (*diag. B, white arrow*). This patient complained tenderness and swelling in relation to tooth # 36 several years after RCT.

Clinical features of Endo–Perio lesions

Endo–perio lesions present a ***mix*** of clinical features of an inflamed-infected pulp and periodontitis. Features of periodontitis have already been discussed earlier (*see Chapter 10,*

'Plaque Induced Gingivitis and Periodontitis' page 147). Clinical features of endo-perio lesions depend on the stage of inflammation and infection in the pulp:

1. Tooth hypersensitivity, i.e. tooth is very sensitive to slight changes in temperature. This suggests pulpal hyperemia (*reversible pulpitis*).
2. Extreme pain on taking anything hot or cold. This suggests setting in of acute pulpitis (*irreversible symptomatic pulpitis*).
3. Tooth tenderness with or without hypersensitivity.
   a. Tenderness suggests formation of periapical abscess (*of pulpal origin; TFO can be a contributing factor*).
   b. If pulp has chronic pulpitis, the tooth may present with tenderness and mild hypersensitivity.
   c. If, however there no sensitivity, pulpal necrosis could have occurred.
4. Radiological picture of endo–perio lesions is variable:
   a. Chronic periapical abscesses present as periapical radiolucencies in a radiograph.
   b. Acute abscesses ***do not*** show up in the radiograph. If, however an acute abscess results from a chronic abscess the radiographic picture is similar to that of a chronic abscess.
   c. Bone and/or root resorption areas (*radiolucency*) may also be seen along lateral surfaces of the root, this suggests opening of the accessory canal in that area.
5. Periodontal pockets in communication with the periapical abscess are ***untreatable*** despite periodontal treatment.

◂ *What causes tooth hypersensitivity?*

◂ *What is the diagnosis if there is extreme sensitivity in a tooth to cold and hot foods?*

◂ *What could be the diagnosis if a tooth is tender?*

◂ *Which of the two, acute or chronic abscesses appear on a radiograph?*

Classification Endo–Perio lesions

1. Primary periodontal lesion
2. Primary endodontic lesion
3. Primary endodontic lesion with secondary periodontal involvement (*retrograde periodontitis*)
4. Primary periodontal lesion with secondary endodontic involvement (*retrograde pulpitis*)
5. True combined lesion

◂ *What is the difference between a primary periodontal and a primary endodontic lesion?*

1. **Primary periodontal lesion:** Only periodontal tissues are involved; pulp is not affected. They heal after periodontal treatment.
2. **Primary endodontic lesion:** Periapical abscess arising from a necrotic pulp and draining through the periodontium (*sulcus/pocket*). They heal after endodontic treatment (*RCT*).
3. **Primary endodontic lesion with secondary periodontal involvement:** If a primary endodontic lesion stays active for a long time, it can cause periodontal inflammation (*periodontitis*) and periodontal tissue destruction surrounding the apical foramen and openings of accessory canals **(Fig. 21.9, diags A and B)**. A similar situation results in areas of perforations that occur during endodontic treatment or restoration of teeth with posts. Such periodontitis arising from infection of pulp is called ***retrograde periodontitis.*** In such cases ***endodontic treatment is done first*** followed by periodontal treatment.
4. **Primary periodontal lesion with secondary endodontic involvement:** Microorganisms from periodontal pockets can gain access to the pulp through accessory canals, apical foramen or dentinal tubules and could then cause pulpitis **(Fig. 21.9, diags A and C)**. This is more likely to occur if the periodontal lesion extends up to the apical foramen. Such pulpitis resulting from infection originating in a periodontal pocket is called ***retrograde pulpitis.*** To treat such teeth, ***endodontic treatment is done first*** followed by periodontal treatment.
5. **True combined lesion:** When true periodontal and true endodontic lesions occur simultaneously, they are called a true combined lesion **(Fig. 21.7, diag. A)**. To treat such lesions ***endodontic treatment is done first*** followed by periodontal treatment.

◂ *How does an endodontic lesion contribute to causing a periodontal lesion?*

◂ *What is retrograde periodontitis?*

◂ *How does a periodontal lesion contribute to causing an endodontic lesion?*

◂ *What is retrograde pulpitis?*

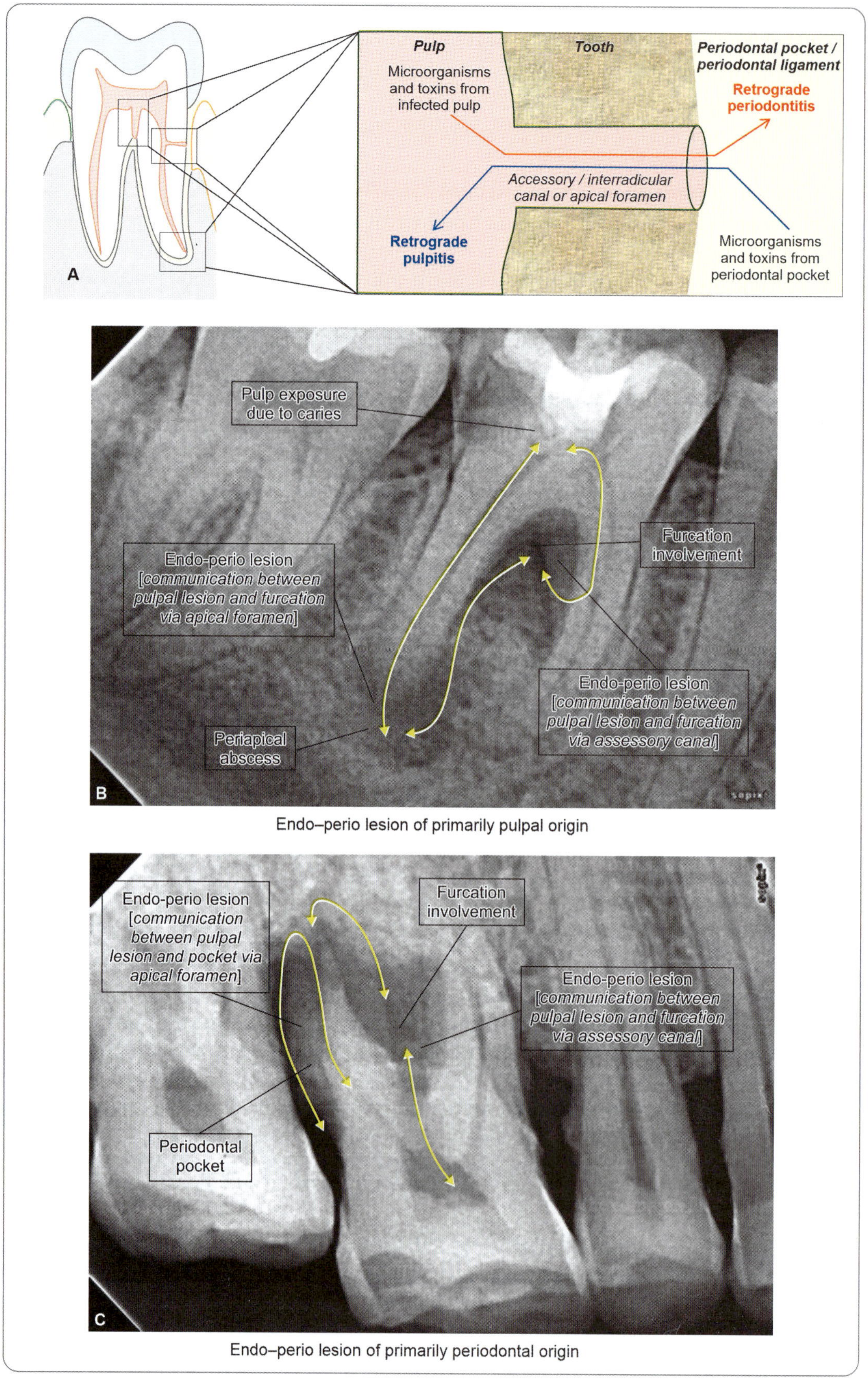

Endo–perio lesion of primarily pulpal origin

Endo–perio lesion of primarily periodontal origin

Fig. 21.9: Schematic diagram and radiographs depicting formation and continuance of retrograde periodontitis and pulpitis. Microorganisms and toxins from infected pulp can infect a periodontal pocket via accessory canals or apical foramen to cause retrograde periodontitis. Microorganisms and toxins from periodontal pockets can similarly infect pulp to cause retrograde pulpitis.

CLINICAL UTILITY AND SHORT ANSWER

How can an endodontically involved tooth be diagnosed? What are its presenting clinical features?

Condition of the pulp can be diagnosed by preforming the following tests and investigations:

1. **Pulp vitality tests:** Electric pulp vitality test is ideal. Thermal vitality can be done but is not recommended as it is inaccurate and can damage the pulp.
2. **Radiographic evaluation:** Radiographs ***do not*** give indication of the present condition of pulp. However, peri-apical radiolucency due to peri-apical abscess, granuloma or cyst formation are ***indicative*** of pulp necrosis or defective endodontic treatment (*RCT*).
   Periapical radiolucency (*similar to one seen in relation to a periapical abscess or granuloma*) may also be there due to initial stage ***cementoma*** (*periapical cemental dysplasia*)—a condition that is ***not*** associated with pulpal condition of a tooth. Teeth with initial stage cementomas have vital pulps; pulp vitality tests help to make a differential diagnosis in such cases.
3. **Presence of pain:** A tooth with pulpitis will have pain and hypersensitivity. Pulpal or periodontal abscess if acute, i.e. non-draining, can present with moderate-severe pain.
4. **Percussion test (*checking tenderness*):** Non-vital teeth with periapical abscesses (*infection*) become tender. Percussing such a tooth lightly produces pain. Teeth can ***also*** be tender due to ***TFO***; such teeth may have either vital or non-vital pulps. Tenderness reduces after acute periapical abscess becomes chronic.

◂ *How can a periapical radiolucency arising from a periapical abscess differentiated form one due to initial stage cementoma?*

◂ *What are the possible causes of pain in teeth?*

◂ *What are the possible causes of tooth tenderness?*

CLINICAL UTILITY AND SHORT ANSWER

What are the differences between endodontic (*pulpal origin*) and periodontal abscesses?

Pure periodontal abscesses	*Pure pulpal abscesses*
1. It usually presents as a mild–***moderate*** local painful and tender swelling in the gingiva. Tooth may be tender.	1. Tooth with an acute periapical abscess has ***severe*** pulsating pain and is tender to touch. If infection spreads to adjoining soft tissue spaces it causes swelling of soft tissues in vicinity of the affected tooth and same side of the face. In severe cases infection can spread to other side of the face also. Chronic abscesses present with milder clinical features.
2. They usually occur in soft tissue of the pocket over the periosteum. Therefore, swelling is produced in the soft tissue outside the alveolar bone. As there is no elevation of the periosteum, therefore the pain is not as severe as that in a periapical abscess of pulpal origin.	2. They usually occur in the periapical region of the affected tooth and may spread there. Because the abscess is in a confined space (*within alveolar bone*), it cannot expand. This produces a lot of pressure on the sensory receptors of the periodontal ligament and periosteum. This results in severe pain.
3. A periodontal abscess may occur in relation to either a vital or non-vital tooth.	3. Pulpal abscess occurs only in relation to an endodontically involved tooth. Tooth may be non-vital or may have chronic pulpitis.
4. Usually drains through the pocket/sulcus.	4. Usually drains through a sinus located a small distance away from free gingiva but may also drain through sulcus/pocket (Fig. 21.10, diag. A).
5. If a warm gutta percha point is gently inserted into the abscess opening it stops inside the periodontal pocket (*as seen on the radiograph*).	5. If a warm gutta percha is gently inserted through the sinus opening it traces the sinus track and stops at the abscess. It thus points at the offending tooth in the radiograph (Fig. 21.10, diags A. A' and A").
6. As a periodontal abscess can form on any side of a tooth, therefore, it may drain on any side of the tooth.	6. Because a tooth's root apex is closer to buccal bone plate than lingual/palatal bone plate, a pulpal/periapical abscess ***usually*** drains on the ***buccal*** side of the tooth.

◂ *Why is pain in a periapical abscess more severe than compared to pain in periodontal abscess?*

◂ *A periodontal abscess is associated with vital or non-vital teeth?*

◂ *Why is a periapical abscess more likely to drain on the buccal side and a periodontal abscess drain on any side of the tooth?*

CLINICAL UTILITY AND SHORT ANSWER

Does a periapical radiolucency always mean there is a periapical abscess?

Periapical radiolucency may also be seen in initial stages of Cementoma (*periapical cemental dysplasia*) that is forming at the apex of a tooth. Cementomas occur more in association with TFO. Periapical radiolucency is also seen around an incompletely formed tooth root. In such cases the tooth vitality tests may be normal.

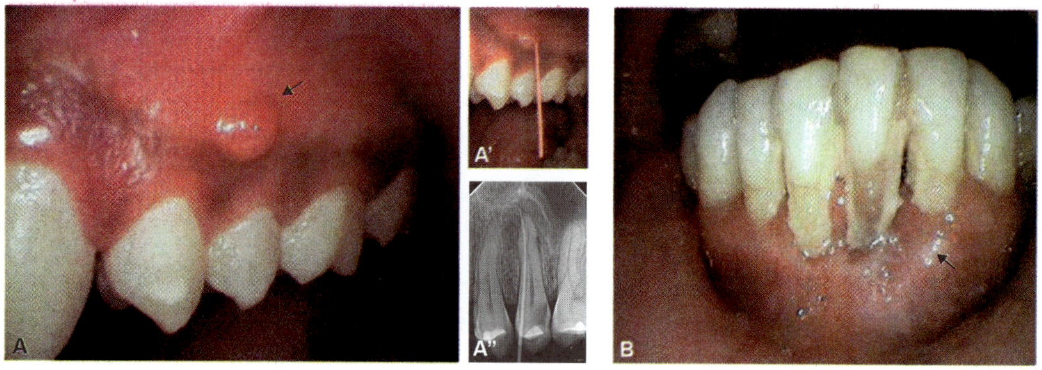

Fig. 21.10: Pupal abscess (*diags A, A' and A''*) and a periodontal abscess (*diag. B*)

Interrelationships between Periodontics and Orthodontics

Orthodontic treatment is done to improve tooth position, arch alignment, overcrowding, malocclusion or as a preparatory treatment prior to mucogingival therapy.

How does orthodontic treatment affect periodontal health? ▶

- Orthodontic bands retainers and appliances increase plaque deposition, decrease plaque removing efficiency of oral cleansing devices (*tooth brushes, etc.*).
- During orthodontic treatment, teeth need to be maintained in good periodontal health with SRP and/or periodontal surgery.
- Frenula may need to be incised or removed and adequate width of attached gingiva has to be maintained (*see Chapter 19 'Mucogingival therapy'*).
- Some periodontal conditions can only be treated with orthodontic correction. For example, teeth in palato-version have thick marginal gingiva on the labial side; the crest of their buccal gingiva is more coronal (*covering more crown than normal*), thicker and is rounded (*see Chapter 2, 'Gingiva', page 22 and Fig. 2.17*). If such gingiva is surgically excised without orthodontic correction of tooth's position, the gingiva will regrow to its original position within a few weeks. In some such cases, gingival margin corrects itself automatically with orthodontic correction alone (*without surgical intervention*).
- Orthodontic correction and shifting of the tooth into curve of the arch improves width of attached gingiva. on the contrary if teeth are moved out of curve of the arch, gingiva and crest of alveolar bone will shift apically **(Fig. 21.11, diag. B)**.

How can alveolar crest be shifted coronally by orthodontic treatment? ▶

- Orthodontic extrusion of teeth can shift crest of alveolar bone coronally. When a tooth is extruded, its alveolar bone crest shifts coronally along with it. This happens due to the coronal pull exerted on the crest of the alveolar bone by alveolar crest and horizontal fibers of the periodontal ligament (*see Chapter 3, 'Periodontal ligament, Cementum and Alveolar bone, page 31 and Fig. 3.3*). Shifting of crest of alveolar bone coronally, while extruding a tooth, can be a good way of treating infra bony defects and can also increase height of alveolar bone for implant placement.

  If coronal shift of bone crest is not desired, e.g. as during crown lengthening for restorative purposes, alveolar crest and horizontal fibers of the periodontal ligament must be incised during extrusion (*see Chapter 19, 'Mucogingival Therapy', section on crown lengthening: 'Forced eruption with fiber resection', pages 353 and 354*).

SUPPORTIVE PERIODONTAL THERAPY FOR MAINTENANCE OF PERIODONTAL HEALTH

(Phase IV/Maintenance Phase of Periodontal Treatment)

What is supportive periodontal therapy? ▶

As periodontitis is caused by oral biofilm/plaque, therefore, after phase I, II and III treatments, patients must be led onto a phase during which health of teeth, periodontium and prosthetic restorations is maintained by the patient by active and effective plaque control **(Fig. 21.12)**. This marks the beginning of phase IV or maintenance phase of treatment plan. As this phase stresses on supporting the ***patient's own efforts*** in controlling periodontal

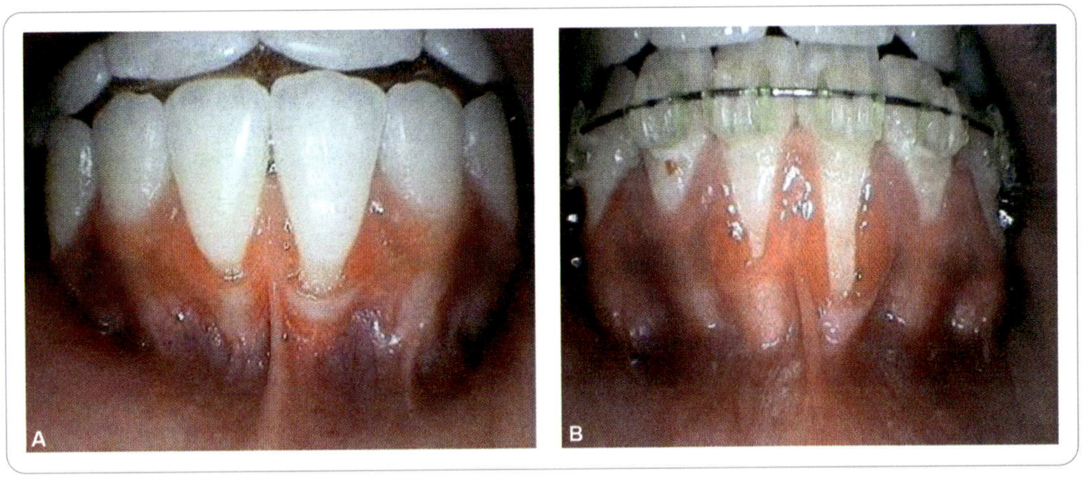

Fig. 21.11: Prominent roots often present with gingival recession and inadequate attached gingiva (*diag. A*); in such cases, root prominence must be reduced by orthodontic treatment if width of attached gingiva has to be increased and coverage of gingival recession has to be done. Improper orthodontic treatment that results in root prominence can cause gingival recession (*diag. B*). Note increased plaque deposits and gingival inflammation caused by improper plaque control due to orthodontic appliances (*diag. B*).

disease and preventing its recurrence, maintenance phase therapy is also called 'Supportive Periodontal Therapy' (*SPT*). Important points for success of maintenance phase are:

- Maintenance phase starts ***after*** completion of all scheduled dental treatment. Therefore, maintenance phase and supportive periodontal therapy may start after completion of either phase I or phase II (*if required*) or phase III (*if required*) treatments (Fig. 21.12).
- At this time a patient is re-educated (*reminded*) about etiology of dental disease, motivated to maintain oral health and then instructed about necessity of good plaque control and plaque control measures. Reminding a patient of the time and cost of dental treatment done so far and the possibility of disease surfacing again helps in motivating patients to undertake plaque control seriously. Plaque control instructions can be given by all staff of the dental clinic.
- ***Systemic health*** of the patient is ***re-assessed at each maintenance visit***. If medical history has changed since the patient's last visit, necessary treatment and changes to the maintenance schedule are advised.
- All patients must be advised a definite and pre-decided schedule of periodic recall visits for preventive (*prophylactic*) treatments especially SRP.

◄ *When does maintenance phase start?*

Maintenance/Periodic Recall Visit (*SPT*)

Repeated scheduled periodic visits of a dental patient for continued periodic assessment for early detection and prophylactic treatment of new and recurring disease is called periodontal maintenance/periodic recall visit.

◄ *What is maintenance/ periodic recall visit?*

Aims of Maintenance/Periodic Recall Visit (SPT)

1. Prevention of new and recurrence of already treated dental and/or periodontal disease, e.g. gingivitis, periodontitis, peri-implantitis, etc.
2. Prevention of tooth loss by maintenance of health of dentition and prosthetic replacements of natural teeth.
3. Diagnosis and timely treatment (*before the disease becomes severe and causes substantial and irreparable damage or other associated illness*) of other diseases and/or conditions of the oral cavity.

◄ *What are the aims of maintenance/periodic recall visit?*

What is done during a Maintenance/Periodic Recall Visit (SPT)

The recall visit must be planned according to the patient's individual needs and his/her personal convenience. The recall visit involves:

1. Re-education and re-motivation of the patient regarding general, oral and periodontal health. ***Disclosing plaque*** with *plaque disclosing solutions* must be done for all patients.

Oral hygiene measures practiced by the patient are re-assessed and if required the patient is re-instructed and re-taught oral hygiene measures, e.g. tooth brushing, flossing, etc.

2. Re-evaluation of the patient's current oral health. This includes assessment and examination of health of the periodontium by assessing probing depth, bleeding on probing, calculus deposition, mobility of teeth, TFO (*trauma from occlusion*), etc.
3. Re-evaluation of systemic health and medication.
4. Taking intra oral radiographs (*IOPA*) for assessment and diagnosis of new or continuing alveolar bone loss, caries, old restorations, etc. (*full mouth bitewing/IOPA radiographs are recommended every two years for all individuals*).
5. Diagnosis of new/secondary caries lesions.
6. Assessment of all old restorations and prostheses.
7. Examination of ***entire*** oral cavity and pharyngeal region for detection and assessment of ***oral lesions*** and ***oral cancer*** screening.
8. All prophylactic treatments like SRP, polishing, minor restorations, fluoridation, etc. may be done. More advanced periodontal therapy, restorative dental procedures, etc. may be performed on subsequent visits.

Planning of a Scheduled Maintenance/Periodic Recall Visit (SPT)

What are the aims of maintenance/periodic recall visit? ▶

Maintenance visits must be scheduled at least ***every 6 months*** for everybody. In individuals who have stage III or IV and grade B or C periodontitis, who for some reason cannot brush their teeth properly or have systemic diseases or conditions that complicate periodontitis, e.g. diabetes, immune deficiency, etc. maintenance visits can be scheduled earlier after every ***1–3 months***.

A recall visit of 45 minutes–1 hour must be scheduled and planned as under:

What is done during the first part of a scheduled periodic recall visit? ▶

Part 1—initial 10 minutes: Examination of entire oral cavity, re-evaluation of the patient's current ***oral and systemic*** health status and maintenance of results of treatments performed earlier.

Is the patient re-educated, re-motivated and re-instructed during a recall visit? ▶

Part 2—next 10 minutes: Re-educate, re-motivate and re-instruct the patient regarding cause, prevention and treatment of oral disease.

Is oral prophylaxis done during a recall visit? ▶

Part 3—next approximately 20–30 minutes: Oral prophylaxis (*scaling, root planing and polishing*) and/or other minor treatments that maybe required and possible, e.g. fluoridation of teeth, minor restorations, etc.

Part 4—next approximately 10 minutes: Re-explaining the need and scheduling the patient's next treatment or recall visit.

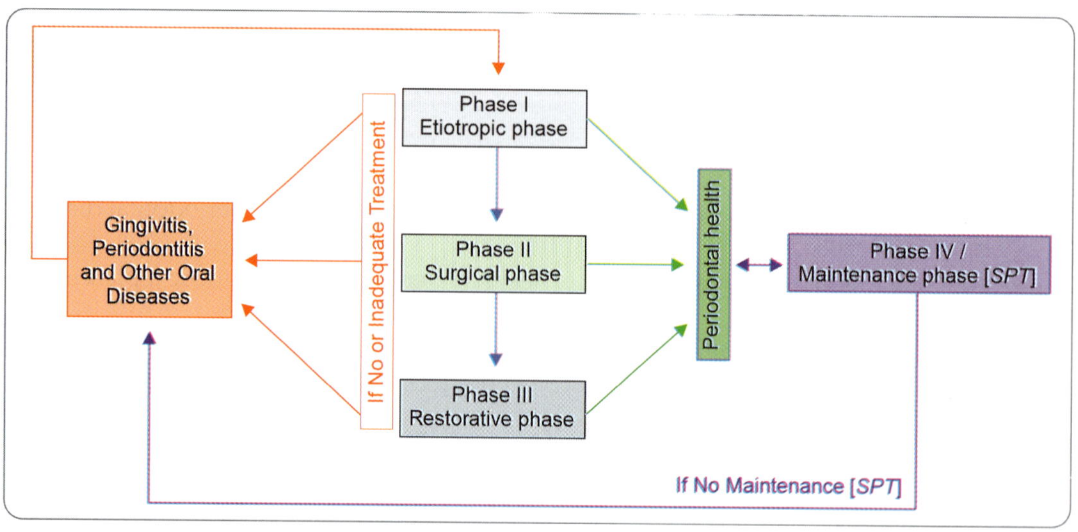

Fig. 21.12: Phase IV or maintenance phase (*supportive periodontal therapy*) must start and continue after all phases of treatment.

CLINICAL UTILITY AND SHORT ANSWER

Should a patient come for prophylactic SRP (*maintenance phase treatment*) even if he/she is following all oral hygiene instructions and has no complaints like bleeding from gingiva, tooth mobility, pain, etc.?

Maintenance phase visits and SPT are based on the fact that most of the ***dental diseases are usually painless to start and that it is at the starting stage that dental diseases are the easiest to treat and chances for successful treatment and recovery are the maximum.***

Therefore, all individuals must report for maintenance therapy (*SRP, etc.*) even if they do not have pain or other symptoms of dental disease.

◂ *What is the reason for scheduling prophylactic SRP even if the patient has no complaints?*

Why do Individuals Avoid Prophylactic Treatment (*Maintenance*)?

Reasons for individuals avoiding prophylactic (*maintenance*) include:

- Ignorance; either the individual was not educated or was not convinced enough about need for maintenance visits.
- Fear of dental treatment.
- Unaffordable cost of dental treatment.
- Dental diseases are recurrent in nature; this fact may lead to the belief that dental disease is untreatable and will recur anyway and therefore getting treatment is useless.
- Fear of diagnosis of serious illness (*cancer, etc.*).

REVIEW QUESTIONS

1. What is meant by the term interdisciplinary interrelationships?
2. How does crown and restoration design affect the health of the periodontium?
3. What is biologic width? What happens if biologic width is violated by crown and restoration margins?
4. What is the ideal location of finish lines of tooth crown preparation?
5. Why is it important to maintain periodontal health in abutment teeth?
6. What is 'endo–perio relationship'? What are the clinical features of endo–perio lesions?
7. What are the clinical features of a tooth with pulpal disease? How can one differentially diagnose stages of pulpal involvement?
8. How can infectious microorganisms reach the pulp from a periodontal pocket?
9. What are accessory canals? Where are they usually located?
10. What are retrograde periodontitis and retrograde pulpitis?
11. How can you differentiate between pulpal and periodontal abscesses?
12. Write a note on periodontic–orthodontic interrelationship.
13. What is supportive periodontal therapy? What are the aims of SPT?
14. What is done during a maintenance visit?
15. At what intervals must maintenance visits be planned?
16. What are the reasons for noncompliance of advised SPT and maintenance visit schedule by the patient?
17. What is the rationale of SPT and periodic maintenance visits?
18. Why must patients come for maintenance phase treatment even if the patient has no complaints like bleeding, etc. and is practicing adequate plaque control?

Chapter

22

Dental Implants

A dental implant is a small cylindrical object (*artificial root*) made of Titanium. It is surgically placed into a natural tooth socket (*after recent extraction*) or a freshly prepared socket like cavity (*osteotomy*) that is drilled into the alveolar bone of the maxilla or mandible. Such implants are called endosseous implants. Implants of different sizes, shapes and designs are available and have a 90–95% success rate (*when evaluated over a 5-year period*). As ***only endosseous dental implants are in wide use today*** therefore, only endosseous implants are described in the under mentioned text.

How successful are dental implants? ▸

COMMONLY USED TERMS THAT DESCRIBE CHARACTERISTICS OF FREQUENTLY USED PRESENT-DAY IMPLANTS

1. **Threaded implant:** Implants have one or more ***threads*** running on their bodies. These threads make them look like screws.
2. **Tapered implant:** Implants are ***conical*** in shape just like roots of teeth.
3. **Single body implant:** Implant body and abutment are ***not*** separable.
4. **Two-part implants:** Implant body and abutment are separate and are joined with a screw.
5. **Internal connection implant:** When abutment body fits ***into*** the implant neck.
6. **External connection implant:** When abutment fits ***over and around*** the implant neck.

What is the difference between a single body and two-part implant? ▸

What is an internal connection implant? ▸

ACCESSORIES AND PARTS OF DENTAL IMPLANT

Name the components of dental implants. ▸

Dental implants have two components:

1. **Implant fixture** (*root component*): It is inserted in the alveolar bone (Fig. 22.1, diag. A).
2. **Abutment** (*crown component*): It is fixed with a screw to body of the implant (Fig. 22.1, diags E and F and Figs 22.3 and 22.4).
   i. In some implant designs, abutments are pre-attached (*pre-fixed by factory*) to the body of the implant.
   ii. Abutments may be straight or angulated (Fig. 22.1 diag. F and Fig. 22.4).
3. **Cover screw:** After an implant is fixed in the bone, a cover screw is fixed on it to prevent bone and soft tissue from growing into the implant body during healing (*usually 2–6 months*) (Fig. 22.1, diag. B).
4. **Healing screw (*also called healing abutment or gingival former*):** At end of healing period (*usually 2–6 months*), cover screw is removed and healing screw is placed in the implant body. The healing screw shapes gingiva during gingival healing so that healed gingiva fits around the abutment body comfortably (Fig. 22.1, diag. C).

What is the difference between a cover screw and healing screw? ▸

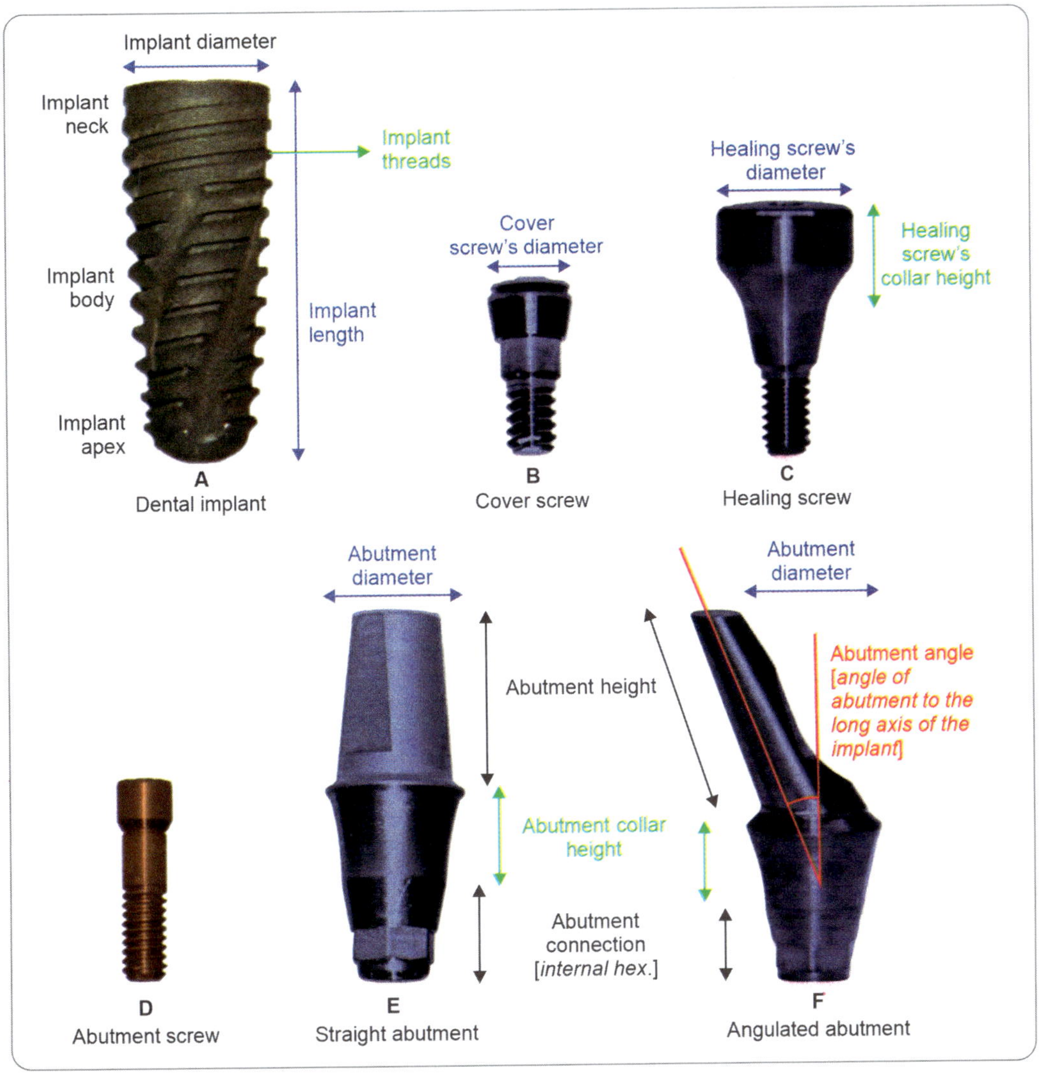

Fig. 22.1: Dental implants and other commonly used implant components

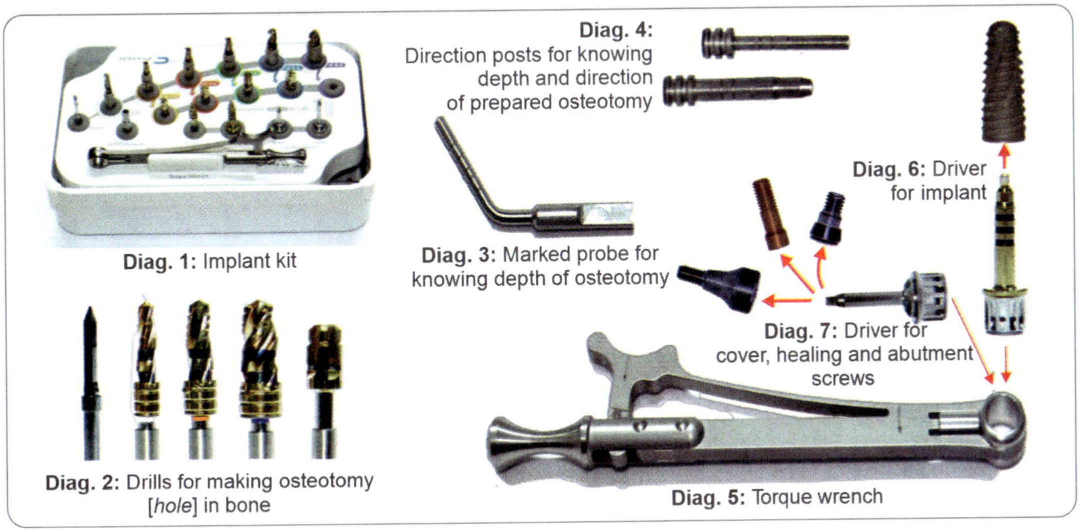

Fig. 22.2: Implant kit and its components. Implant kit (*diag. 1*); Osteotomy drills (*diag. 2*). Marked probe for ascertaining depth of prepared osteotomy (*diag. 3*). Direction posts for knowing direction, parallelism and distance between two or more osteotomies (*diag. 4*). Torque wrench for providing torque for turning implants into and out of the osteotomy (*clockwise and anticlockwise*) and tightening or loosening screws (*diag. 5*). Driver for turning implants into and out of the osteotomy (*diag. 6*). Driver for tightening or loosening screws (*diag. 7*).

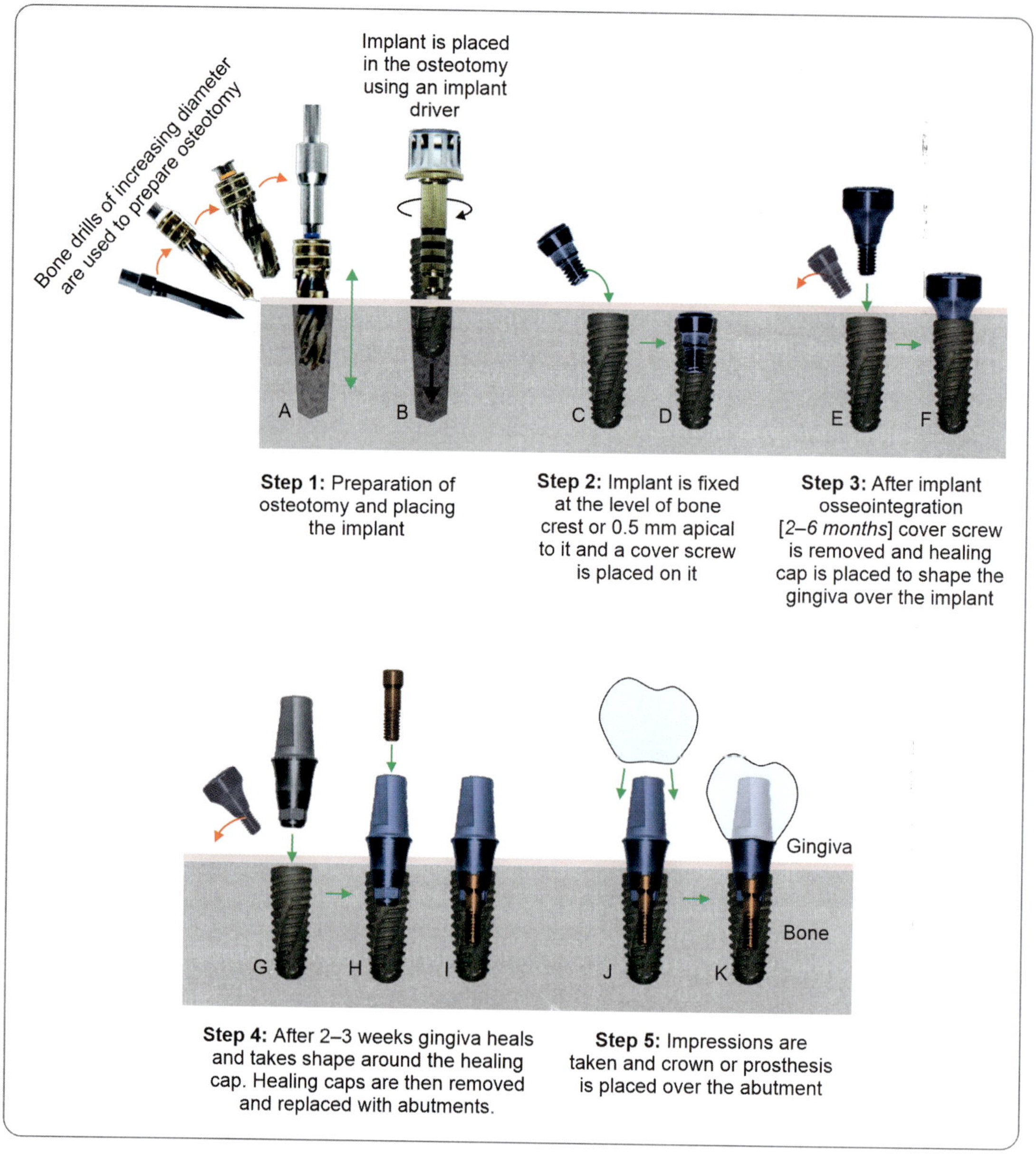

Fig. 22.3: Diagrammatic representation of steps of placing and loading of a dental implant

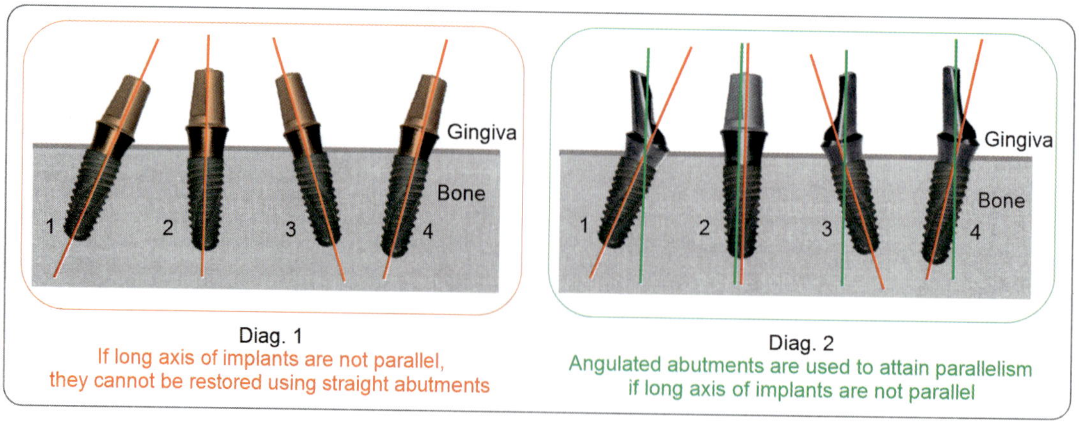

Fig. 22.4: Angulated abutments help attain parallelism when implants are not parallel. In diag. 1, long axis of all implants (*red lines*) are not parallel. These implants therefore cannot be restored with straight abutments. In diag. 2, when a combination of straight and angulated abutments are used over the same implants, the long axis of abutments become parallel ...thesis can now be constructed on it.

PERI-IMPLANT PERIODONTAL TISSUES

What are the characteristics of peri-implant tissues?

- Healthy peri-implant gingiva is ***similar*** to gingiva surrounding a natural tooth (Fig. 22.5, diag. 1). It is tightly adapted to the implant and its abutment.
- Junctional epithelium is about 2 mm long.
- Peri-implant sulcus is lined by sulcular epithelium.
- Gingival fibers are present but they run parallel to implant surface and ***do not*** attach to the implant (*in teeth, gingival fibers attach to the root cementum*).

Do gingival fibers attach to the implant body?

- After an implant is placed, alveolar bone undergoes remodeling. The crest of the alveolar bone may resorb and lie slightly apical to its original position. If a platform shifting implant has been placed and it has been submerged 0.5 mm apical to the bone crest, bone may form over the implant neck (Fig. 22.6, diag. 1).
- After osteointegration, crest of the alveolar bone surrounding the implant body is usually horizontal (Fig. 22.6, diag. 1, green arrows) or saucer shaped (Fig. 22.6, diag. 2, red arrows).

CLINICAL UTILITY AND SHORT ANSWER

What are platform shifting implants?

Platform shifting refers to use of smaller diameter abutment connected to an implant neck (*implant platform*) of larger diameter. Implants with this feature are called platform shifting implants (Fig. 22.3 diags F, I and K). Platform shifting preserves alveolar bone around the neck of the dental implant during and after osseointegration of the implant (Fig. 22.6, diag. 1, green arrows).

Implants in which abutment diameter is the same as the implant neck (*implant platform*) are called platform matching implants (Fig. 22.6, diag. 2, red arrows).

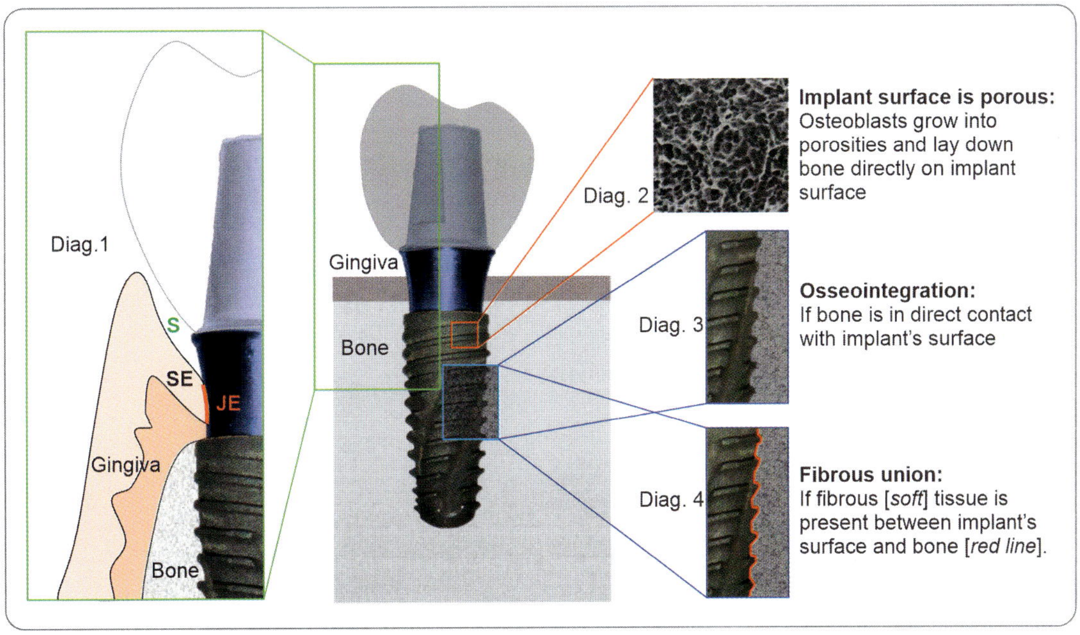

Fig. 22.5: Peri-implant tissues, osseointegration and fibrous union. Diag. 1 shows junctional epithelium (*JE, red line*), sulcular epithelium (*SE*) and sulcus (*S*); Diag. 2 shows electron microscopic view of porosities on surface of a dental implant. Osteoblasts of the surrounding bone grow into these porosities and lay down bone directly on surface of the implant for osseointegration. Diag. 3 shows osseointegrated implant surface where bone is present directly over the surface of the implant. Diag. 4 shows fibrous union where fibrous (*soft*) tissue (*red line*) is present between implant surface and the bone.

INDICATIONS AND CONTRAINDICATIONS OF DENTAL IMPLANTS

Indications

- Any patient who has missing teeth can be a candidate for dental implant surgery.
- Prosthetic replacement of single tooth, multiple teeth or the entire dentition with fixed rigid prosthesis.

- For providing adequate retention and stability to complete dentures by making implant supported dentures that use implant attached components in severely resorbed maxillary or mandibular alveolar ridges (*e.g. ball attachment, etc.*).

Contraindications

In which situations can implants not be placed or are likely to fail? ▶

- Systemic diseases, e.g. uncontrolled diabetes, untreated bleeding and clotting disorders, etc.
- Non-availability of enough volume (*dimensions*) of alveolar bone for implant placement. Height and width of alveolar bone reduce soon after loss of a tooth. If implant placement is delayed for more than a few weeks after tooth loss, height and width of alveolar bone can reduce to an extent that enough bone volume (*bone housing*) for placing implants may not be available to place implants.
- Non-availability of sufficiently dense bone. If bone is too porous (*of very less density, e.g. due to osteoporosis, incompletely healed extraction sockets, etc.*) it will not provide enough hold to the implant (*immediately after implant placement and for osseointegration*).
- Nearness of the implant site to critical anatomical structures. Implants must be placed at least 3–5 mm away from nearby anatomical structures like adjoining roots, mandibular canal, etc.

OSSEOINTEGRATION

(How an Endosseous Dental Implant is Unmovably Fixed in Bone)

How is an implant retained in the bone immediately after insertion? ▶

Immediately after an implant is inserted into the osteotomy prepared in the bone (*cavity prepared in the bone or refined tooth root socket*), it is ***initially*** retained in the alveolar bone by ***physical force*** produced by the tight fit of the implant in the prepared osteotomy/tooth socket. ***Later***, after new bone is laid down over the implant surface, it gets joined with the bone—this process is called ***osseointegration.*** Osseointegrated implants can bear occlusal loads and function like natural teeth.

What is osseointegration? ▶

Definition: Osseointegration is the process of joining of dental implant to the bone by formation of a direct structural and functional connection between normal living bone and surface of a dental implant **(Fig. 22.5, diags 2 and 3)**.

(There is ***no intervening soft tissue*** *(cartilage or ligament) between implant and bone, i.e. implants are* ***ankylosed*** *with the alveolar bone; a natural tooth has periodontal ligament between its root and bone).*

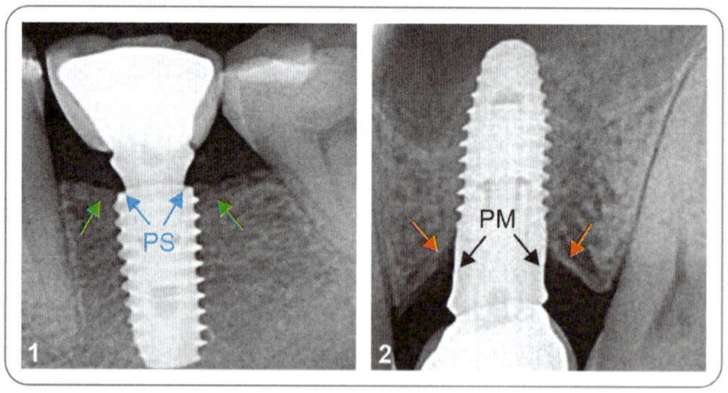

Fig. 22.6: Successfully osseointegrated implants may show no (*diag. 1, green arrows*) or some saucer shaped (*diag. 2, red arrows*) bone loss around neck of the implant (*this usually has no measurable impact on implant health and functioning*). Bone loss is usually not seen in platform shifting implants (*diag. 1, PS*) where abutment diameter is smaller than the implant neck (*implant platform*) (*diag. 1 blue arrows*). It is more common in platform matching (*diag. 2, PM*) implants where abutment diameter is same as the implant neck (*diag. 2, black arrows*).

Density and Quality of the Alveolar Bone Affects Osseointegration

How is bone classified according to its density and resistance to drilling? ▶

Density of bone plays an important role in successful osseointegration of implants. Depending on radiographic appearance and resistance to drilling into bone, bone quality is classified into four categories (*densities*) (*Lekholm and Misch*) **(Fig. 22.7)**.

1. *Type 1 (D1) Bone*

i. ***Very thick dense and compact*** **(cortical)** ***bone*** surrounds a ***thin*** zone of ***trabecular*** bone.
ii. It is feels very hard to drill into (*during osteotomy preparation*).
iii. It provides very good initial stability to implants.
iv. It has ***lesser*** blood supply than other bone types.
v. As blood supply is lesser, bone healing and bone re-formation are ***slower***.
vi. Because of slower healing, osseointegration of dental implants in Type 1/D1 bone is slower.

◄ *What are the benefits and shortcomings of type 1 bone?*

2. *Type 2 (D2) Bone*

i. ***Thick layer of dense and compact*** **(cortical)** ***bone*** surrounds dense trabecular bone.
ii. It is not as hard as type I bone but has better blood supply.
iii. It provides very good initial stability to implants.

3. *Type 3 (D3) Bone*

i. ***Thin layer*** of compact (*cortical*) bone surrounds a ***large core of dense trabecular bone***.
ii. It provides lower initial stability to implants.

◄ *What is the major shortcoming of type 3 bone?*

4. *Type 4 (D4) Bone*

i. ***Thin layer*** of compact (*cortical*) bone surrounds a large core of ***low-density trabecular bone***.
ii. It provides poor initial stability to implants as it has poor strength.
iii. Dental implants may take longer, i.e. usually more than 6 months to osseointegrate in type 4 (*D4*) bone.

◄ *What is the major shortcoming of type 4 bone?*

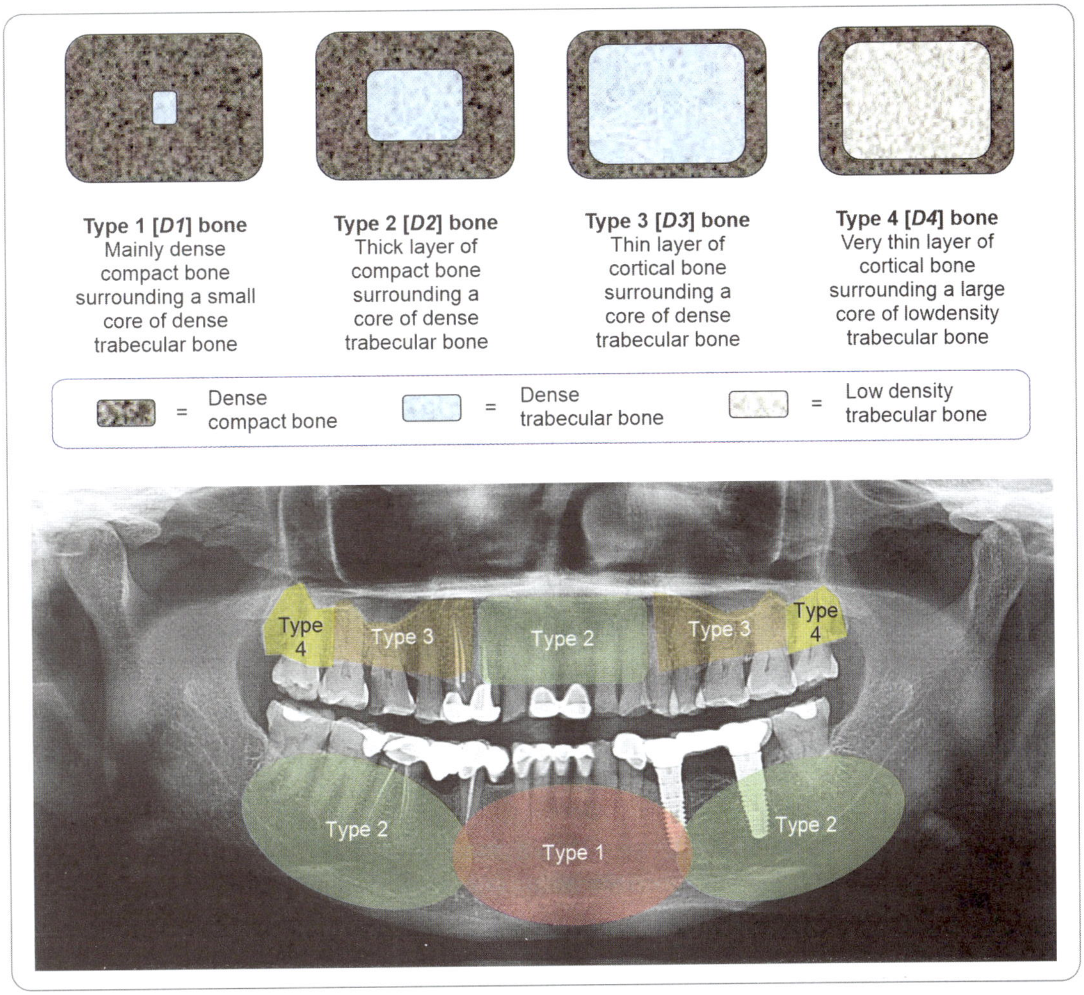

Fig. 22.7: Types of bone quality and distribution of these in maxilla and mandible

CLINICAL UTILITY AND SHORT ANSWER

How is bone density measured?

How is radiographic density of bone measured?

- Tissues have different radiodensities (*density seen in X-ray*) that makes them identifiable on radiograph.
- Density of bone can be accurately known using a medical grade CT scan. Experienced clinicians can have a good estimate of bone density (*of a particular bone*) from a routine radiograph.
- Radiodensity (*at a particular area of a particular bone*) is measured in Hounsfield units (*HU*).
- Radiodensities of human bone on the Hounsfield scale are:

What is the radiographic density of cancellous and cortical bone?

  - Cancellous bone = approximately +700 HU
  - Cortical bone = approximately +3000 HU
- Dense bone appears more radiopaque while osteoporotic and rarefied bone has large radiolucent areas in it and appears more radiolucent.
- To gauge generalized osteoporosis and level of calcification of bones (*bone density*), **DEXA scan** (*Dual energy X-ray absorptiometry*) is done (*usually done for bones of spine and hip region*).

What Happens if Soft Tissue forms between Implant and Bone?

What is fibrous union of implants?

Sometimes, due to several reasons, bone does not form directly over the surface of implant. Rather, soft tissue forms between the implant surface and bone; such a union is called ***Fibrous union*** **(Fig. 22.5, diag. 4, red line)**. Such implants failed to osseointegrate and therefore are mobile and ***cannot*** bear occlusal loads (*also see section on reasons implant failure later in this Chapter*).

PROCEDURE FOR PLACING AND LOADING DENTAL IMPLANTS

There are two methods of placing and loading dental implants:

What is the difference between one- and two-stage implant placing and loading methods?

1. **Two-stage method:** Implants are usually placed using a two-stage method wherein the implant body is first placed in the alveolar bone. Then, after allowing the implant to osseointegrate (*unite*) with the bone for a period of 2–6 months, a suitable implant abutment is attached and a crown is fabricated and placed over the abutment (*osteointegration is slower in maxilla than the mandible; it is also relatively slower in D4 bone*).
2. **One-stage method:** If the alveolar bone is fairly dense (*e.g. type 2/3 bone*) **(Fig. 22.7)** and the implant has ***good initial stability***, i.e. it has been placed into the osteotomy with good torque (*approximately 40 N. cm or more*), the implant can be ***immediately loaded*** (*crown is placed over the implants immediately*).

Immediate loading is usually indicated when a single rigid prosthesis is placed over multiple implants. Single implants can also be immediately loaded if they meet the criteria mentioned above.

CLINICAL UTILITY AND SHORT ANSWER

What is torque?

- Torque is a commonly used term in dental implantology.
- Torque is a measure of the turning force on an object around an axis, e.g. force applied on a wrench to tighten or loosen a screw.
- The SI unit of torque is newton meter (*N.m*), as smaller forces are used for dental implants, newton centimeter (*N.cm*) is used (*N.cm is 1/10th of N.m*).
- Torque (*turning force*) is required for turning bone drills (*to make an osteotomy*), tightening cover screws, healing screw (abutment)s, abutment screws, etc.
- Torque (*turning force*) can be applied manually or by an electrical motor called physiodispenser.

Steps of Two Stage/Delayed Loading Method for Dental Implants

Step 1: Diagnosis and Treatment Planning

Shape of alveolar bone ridge, width and dimensions of edentulous space and position of neighbouring teeth are important determinants for deciding the size, type and number of dental implants to be placed. If bone ridge is too thin or its height is not adequate, dental implants cannot be placed. Guided bone regeneration must be done to increase volume of alveolar bone in such cases. Diagnosis and treatment planning is done by:

◂ *Name the important modalities used in treatment planning for implants.*

1. Physical examination of the edentulous areas/ridges
2. Diagnostic casts
3. Radiographic assessment using IOPA (*intra oral periapical radiographs*), OPG (*orthopantomogram*), CBCT (*cone bean computed tomography*) (*number, type, location and orientation of dental implants and fabrication of surgical templates can also be done digitally by using special software that uses CBCT data to plan implant placement*).
4. Fabrication of surgical template (*optional*)

Step 2: Preparation of Osteotomy

Before starting to prepare the osteotomy, suitable length and diameter of the implant to be placed at a particular site must be known. A prefabricated surgical template is helpful in preparing osteotomy sites.

◂ *What is flapless technique for placing implants?*

1. Alveolar bone crest is ***exposed*** (*minimum*) by raising a full thickness flap or cutting a small window in the gingiva (*through which osteotomy is prepared and implant is placed—flapless technique*).
2. A 1.8/2.0 mm diameter drill rotating at 800–1200 RPM is used to initiate the osteotomy under constant irrigation with normal saline. After drilling to a length of 4–5 mm, a ***direction indicator post*** is inserted into the osteotomy and a radiograph is taken to reconfirm the direction of the osteotomy (Fig. 22.8, diag. 2). Osteotomy is then prepared to the desired length.
3. Diameter of the osteotomy is increased by using sequential drills of wider diameter (*depending on the decided diameter of the implant to be placed*).
4. The implant is then taken out of its sterile packaging, mounted on a suitable driver and placed in the osteotomy using a physio-dispenser (Fig. 22.8, diag. 4).
5. Implants are tightened to the recommended torque (*as recommended by the manufacturer; usually between 35–70 N. cm.*).
   - Higher implant fixation torque (*within recommended torque range*) means higher initial implant stability; this increases the chances of successful osseointegration.
   - Implants placed with initial torque of 40–45 N. cm or above can be immediately loaded (*if other conditions permit; when using immediate loading method*).
   - Exceeding the recommended torque can fracture the implant and causes severe bone compression that leads to excessive bone loss around the implant and implant failure.
6. Position of the implant collar with respect to the bone crest is confirmed with a radiograph and a cover screw or healing screw is placed (Fig. 22.8, diags 5 and 6). Healing screws are tightened to torque of around 5–10 N. cm. using a hand-held key.
7. Flap over the implant is closed with interrupted sutures (*this is not required if flapless technique was used*).

◂ *What is ideal torque for tightening implants in an osteotomy?*

◂ *What are the benefits of higher initial implant fixation torque?*

◂ *What happens if implant tightening torque is exceeded?*

Step 3: Allowing Undisturbed Healing for Osseointegration

After inserting the implant, it must be left '***undisturbed***'/'***unloaded***' in the osteotomy to allow it to osseointegrate with the bone.

◂ *How long does it take for an implant to osseointegrate?*

- Average time taken for osseointegration is:
  - Approximately 3–6 months or more for maxillary implants (*osseointegration is slower in D4 bone*).
  - Approximately 2–3 months or more for mandibular implants
  - If implants are loaded earlier, it may lead to loss of implant stability (*implant becomes loose and mobile*) and ultimately loss of implant.
- If immediate loading method is indicated and used, implants can be loaded immediately within one week after implant placement (*osteointegration will continue while implant is being used*).

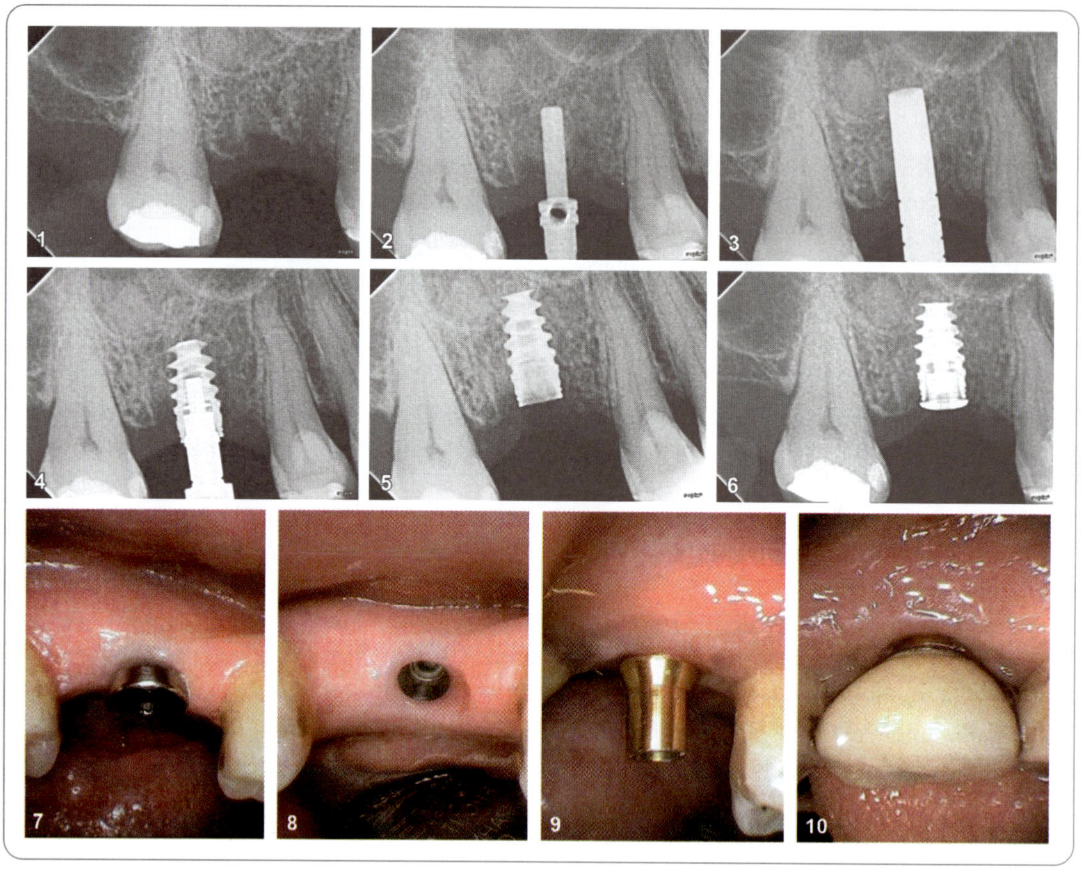

Fig. 22.8: Clinical steps in placing an implant and indirect sinus lift in maxillary posterior area. Diag. 1: Pre-operative radiograph. Diag. 2: After initiating the osteotomy (*1.8–2 mm drill*) and reaching a depth of approximately 5 mm, direction indicating post is inserted into the osteotomy to know the direction of the osteotomy. Osteotomy is prepared to the desired length and diameter using drills of larger diameter in sequence (*base of the maxillary sinus floor in this case*). Diag. 3: Floor of the maxillary sinus at the end of the osteotomy is then fractured and lifted up 2–3 mm by using osteotomes (*indirect sinus lift instruments*). Diag. 4: Implant is then mounted on an implant driver and put into the osteotomy. It is turned clockwise to insert it into the osteotomy with an implant mount (*using physiodispenser and torque wrench*). Diag. 5: Implant is inserted into the osteotomy till the crest of the alveolar bone or just 0.5 mm apical to it. Diag. 6: Cover screw is fixed over the implant to prevent food, plaque and soft tissue growing into it. Diag. 7: Cover screw is replaced with a healing screw. Diag. 8: After allowing gingival healing for about 15 days, gingival collar forms around the healing screw (*abutment*). Diag. 9: Selected abutment is fixed on the implant. Diag. 10: Crown is fabricated and placed on the implant.

Step 4: Re-surfacing the Implant after Healing Period

What does the healing screw (abutment) do? ▶

At the end of the healing phase (*step 4 above*) or any time later, implant is re-surfaced (*exposed*) by making a window in the overlying gingiva. Cover screw placed earlier is replaced with a healing screw (*abutment*) (Fig. 22.8, diag. 7) for 10–15 days to allow shaping and healing of the gingiva around the neck of the implant (Fig. 22.8, diag. 8).

Step 5: Impression Making, Preparation of Plaster Cast and Crown Fabrication

1. **Indirect impression technique**
   i. After 10–15 days, the healing screw (*abutment*) is removed and an impression coping is screwed into the implant body for making an impression with rubber base impression materials.
   ii. After making the impression, the impression coping is removed and healing screw (*abutment*) is put back on the implant body.
   iii. Implant analog (*substitutes for implant body in the plaster cast*) is attached to the impression coping.

iv. Impression coping (*with the attached implant analog*) is now inserted into its impression in the rubber base impression and the impression is poured with plaster (*die stone*) to make a plaster cast.

v. After plaster cast is ready, impression coping is removed. An abutment is then attached to the implant analog that is embedded in the plaster cast.

vi. Crown/prosthesis is fabricated on the abutment.

2. **Direct impression technique**

i. Abutment is attached to the implant body. After making an impression, the abutment is removed and healing screw (*abutment*) is refixed over the implant. Final or temporary crowns are fabricated on the cast made after pouring the impression with die stone.

Step 6: Fixing Abutment to the Implant Body and Restorative Crown to the Abutment

Abutment is fixed to the implant body using an abutment screw that is tightened to approximately 20 N. cm torque **(Fig. 22.8, diag. 9)**. Crowns/prosthesis is then cemented over abutments **(Fig. 22.8, diag. 10)**.

Steps of *Immediate Loading Method* for Dental Implants

When following the immediate loading method, crown/prosthesis is placed over implants ***within one week*** of their placement. All other ***steps remain the same*** as for two stage/delayed loading method.

CLINICAL UTILITY AND SHORT ANSWER

If implants have to be immediately loaded, why must this be done within one week after implant placement?

- Immediate loading of implants is recommended only if they have been placed with at least 40–45 N. cm initial fixation torque. The initial stability/torque is derived from frictional force between the bone and the implant.
- After implant placement, a phase of bone resorption starts in which bone on the periphery of implants is resorbed resulting in lower implant stability. This bone resorption and the resulting lower implant stability reaches its maximum after about two weeks of implant placement and lasts for 2–3 months. New bone also forms during this period and implant gets osseointegrated.
- During the phase when initial stability of the implant is low, an implant can get unscrewed out of the bone due to the torque (*turning force*) from procedures done to place crown or prosthesis over it.
- If such an implant is somehow loaded (*crown placed over it*), it will not be able to bear the occlusal forces and will thus fail if loaded during this time.
- Implants must therefore either be loaded within one week or after 2–6 months (*required for osseointegration; more time is required in case of maxillary bone and D4 bone*) after their placement.

ALERT!

- Medical fitness criteria and diagnostic tests (*blood clotting tests, blood sugar levels and blood sugar control history, complete blood counts, routine urine examination*, etc.) for dental implant surgery are the same as for any other minor oral surgery (*extractions, etc.*).
- Implant treatment must always be ***started with the end in mind***, i.e. before starting it, in addition to the likely surgical challenges, all prosthetic requirements and problems must be kept in mind from the very start. This will allow more convenient implant loading at the end of the treatment.
- Patients who smoke and do not maintain their dental health are also ***not*** likely to maintain their dental implants in plaque free state. This increases chances implant failure (*due to periimplantitis*).

◄ *Are any special blood tests usually required for implant surgery?*

HOW TO INCREASE BONE VOLUME FOR IMPLANT PLACEMENT—GUIDED BONE REGENERATION (*GBR*)

Many times, areas where implants have to be placed do not have sufficient bone for implant placement. This may be due to bone atrophy, resorption, large maxillary sinus, etc. In such cases, bone volume can be increased by guided bone regeneration (*GBR*). GBR can be done along with implant placement or as a first stage surgery to attain bone volume many weeks before implant placement. For GBR to be successful, two requirements have to be met:

What are the major challenges in trying to increase volume of bone for implant placement? ▶

1. Keeping graft material contained in the desired shape (*desired ridge size and shape*) at the designated site.
   This is done by placing a protective 'canopy' (roof), e.g. thin titanium mesh and barrier membrane over the graft material at the GBR site. This prevents de-shaping and dislodging of the graft material by physical forces. Such titanium mesh canopies can be made by contouring and trimming a piece of commercially available at titanium mesh to size at the time of surgery or prior to it on a diagnostic cast.
2. Helping bone marrow cells to enter the graft and preventing ingrowth of fibrous tissue into the healing graft during healing.
   This is done by decortifying bone by drilling several small holes in the bone (piercing the cortical bone) over which graft will be placed and placing a GTR membrane over the graft.

How is bone augmentation done in the mandibular ridge? ▶

Mandibular Ridge Augmentation

- It is done only if there is a severe mandibular ridge deformity.

What is decortication of bone? ▶

- To do this, mandibular bone is ***decortified*** by drilling several small holes in the bone and bone graft is placed over it. Bone graft is covered with a GTR membrane to protect it (*preferably with one that has a reinforcing titanium mesh*).

Is bone graft more successful in improving width or height of bone ridge? ▶

- Bone grafts are most ***successful for increasing width*** of the mandibular alveolar ridge but are ***less effective in improving height*** (*vertical augmentation*) of the mandibular ridge.

Maxillary Ridge Augmentation

- In the maxillary anterior region, ridge augmentation is done in a similar way as it is done for the mandibular ridge.

What is sinus lift surgery? ▶

- The posterior maxillary ridge deficiencies are usually due to an extended maxillary sinus into body of the alveolar ridge. In such cases, width of buccal alveolar ridge is satisfactory but due to deep extension of maxillary sinus into body of the alveolar ridge, bone height (*thickness of maxillary sinus floor*) is not sufficient for implant placement. To increase bone height (*thickness of the sinus floor*), sinus lift surgery is done by placing bone graft material inside the maxillary sinus cavity but under the sinus's membrane. It can be done by:
  1. Indirect sinus lift technique
  2. Direct (*open*) sinus lift technique.

Indirect Sinus Lift Surgery (*Indirect Sinus Floor Augmentation Surgery*)

How is indirect sinus lift surgery for bone augmentation done? ▶

Indirect sinus lift procedure works best if only ***few*** millimetres (*usually 3–4 mm*) of bone augmentation is needed. It is done at the time of implant placement as under:

- Implant osteotomy is made with implant drills just about 1–2 mm short of the sinus floor.

What is an osteotome? ▶

- Osteotomes (*cylindrical instrument with a cup shaped end that scrapes bone from sides of bone cavity and pushes it forward as osteotome progresses*) of increasing sizes are then used to enlarge implant osteotomy progressively.
  - For this, osteotome of small diameter (*just fitting the osteotomy created by drill*) is inserted into the drilled osteotomy and is tapped with a surgical mallet with just enough force to advance the osteotome 1–2 mm with every hit till the floor of the sinus is fractured.
  - This way the osteotome is advanced 3–4 mm into the sinus cavity.
  - Osteotomes of increasing diameter are then used sequentially in the same way till intended implant diameter is reached.
  - As the osteotome is advanced, it scrapes bone pieces from the sides of the osteotomy. These bone pieces and the advancing tip of the osteotome pushes the sinus membrane upward (*elevating it*). In this process, the scrapped bone pieces from osteotomy's wall and apex get deposited into the sinus under the sinus's membrane. The bone pieces act like an autogenous bone graft material and serves to augment the bone volume. If needed, alloplastic bone graft material can be additionally added through the implant osteotomy to provide added bulk to the bone graft.

Direct Sinus Lift Surgery *(Direct Sinus Floor Augmentation Surgery)*

◂ *How is direct sinus lift surgery for bone augmentation done?*

Direct sinus lift bone augmentation surgery is done if more than 5 mm bone augmentation is required.

- This surgery is performed using lateral approach.
- To start, bone on buccal side of the sinus (*bone making the lateral wall of the sinus and alveolar ridge*) is exposed after raising a full thickness flap.
- A window is then cut out in the lateral wall of the sinus to expose the sinus membrane (*Schneiderian membrane*). This window is created at preferably 2–3 mm above the level of the floor of the sinus (*the 2–3 mm lateral wall of the sinus left below the level of the window will retain graft material better in the sinus cavity*).
- The sinus membrane is then gently separated from the floor of the sinus (*using direct sinus lift instruments*) and elevated to the required height (*a little more than the length of the implant to be put in*).
- The cavity created under the elevated sinus membrane is then filled with graft material and the flap is sutured back (*a barrier membrane may or may not be used to cover the graft material*).
- Implants may be inserted at the same time or during a second stage surgery done after at least 3 months (*healing time*).

◂ *What is the name of maxillary sinus membrane?*

◂ *At what level is the window cut out in the lateral wall of the maxillary sinus for direct sinus lift surgery?*

WHY IMPLANTS FAIL

The reasons for implant failure are:

◂ *What are the reasons of implant failure?*

1. Failure to Osseointegrate *(Joining with the Bone the First Time)*

◂ *Why do some implants fail to osseointegrate?*

Implants can fail to osseointegrate due to:

i. Very high drilling speed (*more than 1200 RPM*) and/or using very little irrigation during preparation of osteotomy. Both these factors can raise temperature of bone ***above 37°C***. This causes death of bone cells leading to failure of osseointegration.

ii. Very low implant placement torque leading to very low initial stability of dental implant. This can be due to:

   a. Placement of implant into an osteotomy that is larger than the implant length and diameter.

   b. Too much manipulation during implant placement resulting in a 'spinning' implant (*easily rotating implant in the osteotomy*).

   c. Type 3 (*D3*)/type 4 (*D4*) quality bone.

iii. Too high initial implant fixation torque. Exceeding the manufacturer recommended implant tightening torque can cause bone loss around the implant body leading to loss of implant.

iv. An implant must have at least 2 mm of bone on all its sides. If thinner bone cover is there, the bone in that area will resorb and implant will not osseointegrate in that area. This may lead to implant failure. Causes of thin bone cover over an implant are:

   a. Placement of a larger implant in a smaller volume of bone.

   b. Incorrect design of prepared osteotomy (*location and/or angulation*) will lead to thin bone cover over the implant despite presence of an adequate volume of bone.

v. Loading of implants immediately after placement despite it not being indicated (*especially in D4 bone or healing sockets in which bone healing is not complete and bone density is still low*).

vi. Early loading of dental implants (*before complete osseointegration*).

2. Bone Loss Leading to Implant Mobility after Osseointegration

◂ *Why do some implants fail after successful osseointegration?*

After osseointegration, implants working normally for some time, may become painful, tender, mobile and are ultimately lost. This may happen due to:

i. Peri-implantitis
ii. Overloading of implants
iii. Large cantilever of prosthesis (*extended and unsupported part of the prosthesis*)
iv. Smoking.

3. Rarely Implants may be Rendered Useless due to

What are the other miscellaneous causes of implant failure? ▶

i. **Fracture of implant body**
   a. ***During*** placement (*due to application of more than manufacturer recommended torque which may be up to 70 N.cm*)
   b. ***After*** osseointegration (*due to very high occlusal force*)
ii. **Fracture of abutment retaining screw**
   a. During placement (*due to very high screw tightening torque; screws are usually tightened to 10–25 N.cm*).
   b. During use (*usually due to occlusal overloading*).
iii. **Implant placed in a position where it cannot be restored.**

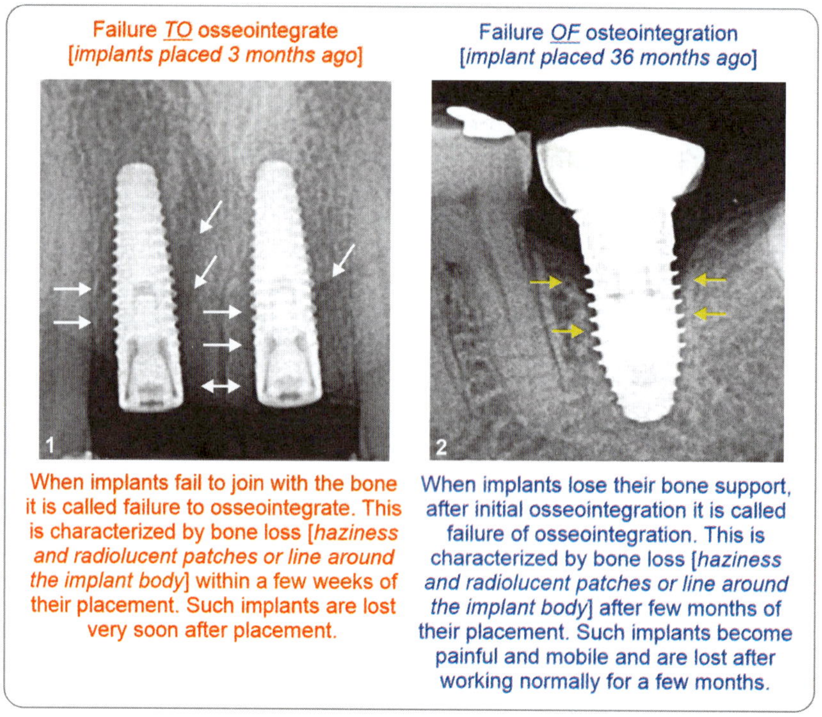

Fig. 22.9: Implant mobility and loss due to failure to osseointegrate (*diag. 1*) and failure of osseointegration (*diag. 2*)

PERI-IMPLANT MUCOSITIS AND PERI-IMPLANTITIS

What are peri-implant mucositis and peri-implantitis? ▶

Peri-implant mucositis is a ***reversible*** inflammation of ***soft*** tissues surrounding the neck of a dental implant.

Peri-implantitis is a site-specific inflammatory disease characterized by peri-implant mucositis and progressive bone loss around a functional (*load bearing*) osseointegrated implant.

Peri-implant mucositis and peri-implantitis affects 5–10% of all osseointegrated implants.

What Causes Peri-implant Mucositis and Peri-implantitis?

What causes peri-implant mucositis and peri-implantitis? ▶

The following factors are thought to be responsible:

1. Inflammation of mucosa around an implant is caused by ***anaerobic and G –ve bacteria plaque microorganisms*** (*P. gingivalis, A. actinomycetemcomitans, T. denticola, etc.*) (*just as gingivitis and periodontitis*).
2. ***Excessive*** and/or ***inadequate distribution*** of occlusal loads on osseointegrated implants. Abnormal occlusal loads cause bone loss and create conditions for pocket formation around an implant. This leads to progressive implant mobility and eventual loss of implant.
3. Other factors that are linked to peri-implantitis are: Diabetes mellitus, smoking, osteoporosis, immune suppressant drugs, e.g. corticosteroids when taken over a long period of time, etc.

ALERT!

Healthy gingiva plays an important role in prevention of peri-implantitis

- Free and attached gingiva act like physical barriers that restrict entry of plaque microorganisms into peri-implant sulcus.
- Implants must preferably be placed at sites where there is an adequate zone of attached gingiva.

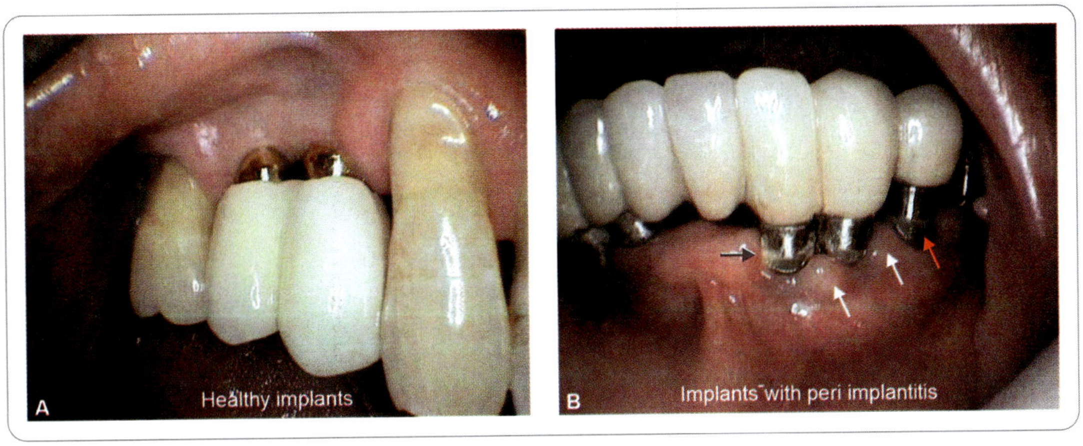

Fig. 22.10: Implant health and Peri-implantitis. Diag. A, healthy implants; note normal gingiva, complete absence of inflammation and excellent maintenance of oral hygiene that contribute to health of implants. In diag. B, note denudation of implants due to bone loss and recession of gingiva (*red arrow*), inflamed gingiva around implants (*white arrow*) and plaque deposits on body of implants (*black arrow*).

Management of Peri-implant Mucositis and Peri-implantitis

How are peri-implant mucositis and peri-implantitis treated?

Peri-implant mucositis and Peri-implantitis have similar etiology as gingivitis, periodontitis and trauma from occlusion. Management of these is therefore ***similar*** to ***management of gingivitis, periodontitis and trauma from occlusion*** and includes:

1. Scaling.
2. Antimicrobial therapy using metronidazole, ornidazole, amoxicillin, etc. to reduce pocket depth.
3. Surgical pocket reduction around the implant.
4. Decontamination of involved implant surface by citric acid, chlorhexidine, lasers therapy, etc.

Review Questions

1. What is a dental implant?
2. What are the indications and contraindications of endosseous implants?
3. What are the parts of a dental implant?
4. How are dental implants retained in the bone? What is osseointegration?
5. What is fibrous union? How is fibrous union different from osseointegration?
6. What is the procedure for placing and loading dental implants using the two-stage method?
7. What are the precautions that must be kept in mind when preparing an osteotomy for placing an endosseous implant?
8. Why is initial stability of an endosseous implant important?
9. Classify alveolar bone according to its density. How does density of bone affect osseointegration?
10. Why is D4 bone less suited for placing endosseous implants?
11. How can density of alveolar bone for placing endosseous implants be measured?
12. What are the causes of failure of dental implants?
13. Why does osseointegration fail?
14. What are peri-implant mucositis and peri-implantitis? How are they treated?

Index

R

S

T

U